PROFESSIONAL GUIDE TO

Complementary & Alternative Therapies

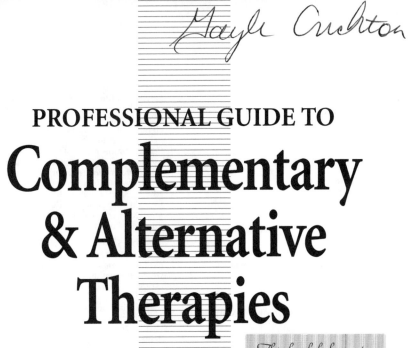

PROFESSIONAL GUIDE TO
Complementary & Alternative Therapies

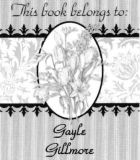

This book belongs to:

Gayle
Gillmore

SPRINGHOUSE
Springhouse, Pennsylvania

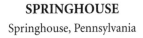

STAFF

Senior publisher
Donna O. Carpenter

Creative director
Jake Smith

Clinical director
Marguerite Ambrose, RN, MSN

Editorial director
H. Nancy Holmes

Clinical project manager
Lisa Morris Bonsall, RN, MSN, CRNP

Editors
Jennifer P. Kowalak (senior associate editor),
Elizabeth Jacqueline Mills

Copy editors
Catherine B. Cramer, Dolores P. Matthews,
Barbara F. Ritter

Clinical editors
Shari A. Regina Cammon, MSN, RN, CCRN;
Elizabeth D. McNeeley, BSN, RN;
Linda Roy, MSN, CRNP

Designers
Arlene Putterman (senior art director),
Susan L. Sheridan (design project manager),
Joseph John Clark, Donna S. Morris

Cover illustration
John Hubbard

Electronic production services
Diane Paluba (manager), Joyce Rossi Biletz

Manufacturing
Patricia K. Dorshaw (manager),
Otto Mezei (book production manager)

Editorial assistants
Danielle Jan Barsky, Carol Caputo,
Arlene Claffee, Beth Janae Orr, Linda Ruhf

Indexer
Ellen Brennan

Printed in the United States of America.

PGCAT – D N O S

03 02 01   10 9 8 7 6 5 4 3 2 1

**Library of Congress
Cataloging-in-Publication Data**

Professional guide to complementary & alternative therapies.
    p. ; cm.
    Includes bibliographical references and index.
    ISBN 1-58255-127-8
    1. Alternative medicine—Handbooks, manuals, etc. I. Title: Professional guide to complementary and alternative therapies. II. Springhouse Corporation.
    [DNLM: 1. Alternative Medicine—Handbooks. WB 39 P9637 2002]
    R733 .P755 2002
    615.5—dc21
                                        2001049079

Contents

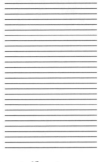

Contributors and consultants

Angella Bascom, MSN, ARNP
Elliot Hospital/Regional Partners in
   Occupational Health
Manchester, N.H.

Mark A. Breiner, DDS, FAGD, FIAOMT
Dentist
Private Practice
Orange, Conn.

Michael Briggs, PharmD
Pharmacist/Co-Owner
Lionville Natural Pharmacy
Exton, Pa.

Michael F. Cantwell, MD, MPH
Medical Director and Coordinator of
   Clinical Research
Health and Healing Clinic/California
   Pacific Medical Center
San Francisco

Elizabeth A. Chester, PharmD, BCPS
Clinical Pharmacy Specialist, Primary Care
Kaiser Permanente
Aurora, Co.

Jeanneane L. Cline, RN, MS, CS, HTP,
   LCDC, LMFT
Instructor
School of Nursing
University of Texas at Arlington

Alan R. Cohen, MD
Medical Director
Harmony Health Care/Alan R. Cohen,
   MD PC
Milford, Conn.

Jason C. Cooper, PharmD
Pharmacist
Bon Secours/St. Frances Hospital
Charleston, S.C.

Ami Dansby, RPh
Pharmacist, Natural Medicine
   Consultant
Bruce's Pharmacy
Charlottesville, Va.

Lana Dvorkin, RPh , PharmD
Assistant Professor, Clinical Pharmacy
Massachusetts College of Pharmacy and
   Health Sciences
Boston

Jacob Farin, ND
Naturopathic Physician
Center for Traditional Medicine
Lake Oswego, Ore.

Hope Farner, NMD, MS
Assistant Professor, Naturopathic
   Medicine
Southwest College of Naturopathic
   Medicine
Tempe, Ariz.

Marie Fasano-Ramos, RN, MA, MN, CMT
Holistic Nurse Practitioner
InterAge
Ventura, Ca.

June M. Ferrari, ND, CNC
Health Revolutions and Holy Redeemer
   Hospital Women's Center
Feasterville, Pa.

Tatyana Gurvich, PharmD
Clinical Pharmacist
GAFPRP
Glendale, Ca

AnhThu Hoang, PharmD
Scientific Associate
IntraMed Educational Group
New York

Susan Simmons Holcomb, RN, MN,
  CCRN, CS, FNP
Nurse Practitioner, Nutritional
  Counseling
Sastun Center of Integrative Healthcare
Mission, Kan.

Julia N. Kleckner, PharmD
Pharmacy Manager
Option Care
Upper Darby, Pa.

Robert J. Krueger, PhD
Professor, Pharmacognosy
College of Pharmacy
Ferris State University
Big Rapids, Mich.

Suzanne C. Lawton, ND
Naturopathic Physician
Private Practice
Tigard, Ore.

Yun Lu, RPh, MN, MS, PharmD
Cardiology/Anticoagulation Clinical
  Specialist
Hennepin County Medical Center
Minneapolis

Susan Luck, RN, BS, MA, CCN, HNC
Holistic Health Education, Clinical
  Nutritionist
Biodoron Immunology Center
Hollywood, Fla.

June H. McDermott, RPh, MBA, MS
  Pharm, FASHP
Clinical Assistant Professor
School of Pharmacy
University of North Carolina at Chapel
  Hill

Thomas M. Motyka, DO
Clinical Assistant Professor
School of Medicine
University of North Carolina at Chapel
  Hill

Jolynne Myers, RNCS, MSEd, MSN, ANP
Clinical Research Coordinator
Life Waves International
Kansas City, Mo.

Scott Olsen, BA, ND
Naturopathic Doctor, Research Writer
Private Practice
Littleton, Co.

Steven G. Ottariano, RPh
Clinical Staff Pharmacist
Veterans Affairs Medical Center
Manchester, N.H.

Robert Lee Page, II, PharmD, BCPS
Assistant Professor
School of Pharmacy
University of Colorado Health Sciences
  Center
Denver

June Riedlinger, RPh, PharmD
Assistant Professor, Clinical Pharmacy
Director, Center for Integrative Therapies
  in Pharmaceutical Care
Massachusetts College of Pharmacy and
  Health Sciences
Boston

Karin K. Roberts, RN, PhD
Associate Professor
Research College of Nursing
Kansas City, Mo.

Alean Royes, MSN, RNC, CNS, APN
Faculty
School of Nursing
University of Texas at Arlington

Anna Russo, NLP Practitioner, Master
Practitioner, NLP International Trainer,
Master Ericksonian Hypnotherapist
Master Trainer and President
Success Strategies NLP of Michigan
Troy, Mich.

Sharon Scandrett-Hibdon, RN, PhD,
CHTI, CS, FNP, HNC
Family Nurse Practitioner
Groff Medical Center
Aubrey, Tx.

Jacob J. Schor, ND
Naturopathic Physician
Denver (Co.) Naturopathic Clinic

Marcia Silkroski, RD, CNSD
President
Nutrition Advantage
Chester Springs, Pa.

H. Robert Silverstein, MD
Medical Director, Preventive Medicine
Center
Clinical Assistant Professor of Medicine
School of Medicine
University of Connecticut
Hartford

Ann McCloud Sneath, MSN, CRNP
Nurse Practitioner, Integrative Medicine
Private Practice
Paoli, Pa.

Katrina A. Steinberger, NMD
Medical Director
Scottsdale (Ariz.) Clinic for Alternative
and Longevity Medicine

Ronald Steriti, NMD, PhD
Naturopathic Physician
Naples, Fla.

Maria A. Summa, RPh, BCPS, PharmD
Assistant Professor of Clinical Pharmacy
Massachusetts College of Pharmacy and
Health Sciences
Boston

Dorota Szarlej, BS, PharmD
Clinical Pharmacist, Drug Use Policy and
Clinical Services
Thomas Jefferson University Hospital
Philadelphia

Timothy Taneda-Brown, ND, DC,
Diplomate Acupuncture, Naturopath
Ocean Pacific Natural Therapies
Surrey, British Columbia, Canada

Gail D. Vanark, RN, BSN
Staff RN
St. Joseph's Hospital/St. Joseph's Family
Medical Center
Merrimack, N.H.

Diane Wind Wardell, PhD, RNC, HNC
Associate Professor
University of Texas at Houston

George L. White, Jr., MSPH, PhD, PA-C
Professor and Director Public Health
Programs
Department of Family and Preventive
Medicine
School of Medicine
University of Utah
Salt Lake City

Laurie Willhite, PharmD
Clinical Pharmacy Specialist
Fairview University Medical Center
Minneapolis

Jared L. Zeff, ND, LA, Licensed in
Acupuncture, Naturopathic Medicine
Naturopathic Physician, Acupuncturist
Professor of Naturopathic Medicine
Bastyr University
Bothell, Wash.

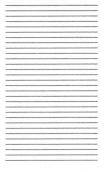

Foreword

Consider the following scenarios: Your patient confides that she's taking ephedra for appetite control; do you know that this herb could counteract the beta blocker prescribed for her hypertension? Another of your patients has read about ginseng on the Internet and thinks it will pep him up; will it do any good? Another drinks 5 cups of rose hip tea daily to help her digestion; do you know that it could aggravate her asthma? Another patient asks you how to find a qualified acupuncturist for his back pain; where do you start? Another points out that the British royal family uses homeopathy, so why shouldn't he? Yet another patient wants to stop his debilitating chemotherapy and, instead, try shark cartilage and a macrobiotic diet for his cancer; how do you counsel him?

The risk of patient silence

Apitherapy for arthritis pain, or chondroitin and glucosamine? Meditation to reduce blood pressure? Echinacea to prevent the common cold? Antioxidants or royal jelly to lower cholesterol? Ginkgo to avert Alzheimer's disease? What do you tell your patients? How do their actions impact the health care *you're* providing? What do you say if you don't even know what your patients are doing?

More and more people are turning to alternative therapies for the treatment of health concerns from minor infections and backache to diabetes and cancer.

Studies indicate that nearly 50% of Americans have used some form of complementary or alternative therapy, and most don't consult their primary care practitioner for advice or even volunteer information about their concurrent treatments.

As a clinician, you need a working knowledge of the alternative options your patients may be using — what's known and unknown about the underlying theory, training of practitioners, treatment recommendations, and risks. This working knowledge will help you formulate questions to elicit information that can directly affect your patients' medical care and allow you to advise them wisely.

The backup you need

Professional Guide to Complementary & Alternative Therapies provides that working background for you — and the answers to the questions your patients raise. Its easy-to-use, A-to-Z format is designed to allow you speedy access to the most up-to-date information on complementary and alternative treatments, from herbs to procedures. With nearly 300 entries devoted to herbal medications and more than 70 entries discussing other therapies, this invaluable reference book provides the clinical backup you need in your practice.

Each *herbal* entry consists of six sections that provide comprehensive, objective information about the treatment covered. It opens with an introduction that includes the herb's generic or common name, its Latin name and other names by which it's known, its appearance, and its useful components (such as dried leaves, flowers, or root). *Reported uses* lists diseases or medical conditions for which the herb is historically or currently used, including whether the use is oral or topical. *Administration* provides typical dosage, including usual methods for preparing teas and infusions. *Hazards* highlights potential adverse effects, contraindications, and interactions with prescribed drugs, foods, or other herbs. *Clinical considerations* informs you of health markers you should monitor if your patient is using the herb. It also presents advice you should offer to your patient — from general suggestions about keeping providers and pharmacists informed about using an herb to precautions about the herb's short- and long-term effects. Each entry ends with a *Research summary*, which provides information about studies into the herb's efficacy.

Using a similar format, each entry devoted to a *therapy* opens with a description of the therapy, the theory underlying its development, a short history of its uses, and often a brief biography of its founder. *Reported uses* describes conditions or diseases for which the therapy is used. *How the treatment is performed* provides a comprehensible explanation of the treatment process, including any special equipment required, such as needles for acupuncture. *Complications* lists potential adverse effects as well as risks for pregnant, pediatric, and geriatric patients. In addition to patient advice, *Clinical considerations* for therapies details contraindications for certain patient groups — for example, deep muscle massage, such as Hellerwork, that might be inappropriate for elderly patients. Therapy entries also conclude with a *Research*

summary that details anecdotal and clinical research studies into a therapy's use and effectiveness.

A wealth of additional information

Professional Guide to Complementary & Alternative Therapies also uses attention-getting graphic devices to highlight important aspects of a therapy's use. *Safety risk* emphasizes potentially serious contraindications or life-threatening side effects related to an herb or therapy. *Training* explains the type of training available for a specific therapy, including any necessary licensing or certification, and provides names, addresses, and often Web addresses for training facilities. *Reimbursement* describes the kinds of third-party payment available for some alternative treatments.

One of the most valuable elements of the *Professional Guide to Complementary & Alternative Therapies* is its appendices, which include selected references, a listing of alternative therapies for specific conditions, monitoring precautions for specific herbs, recommended dosages of supplemental vitamins and minerals, and a list of alternative therapy organizations (including Web sites).

The growing acceptance of complementary and alternative therapies is apparent in the number of agencies and publications that have sprung up — from the U.S. government's own National Center for Complementary and Alternative Medicine (NCCAM) to countless alternative medicine books, journals, and Web sites. It's clear that numerous complementary and alternative therapies are taking their places alongside mainstream medical practices. Ongoing research continues to clarify the role these therapies have in maintaining and improving health.

The *Professional Guide to Complementary & Alternative Therapies* is the perfect solution for health care professionals looking for a wide-ranging, up-to-date,

easy-to-use guide to the alternative
therapies that ever-greater numbers of
patients are using.

Eric Henley, MD, MPH
Assistant Professor and Head
Department of Family and Community
    Medicine
University of Illinois College of Medicine
    at Rockford

Health care comes full circle

In 1997, four out of ten adults in the United States used at least one form of complementary or alternative medicine (CAM), according to Eisenberg et al. (1998). Among people between ages 35 and 49, the numbers increased to one out of two. The most frequently used therapies were relaxation techniques, herbal medicine, massage, and chiropractic manipulation. Eisenberg and colleagues also estimated that visits to alternative health care providers increased from 427 million in 1990 to 629 million in 1997, creating a $21.2 billion industry. In fact, the number of visits to CAM providers exceeded visits to primary care physicians by approximately 243 million, with an estimated $12.2 billion paid out of pocket. Burg's study (1998) found similar usage rates among health care professionals; more than half of his respondents had used at least one type of alternative therapy at some time. A 1998 study by Wetzel et al. revealed that almost two-thirds of medical schools have integrated alternative and complementary approaches into their curricula.

Neck and back problems were the most frequently cited (42%) medical problems for which CAM was sought. People also sought CAM for the treatment of anxiety and depression, headaches, arthritis, GI problems, fatigue, insomnia, sprains and strains, allergies, lung problems, and hypertension. One out of three people who visited a medical doctor also consulted a CAM provider for the same medical problem. Most patients, however, didn't discuss their plans to combine CAM with conventional treatment with their medical doctor (Eisenberg et al., 1998). According to Astin (1998), the following qualities served as indicators of those most likely to use CAM: higher level of education, poorer health status, interest in spirituality or personal growth psychology, history of a transformational experience that altered the individual's world view, and identification with a cultural group committed to environmentalism or feminism.

Why has the use of CAM risen so sharply? To understand the answer to that question, it is first necessary to understand what CAM is and where it came from.

What is CAM?

A 1998 study by Eskinazi proposed that alternative medicine be defined as "a broad set of health care practices that are not readily integrated into the dominant health care model because they pose challenges to diverse societal beliefs and practices (cultural, economic, scientific, medical, and educational)." The National Center for Complementary and Alternative Medicine (NCCAM) defines alternative medicine as "a broad range of healing philosophies (schools of thought), approaches, and therapies that mainstream Western (conventional) medicine does not commonly use, accept, study, understand, or make available." But it was NCCAM that took the definition a step further by adding "complementary" to the general definition to arrive at "complementary and alternative medicine, or CAM." This is an important distinction, because CAM may be used either as an *adjunct* to modern medicine (hence "complementary") or *in place of* conventional therapy (hence "alternative").

History of CAM

Many of the myriad philosophies and therapies falling under the general heading of CAM actually date back thousands of years. Long before university-trained doctors became the providers of healing, a society's religious leaders were also its healers. Shamanism, a spiritual philosophy in which the individual is believed to be a unit composed of equally important physical and spiritual elements, is a system of spiritual practice dating back 40,000 years to the Stone Age. The tie between physical health and spirituality is also at the core of many of the world's spiritual and philosophical practices, including those of Tibet, India, Japan, and the cultures of Native American peoples.

Priest (or shaman) and healer remained the same person for centuries, even into the European society of the early 1600s. It was in this period that French philosopher Rene Descartes proposed that the study of spirit belonged to the discipline of philosophy (or religion), while the study of the physical body was the province of science. This rejection of the relationship between spirit and body set the stage for the division between practitioners of then-traditional medicine and those who believed that science should be the basis for all health care. This concept took some time to catch on, however.

Prior to the Industrial Revolution, which began in the late 1700s and lasted until the mid-1800s, science — particularly medical science — was still primarily viewed through a haze of superstition and suspicion. In fact, some nations had laws forbidding certain forms of research; for example, in Victorian England it was illegal to dissect a human cadaver for research purposes. During the course of the Industrial Revolution, however, a more tolerant view of science began to surface. By the end of the 19th century this newfound tolerance had grown into enthusiastic acceptance as people began to take pride in their willingness to embrace new technologies.

Like many other sciences, modern health care was in its infancy in the early 1900s. Surgical techniques were primitive at best, cellular understanding of disease was very basic, and hospitals were where people went to die. Aside from sulfur, antibiotics were unavailable, making infectious disease the most common cause of death. Although cities were growing, and with them a more impersonal way of life, most people still lived in close proximity to their families, and a strong sense of family responsibility was still the cornerstone of most lives. People still relied on family members or acknowledged healers to provide health care, and treatment typically took the form of traditional home or cultural remedies, herbal preparations, and other methods that supported the body's own recuperative powers.

As the decades passed, though, the modernization of health care gained momentum until it became a revolution. A better understanding of disease and its etiology made treatments more effective. Drugs and immunizations eradicated many infectious diseases, once-fatal illnesses were now curable or at least controllable, and the expected lifespan of Americans lengthened beyond that of individuals in any other country. Whereas local healers, usually trained by their predecessors, once provided most, if not all, of a community's medical care, formally trained physicians became the center of the new health care system. With the increasing availability — and variety — of scientific health care methods and the growing number of practitioners familiar with those methods, modern health care supplanted traditional medicine.

In the past two to three decades, attitudes toward health care issues have started to come full circle. Conventional (or "modern") medicine uses pharmaceuticals, surgery, radiation, chemotherapy, or apparatus such as dialysis machines to treat disease. Many of the methods were developed first in research laboratories rather than by practitioners. There are times when such methods may be preferable to CAM. Often, however, expensive, invasive, or side-effect-fraught treatments are used before other treatments are considered.

Spiraling health care costs, dissatisfaction with the "cost effective" practice methods dictated by insurance companies, and general disillusionment with a high-tech, low-touch health care system that so often treats symptoms without regard for the cause (Eliopoulos, 1999) have caused many people to seek alternatives to the modern form of health care. Information that wasn't previously accessible — for example, therapeutic modalities that are standard in one country, but not in another — is now widely distributed via the Internet and other media. The accessibility of a broader range of options has empowered people to seek alternative treatments for illnesses and chronic conditions unresponsive to conventional treatment, and the result is the resurgence of CAM.

Foundations of CAM

One of the difficulties in defining CAM is the broad range of therapies that the term encompasses. This section describes and defines some of the basic principles and domains of CAM.

Holism

One of the most significant aspects of the resurgence of CAM is the reunion of science and philosophy (or religion) as Western culture once again recognizes the importance of inner experiences to the health of the individual. Nowhere is this concept more apparent than in the notion of holism, which is one of the cornerstones of CAM. Holism is the view that individuals are composed of four interdependent and interrelated elements — physiological, psychological, sociological, and spiritual — which must be addressed as a unit when treating illness and promoting good health. Note that holism isn't a recently formulated concept; before the discovery and development of pharmacotherapeutic treatments for tuberculosis, Canadian physician Sir William Osler (1849-1919) believed that a patient's recovery was more dependent on what went on in his or her mind than in the lungs (Siegel, 1986).

Holism has gained popularity since Osler embraced the concept at the turn of the 20th century, and now many organizations and individuals involved in CAM share a common belief in the importance of the holistic view. The health care model of the American Holistic Nurses Association (AHNA) is framed on a holistic approach. Central to holistic nursing is the necessity to identify the interrelationship of the four elements and the knowledge that the individual is a unitary whole in mutual process with his or her environment (Dossey et al., 2000).

The concept of holism was both expanded and refined by Eliopoulos (1999), and is also a key component of at least one of the five health care domains described by NCCAM, as discussed below.

Five basic principles

Eliopoulos' 1999 study identified five basic principles underlying CAM:
- the body has the ability to heal itself
- health and healing are related to a harmony of mind, body, and spirit
- basic, good health practices build the foundation for healing
- healing practices are individualized
- people are responsible for their own healing (Eliopoulos, 1999).

The notion that mind, body, and spirit are interrelated and that stress on one dimension invariably places stress on the others is reflected in Eliopoulos' principles and, indeed, is the foundation of many CAM therapies. The core of many CAM practices is teaching patients the importance of taking a holistic view of the healing process.

NCCAM's five domains

Because there are almost as many forms of CAM as there are people walking the earth, it is helpful to categorize the various systems into domains based on how they are used. NCCAM has identified CAM practices in five primary domains: alternative medical systems, biologically based treatments, manipulative and body-based methods, energy therapies, and mind-body interventions (NCCAM, 2000).

Alternative medical systems

Alternative medical systems include complete systems of theory and practice that exist outside conventional biomedicine and are frequently practiced by cultures in other parts of the world. The alternative medical systems most familiar to many Westerners are Chinese medicine and Ayurveda, or Indian medicine. Both Chinese medicine and Ayurveda approach healing from a holistic standpoint.

Biologically based therapies

Biologically based therapies include the use of dietary supplements, herbal preparations, special diets, and orthomolecular and biological therapies. Examples of orthomolecular therapies are administration of megadoses of vitamins or other chemical supplements, such as magnesium and melatonin. Biological therapies include the use of preparations derived from nature, such as shark cartilage for cancer or bee pollen for autoimmune and inflammatory disorders.

Manipulative, body-based, and energy therapies

Manipulative and body-based therapies include chiropractic manipulation as well as massage, Rolfing, and the Feldenkrais method. Energy therapies focus on energy fields that either surround or penetrate the body, or consist of outside sources such as electromagnetic fields. Therapeutic Touch is an energy therapy originated in the United States by Dolores Krieger, a registered nurse. It's performed by a trained practitioner who assesses, and subsequently attempts to manipulate and balance, the energy field surrounding the patient (Krieger, 1993).

Mind-body interventions

Mind-body interventions are based on the existence of a mind-body connection and the ability of the mind to affect bodily functions and symptoms. Examples of mind-body therapies are meditation, hypnosis, visual imagery, prayer, and mental healing. Many of these therapies can be said to include a holistic approach.

An overview of CAM systems

This section provides an expanded view of several of the most widely used CAM systems.

Chinese and Indian medicine

Two of the most well known and ancient systems of CAM are Chinese medicine and Indian medicine (or *Ayurveda*), both of which have been in use for thousands of years.

The core of Chinese medicine is the notion of an energy force called *qi* (pronounced "chee"), which flows through the body along paths called *meridians*. The unimpeded flow of qi is necessary for the restoration and maintenance of health. If an individual's qi is stagnant, accumulations occur in the body and can lead to poor health — mental, spiritual, and physical. Physical manifestations of stagnant qi can include obesity, cancers, and other problems that manifest as immune or degenerative diseases.

To understand qi, one should also be familiar with the principles of *yin* and *yang*. The yin-yang symbol may be familiar: it depicts two fish, intertwined head to tail. One fish is dark with a white eye (yin); the other, white with a dark eye

(yang). The intertwined fish form a circle representing a universe that's made up of unlimited pairs of opposites interacting with each other. Qi is a yang force, associated with energy of the body, and yin is considered the "mother of qi" because it's associated with body fluids, specifically blood. One method that facilitates the flow of qi is acupuncture, a practice that has been the mainstay of Chinese medicine for centuries. (Acupuncture is described in detail in the section below devoted to energetic manual healing.) Other methods for maintaining or restoring the balance of qi include diet, exercise, meditation, spiritual practices, and herbal therapy. Qi is synonymous with *prana* in India and *ki* in Japan.

Another complex and ancient system of medicine is *Ayurveda*, practiced in India. Ayurveda means "science of life" and has been practiced as the medical model in India for over 5,000 years. As with Chinese medicine, Ayurvedic medicine is highly individualized, using therapies that bring the body, mind, and spirit back into harmony within the individual and within nature. It's also based on the concept of energy flow, called prana, which is facilitated by a balancing of *doshas* (body types). *Constitution* is the term used to describe an individual's character, temperament, and overall health profile, including strengths and weaknesses. Ayurvedic medicine identifies three major doshas: *vata*, *pitta*, and *kapha*.

The vata dosha is changeable and unpredictable. Vata individuals tend to be erratic in both thought processes and behavior, to be anxious, and to suffer from insomnia. People who are vata tend toward slenderness. Although vatas have a lot of energy, they often fail to follow a project through to completion.

Pitta individuals, as opposed to vatas, tend to be quite predictable. They are of medium build and possess strength and endurance. Pittas tend to be intelligent and so passionate as to be unduly critical or display explosive outbursts.

The kapha individual is relaxed, solid, heavy, and strong. Kaphas have a tendency to be overweight. For kaphas, everything related to thinking and behavior is slow, and for this reason they often procrastinate.

The purpose of Ayurvedic medical treatment is to bring the patient back into harmony within himself and within nature. Disease management in Ayurvedic medicine concentrates on cleansing and detoxifying (*shodan*), palliation (*shaman*), rejuvenation (*rasayana*), and mental hygiene and spiritual healing (*satvajaya*). Specific therapies may include diet, exercise, yoga, meditation, massage, tonics, baths, enemas, or aromatherapy.

Both Chinese medicine and Ayurveda are sophisticated systems based on the assumption of a mind-body connection and the body's innate ability to heal itself if provided the proper tools and environment.

Homeopathic medicine

Homeopathy, derived from the Greek words *homeo*, meaning similar, and *pathos*, meaning suffering, is a form of CAM that has been practiced for only around 200 years. Samuel Hahnemann, a German physician, was the first person to posit the concept of homeopathic medicine. Hahnemann tested hundreds of different minerals and herbs, carefully recording the response or symptoms that each produced. From his findings he drew three primary conclusions: first, that like cures like, a notion first proposed by Hippocrates and termed the Law of Similars; second, that substances gain rather than lose potency as they are diluted, a concept referred to as the Law of Infinitesimal Dose; and third, that illnesses are specific to individuals and can't be treated with a universal panacea.

The Law of Similars manifests in the development of vaccines against illnesses such as measles, influenza, pneumonia, and so forth, and is also the basis for the practice of immunotherapy for allergy patients. According to this ancient principle, giving a patient a very minute quantity of the substance responsible for his disease awakens the immune system, forcing it to produce antibodies against the disease.

Homeopathic medicine, as outlined by Dr. Hahnemann, is widely practiced in Europe, including the United Kingdom, France, and Germany. The British Royal family is known to use homeopathic remedies, and homeopathy is considered a postgraduate medical specialty in Britain. Homeopathy is also practiced in India, Mexico, Argentina, and Brazil. Underscoring the importance of homeopathic medicine worldwide, the World Health Organization called for it to be integrated with conventional medicine by the year 2000 to ensure adequate provision of global health care. Interestingly, however, the reason homeopathic medicine works can't be explained, even by homeopaths—the practice doesn't follow any known laws of chemistry, physics, or pharmacology.

Naturopathic medicine

Naturopathic medicine—cures derived from nature—is based on the principle that disease is a manifestation of natural systems the body uses to heal itself. This philosophy is a derivation of the ancient medical systems, including traditional Chinese medicine, Ayurveda, Native American medicine, and ancient Greek medicine. From these disciplines, naturopathic medicine borrows its basic principles: treat the cause rather than the effect, do no harm, treat the whole person, and prevention is the best cure. Father Sebastian Kneipp, a priest who credited his recovery from tuberculosis to bathing in the Danube, popularized naturopathy. Naturopathy further developed and spread through Kneipp's student, Benedict Lust, who carried the discipline of naturopathy to the United States in the 1890s and founded the first naturopathic college in the United States in New York City in 1902.

Treatment and prevention modalities used by naturopaths include nutrition, homeopathy, acupuncture, electrotherapy, herbal medicine, hydrotherapy, exercise, manipulation, physical therapy, stress reduction, counseling, and pharmacology. Lust's program for curing included elimination of "evil" habits, incorporation of corrective habits, and development of new principles of living. In naturopathic medicine, the physician serves also as teacher and as such is responsible for educating, empowering, and motivating patients.

Diet, nutrition, and lifestyle changes

The type of CAM falling under the heading of diet, nutrition, and lifestyle changes may be considered to overlap with the holistic approach to wellness because its basic premise is that a lack of appropriate diet and lifestyle habits contributes to the development of disease. Subcategories within this broad category include dietary changes; supplemental therapy with vitamins, minerals, or other nutritional supplements; exercise for the mind and body; relaxation for the mind and body; and lifestyle changes.

Diet and nutrition

Throughout history, people have used food to aid the healing process and to promote good health; the Greek physician, Hippocrates, referred to food as medicine. However, it was not until 1988 that the Surgeon General of the United States publicly acknowledged the connection between diet and health. Possible reasons for modern society's failure to recognize the importance of proper nutrition may include a lack of extensive study of the topic in the typical medical school curriculum and the convenience of "fast" and "junk" foods. However, with each passing day, more people recognize the connection between today's poor food sources and disease.

The nutritional value of modern food is affected in two ways: by processing or altering with chemical additives, and by the degeneration of the environment itself. Food is routinely altered by any of over 2,000 additives used for flavoring, coloring, preserving, texturizing, and stabilizing. Adulteration also includes hydrogenation of oils, thereby producing trans fatty acids, which are implicated in the development of degenerative diseases. The very environment in which they're produced also contributes to the poor nutritional value of most modern foods. Minerals in the soil, clean water, and pure air are essential to the growth of whole, healthy foods, but all are in dangerously short supply. Crops are exposed to any of more than four hundred pesticides that are approved for use in the United States. These pesticides penetrate soil, water, and both land and water animals — and thereby pervade much of the food we consume. Irradiation, which is used to combat bacteria, viruses, and fungi, may be effective in destroying these organisms, at the cost of forming toxins such as benzene and formaldehyde.

Dentist Weston A. Price (1997) determined the relationship between eating habits and degenerative diseases. He observed that among primitive tribal populations, those who stuck to their native diets and consumed no processed or otherwise adulterated foods had healthy dentition: straight teeth, no caries, well-developed arches and nasal passages, with no evidence of degenerative diseases or cancers. Individuals who abandoned the tribal foods in favor of modern diets demonstrated poor dental health — as evidenced by crooked teeth, caries, and small arches leading to small nasal passages — and degenerative diseases.

Price's findings, when considered alongside the growing number of people afflicted with cancer, heart disease, obesity, and other diseases or disorders, add to the evidence that the modern diet of refined and processed food not only fails to protect against disease, but may well contribute to the development of many diseases. Recent studies have revealed the role of various foods in causing heart disease, cancer, osteoporosis, and other degenerative diseases.

For thousands of years, practitioners of Chinese medicine have used food to help people maintain health, balance, and well-being. Interestingly, food itself isn't the only important aspect of diet in the Chinese medical model. Preparation, combinations of foods eaten at a given meal, and the thoughts and feelings associated with the preparation and consumption of food are all important aspects of the way food contributes to harmony and health, reflecting the Chinese recognition of the interplay between humans and nature. Specific types of food also reflect this awareness of balance; for example, people who are affected by the summer heat can be brought back into balance by consuming foods considered to be "cooling," while those whose condition indicates the presence of toxins in their system may be given detoxifying foods and food substances to cleanse their bodies. Because food is valued for its harmonizing qualities as well as its nutrients, variety is an important aspect of meal preparation.

For many years, it was accepted practice not to feed patients in a critical care unit. However, systems of CAM that focus on diet and nutrition recognize the importance of nutrients to the healing process. As the use of CAM gains popularity, growing numbers of nutritionists and other health care practitioners are using nutrition to enhance patients' ability to heal.

Food therapies are abundant and include not only philosophies regarding food, such as those seen in Chinese, naturopathic, and Ayurvedic practices, but also specific treatments or cures that employ certain types of food. Treatments or cures for diseases using food include different types of fasts; juice therapies; enzyme therapy; yeast-combating diets; macrobiotic diets; elimination diets; low-fat, high-carbohydrate diets; high-protein or low-protein diets; Mediterranean diets; anticancer diets; cardiovascular diets; and numerous antiobesity diets.

Orthomolecular medicine is the use of vitamins and minerals, generally in the form of nutritional supplements, to prevent or cure diseases. The most well known use of orthomolecular medicine is the vitamin C research conducted by Nobel prizewinner Linus Pauling. Orthomolecular medicine has far-ranging implications, including the effect of antioxidants on cancer, heart disease, and other degenerative diseases; the use of supplements to cure deficiencies seen in psychiatric patients; and the prevention and reversal of osteoporosis. Other potential uses of orthomolecular medicine include the use of amino acids, essential fatty acids, or glucosamine to cure or prevent degenerative diseases.

Lifestyle changes

Lifestyle changes include stimulating and relaxing the body and mind as well as ridding the body of toxic substances such as nicotine, alcohol, and drugs (both medicinal and illegal). Exercise and relaxation may boost the immune system in addition to building stronger bodies and minds. Price (1997) found that many tribal cultures knew the importance of exercise to strengthen the body, mind, and spirit, including the association between strong abdominal muscles and maximal breathing. A key element of Chinese medical and philosophical practice is the importance of breathing, movement, and meditation for overall balance between the individual and nature. Modern authorities are also beginning to recognize the relationship between lifestyle and health. For example, Hans Selye (1974) examined the relationship between stress and the development of degenerative diseases or distress. Norman Cousins' personal experience helped him to discover the stress-relieving benefits of laughter (Cousins, 1981).

Exercise bolsters the immune system and strengthens both body and mind.

Relaxation also boosts the immune system; in addition, it lowers blood pressure and enables people to handle everyday stress. Popular relaxation techniques include tai chi, qigong, yoga, meditation, prayer, and journaling.

Qigong overlaps other therapeutic approaches in its use of movement, breathing, and meditation to enhance the flow of energy in the body for the purpose of enhancing circulation and strengthening the immune system. Both the ill and the well can use qigong, and its wide usefulness has made it the nucleus of the self-care health system of China. So important is qigong in China that it's estimated to be practiced daily by more than 200 million of China's citizens.

Eliminating toxic substances improves the health in myriad ways, including but not limited to improving cardiac and lung functions and perhaps extending life.

Herbal medicine
An herb is a plant or part of a plant used as a food, spice, or medicine. Any part of an herb — the root, bark, leaf, berry, flower, fruit, stem, or seed — may be harvested for use.

Herbal medicine, or the use of herbs for medicinal purposes, is also referred to as phytomedicine or phytotherapy. Some conventional practitioners cringe at the thought of using herbs as medicine, when in fact at least a quarter of the pharmaceuticals used today are derived from plant sources. The very word "drug" is derived from an old Dutch word, *drogge*, meaning "to dry." Early medicines typically consisted of a single dried herb or a combination, usually administered in the form of a tea or sprinkled into some other beverage or on food. Two common examples are digoxin, which is derived from foxglove, and aspirin, which is derived from white willow bark. Because nature's products can't be patented, herbal pharmaceuticals are combined with other, mainly synthetic ingredients,

the preparation is patented, and its herbal origins are forgotten.

Interest in herbal medicine is increasing because of drug interactions and side effects associated with conventional medications. Proponents of herbal medicine stress the decreased likelihood of interactions and untoward effects when such medicines are used properly. In Europe, herbal medicines share the mainstream with modern medications. Commission E in Germany is one notable pharmaceutical agency that produces a well-respected formulary of herbal medicines. As interest in herbs grows in the United States, informational resources for practitioners have become available.

Manual healing
Manual therapy is a small term to describe the large array of therapies that have at their core the use of the practitioner's hands. These therapies use the therapist's hands directly to manipulate the patient, as energy fields to deliver healing to the patient, or in a combination of touch and energy. Manual therapies can be divided into four overlapping categories, including energetic healing, movement repatterning, pressure-based techniques, and adjustment-based techniques. (See *Types of manual healing therapies*, page 10.)

Energetic healing includes techniques such as therapeutic touch and acupuncture. Movement repatterning includes techniques such as the Alexander, Feldenkrais, and Trager methods. Massage, reflexology, and pressure-point therapies are examples of pressure-based techniques. Chiropractic, osteopathic, and craniosacral therapy are forms of manipulative or adjustment-based techniques. Applied kinesiology overlaps the disciplines of pressure-based and adjustment-based techniques. Rolfing may be said to encompass the energetic healing, movement repatterning, and pressure-based categories. Qigong incorporates energetic healing and movement repatterning. The common factor shared by

TYPES OF MANUAL HEALING THERAPIES

The diagram below shows the different types of manual healing therapies and how they can overlap.

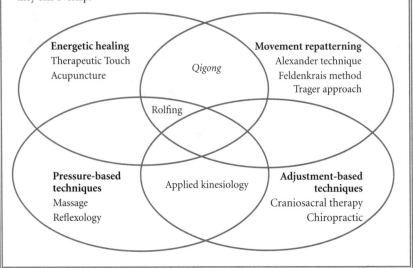

these techniques is that they are all used to reduce pain and stress, to enhance relaxation, and to stimulate circulation in order to promote healing.

Energetic manual healing

The energetic forms of manual healing are similar in that they use touch to transfer energy and healing into the patient. However, energetic healing may be either noninvasive, as in the form of Therapeutic Touch, or invasive, as in the case of acupuncture, which requires the use of needles.

Dolores Krieger, considered the founder of modern Therapeutic Touch, developed this therapy in 1972 as an interpretation of several ancient practices in which the practitioner modulates energy fields to decrease the patient's pain and anxiety. Therapeutic Touch is also used to correct problems with autonomic nervous system dysfunction. Rarely touching the patient, the practitioner's hands are kept approximately two to six inches above the body surface. They

move along the patient to determine the locations of a blockage in the patient's energy fields. As blockages are identified, the practitioner works to relieve congestion and obstruction and to replenish energy flow.

Acupuncture is a complete system of healing that alleviates pain and boosts the immune system to both heal and prevent illness. Acupuncture theory and technique, based on balancing qi (the vital life energy) within the body, was developed in China thousands of years ago. Qi is mapped via meridians along the body and further divided into over 1,000 acupoints that enhance qi when stimulated with needles. The meridian system has been verified using Galvanic skin response, which detects energy flow along the meridians.

Acupuncture is used to treat pain, addictions, and illnesses. It's so effective in relieving pain that many insurance companies identify acupuncture as an accepted treatment intervention. Practitioners of Chinese medicine perform acupuncture in a very traditional style, using only defined meridians and acupoints; this method requires thousands of hours of practice before the practitioner becomes proficient. Chiropractors, anesthesiologists, and others may also practice a form of acupuncture that is similar to pressure-point therapy; in this method the needles are inserted into trigger points and the trigger point is stimulated either with the needle alone or by use of accompanying electrical stimulation.

Movement repatterning

Movement repatterning includes the Alexander, Feldenkrais, and Trager techniques. The Alexander technique was devised by Fredrick Matthias Alexander, a Shakespearean actor who noticed a connection between posture and both physical and emotional problems. This therapy uses body awareness, movement, and touch to bring the posture and the body back into balance. The Alexander technique is especially helpful to those with chronic pain and back disorders.

Physicist Moshe Feldenkrais developed the technique bearing his name following a traumatic injury for which he refused surgical intervention. Studies of the nervous system and human behavior served as a jumping-off point for his method, into which he also incorporated martial arts, physiology, anatomy, psychology, and neurology. Feldenkrais determined that one's self-image is of utmost importance to one's health and well-being and that in order to overcome maladies, one must first redefine this image. The method also includes attention to breathing and movement and, as with the Alexander technique, the Feldenkrais method also considers posture to be the nucleus of movement. The practitioner uses touch to help the patient experience improved self-image and movement.

Milton Trager, a physician, developed the method that bears his name in the 1920s. The Trager method combines gentle and rhythmic touch with movement exercises. This method is also used to teach patients how to recognize posture and movement patterns indicating tension, and how to replace these patterns with healthy patterns. "Mentastics" is the term Trager coined for the increased awareness of movement gained by patients who practice his free-flowing and dancelike exercises.

Pressure-based therapies

Pressure-based therapies include massage, reflexology, and pressure-point therapy. Massage has been shown to be beneficial in the treatment of pain and tension; massage also speeds recovery from illnesses and surgery. Massage therapy is relaxing, speeds recovery from exercise, helps break up scar tissue and adhesions, increases lymphatic drainage, reduces swelling, improves circulation, promotes respiratory drainage, and can increase peristalsis.

Reflexology is approximately 4,000 years old and is believed to have originated in Egypt. The Chinese have also used reflexology in conjunction with acupuncture. The purposes of reflexology include relief of congestion, inflammation, and tension. The modern method of reflexology evolved from zone therapy, which is practiced in Europe; laryngologist William Fitzgerald is credited with having brought reflexology to the United States. The guiding premise behind reflexology is that the hands and feet have reflex points corresponding to every part of the body, including the spine, organs, and glands. Nerve endings in the hands and feet seem to have an extensive interconnection to the spinal cord and brain, and therefore to all areas of the body. Therapy is administered by a practitioner who applies gentle pressure to the reflex points on the patient's hands or feet.

Bonnie Prudden, one of the cofounders of the President's Council on Physical Fitness and Sports, is credited with the development of pressure-point, or trigger-point, therapy. A trigger point is a point within a muscle that was once exposed to trauma. Long after the original trauma heals, the trigger point remains, and may cause spasm and tenderness within the muscle whenever the patient experiences emotional or physical stress. The pain associated with trigger points can be exacerbated by many physical and emotional stressors, including disease, aging, or poor lifestyle habits. In Prudden's method, pressure is applied to the trigger point until discomfort is noted, after which it is maintained for 5 to 7 seconds. Trigger-point therapy is combined with stretching to retrain the muscle into a more relaxed state.

Adjustment-based therapies

Manipulative and adjustment-based therapies include chiropractic, osteopathic, and craniosacral methods. The discipline of chiropractic centers its theory of wellness on the relationship between nervous system, spinal column, and musculoskeletal system. The nervous system is thought to hold the key to health because it has the ability to coordinate and control all tissues of the body. If there is pressure on a nerve caused by subluxation, or misalignment, of a vertebra, pain can result and interfere with body function as well as with the immune system. The discipline of chiropractic was used in ancient Egypt, but the modern form was developed in 1895 by Daniel David Palmer. Palmer's first chiropractic patient reportedly had been deaf since a traumatic back injury. Palmer noted a misaligned vertebra in the patient's back and, after realigning it, the man regained his hearing.

Osteopathy is based on the premise that restoring the structural balance of the musculoskeletal system helps to restore health in the individual because structure equates to function. An osteopathic physician's patient evaluation may include observation of mechanical elements, such as posture, gait, motion, and symmetry, and an inspection of soft tissues. Osteopathic treatment can include mobilization, articulation, positional release methods, muscle energy techniques,

and cranial manipulation. Physician Andrew Taylor Still founded the first school of osteopathy in the United States in 1892. Osteopathic training combines conventional medicine along with osteopathic techniques; however, today many osteopathic schools don't devote the same attention to osteopathic techniques that they do to conventional medicine.

Craniosacral therapy is used to manipulate the bones of the skull in an effort to treat a variety of health concerns, including headache, stroke, upper respiratory infection, and cerebral palsy. The three subdisciplines of craniosacral therapy are sutural, meningeal, and reflex; these approaches may also be combined in various ways. Osteopathic physician William Garner Sutherland developed the sutural approach, in which the practitioner manipulates the skull sutures to bring them back into alignment, thereby easing pressure and increasing the cranial bones' mobility. The meningeal approach was developed by osteopathic physician John Upledger; this method focuses on manipulating not only the cranial sutures but also the underlying meninges. Chiropractor George Goodheart devised the reflex approach, in which the nerve endings in the scalp and between the cranial sutures are stimulated to relieve stress. The sacro-occipital technique was developed by chiropractor M.B. DeJarnette and combines all three approaches — sutural, meningeal, and reflex.

George Goodheart also developed applied kinesiology. This approach is used to explain medical problems as they relate to detected, but often subtle, muscle weaknesses. After the muscles are tested, techniques designed either to stimulate or relax the afflicted muscles are performed to relieve the condition affected by the weakened muscle. Applied kinesiology is also used by many practitioners as a diagnostic tool to reveal a variety of problems, from specific pathology to specific food allergy.

Rolfing was developed in the 1970s by biochemist Ida Rolf and combines the disciplines of osteopathy and Hatha yoga. It is similar to other methods in the category of adjustment-based therapies in that it is based on the premise that proper alignment affects proper body functioning. Rolfing reestablishes alignment through manipulation and stretching of muscle structures, fascial layers, and connective tissue. Ida Rolf's ideas were expanded upon by Judith Aston, developer of Aston-Patterning, and Joseph Heller, creator of Hellerwork. Both Aston and Heller added their own styles of bodywork to Rolf's model, with the common purpose of realigning the body's structures to enhance health and well-being.

Mind-body therapies

Mind-body therapies, like manual therapies, are numerous, and include such methods as art, dance, and music therapy; spirituality or religious practices; meditation, relaxation, and imagery; and hypnosis, biofeedback, and support groups. The interrelationship of mind and body, and how that interrelationship affects the whole person, is an integral element of mind-body therapies.

Importance of attitude

Another important aspect of mind-body therapies is the realization that attitude makes a difference to a person's physical and emotional well-being. Negative feelings beget negative internal workings and promote the development of disease. Positive attitudes and feelings help healing and seem to boost the immune system. Norman Cousins' *Anatomy of an Illness* (1981) is an account of the author's healing process, in which he employed laughter as a recovery tool. Studies have shown that an individual's opinion about his or her health is the best predictor not only of current health status but of future health status as well. Investigation into this relationship between health, the body, and the mind grew into a new field of study, called psychoneuroimmunology, in the 1970s. Psychoneuroimmunologic research has revealed the presence

of neurochemicals such as endorphins and other neuropeptides that link emotions with physical well-being. Mind-body therapies employ a variety of techniques to control stress-related illnesses, such as tension headaches, hypertension, and irritable bowel syndrome. These techniques are also used to treat incontinence, muscle spasms, dyskinesia, and other illnesses. Mind-body therapies empower individuals to become active participants in their health care rather than passive recipients who rely solely on practitioners.

Art, biofeedback, hypnosis

Art forms such as painting or drawing, dancing, or playing a musical instrument can have stimulating or relaxing effects and seem to affect the immune system. Prayer, either for one's self or for others, has been shown to create literal miracles. Recent studies have shown prayer to influence healing even when the person praying was unknown to the person for whom the prayer was intended. Meditation, relaxation, and imagery all employ techniques to slow breathing, improve energy flow, and visualize a positive outcome.

Biofeedback teaches people how to use electronic monitors as an aid to exerting conscious control over various autonomic functions. By observing the fluctuations of a particular body function — such as breathing, heart rate, or blood pressure — on the monitor, patients eventually learn how to adjust their thinking and other mental processes in order to control that function. As with other mind-body techniques, biofeedback gives the individual an active role in self-care management.

Hypnosis uses a more passive approach by having the therapist offer suggestions to patients while they are in an altered level of consciousness. The suggestions are intended to effect positive changes in behavior or enhance well-being; for example, hypnosis may be used to overcome habits such as smoking or overeating. The hypnotic suggestions are used, as with biofeedback, to give the patient control over autonomic or conditioned responses.

Pharmacologic and biological therapies

Pharmacologic and biological therapies use chemically or biologically active entities for treatment of diseases. These treatment modalities include antineoplaston therapy, chelation therapy, oxygen therapy, light therapy, neural therapy, apitherapy, aromatherapy, and biologicals such as shark cartilage.

Pharmacologic therapies

Antineoplaston therapy is used to eradicate cancer by injecting polypeptides into the body that convert cancerous cells into normal cells. This form of cancer therapy was developed by Dr. Stanislaw Burzynski and has been in use for the past 20 years.

Chelation therapy uses I.V. administration of ethylenediaminetetraacetic acid (EDTA) to draw out toxins and metabolic wastes to promote healing. It has been used to rid the body of calcium plaques in heart disease. By removing toxins, chelation acts as an anti-inflammatory agent that removes free radicals in order to reduce the pain and disability associated with degenerative diseases such as arthritis, lupus, and scleroderma. EDTA is not FDA-approved for chelating anything except for heavy metal toxins, such as lead; however, this therapeutic approach has been in use in the United States for almost 50 years.

Oxygen therapy is used primarily to destroy microbes such as viruses, bacteria, fungi, and amoebas in patients with acute myocardial infarction or poor circulation syndromes, such as those seen in diabetes, chronic fatigue syndrome, arthritis, allergies, cancer, and multiple sclerosis. Antioxidant enzymes such as superoxide dismutase, glutathione peroxidase, methionine reductase, and catalase are often recommended for use in combination with hyperoxygenation therapies. Oxygen therapies make use of many oxygen derivatives, such as hydrogen peroxide, ozone, glyoxylide, and stabilized oxygen compounds such as chlorine dioxide, magnesium oxide, and electrolytes of oxygen. Oxygen therapy can also be used in the form of hyperbaric oxygenation.

Ultraviolet (UV) light therapy, which is used to treat skin conditions such as psoriasis, is also based on oxygen therapy techniques because UV light activates oxidation at the dermis level. In the treatment of seasonal affective disorder, UV light is used to stimulate the neurochemical transmitters of the brain that affect depression and mood. Today, light in all its forms — full-spectrum, ultraviolet, colored, and laser — is considered an important source of healing.

Neural therapy uses anesthetic agents that are injected into nerve sites of the autonomic nervous system, acupuncture points, scars, glands, or other tissues to correct blockages present in these areas. Clearing the blockage restores energy, thereby reducing pain and improving function.

Biological therapies

One of the most well-known forms of biological CAM is the use of shark cartilage to arrest cancer. Hypothetically, it works by inhibiting angiogenesis. Proponents of this therapy often claim that shark cartilage may cure almost any illness.

Substances such as the venom and honey produced by honeybees are at the center of apitherapy, a method that has been in use since the time of Hippocrates. The most common modern use of apitherapy is in the treatment of inflammatory conditions such as arthritis.

Aromatherapy is based on the premise that odors stimulate the limbic system to release neurochemicals that affect the autonomic nervous system, help control pain and stress, and may even affect the regulation of hormones such as insulin. The term was coined in the 1930s by

French chemist René-Maurice Gattefosse, who studied plant oils and the beneficial effects they produced when inhaled or rubbed into the skin. Modern aromatherapy is used to reduce stress, thereby helping to prevent disease, and to treat certain illnesses of both mind and body.

Bioelectromagnetic applications

The theory of bioelectromagnetics rests on the fact that every object in nature — earth, heavens, animals, and plants — produces an electric charge and that manipulation of the charge through the use of magnets can redirect the flow of the electrical field and result in diagnostic or healing benefits.

Electromagnetic technology, in the form of magnetic resonance imaging, magnetoencephalography, or positron emission tomography, is used in conventional medicine for the diagnosis of illness. The first application of electromagnetic fields in the treatment of disease occurred in 1974 when Albert Roy Davis, PhD, used magnets to destroy or arrest the growth of cancer cells in animals. Davis suggested that magnets could also be used to treat other diseases including arthritis, glaucoma, and infertility. He theorized that negative magnetic fields have beneficial effects and that positive magnetic fields are stressful to organisms. Negative magnetic fields, then, would be those that arrest disease and promote healing, whereas positive magnetic fields, of the type existing in man-made electromagnetic fields, may contribute to disease.

Magnetic fields, either positive or negative, are believed to affect organisms by increasing metabolism and the amount of oxygen available. Magnetic strength is measured in units of gauss or tesla, with 10,000 gauss equaling 1 tesla. All magnetic devices have a gauss rating; however, a magnet's strength at the skin's surface is often much lower — usually around 75% less — than the gauss rating. If magnets aren't placed directly on the skin, the gauss rating is even lower. Besides strength, magnets also contain a positive and negative pole and, as previously mentioned, negative poles seem to have beneficial effects whereas positive poles may prove to be deleterious. Magnets rated at a strength of 850 gauss or less are believed to reflect more nearly the strength of the earth's natural magnetic field. For this reason, practitioners consider them safe, even for prolonged periods, regardless of the polarity used.

Electromagnetic therapy can be used to reduce pain and speed the healing of fractures. Physician Robert Becker was instrumental in popularizing the use of weak electrical currents to help in the remineralization of orthopedic fractures. Others, including scientists from the Bio-Electro Magnetics Institute and the Institute for Biophysics in Germany, continue to research the efficacy of electromagnetic therapy.

Negative electromagnetic therapy is also being used in the treatment of many other human diseases, including cancer, rheumatoid diseases and other inflammatory processes, infections, headaches (particularly migraine), sleep disorders, and circulatory problems.

CAM today

Despite parents' best efforts to teach their children basic health practices, those basic guidelines may fall by the wayside as children grow. If adults lose sight of the importance of nutrition, exercise, and rest and the avoidance of harmful substances, such as drugs, alcohol, and tobacco, they may rationalize this change in behavior and its subsequent effect on their body as a natural part of aging. Even when they realize it's time for a change, people may opt to use the kind of quick fixes — fad diets and medications for weight loss, analgesics for headache and arthritis pain relief, and anti-anxiety drugs to lessen or suppress the emotional response to chronic stress — that make lifestyle changes seemingly unnecessary. One of the greatest advantages of CAM is its stress on balancing a person's basic lifestyle and using preventive measures to maintain health and treat illness.

Each person's body reacts in its own way to stress and illness. Standardized protocols for specific diagnoses are not always the best treatment for everyone. CAM recognizes that people must be assessed individually, with treatment plans tailored to each person, an approach that is time-consuming and difficult to actualize in many conventional health care systems. Too often, symptoms are treated without identifying the underlying cause, which further delays accurate diagnosis and may even precipitate the evolution of a disease into a chronic state if the cause is an environmental factor or lifestyle-related behavior that isn't corrected.

Personal responsibility is the hub of much of CAM because it requires people to assume an active role in maintaining or restoring their health. While many people still prefer the "quick fix" of conventional medicine, CAM's ability to empower people to make their own health care decisions and lifestyle choices, and to draw on their own innate resources for health, is gaining popularity.

Modern practitioners of CAM

As people become more active participants in their health care, CAM's popularity and that of its more famous practitioners is increasing. Physicians Bernie Siegel, Deepak Chopra, and Andrew Weil, to name only three, have written books that make information about CAM accessible to the public at large.

In *Love, Medicine, and Miracles* (1986), Bernie Siegel describes his transformation from a traditional surgeon to a proponent of the belief that the ability to fight disease and remain healthy resides in one's ability to love oneself and to love life. During the 10 years he practiced conventional modern medicine, Siegel was haunted by feelings of failure when his patients didn't get better and when they died. He said he felt like a "mechanic" because his attention was focused on the physical body with no provision for healing the spirit. Siegel also began to question the worth of his profession's attempts to prolong life unconditionally and to cure disease in the elderly or terminally ill. A shift to a highly personal method of practice, in which he let down his emotional barriers and began to feel for and love his patients, resulted in a feeling that he was able to offer them a deeper dimension of healing. Siegel's revised view is that his role as a surgeon is to buy people time, help them understand why they became ill, and help them learn how to heal themselves. His core philosophy is based on a patient's ability to facilitate the healing process by being an active participant and drawing on the inner energy that resides within every individual.

Deepak Chopra is a physician from India who was trained in Western medicine and served as chief-of-staff at a Boston hospital for several years. According to an interview in *Time* magazine (Van Biema, 1996), Chopra's lifestyle during his early years of practice included consuming pots of coffee on a daily basis, smoking packs of cigarettes, and drinking Scotch every night to relax. He reported feeling like a sort of "legalized drug pusher" who provided short-term cures without concern for long-term prevention. Chopra felt that he was fostering a diseased system — indeed, contributing to a diseased world — with himself in the center like a spider in a web. With the help of the Maharishi Mahesh Yogi, Chopra rediscovered his spirituality and its place in healing. His clinic today offers a combination of Western, Ayurvedic, and East Asian therapies, and he has written several books on Ayurveda, including *Quantum Healing: Exploring the Frontiers of Body-Mind Medicine*, and *Perfect Health*.

Andrew Weil is another traditionally educated physician who became disillusioned with traditional methods. He spent three years in Peru, Ecuador, and Columbia learning about herbal and alternative therapies, after which he established a program of what he calls "integrative medicine" at the University of Arizona. Weil practices both natural and preventive medicine, encouraging well people to come in for preventive health checks and providing advice about diet, exercise, and stress reduction. A critic of the public's blind faith in professional medicine, he believes that most individuals have no sense of their own health or their power to affect it for good or ill (Weil, 1995).

The focus of Weil's health care model is on helping people design a healthy lifestyle and reduce the risk of getting a disease (primarily those that cause premature death, such as heart attack, stroke, and cancer), and on educating people about natural forms of treatments they can use themselves. Weil has also written several books that focus on integrative health care, including *Eight Weeks to Optimum Health*; *Spontaneous Healing*; and *Natural Health, Natural Medicine*.

The influence that the mind and spirit have on health isn't limited to medical practice; those involved in research are also beginning to embrace the holistic notion of healing. In an article in *Time* magazine, David Felton, chairman of the department of neurobiology at Boston University, discussed research findings showing that meditation and controlling one's state of mind can alter hormone activity and potentially affect the immune system (Wallis, 1996). Holmes and Rahe (1967) provided the support for this relationship as far back as the 1960s with their Social Readjustment Scale, which they developed to measure the correlation between amounts of positive and negative stress and the likelihood of becoming sick. Psychoimmunology, the study of this phenomenon, is a growing area of research.

Regulation of CAM

The health care industry is striving to keep pace with the technological advances of the 21st century in a cost-effective manner. While keeping pace and controlling costs may appear to be mutually exclusive, combining the two seemingly disparate aims has nurtured the growing acceptance of CAM in our society. Many health care providers are finding that a combination of both conventional medicine and CAM may be a compatible marriage. Eighty percent of all disease in our society is chronic in nature, and such illnesses often respond better to CAM, which has the added advantages that it may be cheaper and cause fewer side effects over time. CAM has provided consumers a choice of options and, with those options, the opportunity to regain control of their health care. As CAM's popularity and use continue to grow, governments — particularly the United States government — are beginning to acknowledge the importance of alternative medicine and to formulate guidelines for its practice and use.

The National Institutes of Health created the Office of Alternative Medicine (OAM) in response to the U.S. Congress' recognition of the importance of CAM. As its scope and purview increased, the OAM was elevated to the status of "national center" and given its present name, NCCAM. Its modest 1993 budget of $2 million rose to $68.7 million for the year 2000. NCCAM was formed to conduct and support basic and applied clinical research and research training in various forms of CAM. It also houses a scientific database and serves as a central clearinghouse of information for researchers, health care providers, and consumers. Eleven research centers have been set up to evaluate alternative treatments in areas such as addiction, aging, arthritis, cancer, cancer and hyperbaric oxygen therapy, cardiovascular disease, cardiovascular disease and aging in African-Americans, chiropractic, craniofacial disorders, neurological disorders, and pediatrics. (See

NCCAM research sites and current studies.)

Another important aspect of government involvement in the growing use of CAM is the regulation of practitioners, which varies according to the therapy employed. Some therapies are practiced by highly educated, clinically supervised practitioners of conventional medicine who have added some form of CAM to their models of care; such specialists include osteopaths, chiropractors, naturopaths, and medical doctors who have completed programs in acupuncture. Other practitioners may have been trained and certified in the use of a specific form of CAM in accordance with standards set by the certifying body for that form; examples include acupuncturists, massage therapists, or herbalists who received certification from the governing bodies of their respective specialties. Another group may have received training from practitioners within the same discipline, from continuing education, or from self-study without subsequent certification (Eliopoulos, 1999). While all 50 states require licensing for chiropractors, only half do so for acupuncture and massage therapists. Many states do not require licensing for homeopathy, naturopaths, or other CAM providers, allowing practitioners to operate freely (Jonas, 1998).

Medical clinicians committed to holistic practice formed the American Holistic Medical Association (AHMA) in 1978 to unite licensed physicians who practice holistic medicine. AHMA membership is open to licensed medical doctors (MDs), doctors of osteopathic medicine (DOs), and medical students studying for those degrees. Associate membership is also open to those health care practitioners certified, registered, or licensed in the state in which they practice. The mission of the AHMA is to support practitioners in their evolving personal and professional development as healers and to educate physicians about holistic medicine.

The American Holistic Nurses' Association (AHNA) was formed in 1981 to prepare nurses for holistic nursing practice, to standardize holistic nursing practice, and to unify holistic nursing care. The role of the holistic nurse is to incorporate mind-oriented therapies in all areas of nursing in order to treat the physiological, psychological, and spiritual sequelae of illnesses (Dossey et al., 2000). The association has established the underlying principles of holistic nursing practice, and sets standards of practice based on five core values. (See *The five core values of the American Holistic Nurses' Association,* page 22.)

The AHNA certification program provides a credential in holistic nursing to registered nurses who complete courses such as the Holistic Nurse Caring Process; Physical Fitness, Bodywork, and Movement; Energy Systems; Nutrition and Elimination; Communicating with the Whole Person; and Relaxation and Imagery. Information regarding the certification program is available on the AHNA Web site. The AHNA has also published *Holistic Nursing: A Handbook for Practice* (2000), a practice guide that is now in its third edition. The AHNA is also a good resource for locating instructional programs related to therapies such as Therapeutic Touch, imagery, aromatherapy, and so forth.

Each day, more primary care physicians are changing the face of their practices by adding such specialists as acupuncturists, massage therapists, and chiropractic doctors to their staffs. Integration of conventional and CAM services into one office holds promise for combining the best of both worlds. As Andrew Weil wryly observed (1995), "If I'm in a car accident, don't take me to an herbalist. If I have bacterial pneumonia, give me antibiotics. But when it comes to maximizing the body's natural healing potential, a mix of conventional and alternative procedures seems like the only answer." The use of CAM in relation to conventional medicine isn't an either/or

NCCAM RESEARCH SITES AND CURRENT STUDIES

Shown below are studies currently underway at research sites of the National Center for Complementary and Alternative Medicine (NCCAM).

Center	Objective	Current studies
Center for Addiction and Alternative Medicine Research, Minneapolis Medical Research Foundation	To scientifically evaluate complementary and alternative medicine (CAM) treatments for addictions	▪ Herbal compounds to help prevent alcoholic relapse ▪ Electroacupuncture to map the neural substrates of opioids ▪ Herbal compounds to treat hepatitis C symptoms
Center for CAM Research in Aging and Women's Health, Columbia University, New York	To analyze the effect herbal and dietary treatments have in the treatment of postmenopausal women	▪ Black cohosh to treat menopausal complaints ▪ Safety of Chinese herbal preparations for women with or at risk for breast cancer ▪ Comparison of a macrobiotic diet with an American Heart Association diet in relation to hormone and phytoestrogen metabolism, cardiovascular function, and bone metabolism
Center for Alternative Medicine Research on Arthritis, University of Maryland, Baltimore	To explore the potential efficacy, safety, and cost-effectiveness of CAM for arthritis-related illnesses	▪ Acupuncture to treat osteoarthritis of the knee ▪ Mind-body therapies to treat fibromyalgia ▪ Electroacupuncture to treat persistent pain and inflammation ▪ Herbal therapies with possible immunomodulatory properties
The Center for Cancer Complementary Medicine, Johns Hopkins University, Baltimore	To investigate CAM therapies in the treatment of cancer	▪ Antioxidant effects of herbs in cancer cells ▪ Antioxidant and anti-inflammatory properties of soy and tart cherry on aspects of cancer pain ▪ Safety and efficacy of PC-SPES* to treat prostate cancer ▪ Impact of spiritual practices on disease recurrence and immune and neuroendocrine function in African-American women with breast cancer
Center for Research in Hyperbaric Oxygen Therapy, University of Pennsylvania, Philadelphia	To examine the mechanisms of action, safety, and clinical efficacy of hyperbaric oxygen therapy for head and neck tumors	▪ Benefits of hyperbaric oxygen after laryngectomy ▪ Effects of hyperbaric oxygen on growth of blood vessels and tumors ▪ Effects of hyperbaric oxygen on cell adhesion and growth of metastatic tumor cells in the lung ▪ Effects of elevated oxygen pressures on cellular levels of nitric oxide

(continued)

NCCAM RESEARCH SITES AND CURRENT STUDIES *(continued)*

Center	Objective	Current studies
Center for Cardiovascular Diseases, University of Michigan, Ann Arbor	To investigate the use of CAM to treat and prevent cardiovascular disease as well as stressing education and promotion of validated CAM for cardiovascular well-being	▪ Hawthorn extract to treat congestive heart failure ▪ Reiki biofield energy healing technique to treat diabetic peripheral vascular disease and autonomic neuropathy ▪ Effects of spirituality on patients undergoing coronary artery bypass surgery ▪ Effects of qi gong on pain and healing after coronary artery bypass graft
Center for Natural Medicine and Prevention, Maharishi University of Management, Fairfield, Iowa	To evaluate CAM for the prevention of cardiovascular disease in high-risk older African-Americans	▪ Effects of meditation on atherosclerotic cardiovascular disease ▪ Effects of meditation on carotid atherosclerosis, cardiovascular disease risk factors, physiological mechanisms, psychosocial risk factors, and quality of life in older African-American women with cardiovascular disease ▪ Comparison of effects of herbal antioxidants and conventional vitamin supplementation on carotid atherosclerosis, endothelial function, oxidative stress, cardiovascular disease risk factors, and quality of life
Consortial Center for Chiropractic Research, Palmer Center for Chiropractic Research, Davenport, Iowa	To examine the potential effectiveness and validity of chiropractic health care and to provide the appropriate clinical, scientific, and technical assistance to chiropractic researchers in developing high-quality research projects	▪ Development of research workshops and educational materials to provide an institutional focus for formal training in research methodology, bioethics, biostatistics, clinical trial design, epidemiological and health services studies, and basic laboratory methods ▪ Establishment of a network of chiropractic clinicians and investigators in specific topic areas ▪ Prioritization of research topics related to chiropractic treatment of musculoskeletal conditions ▪ Development of a mechanism for scientific and technical merit review of research proposals ▪ Implementation of selected research projects
Center for Complementary and Alternative Medicine Research in Craniofacial Disorders, Kaiser Foundation Hospitals, Portland, Oregon	To research the efficacy, effectiveness, effects on health care resource use, and psychosocial and other health outcomes associated with CAM for craniofacial disorders, as well as the physiological and psychological mechanisms underlying these practices	▪ Alternative approaches to pain management in temporomandibular disorders (TMD) ▪ Alternative medicine approaches to treat TMDs in women ▪ Complementary naturopathic medicine to treat periodontitis

NCCAM RESEARCH SITES AND CURRENT STUDIES *(continued)*

Center	Objective	Current studies
Center for Complementary and Alternative Medicine in Neurological Disorders, Oregon Health Sciences University, Portland	To assess the use of antioxidants and stress reduction as treatments for neurodegenerative and demyelinating diseases	▪ Facilitation of four research projects and maintenance of four core facilities that integrate the research strengths of conventional medicine and CAM practitioners and researchers ▪ Promotion of new areas of CAM research and spearheading of research on CAM therapies for neurologic disorders
Pediatric Center for Complementary and Alternative Medicine, University of Arizona, Tucson	To study integrative approaches in pediatrics	▪ Implementation of three projects to investigate alternative approaches to three common pediatric problems: recurrent abdominal pain, otitis media, and cerebral palsy ▪ Establishment of a pediatric research fellowship in CAM and research methodologies

*PC-SPES is a formulation of seven plants and one fungus. The name is derived from the common abbreviation for prostate cancer (PC) and the Latin word *spes,* meaning hope. Don't confuse PC-SPES with a related herbal combination product called simply SPES, also under development as a potential cancer treatment.

proposition; the greatest benefits to people both healthy and ill may be achieved using a judicious blend of both methods.

The present, inconsistent regulation of CAM dictates that practitioners must become familiar with the recommended certification for each particular treatment modality. They must also know how to access this information to ensure safe referrals. Books on CAM and integrative medicine provide excellent listings of national organizations devoted to CAM and its various specialties. (See Appendix 1, *Herbal resource list,* page 527.) The Internet is another good place to search for information on CAM, as many national organizations' Web sites list the recommended certifying body and certification level for a particular CAM practice.

Consumers and integrated practice
A new generation of consumers is demanding a more informed, active role in their health care. NCCAM established a clearinghouse in 1996 through which consumers can access information about

CAM, NCCAM programs, conferences, and research activities. This information is accessed through a toll-free information line, fact sheets available from the NCCAM Clearing House, and a newsletter available through postal mail or online. While NCCAM provides a plethora of information on CAM, including the newest research findings, consumers can also find information at the library, bookstores, and Internet websites. However, sorting through this information can be challenging for the lay person without help from health care providers familiar with CAM.

In 1998, Eisenberg et al. recommended that "federal agencies, private corporations, foundations, and academic institutions adopt a more proactive posture concerning the implementation of clinical and basic science research, the development of relevant educational curricula, credentialing and referral guidelines, improved quality control of dietary supplements and the establishment of postmarket surveillance of drug-herb (and drug supplement) interactions." In the

---

THE FIVE CORE VALUES OF THE AMERICAN HOLISTIC NURSES' ASSOCIATION

1. Holistic philosophy and education
2. Holistic ethics, theories, and research
3. Holistic nurses' self-care
4. Holistic communication, therapeutic environment, and cultural diversity
5. Holistic caring process

---

meantime, health care providers must become informed about CAM and consider integrating them into conventional practice. Doing so will foster a model of health care, characterized by collaborative practice, that provides patient-focused, individualized care in a cost-efficient, self-responsible manner. The renewed interest in CAM shown by health care consumers and the increased political and financial support offered by the NIH indicate that CAM's resurgence isn't a trend that will pass with time.

Conclusion

It's time to recognize the power of the mind and its effect on the body—for example, studies show that the placebo effect works in 25% of people regardless of what intervention they're undergoing. As increasing numbers of patients turn to CAM, it behooves practitioners to familiarize themselves with these alternative approaches to healing and wellness in order to intelligently direct patients to the best possible care and prevention strategies. Even if no scientific evidence supports a particular therapy, if it produces measurable outcomes in patients, then either the therapy works or the placebo effect is in place.

As we learn about the various forms of CAM, we must remember that conventional Western medicine as it exists today was once viewed with the kind of suspicion with which many modern practitioners now view CAM. Traditional practices that had long been abandoned as archaic—for example, bloodletting by the application of leeches—are now being reassessed and found to have some validity. Perhaps we'll find that the most important aspects of wellness and the prevention of disease, as well as the treatment of disease, are based upon natural elements—foods and food substances, personal lifestyle, interaction with nature, and spiritual well-being—that our ancestors once embraced and later abandoned. We may find that the use of these basic elements affects our physical and emotional well-being more than any conventional medicine ever could.

Not long ago, osteopathy, chiropractic, and naturopathy were not considered accepted disciplines for diagnosing and treating illness, yet now insurance companies reimburse all three. Also, Medicare is considering the use of acupuncture for treating pain. Therapeutic Touch and reflexology are used in well-respected teaching hospitals. Music therapy and prayer are also being mainstreamed into hospitals. So many things about this world still lie beyond our understanding; who can say that what isn't currently considered mainstream lacks credibility?

acacia gum

Acacia senegal, *acacia vera, cape gum, Egyptian thorn, gum acacia, gum arabic, gum Senegal,* Gummae mimosae, Gummi africanum, *Kher, Somali gum, Sudan gum arabic, yellow thorn*

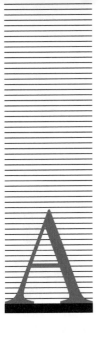

Acacia gum is derived from the sap of the acacia tree, *Acacia senegal.* In its natural form it's an odorless, white or yellow-white to pale amber, brittle solid. The main component of the gum is arabin, which is the calcium salt of arabic acid. It's almost completely soluble in water, but doesn't dissolve in alcohol and is hydrolyzed to form arabinose, galactose, and arabinosic.

Acacia gum is available as flakes, granules, powder, and spray-dried formulations. It's also available in a dry powder form that's commonly used as a stabilizer in drug emulsions and as an additive in various oral combinations. Acacia gum may also be dissolved in water to make a mucilage.

Reported uses
Acacia gum, which is essentially nontoxic, has no significant systemic effects when taken orally.

Although acacia gum is commonly used to reduce cholesterol levels, it may actually elevate these levels in serum and tissue.

Acacia may be used in cough drops to soothe throat and stomach irritation, to treat diarrhea, and to impede absorption of certain substances.

Chewing acacia-based gum may limit development of periodontal disease and may also prevent plaque deposit. Whole gum mixtures of 0.5% to 1% may prevent growth of periodontal bacteria, and mixtures of 0.5% may inhibit bacterial protease enzyme.

Acacia also masks acrid substances such as capsicum and may be used as a treatment for catarrh, a mild stimulant, a food stabilizer, and a film-forming agent in peel-off skin masks. It's also used in some wound-healing preparations.

Administration
- The usual dose of acacia gum in mucilage form is 1 to 4 teaspoons by mouth
- As a component in a drug preparation, the amount of acacia gum varies with the preparation. In periodontal use, for example, concentrations range from 0.5% to 1%.

Hazards
In general, patients with an allergy to acacia gum may develop severe bronchospasm or skin lesions.

When mixed with certain alkaloids, acacia gum may partially degrade them. Acacia gum is insoluble in substances containing ethyl alcohol concentrations of more than 50%. They should not be mixed together.

Ferric iron salt solutions may gelatinize acacia gum. The fiber component of acacia gum may impair absorption of oral drugs. Monitor for loss of therapeutic effect.

 SAFETY RISK *Acacia gum is contraindicated in those with allergy or hypersensitivity to acacia dust. Also, its use in pregnant or breast-feeding women should be avoided because the effects of the herb are unknown.*

Clinical considerations
 SAFETY RISK *Don't confuse acacia gum with sweet acacia (Acacia farnesiana) or products from the tree of the genus Albizia. These products may not be substituted for one another.*

- Monitor for allergic reactions to acacia dust, including severe bronchospasm and skin lesions.
- Warn patient that conditions such as hyperlipidemia, periodontal infection, and GI and throat irritation could worsen if treatment is delayed.
- Advise patient with an allergy to acacia dust not to use acacia gum because severe reactions may occur.
- Advise patient to store dry powder, granule, or flake formulations in tightly closed containers.
- Advise patient that acacia gum may affect the absorption of other oral drugs and that he should notify his health care provider before using the herb.
- Tell patient to remind prescriber and pharmacist of any herbal or dietary supplement he is taking when obtaining a new prescription.

Research summary
The regulatory specifications for *Acacia senegal* are inadequate to ensure that it isn't adulterated with gums from other botanical sources.

acidophilus
Lactobacillus acidophilus

Lactobacillus acidophilus grows naturally in the human GI tract along with *Bacteroides, Escherichia coli, Streptococcus faecalis,* and other microorganisms, each of which prevents the others from overgrowth in the intestine. Acidophilus produces hydrogen peroxide and lactic acid to suppress pathogenic bacteria.

Acidophilus is available as capsules, granules, powders, tablets, and in milk and yogurt, in products such as Bacid, Kala, Lactinex, More-Dophilus, Pro-Bionate, Probiotics, and Superdophilus.

Reported uses
Acidophilus is used to treat lactose intolerance, digestive disorders, or antibiotic-induced diarrhea because it helps replace

intestinal flora. It's also used to ease the pain of a sore mouth caused by oral candidiasis, and to treat fever blisters, canker sores, hives, and acne.

Lactobacillus products are used to treat vaginal yeast or bacterial infections and uncomplicated lower urinary tract infections. They're administered intravaginally to treat bacterial vaginosis in pregnant women in the first trimester, thus restoring normal vaginal flora and acidity.

When antibiotics are given, growth of susceptible bacteria may decline, allowing for overgrowth of other bacteria; acidophilus is then given to restore intestinal flora and, thus, homeostasis.

Some herbal practitioners claim acidophilus may also retard the growth of tumors and reduce cholesterol levels; however, no data support this. Although sometimes used to treat irritable bowel syndrome or inflammatory bowel disease, acidophilus probably isn't effective for these conditions.

Administration
- Bacid: 1 capsule by mouth two to four times a day
- Lactinex: 1 packet added to or taken by mouth with food, milk, juice, or water two to four times a day
- More-Dophilus: 1 teaspoon by mouth every day with liquid
- Pro-Bionate capsules: 1 capsule by mouth every day, up to three times a day
- Pro-Bionate powder: ¼ to 1 teaspoon by mouth every day, up to three times a day
- Superdophilus: ¼ to 1 teaspoon by mouth every day, up to three times a day
- To decrease recurrence of vaginal candidiasis: 1 cup of yogurt containing *L. acidophilus* by mouth
- If dose is quantified as "number of living organisms," 1 to 10 billion viable organisms by mouth three or four times a day.

Hazards
There are no reported drug interactions with acidophilus.

People with sensitivity to dairy products and children under the age of 3 should avoid using acidophilus. Those with high fevers should use acidophilus with caution. The use of acidophilus in pregnant and lactating women should be avoided because the effects are unknown. Acidophilus may cause flatulence.

Clinical considerations
- Inform patient that the potency of acidophilus is reduced by storage conditions and length of time in storage. Acidophilus should be stored in the refrigerator.
- Some products labeled to contain *L. acidophilus* contain little to no active ingredient, whereas others contain contaminants such as *Clostridium sporogenes, Enterococcus faecium,* and *Pseudomonas.*
- Tell patient that flatulence is prevalent with initial dosing but decreases with continued use.
- Inform patient that if he delays seeking medical diagnosis and treatment, conditions such as inflammatory bowel disease, vaginal infections, urinary tract infections, thrush, hyperlipidemia, antibiotic-associated diarrhea, and developing tumors could worsen.
- Advise patient not to use acidophilus for longer than 2 days or while he has a high fever, unless his health care provider has instructed him to do so.
- Advise patient with sensitivity to dairy products to avoid oral use of *L. acidophilus.*
- Tell patient to remind prescriber and pharmacist of any herbal or dietary supplement he is taking when obtaining a new prescription.
- Advise patient to consult his health care provider before using an herbal preparation because a treatment with proven efficacy may be available.

Research summary

According to several studies, regular use of acidophilus and other probiotics can help prevent "traveler's diarrhea" (an illness that usually occurs in developing countries and is caused by contaminated food and drink).

aconite

Aconiti, aconiti tuber,
Aconitum napellus,
blue rocket, friar's cap, helmet flower, monkshood, mousebane, soldier's cap, wolfsbane

Aconite is the dried tuberous root of *Aconitum napellus.* The root contains many alkaloids, with aconitin being the most pharmacologically active; other alkaloids include hypaconitin and mesaconitin. Aconitin increases membrane permeability for sodium ions and slows repolarization. Initially, aconitin is stimulating but later causes paralysis in the central nervous system. In small doses, aconitin causes bradycardia and hypotension; in higher doses, it has an initial positive inotropic effect, then causes tachycardia, cardiac arrhythmias, and cardiac arrest. The other alkaloids have comparable effects, with hypaconitin being the strongest.

Reported uses

Liniments made from aconite are used to treat neuralgia, sciatica, and rheumatism. Aconite is used as a cardiac depressant and as a component in some cough mixtures.

In homeopathic preparations, aconite is used as an analgesic, antipyretic, and antihypertensive.

Administration

For external use, the average dose of aconite tincture is 0.1 to 0.2 g, applied topically with a brush. Maximum daily dose is 0.6 g.

Hazards

SAFETY RISK *All species of the herb aconite are potentially dangerous, even when used topically. Aconite should not be taken by mouth because it's a potent, fast-acting poison, affecting the heart and central nervous system.*

Aconite may cause heart failure, arrhythmias, paralysis of cardiac muscle, paralysis of the respiratory center, hypotension, nausea, vomiting, and paresthesias.

Oral use of aconite isn't recommended, and even aconite-containing liniments absorbed through the skin may produce serious poisoning. Liniments containing aconite should never be applied to wounds or abrasions because of the potential for enhanced absorption, which could cause systemic toxicity.

There are no reported interactions with aconite.

Clinical considerations

- Warn patient that use of this herb isn't recommended because it may have fatal toxic effects.
- Tell patient to remind prescriber and pharmacist of any herbal or dietary supplement he is taking when obtaining a new prescription.
- Advise patient to consult his health care provider before using an herbal preparation because a treatment with proven efficacy may be available.

SAFETY RISK *Because of aconite's toxic effects, it's rarely used in the United States. These effects may be partially decreased by some manufacturing processes; however, inability to predict toxic effects among available products should discourage its use.*

The onset of aconite poisoning is almost immediate, with the delay of symptom onset being as long as one hour. Death from aconite poisoning may occur within minutes to days after ingestion, depending on the dose.

Immediate symptoms of toxic reaction include burning sensation of lips, tongue, mouth, and throat. Numbness of the throat and inability to speak may follow. Numbness of fingers and toes and, eventually, the entire body may progress to a furry sensation. Body temperature may significantly decline. Excessive salivation, nausea, vomiting, urination, hypotension, and blurred vision with yellow-green visual disturbance may also follow initial symptoms.

Treatment of aconite poisoning is symptomatic. Atropine has been used to treat aconite-induced cardiotoxicity in severe cases. Arrhythmias may not respond to procainamide and may worsen with verapamil. Gastric lavage may need to be performed or vomiting induced.

Research summary

Literature on aconite mentions several fatal poisonings and numerous nonfatal toxic effects, perhaps because the herb's therapeutic index is narrow and its potency varies. Even as little as one teaspoon of the root may cause paralysis of the respiratory center and cardiac muscle, leading to death.

Acupressure

Do in, shiatsu, tsubo

Acupressure is an ancient healing art of traditional Chinese medicine that uses finger pressure on key points (called acupoints) on the surface of the skin to stimulate the body's natural self-curative abilities. It's considered a form of massage therapy or bodywork. In acupressure, local symptoms are considered an expression of the condition of the body as a whole (mind, body, and spirit). Acupressure sessions focus not only on relieving discomfort, but also on reducing tensions and toxicities in the body before they develop into an illness.

More than 5,000 years ago, the Chinese discovered that pressing certain points on the body relieved pain where it occurred and also benefited other parts of the body remote from the pain and the pressure point. They also found other points that not only alleviated pain but also influenced the functioning of certain internal organs. The distinction between acupuncture and acupressure (the older of the two techniques) is that needles are used in acupuncture, whereas a firm but gentle pressure of the hands is the basis for acupressure.

The purpose of acupressure is to relax muscular tension and balance the vital energy forces of the body through channels or meridians. The twelve meridians are pathways along the body associated with different internal organs. In theory, obstruction in a meridian causes the energy to flow more slowly, or even stop, resulting in a malfunction or dysfunction in the organ associated with that meridian. Each point along the meridian has a specific purpose and is used for specific health problems. Each point can also be used to help form a diagnosis. Theoretically, a stomach problem arises if an obstruction in the stomach meridian slows down the flow of energy. If the obstruction is removed or dissolved, the energy flow becomes regular and the stomach function returns. However, even though it may be the stomach meridian that is blocked, other areas of the body may also be affected because everything in the body interrelates.

Acupoints are places on the skin that are especially sensitive to bioelectric impulses in the body and conduct these impulses readily. The points follow the body's meridians. Stimulating these points with pressure (or heat or needles) triggers the release of endorphins, the neurochemicals that relieve pain. As a result, the flow of blood and oxygen to the affected area is increased and pain is blocked. Tension tends to concentrate around points. When a muscle is chronically tense or in spasm, the muscle fibers contract due to the secretion of lactic acid caused by fatigue, trauma, stress, chemical imbalance, or poor circulation. As a point is pressed, the muscle tension yields to the finger pressure, enabling the fibers to elongate and relax, blood to flow freely, and toxins to be released and eliminated.

In addition to manipulation of acupoints, a skilled therapist reviews the whole person, taking into account facial and tongue diagnosis, energy pulses, and symptoms, both physical and spiritual. The concepts underlying traditional Chinese medicine and acupressure are *qi* (vital energy), *yin* and *yang*, the five element theory, and the *zang-fu* organ system.

Everything in the universe is composed of and defined by *qi*, sometimes called chi or ki (all pronounced *chee*). Qi, or vital energy, is said to be the basis of life; this concept is a fundamental belief in traditional Chinese medicine. In the human body, the original qi is transmitted from parents to children at conception and is stored in the kidneys. Grain qi is derived from the digestion of food. The lungs extract natural air qi from inhaled air. It all comes together to produce normal qi that permeates the entire body.

The concept of *yin* and *yang* holds that everything in nature has two opposite aspects. The opposition of yin and yang is reflected mainly in their ability to control each other. Warmth and heat (yang) may dispel cold, while coolness and cold (yin) may lower a high temperature. Under normal conditions in the human body, a relative physiologic balance is maintained through the mutual opposition of yin and yang. If an excess or deficiency of either yin or yang occurs, the physiologic balance of the body is affected and illness develops.

In the five element theory, each of the internal organs is linked to one of the five elements in the natural world, namely wood, fire, earth, metal, and water. For example, the heart is linked to fire. Classification according to these elements explains both physiologic and pathologic phenomena and guides clinical diagnosis and treatment. For example, a person with a red complexion accompanied by a bitter taste in the mouth suggests an excess of heart (fire) that must be reduced.

All five elements must exist in balance in the body. If one element predominates, the others will become unbalanced and illness will result.

In the *zang-fu* organ system, the main physiologic functions of the *zang* organs — heart, lungs, spleen, liver, kidneys, and pericardium — are the manufacture and storage of essential substances. The *fu* organs — including gallbladder, stomach, small intestine, large intestine, and bladder — receive and digest food and transmit and excrete wastes. In the Chinese system, the organs are discussed always with reference to their functions and to their relationships with other organs and other parts of the body. There isn't an exact correlate to the anatomy and physiology of Western medicine because of the way Chinese medicine developed over the centuries. The individual is viewed as a whole with interrelationships of the above concepts affecting health and illness.

Other forms of acupressure are *do in*, *tsubo*, and *shiatsu*. *Do in* is stretching and self massage of the acupoints to provide physical energy and mental relaxation. *Tsubo*, developed by K. Serizawa of Tokyo University, refers to key acupoints (or tsubos)on the meridians where energy flow to the zang-fu organs tends to stagnate. *Shiatsu*, the Japanese version of acupressure, also incorporates some gentle manipulation and body stretches along with using the pressure points. Some Swedish massage therapists have also studied acupressure and incorporated it in their treatments.

Reported uses
Acupressure is said to reduce tension, increase circulation, and enable the body to relax deeply. It's reportedly effective in helping to relieve headache, eyestrain, sinus problems, neck pain, lower backache, arthritis, muscle ache, and fatigue. The treatment has also been reported to relieve ulcer pain, menstrual cramps, constipation, and indigestion.

RELIEVING A HEADACHE WITH ACUPRESSURE

Also known as Chinese massage, acupressure is simply acupuncture without the needles. It involves placing firm finger pressure on designated points of the body—known as acupoints—to relieve symptoms such as pain. Each acupoint is believed to be connected to a particular organ system. The acupoint used may be far removed from the site of the patient's symptoms; for example, one of the acupoints for treating headache is located in the hand.

Locating the acupressure points
You can practice acupressure on yourself or your patient with a minimum of training. The diagrams below show useful points to use for releasing a muscle

tension headache. The points known as GB 20 are located at the base of the skull (shown at left); the point known as LI 4 (Hoku point) is located at the base of the thumb and index finger (shown at right).

Breath in, then slowly exhale as you press the designated point. (Use both thumbs to press on both GB 20 points simultaneously.) Press until you feel resistance or pain; then maintain pressure until you finish the exhalation, releasing the pressure as you inhale. Press each point three to five times. Repeat, if needed, after 10 minutes.

Acupressure should not be applied directly over cuts, wounds, sores, scar tissue, or infected areas.

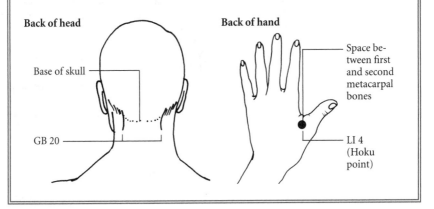

Back of head

Base of skull

GB 20

Back of hand

Space between first and second metacarpal bones

LI 4 (Hoku point)

Acupressure is also a useful self-help therapy and first-aid treatment; for example, it has been shown to reduce the frequency and severity of asthma attacks and promote more effective breathing. The Chinese have used acupressure as a beauty treatment for thousands of years; the points can be used to improve skin condition and tone and relax the facial muscles. By relaxing and toning the back muscles, acupressure makes the spinal adjustments in chiropractic treatment easier and more effective. The deep relaxation promoted by acupressure relieves anxiety and promotes restful sleep. By re-

lieving stress, acupressure strengthens resistance to disease and promotes wellness. (See *Relieving a headache with acupressure.*)

How the treatment is performed
Treatment is performed over light cotton clothing. The practitioner usually works on a mat on the floor, but may use a traditional massage table.

The practitioner uses the thumbs and fingers to press key points on the surface of the skin to locate the stagnation of meridian flow. Pressure is then used to remove the obstruction so that energy can flow as it should and the organ involved can resume its normal function. The pressure releases muscle tension, increases blood circulation, and promotes the function of qi (the body's life force) to aid in healing. Often a point that initially feels sore will improve simply by pressing on it.

In shiatsu and tsubo, practitioners may also use their elbows, knees, and feet to reach the pressure points. Shiatsu also incorporates some stretching movements.

 TRAINING *Because acupressure falls under the auspices of massage therapy, the National Committee Certification for Acupuncture and Traditional Oriental Medicine recently created national examination and credentialing standards for Oriental bodywork and acupressure. A minimum of 500 hours of training, including at least 100 hours of anatomy, is required. While the industry standard is 500 hours, each state has different requirements for licensure.*

Hazards
While shiatsu and tsubo carry little risk if performed correctly, some people object to the pressure. There can be moments where the pressure in a tender spot borders on pain, but this gives way to relief when the pressure is released.

Clinical considerations
■ Acupressure should not be performed on a person who has just eaten or on anyone with a high fever.
■ Pressure should not be applied to areas of inflammation or to wounds. Caution should be used with persons suffering from cancer or heart disease, pregnant women, and the elderly. Gentle pressing techniques can be used in place of the more vigorous ones.
■ Certain points, such as LI 4, must not be used in pregnant women because stimulation of those points can cause premature contractions in the uterus.
■ If pain occurs, the patient should ask the practitioner to adjust the pressure to a more comfortable level.

■ With the self-massage of do in, the individual may tend to work too vigorously and not give the body time to adjust to the stretches.

Research summary
Studies suggest that sensory nerves are probably analogs of meridians because most acupoints are localized near nerve fibers. Pressure can induce a wide array of physiologic responses in nerve fibers and in nerve endings. Dishant Shah's study suggests that some changes in the brain's response to tactile stimuli can be caused by acupressure treatments (Shah, 1999).

Various studies have examined the effectiveness of acupressure in the treatment of morning sickness in pregnant women, post-surgical nausea and vomiting, headaches, motion sickness, backache, and so forth. Research results are mixed.

 REIMBURSEMENT *Insurance companies differ in their coverage for traditional Chinese medicine. Factors that influence these differences include state regulations, licensure of the practitioner, and whether medical supervision is required.*

Acupuncture

A key component of traditional Chinese medicine, acupuncture dates back nearly 5,000 years to around 2700 B.C. *The Yellow Emperor's Classic of Internal Medicine,* a treatise on traditional Chinese medicine believed to have been written in the 2nd or 3rd century BC, contains the first written reference to acupuncture. The "yellow emperor" of the title was actually a composite of numerous Chinese physicians whose medical knowledge was passed down and finally collected in book form.

Acupuncture began to attract widespread attention in the western world after President Richard Nixon's visit to China in 1972. During that trip, *New*

York Times reporter James Reston underwent an emergency appendectomy and wrote an article on the acupuncture anesthesia that was used during the procedure. His article piqued the interest of American doctors, who began traveling to China to observe this procedure firsthand. They discovered a medical practice that was used not only as a substitute for surgical anesthesia but also as a treatment for pain and numerous disorders.

Today, acupuncture is practiced in a variety of mainstream medical settings and is a widely accepted treatment for pain and certain addictions. According to the World Health Organization, there are about 10,000 acupuncture practitioners in the United States, of whom approximately 3,000 are medical doctors. Americans are estimated to spend $500 million and make 9 to 12 million office visits per year for acupuncture treatments.

In November 1997, a National Institutes of Health (NIH) consensus panel reported clear evidence that needle acupuncture is effective in treating postoperative dental pain as well as nausea and vomiting due to surgery, chemotherapy, and pregnancy. The 12-member panel also listed a number of conditions for which acupuncture might be used as an adjunctive therapy or an acceptable alternative therapy. These included (but were not limited to) addiction, stroke rehabilitation, low back pain, menstrual cramps, headache, tennis elbow, fibromyalgia, carpal tunnel syndrome, and asthma.

To promote greater public access to acupuncture, the panel also urged insurance companies and governmental insurance programs, including Medicare and Medicaid, to reimburse for appropriate acupuncture treatments.

In another sign of acupuncture's growing acceptance, the U.S. Food and Drug Administration (FDA) recently removed acupuncture needles from its list of experimental medical devices and now regulates them just as it does scalpels, syringes, and other common medical instruments.

Acupuncture is based on the same principle that underlies traditional Chinese medicine: the existence of a vital life force — qi — that circulates in the body through channels known as meridians. The 12 major meridians are believed to be connected to specific organ systems. (There is also a network of collateral and minor meridians.) The meridians, used in both diagnosis and treatment, act as a road map that allows the practitioner to locate specific acupuncture points (acupoints).

TRAINING *The licensing of acupuncturists varies widely from state to state. A majority of states have laws specifically licensing or registering acupuncture professionals, but the scope of practice varies widely. New Mexico recognizes the Doctor of Oriental Medicine (DOM) as a primary care provider, but a number of states allow only MDs or DOs to practice acupuncture or allow an acupuncturist to practice only under the supervision of an MD.*

Reported uses

According to Chinese theory, an organ that is experiencing an energy imbalance or diseased state may manifest signs or symptoms at its corresponding meridian. Such symptoms may include pain or aching, a change in skin temperature, sensitivity to touch, or alterations in skin texture or color along a portion of the channel. These symptoms help the practitioner determine which organ systems are affected and, thus, which acupoints to use in the treatment. The stimulation of these points by acupuncture needles is believed to balance, release, or enhance the flow of qi and thus relieve pain or restore health.

The World Health Organization has listed more than 100 conditions that may benefit from treatment with acupuncture, including neurologic disorders (migraines, Ménière's disease, trigeminal neuralgia, peripheral neuropathy), GI disorders (colitis, gastritis, ulcers, diarrhea, constipation, hiccups), pulmonary and respiratory conditions (bronchitis, asthma, sinusitis, rhinitis), eye disorders (myopia, conjunctivitis, central retinitis), sciatica, and various rheumatoid and arthritic conditions. In China, acupuncture is commonly used as a surgical anesthetic.

In the United States, acupuncture is used by millions of people primarily to relieve or prevent pain, to relieve nausea and vomiting, and as an adjunctive method to overcome drug and alcohol addictions. (More than 300 substance abuse programs in the United States use acupuncture.) Some practitioners claim acupuncture can improve immune system function and reduce symptoms in patients with acquired immunodeficiency syndrome (AIDS).

How the treatment is performed
Acupuncture as practiced in the United States today isn't a monolithic body of knowledge similar to Western biomedicine; rather, it's based on a number of medical traditions from China, Korea, Japan, England, and France. A practitioner trained in a school following the mainland Chinese model will practice differently from one trained in the Japanese model. The underlying theory of all the schools is identical, but the vast tradition of Chinese medicine allows for quite divergent emphases in practice. Thus, a practitioner may emphasize the five phases theory, the eight principles theory, or the three yin–three yang theory in making a diagnosis. These different diagnostic frameworks result in very different approaches to therapy in each model.

A visit to an acupuncturist is usually similar to a visit to a traditional Chinese medicine practitioner, except that herbs may not be prescribed and the treatment will be done at the time of the visit. Before treatment begins, the practitioner determines the patient's overall condition by the traditional Chinese methods of diagnosis: inspecting, listening, smelling, questioning, and palpating. The assessment includes intensive pulse measurements and questions about eating and sleeping habits, digestive complaints, urine color, and stress.

Treatment is based on the results of the assessment, which indicate the balance of qi flow in the network of channels. However, the particular channels and points chosen for treatment may also be influenced by the practitioner's style and experience as well as the specific school of acupuncture in which he was trained.

The basic technique is similar in all schools of acupuncture. Very fine filiform needles made of solid metal — usually stainless steel — are inserted into the skin. The needles (usually no more than 10 or 12) are placed in designated acupoints on the body, depending on the patient's diagnosis. Although most acupoints are located on a meridian, a number of points located away from any channel have been discovered to have therapeutic effects; these are called miscellaneous points. The needles are typically kept in place for 20 to 30 minutes and may be set in motion or connected to low-voltage electric generators to enhance their intended effects.

Because the needles are so fine and aren't hollow, the patient feels relatively little pain compared to the insertion of tunneling needles used for injections. Strict standards of sterilization are required for nondisposable needles and implements, although it has become customary to use single-use disposable needles.

In addition to inserting needles, acupuncturists commonly use other treatments involving the acupoints, including *moxibustion* and *cupping*. In *moxibustion,* a small piece of an herb called moxa (*Artemisia vulgaris,* commonly known as mugwort) is burned either on the needle tip or on another substance that is then placed over the designated acupoint. This supplementary technique is intended to stimulate or increase the flow of qi in the body. *Cupping* involves the placement of glass or bamboo cups on the skin to create a vacuum suction, which is believed to draw out pathogenic substances.

Some acupuncturists don't use needles at all; instead they substitute electrostimulation, ultrasonic waves, or laser beams for the metal needles. In Chinese massage, or acupressure, the practitioner applies deep finger pressure to the acupoints. A modern variation on acupuncture, called auriculotherapy, was developed in France after World War II and involves inserting needles at specific points on the outer ear that are believed to affect other regions of the body. This method is being used in the United States to treat alcohol, tobacco, and drug addiction.

Hazards
The 1997 NIH consensus panel reported that the incidence of adverse effects from acupuncture treatment is lower than that for many accepted medical procedures used for the same conditions. For example, the steroids and nonsteroidal anti-inflammatory drugs commonly used to treat painful musculoskeletal conditions, such as fibromyalgia and epicondylitis, can cause serious adverse effects, yet the evidence supporting their usefulness is no more compelling than that supporting acupuncture.

Because of the slight chance of life-threatening reactions such as pneumothorax, the NIH panel urged acupuncture practitioners to take appropriate safeguards, including carefully explaining the procedure to their patients and following FDA guidelines on needle sterility.

Bruising from hitting veins and capillaries does occur. Fainting may occur either from fear of needles or vasovagal reactions. Skin infection can occur around the needle site.

Clinical considerations
If your patient is considering acupuncture, inform him that he can obtain a referral from the NCCA.

 REIMBURSEMENT *Some third-party payers have begun providing coverage for acupuncture treatments by qualified practitioners.*

Research summary
Although acupuncture is one of the most widely researched of all the alternative and complementary therapies, most of the published reports have been case studies that don't meet modern scientific standards for assessing efficacy. Double-blind randomized studies are difficult to perform for acupuncture because the treatments are so individualized; two people with the same disease label would probably be treated differently.

Despite these problems, the 1997 NIH consensus panel concluded that "the data in support of acupuncture are as strong as those for many accepted Western medical therapies." The panel also encouraged practitioners to make acupuncture part of a comprehensive management program for asthma, addiction, and smoking cessation.

agar

Agar-agar, Chinese gelatin, colle du Japon, gelatin, Gelidium amansii, gelose, Japanese gelatin, Japanese isinglass, layor carang, vegetable gelatin

Agar is made up of two major polysaccharides: neutral agarose and charged agaropectin. These polysaccharides are extracted from various species of *Rhodophyceae* algae. Agarose is the gelling component of agar.

Agar is available as a dry powder and as thin, odorless, and colorless to pale yellow, orange, or gray translucent strips, flakes, and granules. Dry powder is soluble in boiling water and produces a clear liquid that gels when cooled. Agar strips, flakes, and granules are tough when damp but become brittle when dried.

Agar is also a constituent of various multiple-ingredient preparations including Agarbil, Agarol, Demosvelte N, Diet Fibre Complex 1500, Emulsione, Falqui, Gelogastrine, Lexat, Paragar, and Pseudophage.

Reported uses
Agar aids peristalsis by increasing bulk in the intestines and by swelling the intestines, thus stimulating the intestinal muscles. It's used as an oral bulk laxative to treat chronic constipation.

Agar is also used to make dental impressions and added to other drugs in compounding emulsions, suspensions, gels, and hydrophilic suppositories.

Administration
- As a laxative: 1 to 2 teaspoons of powder by mouth with liquid, fruit, or jam before meals, every day, up to three times a day
- Oral use: 4 to 16 g every day, up to two times a day, with at least 8 oz of water.

Hazards
Agar may cause esophageal or bowel obstruction. It may also cause hypercholesterolemia.

The fiber in agar may impair absorption of oral drugs. Encourage patient to separate administration times.

 SAFETY RISK *Agar is contraindicated in patients with bowel obstruction or difficulty swallowing.*

Clinical considerations
- Monitor patient for chest pain, vomiting, and difficulty swallowing or breathing and advise him to seek immediate medical attention if he experiences these symptoms.
- Advise patient who has difficulty swallowing not to use agar.
- Inform patient that agar may alter the effectiveness of oral drugs, and encourage him to notify his health care provider if he's taking it.
- Advise patient who is using agar to take it with plenty of fluid (at least 8 oz)

to prevent blockage of the throat or esophagus, which could cause choking. chest pain, vomiting, or difficulty swallowing or breathing.
- Tell patient to remind prescriber and pharmacist of any herbal or dietary supplement he is taking when obtaining a new prescription.
- Advise patient to consult his health care provider before using an herbal preparation because a treatment with proven efficacy may be available.

Research summary
The concepts behind the use of agar and the claims made regarding its effects have not yet been validated scientifically.

agrimony

Agrimonia eupatoria, A. procera, *church steeples, cocklebur, common agrimony, fragrant agrimony,* Herba eupatoriae, *liverwort, philanthropos, sticklewort, stickwort*

The dried above-ground parts of agrimony are harvested and dried during flowering season. The herb's astringent properties result from the presence of flavonoids and 4% to 10% condensed tannins. The ethanolic extracts of agrimony are thought to have antiviral properties.

Agrimony is available as a pulverized or powdered herb and as other preparations used to make compresses, gargles, poultices, teas, and various bath preparations. Multiple-ingredient preparations include Rhoival, Gall & Liver Tablets, NeoGallonorm-Dragees, and Potter's Piletabs.

Reported uses
Agrimony is used to treat sore throat, inflammation of the mouth and pharynx, inflammation of the skin, and diabetes. It's also used as an antitumorigenic, cardiotonic, antihistamine, anti-asthmatic, diuretic, sedative, dye or flavoring

agent, and coagulant for skin rashes or cuts.

Agrimony is probably safe and effective as a mild topical antiseptic or astringent. It may be effective for mild, nonspecific acute diarrhea and gastroenteritis.

Historically, agrimony was used to treat gallbladder disorders (in "liver and bile" teas), tuberculosis, corns and warts, and catarrh (mucous membrane inflammation with discharge).

Administration
- External use: Topical poultices using 10% water extract can be made by boiling agrimony at low heat for 10 to 20 minutes. Poultices may be applied several times daily
- Oral use: Average daily dose is 3 g by mouth.

Hazards
Short-term use of agrimony in appropriate doses is considered safe. Adverse effects from agrimony may include hypotension, GI upset, constipation, hypoglycemia, and photodermatitis.

For patients on anticoagulants, high doses of agrimony may influence anticoagulant effects. High doses of agrimony may cause added hypotensive effects in patients taking antihypertensives.

Patients taking both agrimony and either insulin or oral antidiabetics have an increased risk of hypoglycemia.

Sun exposure increases the risk of photosensitivity reactions.

 SAFETY RISK *Oral use of agrimony may be unsafe in pregnant women. Also, because of the tannin content, agrimony use may be unsafe in high topical or oral doses.*

Clinical considerations
- Monitor patient taking supratherapeutic doses for GI upset and constipation.
- Monitor diabetic patient for hypoglycemia. Inform him that agrimony may cause hypoglycemia; if he's taking a conventional antidiabetic, the dosage of that drug may need to be adjusted.

- Monitor blood pressure in patient taking an antihypertensive and high doses of agrimony. Caution him not to exceed recommended doses because high doses may cause hypotension.
- Caution patient that if he delays seeking medical diagnosis and treatment, his condition could worsen.
- Inform female patient that agrimony may affect the menstrual cycle.
- Advise patient that subtherapeutic doses may cause GI upset and constipation.
- Advise patient that long-term use isn't recommended because of the risk of adverse reactions.
- Tell patient to remind prescriber and pharmacist of any herbal or dietary supplement that he's taking when obtaining a new prescription.
- Advise patient to consult his health care provider before using an herbal preparation because a treatment with proven efficacy may be available.

Research summary
The concepts behind the use of agrimony and the claims made regarding its effects have not yet been validated scientifically.

Alexander technique

The Alexander technique is a form of bodywork that focuses on the dynamic interaction of the head, neck, and trunk based on the belief that a variety of physical ailments can be linked to faulty posture. The goal of this therapy is to learn improved balance, posture, coordination, and proper use of the body in order to prevent injury and maximize pleasure in work and leisure.

Frederick M. Alexander (1869-1955), an Australian actor, developed his theory while trying to determine why he frequently lost his voice during performances. Medical doctors were unable to cure his problem with medication and rest, nor could they explain what might be causing the condition, which threatened his livelihood.

Alexander was convinced that something he did while using his voice caused the problem and that if he could uncover that habit, he could work to alter it. By observing himself in mirrors, he saw that he unconsciously moved his head a certain way and sucked in his breath whenever he began to speak. When he made this unconscious movement, the muscles at the back of his neck contracted in such a way as to pull his head down and back. He concluded that this movement also strained his vocal cords and affected his voice.

Experimenting with his body over several years, Alexander practiced postures that were the opposite of the unconscious ones he had observed. In time his voice problem disappeared. He began helping others with posture and movement problems and eventually abandoned the stage to teach his posture technique around the world.

The core of Alexander's teaching was that people use their bodies incorrectly for such routine activities as sitting and standing and that the stresses and strains placed on the body through this faulty posture are the root of many medical problems. By changing the way the body moves when sitting, standing, walking, and talking — specifically, by proper alignment of the head, neck, and trunk — Alexander believed that people could treat a variety of ills and improve overall health.

 TRAINING *The North American Society of Teachers of the Alexander Technique has approved 17 teacher-training programs in the United States. To become certified, teachers must complete 1,600 hours of training over 3 years. There are currently about 600 certified teachers in the United States.*

Reported uses
The Alexander technique has been used for nearly a century for a broad range of physical complaints, from asthma to paralysis, but there are few scientific studies in mainstream medical literature evaluating its efficacy for such disorders. The technique is taught primarily as a preventive method to promote relaxation and enhance movement and posture; actors, musicians, and athletes use it to improve their performance.

Proponents claim the technique is useful in treating chronic conditions, such as neck and back pain, postural disorders, myalgia, breathing problems, hypertension, and anxiety, and in preventing repetitive stress injuries.

How the treatment is performed
The basic elements of the Alexander technique can be learned from books. Ideally, however, one should learn from a teacher because the technique must be specifically tailored to the individual based on an assessment of his movement patterns. A teacher usually begins by simply observing a student as he sits, gets up from a chair, and walks around the room. The teacher will offer suggestions on making proper use of the body, guiding the student's movements with his hands. The focus is on slow, steady development of habits of tension-free movement, which the student practices in everyday life.

Hazards
This gentle technique should cause no complications if performed and taught correctly.

Clinical considerations
■ Advise patient with chronic muscle or joint problems to seek medical advice to make sure this technique won't exacerbate his condition or interfere with any treatment.
■ Make sure that the patient closely follows the teacher's recommendations — as in other areas, a misapplied technique is often worse than none at all.

Research summary

Although many articles have been written about the Alexander technique, most of them don't meet the scientific community's standards for proving a treatment's efficacy. Despite this lack of mainstream research, Barrie Cassileth, a member of the Advisory Council to the NIH's Office of Alternative Medicine, says those who are curious may want to try the technique because it's gentle and unlikely to cause harm. "It may indeed work for you, bringing pain relief, relaxation, and the more efficient body function it claims to bestow."

RESEARCH *The studies reported in Alexander's book* The Use of Self *indicate that respiratory function improves in adults who practice the Alexander technique, as indicted by significant increases in all spirometry test parameters.*

allspice

Clove pepper, Jamaica pepper, pimenta, Pimenta dioica, *pimento, West Indian bay*

Allspice berries and leaves contain a volatile oil that's 60% to 80% eugenol. The leaves contain more eugenol than the berries (up to 96%). The oil also contains caryophyllene, cineole, levophellandrene, and palmitic acid.

Eugenol is responsible for the herb's effects on the GI system and its analgesic properties. It works by depressing the central nervous system (CNS) and inhibiting prostaglandin activity in the colon mucosa. It also increases the activity of some digestive enzymes such as trypsin. Eugenol has antioxidant properties and in vitro activity against yeast and fungi. Eugenol inhibits platelet activity.

Allspice is available as aqueous extract, oil, and powder (consists of ground dried fruit).

Reported uses

Allspice is commonly used to enhance the taste of food and toothpaste and the smell of cosmetics. In herbal medicine, it's used to treat GI problems such as indigestion, stomachache, and flatulence; it's also used as a purgative. Topically, it's used as an analgesic for muscle pain or toothache and as an antiseptic for teeth and gums.

Administration

- As an antiflatulent: 0.05 to 0.2 ml allspice oil by mouth
- Topical use: Oil or paste applied to painful area.

Hazards

Adverse effects associated with allspice may include CNS depression, seizures (with high doses), mucous membrane irritation (with topical use), nausea, and vomiting.

Patients with intestinal disorders should avoid use because allspice and its extracts stimulate the GI tract and may irritate mucous membranes.

Allspice may enhance the effect of anticoagulants and antiplatelet drugs.

SAFETY RISK *Ingestion of large quantities of allspice may cause toxic reaction. Ingestion of more than 5 ml of allspice oil can cause nausea, vomiting, CNS depression, and seizures.*

Clinical considerations

- Monitor patient for bleeding if he's also on anticoagulant or antiplatelet therapy.
- Advise patient not to ingest large quantities of allspice.
- Advise patient not to delay medical treatment for an illness that doesn't resolve after taking allspice.
- Tell patient to remind prescriber and pharmacist of any herbal or dietary supplement that he's taking when obtaining a new prescription.
- Advise patient to consult his health care provider before using an herbal

preparation because a treatment with proven efficacy may be available.

Research summary

The concepts behind the use of allspice and the claims made regarding its effects have not yet been validated scientifically.

aloe

Aloe barbadensis, A. capensis, A. vera, *Barbados aloes, burn plant, cape, curaçao, elephant's gall, first-aid plant, Hsiang-dan, lily of the desert, lu-hui, socotrine, Zanzibar*

Aloe gel is a clear, thin, viscous material obtained by crushing the mucilaginous cells found in the aloe vera leaf. The gel contains a polysaccharide similar to guar gum. Aloe gel's wound healing ability comes from its moisturizing effect, which prevents air from drying the wound. Mucopolysaccharides and sulfur and nitrogen compounds also stimulate healing. Aloe gel may work as an antibacterial against *Staphylococcus aureus, Escherichia coli,* and *Mycobacterium tuberculosis,* but information is conflicting.

A solid residue is obtained by evaporating aloe latex. It contains aloinosides, which irritate the large intestine, increasing peristalsis, thereby producing a laxative effect. Water and electrolyte reabsorption is inhibited. Aloe can cause potassium loss.

Aloe also contains bradykinase, which is a protease inhibitor that relieves pain and decreases swelling and redness. The antipruritic effect of aloe may be related to the antihistamine properties of magnesium lactate.

Aloe is available as dried latex for internal use, extract capsules, juice (99.7% of whole leaf aloe vera juice), tincture (1:10, 50% alcohol), and topical gel.

Reported uses

Used orally, aloe latex is a potent cathartic. It's used to treat constipation; to provide evacuation relief for patients with anal fissures, hemorrhoids, or recent anorectal surgery; and to prepare a patient for diagnostic testing of the GI tract.

Aloe gel is used to treat minor burns and skin irritation and to aid in wound healing. It may also be effective as an antibacterial.

Administration

- As a laxative: 100 to 200 mg of aloe capsules, 50 mg of aloe extract, or 1 to 8 oz of juice taken by mouth at bedtime; or, 30 ml of aloe gel or 15 to 60 gtt of aloe tincture (1:10, 50% alcohol), taken by mouth as needed
- Topical use: Apply liberally to the affected area, three to five times daily as needed.

Hazards

Adverse effects associated with aloe may include: arrhythmias, edema, cramps, diarrhea, albuminuria, hematuria, nephropathy, electrolyte abnormalities, weight loss, muscle weakness, accelerated bone deterioration, and nummular eczematous or papular dermatitis.

Oral administration of aloe to patients taking antiarrhythmic or cardiac glycosides, such as digoxin, may lead to toxic reaction. Concomitant use of aloe and corticosteroids or diuretics can enhance potassium loss. Any herbal preparation that contains alcohol can precipitate a disulfiram-like reaction. Risk of potassium deficiency increases when a patient is taking both aloe and licorice.

Persons with intestinal obstruction, Crohn's disease, ulcerative colitis, appendicitis, or abdominal pain of unknown origin; those who are pregnant; and children younger than age 12 should avoid taking aloe orally.

Products derived from the latex of aloe's outer skin should be used with caution.

Clinical considerations

- Monitor patient for signs of dehydration. Geriatric patients are particularly at risk.
- Monitor electrolyte levels, especially potassium, after long-term use.
- If patient is using aloe topically, monitor wound for healing.
- Laxative effects are apparent within 10 hours of taking aloe.
- Caution patient that if he delays seeking medical diagnosis and treatment, his condition could worsen.
- If patient is taking digoxin or another drug to control his heart rate, a diuretic, or a corticosteroid, warn him not to take aloe without consulting his health care provider.
- Advise patient to reduce dose if cramping occurs after a single dose and not to take aloe for longer than one to two weeks at a time without consulting his health care provider.
- Advise patient to notify his health care provider immediately if he experiences feelings of dehydration, weakness, or confusion, especially if he has been using aloe for a prolonged period.
- Be aware that patients taking insulin or oral antidiabetic agents concomitantly with aloe may have improved blood sugar control, requiring a reduction of antidiabetic drugs.
- Tell patient to remind prescriber and pharmacist of any herbal or dietary supplement that he's taking when obtaining a new prescription.
- Advise patient to consult his health care provider before using an herbal preparation because a treatment with proven efficacy may be available.

Research summary

Evidence from some studies suggests that aloe gel can improve blood sugar control in individuals with type 2 diabetes.

 RESEARCH *A 2-week, double-blind, placebo-controlled trial of 60 men with active genital herpes found that participants who applied aloe cream (0.5% aloe three times daily for five days) healed faster than those who used a placebo. Use of aloe cream reduced the time necessary for lesions to heal (4.9 days vs. 12 days), and also increased the percentage of individuals who were fully healed by the end of 2 weeks (66.7% vs. 6.7%). (Syed, et al., 1997).*

American cranesbill

Alum bloom, alumroot, American kino, chocolate flower, cranesbill, crowfoot, dove's-foot, Geranium maculatum, *old maid's nightcap, shameface, spotted cranesbill, stinking cranesbill, storkbill, wild cranesbill, wild geranium*

American cranesbill is high in tannins, which likely accounts for its antidiarrheal activity. It may have some antiviral and antibacterial properties. A preparation with extract and 80% ethanol may inhibit the growth of some gram-negative bacteria.

American cranesbill is available as dried herb, essential oil, liquid extract, mouthwash, and tincture.

Reported uses

American cranesbill is used to treat diarrhea, dysentery, stomach ulcers, hemorrhoids, dysmenorrhea, Crohn's disease, liver and gallbladder disease, calculosis, and inflammation of the mouth, kidney, and bladder.

Administration

American cranesbill is used as a gargle or mouthwash. Fresh leaves are commonly chewed.

- Liquid extract: 1 to 2 ml by mouth three times a day
- Tea: 1 to 2 g by mouth (prepared by adding 1 teaspoon of herb to 1 pint of cold water, bringing mixture to a boil and leaving it to draw); 2 to 3 cups daily, between meals
- Tincture: 2 to 4 ml by mouth three times a day.

Hazards
American cranesbill may cause stomach upset.

Any herbal preparation that contains alcohol can precipitate a disulfiram-like reaction. Persons with digestive disorders should avoid use because of the herb's high tannin content.

Clinical considerations
- Caution patient not to delay seeking medical evaluation of symptoms that may indicate a serious medical condition.
- Inform patient with a sensitive stomach that American cranesbill could cause nausea or vomiting.
- Tell patient not to exceed recommended dose.
- Advise patient not to take American cranesbill for longer than 1 to 2 weeks at a time without consulting his health care provider.
- Tell patient to remind prescriber and pharmacist of any herbal or dietary supplement that he's taking when obtaining a new prescription.
- Advise patient to consult his health care provider before using an herbal preparation because a treatment with proven efficacy may be available.

Research summary
The concepts behind the use of American cranesbill and the claims made regarding its effects have not yet been validated scientifically.

angelica

Angelica archangelica, *angelique,*
dong quai, engelwurzel,
European angelica,
garden angelica, heiligenwurzel,
oot of the Holy Ghost, tang-kuei

The medicinally active substances of angelica are extracted from the root and fruit seeds of the plant. Angelica seed contains alpha-angelica lactone, which augments calcium binding and calcium turnover. Its action may involve increasing the contraction-dependent calcium pool to be released upon systolic depolarization. The coumarins and furanocoumarins may induce photosensitivity and may be photocarcinogenic and mutagenic.

Angelica is available as liquid extract, tincture, and essential oil. One product containing angelica is Nature's Answer Angelica Root Liquid.

Reported uses
Angelica seed is used as a diuretic and diaphoretic. It's also used to treat conditions of the kidneys and the urinary, GI, and respiratory tracts as well as rheumatic and neuralgic symptoms.

Angelica root is used orally for loss of appetite, GI spasm, and flatulence. It's used topically to treat neuralgia. Other uses include treatment for cough, bronchitis, anorexia, dyspepsia with intestinal cramping, and menstrual, liver, and gallbladder complaints.

Angelica seed has also been used as a flavoring in gin, some regional wines, candied leaves, and cake and pastry decorations.

Administration
- Crude root: 4.5 g by mouth every day
- Essential oil: 10 to 20 gtt by mouth every day
- Liquid extract (1:1): 0.5 to 3 g by mouth every day
- Tincture (1:5): 1.5 g by mouth every day.

Hazards
Angelica may increase acid production in the stomach and so may interfere with absorption of antacids, H_2 blockers, proton pump inhibitors, and sucralfate.

High doses of angelica may potentiate the effects of anticoagulants. There is an increased risk of photosensitivity reactions with sun exposure associated with angelica. Angelica may cause photodermatosis.

SAFETY RISK *Pregnant and breast-feeding patients should avoid use because angelica appears to stimulate menstruation and the uterus.*

Clinical considerations
- Monitor patient for persistent diarrhea, which may be a symptom of underlying illness.
- Monitor patient for dermatologic reactions.
- Photodermatosis is possible after contact with the plant juice or plant extract.
- Caution patient not to delay seeking medical treatment for symptoms that may be related to a serious medical condition.
- Advise patient not to take angelica if pregnant or if taking a gastric acid blocker or anticoagulant.
- Tell patient to remind prescriber and pharmacist of any herbal or dietary supplement that he's taking when obtaining a new prescription.
- Advise patient to consult his health care provider before using an herbal preparation because a treatment with proven efficacy may be available.

Research summary
The concepts behind the use of angelica and the claims made regarding its effects have not yet been validated scientifically.

anise

Aniseed, Pimpinella anisum,
semen anisi, sweet cumin

Anise oil is obtained from fruits of the herb. The highest quality oil comes from anise seeds. The oil's major component is trans-anethole, which is responsible for the taste, smell, and medicinal properties of anise. Anise is rich in calcium and iron.

Structurally, anise is comparable to catecholamines (such as dopamine, epinephrine, and norepinephrine) and the hallucinogenic compound myristicin. It also possesses some estrogenic activity. Bergapten, another component of anise, may cause photosensitivity reactions and may be carcinogenic.

Anise is available as dried fruit, essential oil, and tea.

Reported uses
Anise is used to treat coughs and colds and to decrease bloating and gas. In higher doses, anise is used as an antispasmodic and antiseptic for cough, asthma, and bronchitis, as it has expectorant properties.

Anise also has weak antibacterial effects against gram-positive and gram-negative organisms. The oil has been used to treat lice, scabies, and psoriasis.

Anise has also been used as flavoring in alcohols, various foods, perfumes, and soaps.

In folk medicine, anise has been used to increase lactation, induce menstruation, facilitate birth, increase libido, and alleviate menopausal symptoms.

Administration
- As an antiflatulent: For adults, 1 tablespoon of tea several times every day; for breast-feeding babies, 1 teaspoon of tea by mouth as needed
- Dried fruit: 0.5 to 1 g (3 g maximum) by mouth every day
- Essential oil: 50 to 200 ml by mouth every day
- As an expectorant: 1 cup of tea by mouth in the morning or the evening
- Tea (1 to 2 teaspoons of crushed seed steeped in hot water for 10 to 15 minutes): 1 cup three times a day.

Hazards
Adverse effects associated with anise include seizures, nausea, vomiting, stomatitis, pulmonary edema, erythema, scaling, vesiculation, and photosensitivity reactions.

High doses of anise can interfere with anticoagulants, monoamine oxidase (MAO) inhibitors, oral contraceptives, and other hormone therapy.

There is an increased risk of photosensitivity reactions for patients taking anise. Those with dermatitis or inflammatory or allergic skin reactions should avoid using anise.

Those allergic to anise or anethole should avoid use. Those with coagulation problems should use anise with caution.

 SAFETY RISK *Pregnant patients should avoid using anise because it may cause abortion.*

Clinical considerations

 SAFETY RISK *Don't confuse anise with Chinese star anise.*

■ Preparations containing 5% to 10% essential oil can be used externally.

■ If overdose occurs, monitor patient for neurologic changes and provide supportive measures for nausea and vomiting.

■ If patient is pregnant, instruct her not to use anise.

■ If patient is taking an anticoagulant or an antiplatelet drug, advise him not to take anise.

■ If patient is taking MAO inhibitors or hormones, tell him to seek medical advice before taking anise.

■ Instruct patient not to exceed the daily recommended dose.

■ Advise patient to report any skin changes to his health care provider.

■ Tell patient to remind prescriber and pharmacist of any herbal or dietary supplement that he's taking when obtaining a new prescription.

■ Advise patient to consult his health care provider before using an herbal preparation because a treatment with proven efficacy may be available.

Research summary

The concepts behind the use of anise and the claims made regarding its effects have not yet been validated scientifically.

Antineoplastons

Antineoplastons, a group of synthetic compounds that were originally isolated from human blood and urine, are used as an alternative therapy for cancer treatment. The treatment was developed by Stanislaw Burzynski, a physician and biochemist in Houston, Texas. Burzynski began working with the compounds in 1967, and in 1977 he reported that he had isolated certain peptides in human urine that could reverse activity in cancer cells. It was his belief that the peptides may represent a biomedical communication system in the body and act as a supplemental body defense system. Cancer cells keep multiplying uncontrollably and are, in effect, indestructible, while healthy cells die after a specific number of divisions. Antineoplastons supposedly function by reprogramming cancer cells to die as do normal cells. Healthy cells aren't affected. Two main groups of antineoplastons have been isolated: Antineoplaston A10 (3-phenylacetyamino-2, 6-piperidinedione), with a broad spectrum of activity in many different cell lines; and antineoplaston AS2-1 (phenylacetyglutamine and phenylacetic acid 1:4), with a narrow spectrum of activity against single cell lines.

Burzynski has used antineoplastons to treat patients with a variety of cancers. In 1991, the National Cancer Institute (NCI) reviewed the medical records of seven brain tumor patients from the Burzynski Research Institute (BRI) in Houston to evaluate the clinical responses of patients treated with antineoplastons. All seven patients were thought to have benefited from treatment, so the review didn't constitute a clinical trial, but was, rather, a retrospective of medical records of "best case series." Evidence of antitumor activity was found by the reviewers, and NCI proposed that clinical trials be conducted to evaluate the response rate and toxicity of antineoplastons in adults with advanced brain tumors.

Investigators at several cancer centers developed protocols for phase II clinical trials with review and input from NCI and Burzynski. These began in 1993 at

Memorial Sloan-Kettering Cancer Center, the Mayo Clinic, and the Warren Grant Magnussen Clinical Center at the National Institutes of Health. Patient enrollment in these studies was slow, and by August 1995, only nine patients had entered trials. Investigators could not reach a consensus on changes to increase accrual and studies were closed prior to completion. Because of the small number of patients in these trials, no definitive conclusion could be drawn about the effectiveness of treatment with antineoplastons. Of the nine patients treated, six had responses that were assessable in accordance with protocol stipulations. No patient demonstrated tumor regression.

In February 1998, the state of Texas ordered Burzynski to stop soliciting cancer patients for treatments with antineoplastons because of their status as an unapproved drug. Under the court order, until the FDA rules on antineoplastons, Burzynski and BRI can't distribute them to patients unless the patients are enrolled in FDA-approved clinical trials. Burzynski is prohibited from advertising antineoplastons for the treatment of cancer and must place a disclaimer on his website and in any promotional material and ads stating that the safety and effectiveness of antineoplastons have not yet been established.

Reported uses
Antineoplastons may be used in patients who have not had curative responses to existing therapeutic regimens, including patients with advanced stages of carcinoma of the adrenal gland, cancer of the bladder, breast cancer, lymphoma, leukemia, bone cancer, brain tumors, osteosarcoma, esophageal cancer, and human immunodeficiency virus infection.

How the treatment is performed
Pretreatment evaluation is required before a patient can become eligible to participate in clinical trial treatments using antineoplastons. The evaluation includes complete history and physical examinations; weight and performance status using the Karnofsky performance scale (rating a patient's performance on a scale of 10 to 100, with 10 being fatal processes progressing rapidly and 100 being normal with no evidence of disease); laboratory studies including urinalysis, complete blood count, prothrombin time, partial thromboplastin time, blood urea nitrogen, creatinine level, uric acid level, serum electrolyte studies, glucose, liver function test, tumor markers, and laboratory values on levels of anti-epileptic drugs for a patient who is taking such drugs; and radiology studies, including magnetic resonance imaging or computed tomography scan, chest X-ray, intravenous pyelogram, and bone scan for area of tumor involvement.

The initial 2 weeks of treatment must be administered at the Burzynski clinic in Houston. Patients who agree and are authorized to receive treatment must also receive full supportive care including blood and blood products, antibiotics as needed, nutritional support, and aggressive pain management and end-stage palliative care.

Antineoplastons are available in oral capsules and I.V. preparations. Dosage is determined by the particular clinical trial for a specific cancer. Antineoplaston A10 oral preparations are mainly used in maintenance phases of the protocols. They come in 500-mg capsules and are issued in bottles of 20 capsules. They must be stored at room temperature between 15° C and 30° C (59° F to 86° F) in airtight plastic containers. They are stable for 15 months. All unused capsules must be returned to the Burzynski clinic.

I.V. preparations of both antineoplaston A10 and antineoplaston AS2-1 must be stored at room temperature between 15° C and 30° C (59° F to 86° F). Antineoplaston I.V. therapy must be administered continually over an extended period to allow cancerous cells to go through their life cycle to cellular death. Therefore, stable I.V. access is a necessity and a central venous access device is generally inserted for use in I.V. infusion of the medications.

To maintain the daily dose of medication dictated by the clinical trial protocol, a portable, programmable pump may be used to give escalated doses of multiple, intermittent I.V. injections of antineoplaston A10 and antineoplaston AS2-1. Daily doses vary according to clinical trial guidelines, but the recommended targeted therapeutic daily dose of antineoplaston A10 is 1.0 g/kg; of antineoplaston AS2-1, 0.4 g/kg. Both compounds are absorbed rapidly; antineoplastons can't be detected in the blood approximately 2 hours after I.V. administration. Thus, frequent dosing or continuous infusion is indicated for most clinical trials. Oral doses are absorbed somewhat slower, reaching the highest concentration 3 hours after administration.

TRAINING *Staff involved in assisting with antineoplastons must be familiar with the particular treatment protocol. They must also be familiar with all laboratory values to be monitored during treatment, including neutrophil and platelet counts. All guidelines required by the FDA and protocol must be followed.*

Hazards

As of November 2000, BRI was continuing to conduct clinical trials on a variety of cancers using antineoplastons under FDA supervision. To date, no definitive conclusions have been drawn about the effectiveness of antineoplastons in the treatment of the cancers under study.

Adverse effects reported with use of antineoplastons include reversible grade 2 or 3 neurocortical toxicity, transient somnolence, confusion, central nervous system toxicity, depression, lethargy, agitation, polyneuropathy, increased epidermization, arrhythmia (atrial fibrillation), dizziness, nausea and vomiting, hypernatremia, anemia, hypertension, and edema as well as weakness, fever, skin rash, muscle ache, and abdominal pain. Antineoplastons can affect laboratory values—

specifically, sodium, calcium, potassium, magnesium, and glutamic acid. Additionally, they may cause hepatic toxicity, hypovolemia, polyuria, thirst, and increased fluid retention may occur. Prolonged use of a central venous access device for administration of I.V. treatment carries a risk of infection at the site of the device and phlebitis of infused blood vessels.

Clinical considerations

- All unused medications must be returned to BRI.
- The health care team must provide accurate and up-to-date information to patients considering an alternative therapy for cancer and make sure that they understand the risks involved.
- A patient's cultural beliefs related to death and dying must be assessed because only patients with advanced disease are considered for antineoplaston treatment.
- Practitioners assisting patients in antineoplaston treatment must sign a special form (1572) along with a copy of the investigation brochure. They should be familiar with all aspects of the treatment protocol and make certain that the patient and family have been given adequate information to make an informed decision.
- Aggressive pain management is necessary and may require regular scheduled therapy.
- Nutritional assessment and aggressive support must not be overlooked. Maintaining oral intake may involve trying various food combinations and feeding schedules.
- As long as parents or legal guardians sign an informed consent form, children are eligible for enrollment in some clinical trials; however, caution is advised because parents often have unrealistic expectations of a positive outcome.
- Patients with liver failure, those who are pregnant or breast-feeding, or who have uncontrolled hypertension are ex-

cluded from participating in clinical trials.

■ There are no exclusions based on tumor size or systemic metastases for the studies.

REIMBURSEMENT *Antineoplastons are experimental medications and aren't covered by most insurance companies. However, patients who agree to participate in clinical trials should receive any treatment pertaining to or required for the trial free of charge.*

Research summary

Currently, 75 clinical trials using antineoplastons are in process. For more information, call BRI at 713-335-5687. Also, check with the FDA consumer information line at 1-800-FDA-4010 or www.fda.gov.

RESEARCH *The Mayo Clinic participated in a phase II study of antineoplastons A10 and AS2-1 in patients with recurrent glioma. The objective was to assess antineoplaston pharmacokinetics, toxicity, and efficacy to determine whether evidence of antitumor activity could be documented. Nine patients were treated; in six, the treatment response was assessable in accordance with protocol stipulations.*

antioxidants

Beta-carotene, selenium, vitamin C, vitamin E

Antioxidants are chemicals or other agents that inhibit or retard oxidation of a substance to which they're added. In the body, they're believed to help prevent many diseases, including cancer, heart disease, Alzheimer's disease, Parkinson's disease, and diabetes. They're also alleged to increase longevity, give skin a youthful glow, and prevent cataracts. Vitamins C, E, beta-carotene, and other carotenoids (chemicals that give plants their red, orange, or yellow color) and the mineral selenium are the most studied antioxidants

and the ones most commonly taken by millions of Americans. Although they act on cells in similar ways, they aren't interchangeable or uniformly beneficial.

Linus Pauling (1901-1994) pioneered the role of antioxidants and nutrient therapy. His work and the work of many others has opened new doors in the prevention and treatment of illness as it pertains to oxidative stress.

At the molecular and cellular levels, antioxidants serve to deactivate particles called radicals. In humans, free radicals usually come in the form of O_2, the oxygen molecule. As the body goes through its normal processes and O_2 is used to provide cellular fuel, some of the O_2 molecules lose one of their pair of electrons. They then become free radicals that try to stabilize by stealing an electron from stable molecules, thus creating more free radicals. These free radicals react easily with other compounds and can effect significant changes in the body.

Internal sources that can lead to free radical production in addition to O_2 consumption include emotional stress and strenuous exercise. Numerous external factors include air pollution, cigarette smoke, factory and car exhaust, pesticides, smog, food contaminants, chemotherapy, and radiation.

Under most conditions, cells produce a variety of antioxidants that protect key cell components from damage by neutralizing the free radicals. Antioxidants may also be replenished by consuming foods rich in these substances. Stress and the aging process, however, cause the body to produce fewer antioxidants. Dietary supplements containing antioxidants may then be of some benefit.

Reported uses

There is growing evidence that antioxidants may help thwart some chronic conditions, including heart disease, cancer, vision problems, Alzheimer's disease, Parkinson's disease, and diabetes.

Administration

Currently, the best source of antioxidants is a well-balanced diet including the best sources of these substances, namely, fruits and vegetables. The Food and Nutrition Board of the National Academy of Sciences hasn't issued a report listing recommended intake of antioxidants.

Patients should follow the instructions on the supplement label and not exceed the recommended dosage. Children ages 1 to 6 typically tolerate ⅓ of the adult dose; children ages 6 to 12 tolerate approximately ½ the adult dose. People over age 65 may also need to reduce dosage.

Hazards

Adverse effects can include allergies, rashes, heart palpations, headaches, and stomach pain and bleeding. Such effects aren't common unless dosage is excessive or supplement is taken over a prolonged period of time.

Recommended daily allowances for antioxidants are available through the National Cancer Institute at 1-800-4-CANCER and the National Institute of Health at 301-251-1222.

Pregnant women should not take large doses of antioxidants. Prenatal vitamins with standard dosing among commonly used brands should be checked for labeling and Dietary Reference Intakes (DRI; formerly Recommended Dietary Allowances [RDA]) recommendations. All supplements should be approved by their health care provider.

People taking warfarin and other anticoagulant medications should check with their health care provider before taking vitamin E supplements. Large doses can amplify the risk of internal bleeding.

Clinical considerations

■ Urge patient to consume a healthy diet of natural antioxidant foods before considering supplements. A good rule of thumb for patients who prefer to get their antioxidants from food is to consume at least three colors (for example, orange carrots, yellow fruit, and green leafy vegetable) each day because fruits and vegetables with different pigments are thought to contain different antioxidants.

■ Advise patient to select a name brand and to read the label carefully before purchasing.

■ Counsel patient to consider whether a supplement's claims are reasonable and to be wary of ultra-combination products.

SAFETY RISK *Caution pregnant women not to take large doses of antioxidants and to check labels and Dietary Reference Intakes (DRI; formerly Recommended Dietary Allowances [RDA]) recommendations on prenatal vitamins, with standard dosing among commonly used brands. Tell her that all supplements should be approved by her health care provider.*

■ Older patients may benefit from vitamin E supplementation, although the best source of vitamin E comes from a balanced diet. Sources such as nuts, seeds, wheat germ, lima beans, wheat bran, and most vegetable oils contain high amounts of vitamin E.

■ Educate patient about potential interactions of medications and antioxidant supplements.

■ Although vitamin supplements can be effective, caution patient about becoming fanatical. Benign symptoms that occur when taking antioxidants and last for more than a few days should be reported to his health care provider.

■ Caution patient against abruptly stopping a prescribed medication in favor of self-treatment with a supplement because doing so can pose a significant danger.

 REIMBURSEMENT *Some insurance companies will reimburse prescriptions for supplemental vitamins for cardiac disease, but usually not for other indications. Supplements are provided without charge to patients participating in clinical trials.*

Research summary

A consistent body of research indicates that vitamin E may protect people from heart disease, possibly by preventing free radicals from damaging low-density lipoprotein particles. The studies in question focused on individuals who received vitamin E through supplements rather than through diet. Data generally indicate that taking doses of 100 to 800 International Units (IU) per day may lower the risk of heart disease by 30% to 40%. No consensus exists about the optimal vitamin E dosage. Doses up to 800 IU are considered safe for most individuals. Observational studies of patients who took vitamin C and beta-carotene supplements don't support the belief that these substances also prevent heart disease.

Although evidence suggests that selenium may protect against prostate, lung, colon, and esophageal malignancies, experts believe that it's too early to recommend supplements. Scientists do theorize that the vitamins C and E and beta-carotene may reduce the risk of cataracts. Carotenoids appear to be the key antioxidant in preventing macular degeneration. Recent studies also suggest that vitamins C and E and beta-carotene may slow the aging process.

Strong evidence that antioxidants may prevent cancer comes from studies comparing people whose diets included significant amounts of fruits and vegetables rich in antioxidants. These individuals showed a lower risk for breast, stomach, lung, colon, and prostate cancers.

RESEARCH *Experimental studies have indicated that antioxidant treatment prevents nerve dysfunction in diabetics. One study showed a potential therapeutic value in treatment of diabetic patients. The effects of the antioxidant alpha-lipoic (thioctic) acid were studied in two multicenter, randomized, double-blind, placebo-controlled trials. Intravenous treatment with alpha-lipoic acid (600 mg/day) over 2 weeks proved safe and effective in reducing symptoms of diabetic neuropathy. Oral treatment (800 mg/day) for 4 months may improve cardiac autonomic dysfunction in type 2 diabetes mellitus (Gries and Zieglar, 1997).*

Another study showed the effect of water-soluble antioxidants in rats in response to third-degree burn injuries of 20% of total body surface area. Given after the burn injury, the antioxidants seemed to protect lung tissues from alterations in cell energetics (LaLonde, et al., 1996)

Cigarette smoking is a major risk factor in cardiovascular disease (especially arteriosclerosis), lung cancer, and chronic obstructive pulmonary disease. Many studies suggest that a diet rich in fruit and vegetables is associated with decreased risk for arteriosclerosis and cancer. Dietary intake of fruits and vegetables is reportedly lower in smokers than in nonsmokers. Also, evidence of increased utilization of ascorbic acid, possibly due to oxidative stress, contributes to low plasma antioxidant concentration in many smokers (Cross, et al., 1999).

Apitherapy

Products derived from honeybees — including bee venom and raw honey — have been used for therapeutic purposes since ancient times. The Greek doctor Hippocrates is said to have treated joint problems with bee venom. Today, proponents of apitherapy claim that it can be used to treat a wide range of disorders, including arthritis and multiple sclerosis.

The most popular form of apitherapy used today is bee venom, administered either by injection or live bee stings, to treat chronic inflammatory disorders such as arthritis. Proponents claim that the venom works by stimulating the immune system to trigger the production of anti-inflammatory substances that help relieve the pain and swelling from the venom and, simultaneously, the pain and inflammation from the arthritis. Other bee products available as pills or capsules are bee pollen, raw honey, royal jelly, beeswax, and propolis (the substance used to hold the hive together).

The American Apitherapy Society in Red Bank, NJ, collects and disseminates information on this treatment and provides a forum for researchers to present their findings in a quarterly newsletter.

Reported uses
Apitherapy advocates claim that bee venom can alleviate low back pain; chronic pain associated with arthritis, tendinitis, and fibromyalgia; migraine headache; and the symptoms of multiple sclerosis and dermatologic conditions such as psoriasis and eczema. It's also said to desensitize people to bee stings. Ingesting bee pollen and raw honey is said to increase energy and endurance. In China, raw honey is applied to burns as an analgesic and antiseptic. Other claims made for bee pollen include its ability to fight infection, relieve allergies, and slow the aging process.

Royal jelly is the substance that worker bees secrete and then feed to a female bee, which then becomes the hive's queen. After ingesting the royal jelly, the queen becomes twice as large as the other bees, is able to lay 2,000 eggs a day, and her life span increases from 3 months to 5 years. Based on its effects on the queen bee, proponents and marketers of royal jelly claim it can increase energy and stimulate immune function in humans.

Beeswax is claimed to help lower lipids and relieve ulcers. It's also a common ingredient in soaps, cosmetics, and foods.

Propolis is used orally for tuberculosis, infections, and anti-inflammatory effects and topically for cleaning wounds.

How the treatment is performed
Some apitherapists inject bee venom using a hypodermic needle, but most prefer to use live bee stings. (Alcohol or iodine tincture used to cleanse the site may destroy the activity of the bee venom.) Treatment involves repeated bee stings administered at specific sites (depending on the disorder) over a given time period—for example, 4 to 8 weeks for arthritis. Some practitioners use electrophoresis or ultrasonophoresis to administer the venom.

Other bee products are usually taken orally as capsules, pills, powder, or liquid.

Propolis and beeswax are used topically on the skin or mucous membranes as well as being taken by mouth. Bee pollen is taken by mouth in capsule form.

Hazards
Bee pollen and royal jelly can cause life-threatening allergic reactions in sensitive individuals. There have also been reports of infants developing botulism after eating raw honey. Bee venom can cause inflammation, itching, and swelling, as well as nausea, vomiting, headache, hypotension, and anaphylaxis.

Clinical considerations
- If a patient is considering using bee products, warn about the possibility of allergic reactions.
- Inform patient that bee pollen may contain bee feces and larvae, fungi, and bacteria.
- Explain that the bee venom used in apitherapy comes from honeybees; caution against venom from other related insects.

Research summary
Most of the evidence in support of bee products for therapeutic purposes consists of anecdotal reports collected by the American Apitherapy Society rather than the results of controlled scientific experiments.

Bee venom may be effective for rheumatoid arthritis and other inflammatory musculoskeletal conditions, but conclusive evidence either way is lacking. It's probably not effective for multiple sclerosis or desensitization to future bee stings. Insufficient evidence exists for claims that bee pollen or royal jelly have any beneficial effects aside from royal jelly's possible beneficial effect on lipids. Nor does sufficient evidence exist for the effectiveness of beeswax. Propolis shows anti-inflammatory and antimicrobial activity that may make it useful in dental applications.

Applied kinesiology

Kinesiology is the scientific study of the movement of body parts: how the body moves through space as a unit and the relationships of the body's parts to each other. Applied kinesiology, a method of assessment and evaluation also known as muscle testing, focuses on the relationship of muscle strength and energy flow. George Goodheart, Jr., an American chiropractor, developed this system in the 1960s based on the theory that particular muscles correlate to specific body systems or organs and can therefore be used to diagnose a wide range of disorders.

According to applied kinesiologists, health is a balance among three major factors. The first, the chemical factor, includes nutrition as well as the effects of drugs and other chemicals, such as environmental toxins. The second, the structural factor, includes anatomy and physiology—the structural relationships of bones, muscles, and organs. The third, the mental factor, includes attitudes, moods, and emotions. Practitioners of applied kinesiology believe that these three factors are interdependent; for example, an alteration in body chemistry from poor diet or environmental pollution can affect a person's mood and body organs. This effect will be apparent as decreased functioning of the whole person, which can manifest as a frank disease state or as a chronic condition of low energy and malaise with no apparent cause.

The type of therapy chosen depends on the cause of the disorder, as determined by the practitioner's assessment. After muscle testing, two persons with what appear to be the same symptom— for instance, neck pain resistant to standard therapies— might receive different treatments. One might be treated with spinal adjustment, based on the structural factor, but the other might be treated primarily with dietary supplements, based on the chemical factor. Most treatments are aimed at restoring neuromuscular function. They include joint manipulation and mobilization, spinal and cranial adjustments, myofascial therapies, stimulation of acupuncture points, and reflex procedures. Dietary and nutritional measures may also be used.

The International College of Applied Kinesiology in Shawnee Mission, Kansas, offers information, publishes a newsletter, and provides referrals to applied kinesiology practitioners.

Reported uses

Applied kinesiology is commonly used to assess and treat chronic problems such as musculoskeletal imbalances, joint problems, and structural imbalances. It's especially popular in assessing athletic injuries. People with vague symptoms, such as malaise and tiredness, or illnesses that seem to have no identifiable cause or that are unresponsive to standard treatments may be good candidates for this method.

How the treatment is performed

After taking the patient's history, including diet and lifestyle, the practitioner examines the patient's posture, gait, and any obvious physical problems, such as a limp or drooping shoulder. Then he methodically assesses the strength of various muscles and muscle groups. He does this by placing the patient's limbs in various positions and asking the patient to resist as the practitioner attempts to push against the resistance. By comparing the left and right sides as well as the relative strength of muscles, the practitioner identifies muscles that are weak. (See *Assessing muscle strength,* page 50.)

Because the theory behind applied kinesiology is that each muscle is associated with specific diseases or organ conditions, once the practitioner identifies the weak muscles, he knows where the patient's problem originates— for instance, a weak psoas muscle indicates kidney disease. Depending on the cause, he then prescribes a treatment, such as spinal manipulation, a change in diet, or dietary supplements.

ASSESSING MUSCLE STRENGTH

An applied kinesiology practitioner tests the strength of the patient's deltoid muscles by holding the arm firmly and asking the patient to resist the practitioner's pulling action.

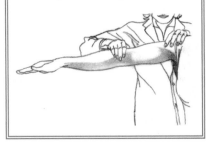

Hazards

When performed by a properly trained practitioner, applied kinesiology shouldn't result in any complications.

Clinical considerations

- If a patient expresses an interest in applied kinesiology, inform him that this technique isn't intended to replace conventional physical examinations and diagnostic measures.
- Be aware that applied kinesiology is a highly specialized technique that should be performed only by a licensed professional trained in differential diagnosis. Despite the existence of several self-help systems for muscle testing, most patients lack the knowledge to interpret the tests properly and reach appropriate diagnostic conclusions.
- Advise patient to seek medical advice before undergoing applied kinesiology to make sure the technique won't exacerbate his condition or interfere with other treatment.

TRAINING *The International College of Applied Kinesiology provides various levels of certification for physicians. Approved courses must be taken from certified teachers approved by the Board of Certified Teachers. The essential program is Basic Applied Kinesiology, a 100-hour course.*

Research summary

Froehle (1996) did a retrospective study showing that applied kinesiology is a successful complementary approach to treating children with ear infections.

arnica

Arnica montana, *common arnica, leopard's bane, mountain snuff, mountain tobacco, sneezewort, wolfsbane*

Arnica is a yellow to orange-yellow flowering plant from which various compounds are harvested. The heads of the plant are dried to extract the active compounds, and parts of the rhizome at the base of the plant may also be used.

The plant contains many chemical compounds, including oils and fatty acids. Its sesquiterpene lactones have mild analgesic and anti-inflammatory effects. Helenalin and dihydrohelenalin, additional sesquiterpenes, may also have antibacterial and additional anti-inflammatory effects. Some components may reduce bleeding times and inhibit platelet function. It may also have antifungal effects. Arnica has some immunostimulatory activity and contains a group of polysaccharides that can modify the immune response.

Arnica is available for external use as an ointment, semisolid cream, and tincture for poultice preparation. For homeopathic preparations, it's available in tablet form. Arnica products include Arnicalm, Arnica Ointment, Arnica-Si, and Weleda Massage Balm.

Reported uses

Arnica poultices and ointments have been used topically to treat skin inflammation, acne, bruises, sprains, blunt trauma injuries, and rheumatic muscle and joint problems. Arnica is also used in hair tonics as an antidandruff preparation.

Oral rinses have been used to treat inflammation of the mouth and pharynx; however, ingestion of arnica can cause severe toxic reaction, including death, so its use as an oral rinse should be avoided or carefully monitored.

Arnica has also been used to treat heart problems, improve circulation, stimulate the central nervous system, provide analgesia, and treat surgical or accidental trauma and postoperative thrombophlebitis and pulmonary emboli.

Administration
- Oral rinse: Tincture diluted 10 times with water.
- Poultice preparation: Tincture diluted 3 to 10 times with water.

Hazards
 SAFETY RISK *Ingestion of arnica may result in severe toxic reaction, coma, or cardiac arrest.*

Other adverse effects associated with arnica include drowsiness, stomach pain, diarrhea, vomiting, gastroenteritis, dyspnea, contact dermatitis, irritation of mucous membranes, and eczema (with prolonged use of topical preparation).

Use of arnica concomitantly with aspirin, heparin, or warfarin may increase the risk of bleeding. Arnica is also associated with possible increased bleeding times or altered platelet function when taken with any of the following: angelica, anise, asafoetida, bogbean, boldo, capsicum, celery, chamomile, clove, danshen, fenugreek, feverfew, garlic, ginger, ginkgo, ginseng, horse chestnut, horseradish, licorice, meadowsweet, onion, papain, passion flower, poplar bark, prickly ash, quassia wood, red clover, turmeric, wild carrot, wild lettuce, or willow.

Pregnant and breast-feeding patients and those allergic to arnica, tansy, sunflowers, or chrysanthemums should avoid use. Any patient taking a drug that affects coagulation or platelet function should use arnica with caution.

Clinical considerations
- Arnica oil is usually made with 1 part herb extract to 5 parts vegetable-fixed oil.
- In tablet form, the active ingredient is extremely diluted.
- Warn patient that arnica should only be used externally.
- Frequent topical use of arnica increases the likelihood of contact dermatitis reactions. Eczema may also result from prolonged contact of arnica-containing external dressings. Advise patient that prolonged or frequent use of arnica dressings can increase the risk of skin reactions.
- Signs and symptoms of overdose include vomiting, diarrhea, drowsiness, dyspnea, and cardiac arrest. If overdose occurs, perform gastric lavage or induce vomiting, and follow with supportive treatment.
- Advise patient with history of dermatologic reactions to perfumes, cosmetics, hair tonics, and antidandruff preparations to use arnica with caution because many of these products contain arnica, and the reactions may indicate an allergy.
- If patient is taking an anticoagulant or using long-term aspirin therapy, instruct him to use arnica with caution and to notify his health care provider of any unusual bleeding or bruising.
- Warn patient that only diluted tincture should be used as a dressing.
- Advise patient to store ointment and undiluted tincture out of children's reach.
- Tell patient to remind prescriber and pharmacist of any herbal or dietary supplement that he's taking when obtaining a new prescription.
- Advise patient to consult his health care provider before using an herbal preparation because a treatment with proven efficacy may be available.

Research summary
The concepts behind the use of arnica and the claims made regarding its effects have not yet been validated scientifically.

Aromatherapy

Used since ancient times to heal the body, mind, and spirit, aromatherapy refers to the inhalation or application of essential oils distilled from various plants. Those who use aromatherapy today say it's effective in reducing stress, preventing disease, and even treating certain illnesses, both physical and psychological.

Modern aromatherapy dates to the work of French chemist René-Maurice Gattefosse in the 1930s. Gattefosse began to study the healing effects of plant oils after burning his hand in his family's perfume factory. He plunged his hand in a nearby container of lavender oil for quick relief and found that his wound healed quickly and without a scar. This incident sparked his interest in the possible therapeutic effects of plant oils, a field he called *aromatherapy.*

Today, aromatherapy is still popular in Europe, where essential oils are inhaled, massaged into the skin, or placed in bath water for specific therapeutic purposes. Specific oils are believed to have either relaxing or stimulating effects. When absorbed by body tissues, they're thought to interact with hormones and enzymes to produce changes in blood pressure, pulse rate, and other physiologic functions.

TRAINING *Aromatherapy may be self-administered or administered by a practitioner trained in the field. In the United States, where interest in aromatherapy has burgeoned in the past decade, several organizations train and certify aromatherapists, including the Pacific Institute of Aromatherapy in San Rafael, California, and the National Association of Holistic Aromatherapy in St. Louis, Missouri. These organizations can also provide information to health care providers and the public, referrals to aromatherapists, and sources for obtaining essential oils.*

Reported uses

Aromatherapists use specific oils, either alone or in conjunction with other therapies such as massage or herbal therapy, to treat specific ailments. Proponents claim that aside from creating pleasant sensations and promoting relaxation, aromatherapy can be used to treat bacterial and viral infections, anxiety, pain, muscle disorders, arthritis, herpes simplex, herpes zoster, skin disorders such as acne, premenstrual syndrome, headaches, and indigestion.

How the treatment is performed

In addition to the appropriate essential oil, aromatherapy may require other supplies, depending on the administration method being used. Massage requires a carrier oil and, for a full-body massage, a massage table. Inhalation requires a bowl of hot water and a large towel. An aromatherapy bath requires a tub filled with warm water. Diffusion requires a micromist, a candle diffuser, or a ceramic ring that can be placed on a light bulb.

Massage involves diluting the essential oil in the appropriate carrier oil and applying it to the exposed body part or the entire body using massage techniques. Bergamot, lemon, orange, grapefruit, and other citrus oils should not be applied before exposure to the sun.

For inhalation therapy, patient leans over a bowl of steaming water that contains a few drops of the essential oil, keeping his face far enough from the water's surface to avoid a burn injury. With towel draped over his head and the bowl to concentrate the steam, the patient inhales the vapors for a few minutes.

For a bath, patient adds a few drops of essential oil to the surface of the water and then soaks in the tub for 10 to 20 minutes, inhaling the vapors as he soaks.

Diffusion involves placing a few drops of the essential oil in the diffuser and turning on the heat source to diffuse microparticles of the oil into the air. The patient should be at least 3 feet (1 m) away from the diffuser. The average treatment time is 30 minutes.

Hazards
Basil, fennel, lemon grass, rosemary, and verbena oils may cause irritation in people with sensitive skin. Very high doses (10 to 20 ml) of certain oils (wintergreen, sage, aniseed, thyme, lemon, fennel, clove, cinnamon, camphor, and cedar wood) can result in nonlethal poisoning.

 SAFETY RISK *Aromatherapy is contraindicated during pregnancy because many essential oils can pose a toxic risk to the mother and fetus or, rarely, trigger spontaneous abortion.*

Aromatherapy should be used with caution in infants and children under age 5 because many essential oils are toxic to this age group. Among these are oils with a high level of terpene, such as rosemary and eucalyptus.

Origanum, sage, savory, thyme, and wintergreen oils aren't safe for home use.

Clinical considerations
■ Advise patient to avoid applying cinnamon or clove oil on the skin and to stop using basil, fennel, lemon grass, rosemary, and verbena oils if skin irritation develops.
■ Caution patient to keep essential oils away from the eyes and mucous membranes to avoid irritation. If contact occurs, the patient should flush copiously with water; if flushing doesn't relieve the pain, he should seek medical attention.

Research summary
Because there's no scientific evidence indicating that aromatherapy prevents or cures disease, it's typically used strictly as a complementary therapy to conventional treatments.

artichoke

Cynara scolymus, *garden artichoke, globe artichoke*

Although the active component of artichoke hasn't been identified, cynarin or a mono-caffeoylquinic acid may have some cholesterol-lowering effects. Cynarin may also have some liver-protective qualities, and it increases bile production.

Artichoke is available as fresh pressed juice or fresh or dried leaf, stem, root, and capsules. Products containing artichoke include Artichoke Ha, Artichoke Power, and Cynara-SI Artichoke.

Reported uses
Artichoke is used to treat dyspepsia, abdominal and gallbladder problems, and nausea. It can also be used as an antidiabetic, antilipemic, diuretic, and liver protectant. However, it's unknown whether artichoke reduces cholesterol in patients with type IIa or IIb familial hypercholesterolemia. Artichoke has also been used to prevent the return of gallstones.

Administration
■ Dried leaf, stem, or root: 1 to 4 g by mouth every day
■ Dry extract: 500 mg by mouth every day in a single dose.

Hazards
Patients who take herbal artichoke and also take insulin or an oral antidiabetic may have an increased risk of hypoglycemia because both the herb and the drugs have glucose-lowering effects.

Contact dermatitis may be associated with use of artichoke.

Those allergic to artichokes, marigolds, daisies, or chrysanthemums and those with bile duct obstruction should avoid using artichoke. Those with gallstones should use artichoke with caution.

Clinical considerations

- Bile duct obstruction should be ruled out before artichoke is used medicinally.
- Monitor blood glucose level in those with diabetes. Advise diabetic patient that artichoke may have a hypoglycemic effect. If he's taking an antidiabetic, his dosage may need to be adjusted.
- Advise patient to avoid medicinal use of artichoke if he's allergic to artichokes, marigolds, daisies, or chrysanthemums.
- If patient has gallstones, advise him to consult his health care provider before using artichoke medicinally.
- Advise patient to store artichoke preparations in a tightly closed container away from light.
- Tell patient to remind prescriber and pharmacist of any herbal or dietary supplement that he's taking when obtaining a new prescription.
- Advise patient to consult his health care provider before using an herbal preparation because a treatment with proven efficacy may be available.

Research summary

Artichoke leaf may work by interfering with cholesterol synthesis. Besides cynarin, a compound in artichoke called luteolin may play a role in reducing cholesterol.

 RESEARCH *According to a double-blind, placebo-controlled study of 143 individuals with elevated cholesterol, artichoke leaf extract significantly improved cholesterol readings (Englisch, et al., 2000). Total cholesterol fell by 18.5% as compared to 8.6% in the placebo group; LDL cholesterol by 23% versus 6%; and LDL to HDL ratio decreased by 20% versus 7%.*

Art therapy

Art therapists believe that the release of creative energy associated with artistic expression can lead to physical, emotional, and spiritual healing. They believe that the act of drawing, painting, or sculpting helps patients by promoting self-awareness, and allowing patients to express feelings that they can't verbalize. Art therapy by itself can't cure disease; rather, it's used to complement the overall health care plan.

Art therapy can use any artistic medium and can occur in any setting, from a hospital bed to the patient's home or an artist's studio. Patients who are unable to create art may benefit by viewing the art of others.

In addition to providing the patient with a means of self-expression and a pleasant diversion, art therapy also helps health care providers understand the patient. A patient's drawings may reveal his state of mind, including his feelings about his health problem and his subconscious concerns. Such insight can help the practitioner or art therapist develop or refine a diagnosis and formulate a plan to help the patient with his specific health problem.

The concept of using art as therapy began in the 1800s in mental institutions. The art of mental patients was seen as valuable, not only in assisting with a diagnosis but also as a tool for rehabilitation. In the 1940s, art and psychoanalysis were combined as a method of helping patients release thoughts and feelings buried in the subconscious.

TRAINING *With the formation of the American Art Therapy Association (AATA) and the Art Therapy Credentials Board (ATCB) in 1969, a code of ethics and standards for the profession were developed. The AATA approves educational programs and works to educate the public about the field. The ATCB offers two levels of credentials. A registered art therapist (ATR) must have a master's degree in art therapy, complete a supervised internship, and meet contact hour requirements. Once registered, an ATR has the option of becoming board-certified in art therapy (ATRBC) by sitting for a certification exam.*

Reported uses

Art therapy can be used in a variety of clinical situations. It's especially useful in dealing with children, who often can't express their feelings or physical sensations verbally. Many survivors of physical or sexual abuse also benefit from art therapy. These patients commonly have feelings of anger, rage, shame, guilt, and fear that they have difficulty expressing verbally. Art therapy provides them with a safe means of expressing those feelings. (See *Indications for art therapy*.)

Art therapy is also useful as a follow-up to other image-evoking mind-body therapies, such as relaxation, guided imagery, and hypnotherapy. It allows the patient to externalize mental images and emotions that form during the session and helps to ground their experience.

Art therapy is practiced in psychiatric centers, drug and alcohol rehabilitation programs, prisons, day care treatment centers, children's hospitals, schools for people with mental retardation, residences for the developmentally delayed, geriatric centers, and hospices, among others.

How the treatment is performed

Almost any medium the patient is physically capable of handling can be used for art therapy: paints, pens, pencils, felt markers, chalks, clay, or crayons. Natural objects such as flowers, grasses, seeds, shells, nuts, stones, feathers, or bones may also be used. The artwork can range from drawings, paintings, or collages to wood or soap carving, papier mâché, or metal or plaster sculptures.

Mask making is another powerful and popular form of art therapy used for both individuals and groups. Masks can be made from many materials, including paper bags, cardboard, Styrofoam, leather, wood, plaster, papier mâché, and metal. Ready-made masks can be purchased and decorated. Masks may be used to mark a life passage, such as adolescence, adulthood, or elderhood, or to celebrate the successful completion of a

---

INDICATIONS FOR ART THERAPY

Art therapy can be used to treat the following types of conditions:
- Age-related role changes
- Attention deficit hyperactivity disorder
- Catastrophic illness (such as AIDS or cancer)
- Chronic disease
- Chronic fatigue syndrome
- Chronic pain
- Chronic stress disorders
- Extensive surgery
- Learning disabilities
- Loss of voice
- Posttraumatic stress disorder
- Prolonged hospitalization or treatment
- Psychiatric disorders
- Spinal cord injuries
- Substance abuse and addiction
- Terminal illness.

Art therapy is also effective in couple and family therapies and for treating children who have been abused or neglected or come from homes in which there were drug abusers.

---

healing process, such as a substance abuse program, chemotherapy regimen, or organ transplantation.

Another form of art therapy, puppetry, can be as simple as the creation of hand puppets from socks, or it can involve the construction of marionettes, a stage, scenery, and a puppet theater. Cameras and computers are also being used as forms of art therapy.

Structuring the environment is an important component of art therapy. The patient should be as comfortable as possible, and surroundings should be free from distractions. Feedback is supportive, never critical or judgmental. Only when the patient feels safe will he allow his feelings to surface in his artwork.

Young children and patients with impaired fine motor skills may work better with larger crayons and markers, finger paints, or modeling clay. Small shells or seeds and projects involving scissors aren't a good choice for very young patients. The patient should be provided with a variety of colors regardless of the medium he's using to ensure that he's able to choose just the right color to express his mood, feeling, or memory.

Art therapy sessions are usually run by a facilitator. The AATA recommends that the facilitator be someone who is sensitive to human needs and expressions, emotionally stable, and patient. In addition, the facilitator should have insight into the psychological process, attentive listening skills, keen observation skills, flexibility, a sense of humor, and an understanding of art media.

The facilitation process begins with an explanation of the procedure and a request for the patient's participation. The patient is asked whether he prefers a particular medium and a determination is made regarding his need for special equipment (such as large crayons for a patient with limited motor skills). The necessary materials are assembled and a quiet, comfortable work area is provided. Ideally, the work surface should be large and flat, but some patients may require an over-bed table or a large clipboard. The patient is reassured that he doesn't need any special drawing talent and that stick figures can convey a message effectively. All the patient's efforts are praised without judgment.

The patient may be encouraged to draw a picture representing himself in relation to his disease. For example, he might be asked to draw himself in the past (before the disease), now (with the disease), and in the future (after treatment). He may be asked to draw the disease itself; this method is commonly used with cancer patients to help them visually express the way they see their disease.

The patient is permitted to complete the drawing to his satisfaction. Some patients may need to draw in minute detail and search for just the right color. Once the drawing is finished, the patient is asked to show and talk about it. The facilitator reflects back to the patient what he has said to validate the meaning of his artwork and help the patient summarize the creative experience.

The facilitator should be alert for clues to the patient's feelings. How did he represent himself in relation to other figures or objects in the drawing. Is the size proportional? Did he draw his entire body? Does his face have a smile or a frown? The overall mood of the drawing — including the way the patient used color — is noted. Even without formal training in art therapy, a great deal of insight can be gained by assessing a patient's artwork.

Hazards

Before beginning a project, the therapist determines whether the patient is physically capable of carrying it out. Some medications, a weakened condition, or inflamed or painful hand joints can interfere with a patient's ability to perform or complete an artistic task. Although no patient should be discouraged from trying, the inability to finish an art project may diminish the patient's self-esteem.

Strong emotions may surface as the patient explores his feelings about an illness through his artwork. If the patient shows signs of agitation or uncontrolled emotion, the session should be ended. The facilitator should stay with the patient and be empathetic. The patient should be reassured that it's normal to have strong feelings and encouraged to express them. The appropriate member of the health care team — physician, social worker, or psychotherapist — should be involved and any referrals documented.

Clinical considerations

■ If the patient doesn't want to participate in an art session, don't insist; instead, work on building a trusting therapeutic relationship. The patient may be open to participating in the future.

- Patients who are physically unable to manipulate a crayon or paintbrush may be able to put together a collage. Allow them to choose pictures, words, colors, and placement to express their feelings.
- Although art therapy can be used with individuals, couples, families, and groups, it's particularly valuable with children, who often can't talk about their most painful and important concerns. Obtain permission from the child's parents before beginning any art sessions.
- Use art supplies that are age-specific — for example, nontoxic crayons and markers for young children prone to putting objects in the mouth.
- The patient's images may change over time. Initially, they may be dark, strong, or heavy, with hard geometric shapes. As healing begins and the patient establishes trust with the therapist and the environment, images typically become softer and more rounded, with less severe boundaries. Colors become lighter, and the drawings may contain representations of hope, freedom, or release, such as suns or rainbows.
- A patient who's especially proud of a piece of art may agree to have it displayed so that others may admire it, another source of acknowledgment for the patient.
- Encourage patient to keep a journal or log of his drawings as a personal record and a coping mechanism for voicing negative or positive thoughts and feelings.

Research summary

Little scientific research has been done on this form of therapy, but some studies have reported benefits for patients with psychiatric illnesses, spinal cord injury and other disabilities, chronic stress disorders, and Alzheimer's disease.

asparagus

Asparagus officinalis, *sparrow grass*

Asparagus is rich in vitamins A and E and contains folic acid. It has saponin components that act as mucous membrane irritants. The shoots have several sulfur-containing acids that can cause urine to become strong smelling.

Asparagus is available as cut rhizome or root, fresh stalks, root powder, and tea. Products containing asparagus include ClearLung (combination product), Hy-C (Bu Yin), Tian Men Dong, and Ultimate Urinary Cleanse.

Reported uses

Asparagus is used with large amounts of liquid as irrigation therapy. It can also be used to treat urinary tract infections and rheumatic joint pain and swelling, to prevent kidney or bladder stones, and to provide contraception.

The seeds and root extracts are used in the production of alcoholic beverages. The seeds are also used in coffee substitutes, diuretic preparations, laxatives, and remedies for neuritis and rheumatism. The seeds may relieve toothaches, stimulate hair growth, and treat cancer. Topical preparations may have drying effects on acne.

Despite the varied uses, irrigation therapy is the only use with clinical supporting evidence.

Administration

- Daily dose: 45 to 80 g by mouth every day
- Root powder: 10 to 50 g mixed with milk and sugar by mouth twice a day
- Tea: 40 to 60 g of cut rhizome or root steeped in 5 oz of boiling water for 5 to 10 minutes, then strained, by mouth every day.

Hazards

Use of asparagus may be associated with mucous membrane irritation, malodorous urine, and contact dermatitis (with external use). Asparagus possibly increases the effects of diuretics.

Those with inflammatory kidney diseases should avoid use. Those with edema caused by heart or kidney disorders shouldn't use asparagus as an irrigant. Pregnant patients should avoid medicinal use of asparagus because the effects on the developing fetus are unknown.

Clinical considerations

■ Using asparagus as a urinary irrigant requires adequate fluid intake. Encourage patient to drink plenty of fluids while taking asparagus.

■ Asparagus may also be applied topically; however, no guidelines for concentration or dosing exist.

■ Inform patient that asparagus may cause urine to develop a strong odor and that the odor may be more pronounced after eating fresh asparagus as opposed to taking the rhizome or root as a tea.

■ Advise a pregnant patient to avoid using asparagus medicinally, but assure her that consuming fresh asparagus should be safe.

■ Tell patient to remind prescriber and pharmacist of any herbal or dietary supplement that he's taking when obtaining a new prescription.

■ Advise patient to consult his health care provider before using an herbal preparation because a treatment with proven efficacy may be available.

Research summary

Of the varied uses for asparagus, irrigation therapy is the only one with clinical supporting evidence.

Aston-Patterning

Aston-Patterning is an integrated system of movement education, bodywork, ergonomics, and fitness training. It assists individuals with using their bodies more efficiently to release tension and pain and to improve posture and movement.

The premise is that an injury or dysfunction in one part of the body causes the rest of the body to compensate in ways that reinforce the original symptoms. All movement is considered a three-dimensional, ascending or descending, asymmetrical spiral, due to the body's asymmetries and the play of gravity and ground reaction force. For any activity, an optimal base of support comes from the legs while standing and the pelvis while sitting. The width, depth, and length of this base of support vary according to the task, ensuring an adequate foundation for the body segments above to prevent strain or injury.

Aston-Patterning teaches that the basic components of all movements are weight transfer, rocking across the hinge joints of the legs and pelvis, and matching flexion and extension of the spine, arms, and legs. Understanding these movements and how to combine and sequence them for a given activity results in added support for the whole body, better use of momentum, better shock absorption, and more stability and mobility.

In 1963, with a B.A. and M.F.A. in dance from the University of California, Los Angeles, Aston started a movement education program for athletes, dancers, and actors at Long Beach City College in California. Exploring the way movement communicates emotion, she worked with psychotherapists to develop a format of body consciousness to assist in the therapy process.

Needing rehabilitation after two car accidents, Aston sought treatment with Ida Rolf in 1968. Rolf's myofascial treatment, called Rolfing, facilitated Aston's recovery and expanded her understanding of how the body can change. Rolf asked Aston to develop a movement education counterpart to Rolfing to help patients preserve the changes they achieved. Aston taught students how to make patients aware of and change the ways they move their bodies in work and play and how to use their bodies with minimum effort and maximum precision. These contributions to Rolfing became known as Rolf-Aston Structural Patterning.

By the mid-1970s, Aston had added environmental modification to her work. She maximized patient comfort by adjusting their chairs at work, using pillows in sleep postures, and modifying their use of sports equipment. This work developed into a line of products designed to help maintain alignment while sitting or exercising.

Aston abandoned her linear viewpoint of bodywork in favor of three-dimensional spiral patterns, in which she perceived retained tension. She taught patients to release this tension by incorporating their asymmetries into their movements, rather than resisting their nature by moving in straight lines. Increasingly aware that her paradigm differed from Rolfing, she dissolved the Patterning Institute associated with Rolfing in 1977 and continued to develop her work as Aston-Patterning.

There are three aspects to Aston-Patterning: neurokinetics, bodywork, and ergonomics. Neurokinetics, the movement education aspect, begins with learning more efficient and less stressful ways of performing the simple movements of everyday life and progresses to more complex activities. All aspects of the movement work aim to evoke easy and efficient activity.

The bodywork aspect consists of Aston massage, myokinetics, and arthrokinetics. The massage uses noncompressive touch to help release functional holding patterns (patterns of tension that are maintained by the nervous system and have not yet created physiologic change in connective tissue) from both superficial and deep layers. Myokinetics uses precise strokes to release structural (more strongly held) holding patterns in the fascial network. Arthrokinetics addresses structural holding patterns at bone and joint surfaces.

The ergonomics aspect of Aston-Patterning identifies environmental factors (such as seating conditions and shoe type) that may be compromising body structure. The practitioner then suggests ways of changing body usage or modifying objects to make them more "body friendly."

Another aspect of Aston-Patterning is Aston fitness training, which includes vertical and horizontal loosening (self-massage techniques), toning, stretching, and cardiovascular fitness.

Aston-Patterning draws on all of these tools as needed. Patients are taught to be more self-aware, so that they can understand the source of their tension and movement. The diversity of techniques available helps them neutralize the negative effects of past history on their body and move into more knowledgeable and comfortable patterns.

Reported uses

Aston-Patterning is a noninvasive technique used in people with injuries involving the spinal axis, peripheral joints, and multiple pain sites. It can be an adjunct to physical therapy and medication or can be used in place of other treatment for an active rehabilitation approach. When the body's segments — legs, pelvis, spine, shoulder girdle, head, and neck — are optimally aligned, movement becomes easier and more natural.

This treatment is considered useful in clients such as dancers or runners who encounter chronic overuse problems. It's considered particularly helpful in individuals who have anterior knee pain (chondromalacia), chronic piriformis syndrome, chronic adductor strains, and a variety of lumbar and sacroiliac joint problems. There may be potential for using Aston work for the prevention of pain, joint wear and tear, and so forth, caused by stressful body use.

How the treatment is performed

An Aston-Patterning session begins with a patient history (physical, psychological, and emotional), a review of everyday activities (work, home, sports, and leisure activities), and a discussion of when or where the patient feels fatigue or pain.

A baseline pretest follows — usually a basic activity, such as walking, sitting, standing, reaching, bending, or lifting, or a particular problem activity such as using a keyboard. This enables the practitioner to visualize some aspect of the client's movement abilities and potential for improvement. To make the patient aware of his movements during the activity, the practitioner may call attention to details, such as how the hand is held when keyboarding, what position the shoulders take as they move, or how the foot is planted on the ground. Movement education or bodywork is included in virtually every session to release unnecessary tension and make the new movement easier and more efficient. Continual emphasis on self-awareness gives the patient the knowledge to keep the changes as part of future patterns of movement. During pretesting, the practitioner makes a chart of the client's postural alignment and tension holding patterns. A new chart is made at each session to document the patient's progress.

Posttesting essentially repeats the pretesting movements, allowing the patient to see and feel the changes that have taken place and to integrate them into daily life. If the session focused on arm and shoulder movements, the client may apply the new movements to a golf swing or to computer keyboarding.

Hazards

Aston-Patterning drills and exercises can be extremely demanding. A client with a heart condition or respiratory problems should check with his health care provider before undertaking this form of therapy. The program can be adjusted to meet the needs of older adults, those in poor health, and patients with special rehabilitation requirements.

The deep massage employed in Aston-Patterning could be an issue if the patient has osteoporosis or a tendency to bruise easily. If the client has a bleeding disorder, takes anticoagulants, or is undergoing long-term steroid therapy, which can make the tissues fragile, Aston-Patterning may not be an appropriate therapy.

For people in good physical condition, most complications are the result of overly intensive training. Exhaustion and pain are the principal problems.

Clinical considerations

- Ask patient if he has a heart condition or respiratory problems before he begins this form of therapy.
- Advise patient to voice any pain or discomfort during the sessions. The experienced practitioner will know how hard to push and when it's best to stop.
- Counsel patient with circulation problems, such as those resulting from diabetes or varicose veins, not to receive deep massage in the legs and feet.
- The Aston Fitness Program may be a useful approach to physical fitness training for the elderly.

TRAINING   *The Aston-Patterning Practitioner Program, a continuing education program for health professionals, includes training in neurokinetics, myokinetics, and ergonomic evaluation plus advanced massage techniques and fitness. The 84-day program is scheduled in five 3-week segments over a period of 1½ to 2 years. Blocks of time between the levels allow the student to apply and practice the skills in work situations. The training is intended to prepare the practitioner to address a wide range of situations, from athletic endeavors to rehabilitation.*

Research summary

The concepts behind the use of Aston-Patterning and the claims made regarding its effects have not yet been validated scientifically.

autumn crocus

Colchicum autumnale, *crocus,*
fall crocus, meadow saffron, mysteria,
naked ladies, vellorita, wonder bulb

Autumn crocus contains colchicine and
other alkaloids. These components act as
antichemotactics, antiphlogistics, and an-
timitotics. Overall, the herb decreases inflammation and collagen synthesis and
inhibits cell division. It's available as pulverized herb, freshly pressed juice, and
other preparations for oral use.

Reported uses

Autumn crocus extracts have been used
to treat arthritis, rheumatism, prostate
enlargement, and gonorrhea. Extracts
have also been used to treat cancer.

The FDA has approved the use of
colchicine, the active ingredient in autumn crocus, for the treatment of gout.
Colchicine has also been used to treat
multiple sclerosis, familial Mediterranean
fever, hepatic cirrhosis, and primary biliary cirrhosis and as an adjunct therapy
in primary amyloidosis, Behcet's disease,
pseudogout, skin manifestations of scleroderma, psoriasis, palmoplantar pustu-
losis, and dermatitis herpetiformis.

Administration

■ For acute gout attack: One dose equivalent to 1 mg of colchicine by mouth, followed by 0.5 mg to 1.5 mg every 1 to 2
hours until pain diminishes (daily maximum 8 mg of colchicine equivalent)
■ For Mediterranean fever: 0.5 mg to
1.5 mg of colchicine equivalent by mouth
as a single dose.

Hazards

SAFETY RISK *Because of the*
plant's toxicity, internal use isn't
recommended. Patients should
consult a knowledgeable practitioner before
use.

Use of autumn crocus may be associated with peripheral neuritis, numbness of
fingertips, irritation of the nose and
throat, GI disturbances, nausea, liver
necrosis, agranulocytosis, aplastic anemia, kidney impairment, and multiple
organ failure.

Autumn crocus may be associated with
additive adverse and toxic effects when
used concomitantly with colchicine.

Pregnant and breast-feeding patients
should avoid using autumn crocus because of its potential teratogenic effects
and antimitotic properties.

Clinical considerations

■ Because many autumn crocus preparations aren't evaluated for colchicine content the way prescription colchicine
products are, overdose is a concern.
■ If patient insists on taking autumn
crocus, advise him to alert his health care
provider first and then to obtain the
product from a reputable source.
■ Monitor patient for agranulocytosis,
aplastic anemia, and peripheral neuritis
with prolonged use.
■ Any patient who experiences nausea,
vomiting, intense thirst, burning in the
mouth, abdominal pain, or diarrhea after
taking autumn crocus should immediately contact the poison control center. Diarrhea may be persistent and may lead to
hypovolemic shock, renal impairment,
and oliguria. Treatment for toxic reaction
includes fluid replacement, induction of
vomiting, and gastric lavage.
■ Advise patient who's pregnant or
breast-feeding not to use autumn crocus.
■ A patient who may become pregnant
should perform a pregnancy test before
beginning therapy. Further, instruct her
to immediately discontinue use and notify her health care provider if pregnancy
occurs.
■ Postmenopausal women and those using adequate contraceptive measures are
the only women who should use autumn
crocus.
■ Slicing the fresh corm can irritate the
nose and throat and cause numbness of
the fingers holding the corm.

- Advise patient who's taking colchicine to avoid using autumn crocus.
- Warn patient that the entire plant is toxic and that he shouldn't take it orally, unless his health care provider has instructed him to do so.
- Advise patient who's using autumn crocus to obtain it from a reputable source that clearly identifies the amount of colchicine that each dose contains.
- Tell patient to remind prescriber and pharmacist of any herbal or dietary supplement that he's taking when obtaining a new prescription.
- Advise patient to consult his health care provider before using an herbal preparation because a treatment with proven efficacy may be available.

Research summary
The concepts behind the use of autumn crocus and the claims made regarding its effects have not yet been validated scientifically.

avens

Benedict's herb, Bennet's root, blessed herb, city avens, colewort, European avens, geum, Geum urbanum, goldy star, herb Bennet, star of the earth, way Bennet, wild rye, yellow avens

Avens contains tannins and phenolic glycosides, including eugenol, which give avens root a clove-like odor. Both components have astringent properties that cause tissues to contract.

Avens is available as aerial parts and root, dried and made into a tea for oral consumption, and liquid extract containing alcohol for oral consumption.

Reported uses
Avens is used to treat diarrhea, digestive complaints, ulcerative colitis, intermittent fevers, sore throats, gingivitis, and halitosis.

Administration
- Extract (containing 25% alcohol): 1 to 4 ml by mouth three times a day
- Tea: 1 to 4 g in boiling water, by mouth three times a day.

Hazards
There are no known adverse effects or interactions associated with use of avens.

Pregnant and breast-feeding patients should avoid use because of a possible effect on the menstrual cycle.

Clinical considerations

 SAFETY RISK *Don't confuse avens with water avens (Geum rivale, chocolate root).*

- Avens is rarely used in herbal medicine.
- If patient is pregnant, breast-feeding, or planning pregnancy, advise her not to use avens and to notify her health care provider if she becomes pregnant during therapy.
- If patient is using avens to treat diarrhea, advise him to contact his health care professional if the diarrhea persists.
- Tell patient to remind prescriber and pharmacist of any herbal or dietary supplement that he's taking when obtaining a new prescription.
- Advise patient to consult his health care provider before using an herbal preparation because a treatment with proven efficacy may be available.

Research summary
The concepts behind the use of avens and the claims made regarding its effects have not yet been validated scientifically.

Ayurvedic medicine

India's ancient healing system, *Ayurveda* (meaning "science of life" in Sanskrit) is an integrated approach to the prevention and treatment of illness that combines philosophical, spiritual, and scientific principles dating back thousands of years. Derived from the Vedas, the ancient body of literature, prayers, and teachings that forms the foundation of Hinduism and Indian culture, Ayurveda is a philosophy of living that encompasses the whole of human life, including the individual's place in the cosmos. In Ayurvedic medicine, concern isn't limited to the curing of disease; the promotion of positive and vital health and longevity is important as well. The books of Deepak Chopra have helped to popularize Ayurvedic beliefs in the West in recent years.

In its basic concepts, Ayurvedic medicine is similar to traditional Chinese medicine. Both systems stress the interconnectedness of body, mind, and spirit and of the individual to the environment, and both espouse the need for balance and harmony among these elements. Both cite a cosmos composed of five basic elements — in the Ayurvedic system, earth, air, fire, water, and space. Both also place great emphasis on the prevention of disease and on the individual's responsibility for achieving that goal through proper diet, exercise, sleep patterns, and other lifestyle interventions.

Determining a person's metabolic body type, or *dosha,* is the cornerstone of Ayurvedic medicine. The three *doshas,* known as *vata, pitta,* and *kapha,* loosely correspond to the Western categories of body physique (thin, muscular, and fat), but they're believed to have more far-reaching effects on a person's health, personality, and susceptibility to illness. Each *dosha* is associated with specific body organs and with two of the five environmental elements.

Most people are a combination of doshas, but one type usually predominates. The predominant dosha is believed to determine not only the person's metabolic body type but also his personality traits and the types of illness he's likely to develop. It also serves as a guideline for the types of food he should eat, the types of exercise he should practice and, in general, how he should conduct his life.

For instance, *vata's* natural element is air, which is constantly moving, so *vata* characteristics pertain to motion, movement, lightness, and changeability. *Pitta's* element is fire, so its qualities are associated with heat, such as anger, redness, and inflammation. *Kapha's* element is earth, so its characteristics signify solidity, slowness, and strength. (See *Characteristics of the three doshas,* page 64.)

According to Ayurvedic beliefs, good health requires a balance between the doshas within each individual; between body, mind, and spirit; and between the individual and the environment. Disease results from an imbalance of the doshas, which can be influenced by an unhealthy lifestyle, internal and external stressors, emotions, seasonal influences, genetic predisposition, and an accumulation of toxic substances in the body.

Once people are aware of their predominant dosha type and its characteristics, they can make appropriate lifestyle changes designed to restore the balance of doshas and thus maintain well-being.

Reported uses
As Ayurveda includes protocols for the care of every system of the body, it can play a role in the management of any disorder. It's being used most effectively on patients with chronic and acute disease; however, Ayurvedic therapies may also be effective in enhancing wellness and preventing disease.

How the treatment is performed
Diagnosis involves determining the patient's predominant dosha, obtaining a detailed history (including interpersonal and family relationships and job situation), performing a physical examination, determining the illness and its causes, and establishing a prognosis. (Because the Ayurvedic practitioner typically doesn't treat incurable disease, it's important to know the patient's chances of recovery.)

The Ayurvedic practitioner uses observation, questioning, palpation, and aus-

CHARACTERISTICS OF THE THREE DOSHAS

The three doshas of Ayurvedic medicine are believed to control all body functions. Each dosha is associated with specific body organs, personality traits, physiologic functions, and natural elements, as shown in the chart below.

Vata	Pitta	Kapha
Body type		
Slender	Medium build, well proportioned	Heavy build
Physical characteristics		
Cool, dry skin; prominent features	Fair or red hair, ruddy complexion, freckles, tendency to perspire heavily	Oily skin, thick hair, slow moving
Personality traits		
Hyperactive, unpredictable, nervous, moody, energetic, intuitive, imaginative, impulsive, eats and sleeps erratically	Predictable, moderate in daily habits, intelligent, articulate, warm and loving, explosive temper, eats and sleeps regularly	Relaxed, slow to anger, slow to eat, slow to act, tolerant, affectionate, obstinate; procrastinates, sleeps long and deeply
Metabolic tendencies		
Prone to nervous disorders, energy and weight fluctuations, anxiety, insomnia, constipation; women prone to premenstrual syndrome	Prone to heartburn, ulcers, and other GI complaints; acne, and hemorrhoids	Prone to obesity, high cholesterol, allergies, and sinus problems
Associated internal organs		
Large intestine, pelvic cavity, bones, ears	Stomach, small intestine, blood, skin, sweat glands, eyes	Lungs, chest, spinal cord, and spinal fluid
Associated natural elements		
Air and ether (space)	Fire and water	Water and earth
Physiologic function		
Breathing, blood circulation, movement	Digestion, metabolism	Nourishment

cultation (of the heart, lungs, and intestines), paying special attention to the pulse, tongue, eyes, nails, and urine. As in traditional Chinese medicine, pulse measurement is much more detailed and significant than in Western medicine. Like their Chinese counterparts, Ayurvedic practitioners can distinguish 12 distinct radial pulses, which help them assess the functioning of specific body organs and the interaction of the three doshas. Observing the tongue surface provides insight into organ function and dosha imbalances. Examining the urine for unusual colors or odors can also help the practitioner detect any dosha imbalances.

Once the Ayurvedic practitioner has determined the patient's particular dosha imbalance, he'll recommend an individualized treatment plan aimed at restoring equilibrium. The regimen typically includes some combination of dietary and lifestyle changes, purification therapy, and mental exercises.

Lifestyle interventions are prescribed according to the person's constitutional type. They may include changes in diet and eating patterns, sleeping and waking times, and sexual activity. Specific foods and condiments are selected not because of their nutritional value but because of their taste (sweet, sour, salty), their tendency to produce heat or cold, and other factors believed to affect dosha balance. The practitioner may also recommend chanting or sitting in the sun for a specified period.

Purification of the body, known as *panchakarma,* is a complex series of steps undertaken to rid the body of physical impurities, or "toxins." The process, which usually takes about a week, includes herbal oil massage to loosen the excess doshas, steam treatments to open up the pores, therapeutic vomiting to cleanse the stomach, bowel purging and enemas to flush out the GI tract, and nasal inhalation of herbal potions to drain excess mucus. The Vedic texts recommend undergoing purification three times a year, ideally at the beginning of spring, fall, and winter.

Meditation, yoga, and breathing exercises are believed to do for the mind what panchakarma does for the body: rid the mind of negative thoughts and emotions, such as fear, anger, greed, and doubt, and generally help the mind achieve a higher level of functioning. As with the other measures, they're recommended not only to treat various disorders but also to maintain good health and prevent disease.

Hazards
The patient's medication history should be obtained to ensure that herbal compounds don't interact with other prescribed herbs or drugs.

Colonic equipment must be sterilized or disposable to avoid the spread of communicable disease. Rectal insertion of hydrotherapy equipment requires caution; vagal stimulation with hypotension and bradycardia may occur.

Clinical considerations
- Help patient understand that he'll need to cooperate in making recommended changes in diet and lifestyle.
- Tell patient not to share Ayurvedic compounds with anyone else.

Research summary
Although many people practice meditation and yoga simply to achieve a sense of serenity and relaxation, extensive research in India and the West has revealed clear physiologic benefits from these two practices. Harvard Medical School Professor Herbert Benson's studies of people who practiced transcendental meditation in the 1970s showed that meditation decreases oxygen consumption and metabolism; lowers blood pressure, heart rate, and respiratory rate; increases the production of alpha brain waves (associated with feelings of well-being); relieves stress; and enhances overall well-being. In fact, research on meditation practice led to the development in the West of biofeedback and relaxation training.

Yoga has been practiced in India for thousands of years as part of an integrated approach to good health. In the West, it has recently been incorporated into a number of programs aimed at treating chronic diseases. One example is Dean Ornish's successful program to reverse coronary artery disease by combining yoga with dietary changes, moderate exercise, and support groups. Numerous research studies on yoga have shown that regular practice can help patients learn to control blood pressure, heart rate, respiratory function, metabolic rate, body temperature, and brain waves as well as improve circulation, flexibility, and stamina.

A 1989 Dutch study of patients using a combination of Ayurvedic therapies for certain chronic conditions (asthma, hypertension, arthritis, constipation, headache, eczema, bronchitis, and non-insulin-dependent diabetes) documented improvements in 79% of patients.

Laboratory studies of certain Ayurvedic herbal preparations have demonstrated potentially beneficial effects for certain cancers, including colon, breast, and lung cancer. The National Cancer Institute has included Ayurvedic compounds on its list of potential chemopreventive agents. The 1994 report to the National Institutes of Health entitled *Alternative Medicine: Expanding Medical Horizons* concluded: "Because of the potential of Ayurvedic therapies for treating conditions for which modern medicine has few, if any, effective treatments, this area is a fertile one for research opportunities."

TRAINING *The only place in the United States where practitioners can receive complete clinical training is the California College of Ayurveda in Grass Valley, California.*

balsam of Peru

Balsam tree, Myroxylon balsamum,
Peruvian balsam, tolu balsam

Balsam of Peru contains 50% to 70% ester mixtures, the greatest quantity being
benzyl ester of benzoic, cinnamein, and
cinnamic acid. It's available in shampoo,
lotions, and syrups.

Reported uses
Balsam of Peru is used topically to help
heal infected and poorly healing wounds,
burns, pressure ulcers, frostbite, sore nipples, leg ulcers, bruises from prostheses,
and hemorrhoids. It's also used topically
to stimulate the heart, increase blood
pressure, and reduce mucous secretions.
Balsam is used as an antiparasitic to treat
scabies and for fevers, colds, cough,
bronchitis, tendency to infection, and
mouth and pharynx inflammation. It's
used to treat pruritus and advanced
stages of acute eczema. All uses are topical.

Administration
■ Topical: 5% to 20% Peruvian balsam
applied daily for up to 1 week
■ Tolu balsam for internal use: 0.5 g by
mouth every day.

Hazards
Balsam of Peru may be associated with
aphthoid oral ulcers, renal damage, allergic skin reactions, urticaria, purpura,
photodermatosis, phototoxicity, and
Quincke's disease.

Use of balsam of Peru along with sulfur-containing products may produce additive effects. Advise patient to use with caution.

Use of balsam of Peru in conjunction with sun exposure increases the risk of photosensitivity reactions.

Balsam of Peru is contraindicated in persons with a propensity for allergies.

Those with hypertension should use balsam of Peru with caution because it may increase blood pressure if ingested.

Clinical considerations
- Caution patient to discontinue use if skin reaction occurs.
- Advise wearing protective clothing and sunscreen and limiting exposure to direct sunlight.
- Warn patient to seek appropriate medical evaluation before using balsam of Peru to treat wound infection or pressure ulcers to avoid a delay in healing and a worsening of the condition.
- Advise him not to use herb with products containing sulfur.
- Instruct female patient who's using the herb externally to treat sore nipples to remove residue from her breasts before breast-feeding an infant.
- Advise patient to limit external application to 1 week or less.
- Tell patient to remind prescriber and pharmacist of any herbal or dietary supplement that he's taking when obtaining a new prescription.
- Advise patient to consult his health care provider before using an herbal preparation because a treatment with proven efficacy may be available.

Research summary
The concepts behind the use of balsam of Peru and the claims made regarding its effects have not yet been validated scientifically.

barberry

Barberry-Berberis vulgaris, B. aquifolium *Pursh, berberis, berberry, jaundice berry,* Mahonia aquifolium *Nutt, mountain grape, Oregon grape, pepperidge bush, pipperidge, sour-spine, sowberry, trailing mahonia, woodsour*

Barberry contains isoquinolone alkaloids in the root and bark, including the widely studied alkaloid berberine. It's a source of vitamin C and is available as liquid extract, tablets, and tea.

Reported uses
Berberine is effective in managing bacterial-induced diarrhea. In small doses, it stimulates the respiratory system. Barberry is also believed to stimulate the immune system, increase iron absorption, and act as a mild diuretic.

Barberry is used to dilate blood vessels and stimulate the circulatory system, to treat GI ailments, and to relieve or reduce fever. It may be beneficial as a bactericidal and for cholera-induced diarrhea, to stimulate uterine contractions, and for its laxative effects.

Administration
- Dried root: 2 to 4 g by mouth
- Fluid extract (1:1): 2 to 4 ml by mouth
- Solid (powdered dry) extract (4:1) or 8% to 12% alkaloid content: 250 to 500 mg by mouth
- Tea (1 to 2 teaspoons whole or crushed barberries steeped 10 to 15 minutes in 5 oz of hot water): 2 to 4 g by mouth or 2 g in 8 oz of water
- Tincture (1:5): 6 to 12 ml by mouth
- Tincture (1:10): 20 to 40 gtt by mouth every day
- For cholera-induced diarrhea: 100 mg of berberine by mouth four times a day or 400 mg by mouth every day, alone or with tetracycline; 500 mg maximum daily dose.

Hazards

Adverse effects of barberry may include stupor, lethargy, hypotension, epistaxis, eye irritation, diarrhea, nephritis, dyspnea, and skin irritation.

 SAFETY RISK *In large doses, barberry may produce dyspnea and lethal respiratory system paralysis.*

Barberry may potentiate the effects of antihypertensive drugs.

Pregnant women should avoid use of barberry because it may stimulate uterine contractions. Patients with heart failure and those with respiratory diseases should use barberry with caution.

Clinical considerations

■ Patient using barberry to treat diarrhea should be monitored to ensure the therapy is working.

■ Ingestion of berberine in doses exceeding 500 mg can produce lethargy, nosebleed, dyspnea, and skin and eye irritation.

SAFETY RISK *Signs of toxic reaction include stupor, diarrhea, and nephritis. If signs or symptoms of toxic reaction occur, patient should stop using barberry and notify his health care provider.*

■ Advise female patient to avoid use during pregnancy and to discontinue use if she becomes pregnant during barberry therapy.

■ If patient is taking an antihypertensive, advise him to contact his health care provider before taking barberry.

■ Caution patient that barberry may be useful in treating bacteria-induced diarrhea only, so he shouldn't delay seeking appropriate medical evaluation for persistent diarrhea or diarrhea of unknown cause.

■ Tell patient to remind prescriber and pharmacist of any herbal or dietary supplement that he's taking when obtaining a new prescription.

■ Advise patient to consult his health care provider before using an herbal preparation because a treatment with proven efficacy may be available.

Research summary

The concepts behind the use of barberry and the claims made regarding its effects have not yet been validated scientifically.

basil

Common basil, holy basil,
Ocimum basilicum,
St. Josephwort, sweet basil

Basil's leaves are harvested and crushed for use fresh or dried. It contains estragole (70% to 85% of essential oil) as a major component and smaller amounts of safrole. Estragole may possess mutagenic effects if taken internally in massive quantities. It's available as an oil and a spice.

Reported uses

Basil is used as an antiseptic, antimicrobial, diuretic, insect repellent, and antihypertensive. It's also used to stimulate digestion and treat halitosis, as a cure for warts, and as an appetite stimulant. Basil is a key seasoning in many foods.

Administration

■ As insect repellent: Oil rubbed on exposed areas before going outdoors.

Hazards

Adverse effects associated with basil include dizziness, confusion, headache, trembling, palpitations, hepatocarcinoma, hypoglycemia, and diaphoresis.

Basil may cause hypotension when used in conjunction with antihypertensives, and hypoglycemia when used along with insulin or oral antidiabetics. Patients should use caution to avoid additive effects.

Pregnant or breast-feeding women, infants, and young children should avoid use.

Clinical considerations

■ Estragole and safrole are procarcinogens with weak carcinogenic effects in the liver. Although the risk of developing cancer from use of basil is minimal, long-term or high-dose therapy isn't recommended.

■ If patient is taking an antihypertensive, inform him that basil may also lower blood pressure, causing an additive effect. If he's taking both and his blood pressure stabilizes, the dosage of the conventional antihypertensive may need to be adjusted when he stops taking basil.

■ Taking medicinal doses of basil may disrupt a previously stable antidiabetic regimen.

■ Monitor patient for signs and symptoms of hypoglycemia, such as dizziness, weakness, sweating, tachycardia, headache, confusion, and trembling.

■ Advise patient that the herb isn't recommended for use in large quantities because it may cause cancer; however, the amounts used in cooking appear to be safe.

■ Advise female patient who is pregnant or breast-feeding to avoid medicinal use of basil.

■ Use in infants and children isn't recommended.

■ Tell patient to remind prescriber and pharmacist of any herbal or dietary supplement that he's taking when obtaining a new prescription.

■ Advise patient to consult his health care provider before using an herbal preparation because a treatment with proven efficacy may be available.

Research summary
Few human studies have examined the effectiveness of basil for medicinal purposes. In vitro, basil is antimicrobial.

 RESEARCH *Agrawal, et al. (1996) found significant reductions in blood glucose levels in patients who used basil, illustrating the usefulness of basil in treating type 2 diabetes mellitus. A larger, controlled study is needed to validate this claim.*

bay

Bay laurel, bay leaf, bay tree, daphne, Grecian laurel, Indian bay, laurel, Laurus nobilis, *noble laurel, Roman laurel, sweet bay, true laurel*

Bay is derived from the dried leaves of the bay laurel, or laurel, tree. It contains 1,8-cineol, which may be bactericidal, and parthenolides, which may help prevent migraine. Bay lowers the blood glucose level by helping the body use insulin more effectively. It's available as berries, extracts, leaves, oils, ointments, and soaps.

Reported uses
Bay is used as an antiseptic and a skin stimulant. It's also used to treat the common cold, muscle spasms, and rheumatic conditions. Bay has an insect repellent effect. It's found in some toothpastes because it may help prevent tooth decay.

Administration
Administration of bay isn't well documented.

Hazards
Although bay is primarily used topically, ingestion may be associated with hypoglycemia and asthma. Allergic reactions, which may be severe, may also occur with any mode of administration. Bay may exacerbate the intended therapeutic effects of conventional antidiabetic drugs.

Bay shouldn't be used internally. Pregnant and breast-feeding patients should avoid use. Patients who are taking an antidiabetic should use bay with caution because it may exacerbate hypoglycemia, disrupting a previously stable antidiabetic regimen.

Clinical considerations
■ Internal use may result in allergic reactions, including asthma.

■ Monitor patient for signs and symptoms of hypoglycemia, such as confusion, dizziness, sweating, and trembling.

■ If patient has diabetes, advise him to consult his health care provider before using bay because it can cause hypoglycemia.

■ Advise female patient not to use if she's pregnant or breast-feeding and to notify her health care provider if she becomes pregnant during bay therapy.

■ Tell patient to remind prescriber and pharmacist of any herbal or dietary supplement that he's taking when obtaining a new prescription.

■ Advise patient to consult his health care provider before using an herbal preparation because a treatment with proven efficacy may be available.

Research summary
The concepts behind the use of bay and the claims made regarding its effects have not yet been validated scientifically.

bayberry

Bayberry bark, bayberry root bark, bog myrtle, candleberry, Dutch myrtle, Myrica cerifera, M. cortex, *sweet gale, tallow shrub, vegetable tallow, wachsgagle, waxberry, wax myrtle*

Bayberry contains tannins, triterpenes, myricadiol, taraxerol, taraxerone, and flavonoid glycoside myricitrin. Tannins give bayberry its astringent properties. Myricadiol may have mineralocorticoid activity, myricitrin may stimulate the flow of bile, and the dried root may be antipyretic. Bayberry is available as capsules, liquid extract, powder, and tea.

Reported uses
Bayberry is used as a tea to treat diarrhea and as a gargle to treat sore throats. It's also used internally for coughs and colds and for its antipyretic and circulatory stimulant properties. Bayberry is also used topically for its astringent properties.

Administration
■ Liquid extract (1:1) in 45% alcohol: 0.6 to 2 ml or 10 to 90 gtt by mouth three times a day

■ Powdered bark: 600 mg to 2 g by mouth three times a day by infusion or decoction.

Hazards
Adverse effects associated with the use of bayberry may include sneezing, cough, stomach upset, and vomiting.

Bayberry may cause additive effects when used in conjunction with antihypertensives and corticosteroids. It may interfere with the intended therapeutic effects of conventional drugs.

Bayberry decreases absorption of iron; patients using both should be advised to separate the administration times by 2 hours.

Patients shouldn't use bayberry internally.

Pregnant patients, breast-feeding patients, and patients allergic to bayberry should avoid use. Patients taking a corticosteroid and those with hypertension, peripheral edema, heart failure, and other conditions in which mineralocorticoid use isn't advised should also avoid use.

Clinical considerations
■ Bayberry has a high tannin content and commonly causes gastric distress and liver damage after long-term use.

■ Long-term use of bark extract may result in malignant tumors.

■ Bayberry should be stored in a cool, dry, dark place because heat, moisture, and light may cause it to break down.

■ Large doses have mineralocorticoid effects such as sodium and water retention and hypertension.

■ Advise female patient to avoid use if she's pregnant or breast-feeding and to notify her health care provider if she becomes pregnant during bayberry therapy.

- Caution patient that internal use of bayberry isn't recommended and that such use can cause stomach upset and vomiting.
- Tell patient to remind prescriber and pharmacist of any herbal or dietary supplement that he's taking when obtaining a new prescription.
- Advise patient to consult his health care provider before using an herbal preparation because a treatment with proven efficacy may be available.

Research summary
The concepts behind the use of bayberry and the claims made regarding its effects have not yet been validated scientifically.

bearberry

Arberry, Arctostaphylos uva-ursi, *bearsgrape, kinnikinnick, manzanita, mealberry, mountain box, mountain cranberry, redberry leaves, rockberry, sagackhomi, sandberry, uva-ursi*

Bearberry leaves contain the hydroquinone derivatives arbutin and methyl arbutin in levels ranging from 5% to 15%. Arbutin is hydrolyzed to hydroquinone when it comes in contact with gastric fluid, which acts as a mild astringent and antimicrobial in alkaline urine. Large amounts of bearberry must be ingested to achieve a significant antiseptic effect. The herb is effective against *Escherichia coli, Proteus mirabilis, P. vulgaris, Pseudomonas aeruginosa, Staphylococcus aureus,* and 70 other urinary tract bacteria.

Bearberry also contains ursolic acid and isoquercetin, which contribute to the plant's mild diuretic effect.

Bearberry may help treat hepatitis; reduce polyphagia, polydipsia, and weight gain resulting from diabetes; and inhibit melanin production. It may also have anti-inflammatory effects. Bearberry is

available as capsules, dried leaves, liquid extract, and tea bags.

Reported uses
Bearberry is used as a urinary antiseptic and a mild diuretic. It's also used to treat contact dermatitis, allergic-type hypersensitivity reactions, and arthritis.

Administration
- Capsules: varies depending on formulation; taken with a meal or a glass of water
- Cold maceration: 3 g in 5 oz of water by mouth up to four times a day or 400 to 840 mg of hydroquinone derivatives calculated as water-free arbutin
- Concentrated infusion: 2 to 4 ml by mouth
- Dried leaves infusion: 2.5 g (1 teaspoon) of finely cut or coarse powdered herb in cold water, rapidly brought to a boil, then strained after 15 minutes
- Liquid extract: 1.5 to 4 ml (1:1 in 25% alcohol) by mouth three times a day or 5 to 10 gtt of extract mixed in a small amount of spring or purified water two to three times a day
- Tea (1 tea bag in 6 oz of boiling water steeped for 3 minutes): 1.5 to 4 g three times a day.

For infusions, cold water may be used instead of hot water to minimize the tannin content; the tea is steeped for 12 to 24 hours before the patient drinks it.

Hazards
Adverse effects associated with bearberry include seizures, tinnitus, nausea, vomiting, inflammation and irritation of the bladder and urinary tract mucous membranes, green-brown urine, hepatotoxicity, cyanosis, and collapse.

Arbutin increases the inhibitory action of prednisolone and dexamethasone on contact dermatitis, allergic-type hypersensitivity reactions, and arthritis. Bearberry may enhance the effect of diuretics. Drugs known to acidify urine, such as ascorbic acid or methenamine, or to increase uric acid levels, such as diazoxide, diuretics, or pyrazinamide, may inhibit bearberry's effects because bearberry needs an alkaline environment. Foods known to increase uric acid levels in the bladder, such as those rich in vitamin C, may inhibit bearberry's effects because bearberry needs an alkaline environment and the urinary acidifier may inhibit the conversion of herb's arbutin to the active hydroquinone component.

 SAFETY RISK *Pregnant patients should avoid use because of bearberry's oxytocic effects, such as induction of labor.*

Patients with kidney disease should avoid use of bearberry because tannin components are believed to be excreted in the urine. Breast-feeding patients and children younger than age 12 should also avoid use.

Clinical considerations

■ Caution patient not to use bearberry for longer than 10 days at a time or more than five times per year.
■ Bearberry contains 15% to 20% tannin, which may produce nausea and vomiting.
■ Bearberry 9 g is equivalent to 400 to 700 mg of arbutin.
■ Signs and symptoms of overdose include inflammation and irritation of the bladder and urinary tract mucous membranes.
■ Tinctures containing alcohol may cause a disulfiram-like reaction.

 SAFETY RISK *Ingestion of 1 g can cause nausea, vomiting, tinnitus, cyanosis, seizures, and collapse. Ingestion of 5 g of hydroquinone can result in death.*

■ Hepatotoxicity may occur with prolonged use, especially in children.
■ If patient has kidney disease or is pregnant or breast-feeding, advise against using bearberry.
■ Advise patient to take bearberry with a meal or a glass of water.
■ Inform patient that urine pH must be alkaline for bearberry to be effective and that a diet high in milk, vegetables (especially tomatoes), fruit, fruit juice, and potatoes can help keep urine alkaline. Tell him that he may also take 6 to 8 g of sodium bicarbonate a day to help keep his urine alkaline.
■ Inform patient that the hydroquinone in the herb may discolor urine greenbrown.
■ Advise patient to consult his health care provider if symptoms persist for more than 7 days or if high fever, chills, nausea, vomiting, diarrhea, or severe back pain occurs.
■ Inform patient that pouring hot water over the leaves when preparing a bearberry beverage may increase the tannin content of the infusion and, thus, increase the risk of stomach discomfort. Instead, advise pouring cold water over the leaves and allowing the mixture to steep for 12 to 24 hours before drinking it.
■ Tell patient to remind prescriber and pharmacist of any herbal or dietary supplement that he's taking when obtaining a new prescription.
■ Advise patient to consult his health care provider before using an herbal preparation because a treatment with proven efficacy may be available.

Research summary

No double-blind studies have evaluated the clinical effectiveness of bearberry. However, two studies have evaluated the antibacterial power on the urine of study participants and found activity against most major bacteria that infect the urinary tract.

bee pollen

Bee pollen, buckwheat pollen, maize pollen

Bee pollen contains about 30% protein, 55% carbohydrates, 1% to 2% fat, 3% minerals, and trace vitamins. Components vary depending on plant source, geographic region, harvest methods, and season of the year. It may contain up to

100 vitamins, minerals, enzymes, amino acids, and other substances, but the physiologic benefit of many of these components is unclear. Some bee pollen supplements also contain 3.6% to 5.9% vitamin C.

Bee pollen is available as capsules, chewable tablets, topical creams (in combination with other moisturizers), jelly, liquid (manufactured bee pollen extract, vegetable glycerin, and grain-neutral spirits), powder, raw granules, soft gel caps, and tablets. It's available in products such as Health Honey and Super Bee Pollen Complex.

Reported uses
Bee pollen is used to enhance athletic performance, minimize fatigue, and improve energy.

It may relieve or cure cerebral hemorrhage, brain damage, body weakness, anemia, enteritis, colitis, constipation, and indigestion. Bee pollen may be beneficial in treating chronic prostatism and relieving symptoms of radiation sickness in those being treated for cervical cancer. It may also be an effective prenatal vitamin, and may aid in weight loss.

Although bee pollen is used to treat allergic disorders, such use isn't recommended because bee pollen commonly causes allergic reactions.

Administration
- Granules: One manufacturer recommends taking 1 teaspoon or more by mouth every day; another recommends starting with 1 granule at lunchtime and increasing by 1 granule with each meal until 1 teaspoon is taken at every meal (may be sprinkled on food or mixed in a drink)
- Liquid: 10 to 12 gtt of extract may be added to 8 oz of water and taken by mouth two to three times a day
- Oral use: 1 to 3 g may be taken by mouth every day
- Powder: 1 to 2 teaspoons (5 to 10 g) by mouth every day; may be consumed as

sold or may be blended or mixed with other foods
- Soft gel cap: 1 cap or more may be taken by mouth every day
- Tablets: Dosage varies depending on the formulation and manufacturer. Tablets may be swallowed whole or taken dissolved in a mixture with warm water and honey.

Hazards
SAFETY RISK *Bee pollen may be associated with acute anaphylactic reactions, including sneezing, generalized angioedema, itching, dyspnea, and light-headedness; chronic allergic symptoms, including hypereosinophilia; and neurologic and GI complaints.*

Those with sensitivity or allergies to pollen should avoid use. Those with allergies to apples, carrots, or celery should use with caution because of the potential for adverse reaction.

No known interactions are reported with bee pollen.

Clinical considerations
- Overall, bee pollen hasn't been found to have significant nutritional or therapeutic benefit over more easily and safely administered nutritional products.
- Some bee pollen products also contain bee propolis extract, vitamins, and numerous other ingredients.
- Doses as low as 1 tablespoon can cause acute anaphylactic reactions. Ask patient how much herb he uses daily.
- Patients taking bee pollen for longer than 3 weeks may experience chronic allergic symptoms such as hypereosinophilia and neurologic and GI complaints; however, such symptoms are likely to resolve after the patient stops taking the bee pollen.
- Inform patient that bee pollen should be taken between meals, with a full glass of water.
- Tell patient to remind prescriber and pharmacist of any herbal or dietary supplement that he's taking when obtaining a new prescription.

■ Advise patient to consult his health care provider before using an herbal preparation because a treatment with proven efficacy may be available.

Research summary

The effects of pure bee pollen on memory have not been investigated, but clinical trials of a Chinese herbal medicine containing bee pollen have been conducted in China and Denmark. The improvements in memory seen in the Chinese study were not significant, and in the more recent double-blind placebo-controlled crossover study in Denmark, no improvements were found.

benzoin

Benjamin tree, gum Benjamin, gum benzoin, Siam benzoin, Styrax benzoin, S. paralleloneurus, *Sumatra benzoin*

Siam benzoin contains benzoate, alcohol, benzoic acid, d-siaresinolic acid, and cinnamyl benzoate. Sumatra benzoin contains benzoic acid and cinnamic esters of benzoresorcinol and coniferyl alcohol, free benzoic acid, cinnamic acids, and other ingredients. These components give benzoin its skin protectant, expectorant, and soothing properties. Benzoic acid also has antifungal and antibacterial properties.

Benzoin is available as compound tincture of benzoin and tincture of benzoin spray, and in various ointment combinations.

Reported uses

Benzoin is used topically as a skin protectant. It's mixed with glycerin and water and applied to cutaneous ulcers, bedsores, cracked nipples, and fissures of the lips or anus. It's also combined with zinc oxide in baby ointments.

Benzoin may be added to hot water and inhaled as a vapor to treat throat and bronchial inflammation, acute laryngitis, or croup.

Administration

■ Topically for the treatment of wounds or lesions
■ As an inhalant, 1% in very hot water.

Hazards

Benzoin may cause skin irritation or urticaria at application site. There are no reported interactions with benzoin.

Those with hypersensitivity to benzoin should avoid use.

Clinical considerations

■ Mild irritation may occur at the application site.
■ Benzoin should be stored in a cool, dry place, away from excessive heat.
■ Tell patient to remind prescriber and pharmacist of any herbal or dietary supplement that he's taking when obtaining a new prescription.
■ Advise patient to consult his health care provider before using an herbal preparation because a treatment with proven efficacy may be available.

Research summary

The concepts behind the use of benzoin and the claims made regarding its effects have not yet been validated scientifically.

betel palm

Areca catechu, *areca nut, betel nut, pinang, pinlang,* Piper betle

Betel palm contains arecoline, arecaidine, arecaine, arecolidine, guvacine, isoguvacine, and guvacoline, which cause central nervous system stimulation. Chewing the nut increases salivary flow and aids digestion.

Betel palm is available as quids, which are made from powdered or sliced areca (betel) nut, tobacco, and slaked lime (calcium hydroxide) obtained from powdered snail shells. These ingredients are wrapped in the betel vine leaf and chewed, thereby increasing salivary flow and aiding digestion.

Reported uses
Betel palm is used as a mild CNS stimulant and a digestive aid. It's used to treat coughs, stomach complaints, diphtheria, middle ear inflammation, and worm infestation.

Some patients steam the leaves and apply them as a facial dressing, but such use isn't recommended because of adverse dermatologic reactions.

Administration
■ Orally: 4 to 15 quids chewed every day, for 15 minutes each.

Hazards
SAFETY RISK *Arecaine, a compound of the betel palm, is poisonous. It affects respiration and heart rate and may cause seizures. Seed doses of 8 g can be fatal.*

Adverse effects associated with betel palm include seizures, tooth discoloration, gingivitis, oral lichen planus-like lesion, oral cancer including leukoplakia and squamous cell carcinoma, periodontitis, resorption of oral calcium, chronic osteomyelitis, asthma exacerbation, and contact leukomelanosis characterized by immediate bleaching, hyperpigmentation, and confetti-like depigmentation.

Betel palm and fluphenazine or procyclidine may cause tremor, stiffness, akathisia because of decreased effectiveness of the drugs in the presence of herb's cholinergic alkaloid, arecoline. Using betel palm with prednisone or albuterol may exacerbate asthma.

Those with a history of asthma should avoid using betel palm because of bronchoconstriction. Those who are pregnant should avoid using betel palm because of possible teratogenic effects.

Clinical considerations
■ Chewing betel palm can cause severe oral mucosal changes, including cancerous lesions. Chewing the betel palm-slaked lime mixture may place patient at higher risk for oral lesions than chewing betel palm alone.
■ Monitor patient for asthma-like symptoms.
■ Betel palm leaf facial dressings can cause severe dermatologic reactions, such as contact leukomelanosis, which occurs in three stages — immediate bleaching, hyperpigmentation, and confetti-like depigmentation.
■ Tell patient to remind prescriber and pharmacist of any herbal or dietary supplement that he's taking when obtaining a new prescription.
■ Advise patient to consult his health care provider before using an herbal preparation because a treatment with proven efficacy may be available.

Research summary
The concepts behind the use of betel palm and the claims made regarding its effects have not yet been validated scientifically.

bethroot

Birthroot, coughroot, ground lily, Indian balm, Indian shamrock, jew's-harp plant, lamb's quarters, milk ipecac, nightshade, Pariswort, purple trillium, rattlesnake root, snakebite, stinking Benjamin, three-leaved Trillium erectum, T. pendulum, *wake-robin*

Bethroot contains a fixed oil, a volatile oil, a saponin called trillarin, a glycoside, tannic acid, and starch. The saponin glycosides have antifungal activity. Bethroot is available as ground drug and liquid extract.

Reported uses
Bethroot is used orally to treat long, heavy menstrual periods, to relieve pain, control postpartum bleeding, and man-

age diarrhea. It's also used as an expectorant.

Bethroot is used externally for varicose veins and ulcers, hematomas, and hemorrhoids, and as an astringent to minimize topical bleeding and irritation.

Administration
Ground bethroot and liquid extract are used for infusions and poultices.

Hazards
Bethroot may be associated with nausea, vomiting, and irritation at the application site. No interactions with bethroot are reported.

Bethroot promotes menstruation and promotes labor in pregnancy. Pregnant patients should avoid use because it stimulates the uterus.

Clinical considerations
- Monitor application site for irritation.
- Advise patient to avoid use during pregnancy.
- Inform patient that high doses of bethroot can cause nausea.
- Tell patient to remind prescriber and pharmacist of any herbal or dietary supplement that he's taking when obtaining a new prescription.
- Advise patient to consult his health care provider before using an herbal preparation because a treatment with proven efficacy may be available.

Research summary
The concepts behind the use of bethroot and the claims made regarding its effects have not yet been validated scientifically.

betony

Betonica officinalis, *betony,*
bishopswort, hedge-nettles,
Stachys officinalis, *wood betony*

The basal leaves of the betony, which contain betaine, caffeic acid derivatives, and flavonoids, are the medicinal part of the herb. They're collected and dried in shade at a maximum temperature of 40° F (4.4° C).

Betony contains 15% tannins, which give the herb its astringent effects. Mixtures of flavonoid glycosides have hypotensive and sedative effects. Stachydrine is a systolic depressant and acts to decrease rheumatic pain.

Betony is available as a tincture, powder, or in 450 mg capsules.

Reported uses
Betony is used as an antidiarrheal, a sedative, and an expectorant for coughs, bronchitis, and asthma. It's also used to treat catarrh, heartburn, gout, nervousness, kidney stones, and inflammation of the bladder.

Betony is used with other herbs such as comfrey or linden as a sedative, a mild hypotensive for treating neuralgia and anxiety, and a decongestant for treating sinus headache and congestion.

Administration
- Oral use: 1 to 2 g every day in three divided doses
- Topical use: Extract or infusion applied to skin as an astringent or as a treatment for wounds.

Hazards
Betony may increase the intended therapeutic effect of antihypertensives and sedatives. It produces additive effects when used with central nervous system depressants. The tincture contains up to 40% ethyl alcohol and may cause a disulfiram-like reaction if used with disulfiram or metronidazole. Betony is associated with additive effects when used with alcohol.

Betony may be associated with GI irritation.

Patients who are pregnant or breastfeeding should avoid use.

Clinical considerations
- Large oral dosage may cause GI irritation because of the tannin content.

- Don't confuse betony (*Stachys officinalis*) with limestone woundwort (*Stachys alpina*).
- Warn patient not to exceed the recommended dosage.
- Caution patient that internal use of betony may cause drowsiness.
- If patient is taking betony to treat diarrhea, advise him to consult his health care provider if the diarrhea continues for longer than 2 days.
- If patient is taking betony to treat headache and it doesn't improve, advise him to discontinue use and consult his health care provider.
- Tell patient to remind prescriber and pharmacist of any herbal or dietary supplement that he's taking when obtaining a new prescription.
- Advise patient to consult his health care provider before using an herbal preparation because a treatment with proven efficacy may be available.

Research summary

The concepts behind the use of betony and the claims made regarding its effects have not yet been validated scientifically.

bilberry

Airelle, bilberry, black whortles, bleaberry, bog bilberry, burren myrtle, dwarf bilberry, dyeberry, European blueberry, huckleberry, hurtleberry, hurts, trackleberry, Vaccinium myrtillus, *whortleberry, wineberry*

The dried fruit of the bilberry contains 5% to 10% tannins, which act as an astringent; these tannins may help target the bowel and help treat diarrhea. The anthocyanidins in bilberry help prevent angina episodes, reduce capillary fragility, and stabilize tissues that have collagen-like tendons and ligaments. They also inhibit platelet aggregation and thrombus formation by interacting with vascular prostaglandins. The anthocyanidins also help regenerate rhodopsin, a light-sensitive pigment found on the rods of the retina, so bilberry may help treat degenerative retinal conditions, macular degeneration, poor night vision, glaucoma, and cataracts.

The antioxidant effects of anthocyanidins may also give bilberry vasoprotective and hepatoprotective properties. The anthocyanidin pigment in the herb may increase the gastric mucosal release of prostaglandin E_2, accounting for the antiulcerative and gastroprotective effects. Bilberry is available as a dried fruit, a 10% decoction for topical use, a dry extract (25% anthocyanosides) in 80 mg capsules, and a 1:1 fluid extract. It's available in products such as Bilberry Power.

Reported uses

Bilberry is used to treat acute diarrhea and mild inflammation of the mucous membranes of the mouth and throat. It's also used to provide symptomatic relief from vascular disorders (including capillary weakness, venous insufficiency, and hemorrhoids), to prevent macular degeneration, and for its potential hepatoprotective properties.

Administration

- Dried fruit: 4 to 8 g by mouth with water several times every day
- Fluid extract: 2 to 4 ml by mouth three times a day
- For eye disorders: 80 to 160 mg dry extract (25% anthocyanosides) by mouth three times a day
- For inflammation: 10% decoction prepared by adding 5 to 10 g of crushed dried fruit to 5 oz of cold water, boiling for 10 minutes, then straining while hot, applied topically as an astringent
- For acute diarrhea: 20 to 60 g of dried fruit by mouth every day.

Hazards

Because the herb may inhibit platelet aggregation, it may be unsuitable for those with a bleeding disorder.

Bilberry may have additive effects when used with the drug warfarin.

Clinical considerations

- Because bilberry may reduce a diabetic patient's blood glucose level, dosage of his conventional antidiabetic may need to be adjusted.
- Consistent dosing of bilberry is needed when using the herb to treat vascular or ocular conditions.
- Advise patient who's using the dried fruit to take each dose with a full glass of water.
- If patient is using bilberry to treat diarrhea, advise him to consult his health care provider if it doesn't improve in 3 to 4 days.
- Tell patient to remind prescriber and pharmacist of any herbal or dietary supplement that he's taking when obtaining a new prescription.
- Advise patient to consult his health care provider before using an herbal preparation because a treatment with proven efficacy may be available.

Research summary

A double-blind, placebo-controlled trial of bilberry extract in 14 people with damage to the retina caused by diabetes and/or hypertension found significant improvements observable by ophthalmoscopic examination and angiography. However, this was a very preliminary study.

Bioelectrical acupuncture

Bioelectrical acupuncture, or electroacupuncture, involves application of electrostimulation to acupuncture needles during traditional acupuncture treatment. Another form of bioelectrical acupuncture uses direct electrostimulation of acupuncture points in place of needles.

Licensed acupuncturists can apply electrostimulation to acupuncture needles during acupuncture. Direct electrostimulation of acupuncture points can be performed by licensed acupuncturists or trained health care workers, or self-administered by a layperson under the supervision of a practitioner. Nurses who work in massage or pain clinics, those trained in acupressure and the acupuncture energy channels (meridians), or those who do bodywork with their patients may also be practitioners of this therapy.

A concept developed by German Dr. Reinhold Voll, called electroacupuncture according to Voll (EAV), is the basis of subsequent bioelectrical acupuncture biofeedback devices, also called electrodermal screening devices. In the United States, these devices are approved only for use as experimental screening devices. They are not yet approved for treatment. Using low frequencies, these devices provide information that can be used to treat conditions that are identified by bioelectrical acupuncture assessment.

Reported uses

As with traditional acupuncture, there are numerous therapeutic applications of bioelectrical acupuncture, depending on the ability and experience of the practitioner. It's reported to be particularly effective for treating physical injury and acute and chronic pain.

How the treatment is performed

Like traditional Chinese acupuncture, bioelectrical acupuncture devices can be used both to assess and to provide treatment for a patient's condition. These devices measure the flow of energy along the meridians at specific acupoints (points along a meridian where energy flow can best be measured and manipulated). A steady flow indicates health, while an impaired flow suggests disease, with different organs associated with specific meridians. Some acupoints, called control measurement points (CMPs), give an overall indication of health in an organ or tissue. Other acupoints relate to specific parts of the organ and can show the specific site of the imbalance in that organ. Over 2,000 CMPs have been identified with this type of meter. Each acupoint has a standard measure that represents health. With deteriorating health, the measurement changes.

Various bioelectrical acupuncture devices are available. They range in sophistication from simple handheld, battery-operated, point-locator treatment devices to multifaceted, computerized units. Computerized bioelectrical acupuncture devices can be used quickly to perform multiple screenings, and they support research with a detailed patient database. Most of these bioelectrical acupuncture devices are battery-operated, using direct current to avoid introducing the possible adverse effects of a pulsating or fluctuating alternating current into the system. Some of the devices are assessment tools; others deliver treatments; and still others do both.

Dermatron

Assessment devices such as the Dermatron, developed by Voll, use sensors to measure the electrical resistance at acupoints. Higher than normal resistance at a specific acupoint indicates irritation or inflammation in the corresponding organ, while lower than normal resistance at the acupoint is indicative of degeneration or fatigue. In this way, the Dermatron provides a means of screening for the existence of disease. It can also test the energetic effects of certain remedies. For example, when a patient takes a homeopathic dilution prescribed for his disease, the EAV reading returns to normal. EAV screening resembles an electronic version of kinesiology, a muscle-testing method that assists the therapist to identify what weakens or strengthens the muscular system.

Locator-stimulator

The locator-stimulator is another example of a bioelectrical acupuncture assessment tool. This simple, battery-operated device is used to locate and treat acupoints and trigger points (any point re-

sponding with pain upon palpation). One dial adjusts to location, emitting a flashing light and sound when a point is located. The stimulation control delivers a fixed frequency signal (10 Hz) for treating the point. For self-treatment, a metal plate on the side of the device can be used to complete the necessary grounding circuit. A separate grounding pole is used to complete this circuit when being used by a practitioner. (See *Locator-stimulator*.)

SOLITENS device

The SOLITENS is a treatment unit that's categorized as a transcutaneous electric nerve stimulator (TENS) device. TENS units were originally developed to block pain by directing a stimulating current into local nerves, using a relatively high-frequency signal. This sometimes created muscle spasm instead of the intended pain relief. Used at low frequencies, TENS devices have been found effective for reducing pain by stimulating acupuncture and trigger points without the use of needles.

The SOLITENS has point location abilities, a timer, a ground, and the capability of delivering a stimulation pulse rate of 15 Hz for treating acupoints and trigger points. Therapeutic applications include symptomatic relief of chronic intractable pain, post-traumatic acute pain (in athletic injuries, for example), and post-surgical pain.

MORA

A combination assessment and treatment device developed by Dr. Franz Morrel, the MORA works under the assumption that all biological processes are bioelectromagnetic and can be recognized by a distinctive, complex waveform. A smooth wave indicates health, and higher or lower wave deviations indicate disease. The MORA collects electromagnetic signals directly from the acupoints, manipulates and adjusts any aberrant wave forms to create normal waves, and then feeds these corrected waves back into the patient

LOCATOR-STIMULATOR

The locator-stimulator is a simple, battery-operated device that can be used by the practitioner or the patient to find and stimulate trigger points. When a point responds with pain to palpation, a dial on the device emits a flashing light and a sound and the stimulation control delivers a fixed-frequency signal (10 Hz), thereby treating the point. For the practitioner's use, a separate grounding pole completes the circuit; for the patient's use, a metal plate on the side of the device completes the grounding circuit.

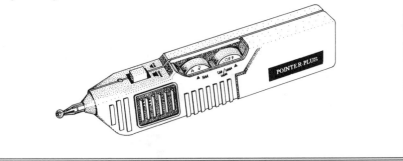

through the same acupoints. Proponents of this device describe it as a truly natural therapy because it uses specific wave information from the patient without introducing any artificial electrical signal.

Therapeutic applications of the MORA include treatment of skin disease and circulation problems; relief of headaches, migraines, and muscular aches and pains; and treatment in conjunction with homeopathy. The MORA doubles as an EAV diagnostic instrument. It can also be used in color therapy to transmit individual color frequencies of the spectrum of electromagnetic fields (EMFs), a treatment believed to impart beneficial effects.

Electro-Acuscope

The Electro-Acuscope is a treatment device that uses extremely low-frequency current — microamperage — rather than the milliamperage used by standard TENS devices. Microamperage is used to stimulate tissue repair. Rather than delivering a premeasured current, the device matches current delivery to the resistance

sensed in the damaged tissue; such self-regulation facilitates the repair process.

This treatment works at the cellular level. Microcurrent stimulation is believed to induce extracellular calcium ions to enter the cell through pores in the cell membrane (called voltage-sensitive calcium ion channels). Higher levels of calcium, in turn, encourage increased synthesis of adenosine triphosphate, which activates mechanisms that control deoxyribonucleic acid and protein synthesis. The result is an increase in the rate of cellular repair and replication.

Treatment with this device calls for a high degree of interaction between the patient and a well-trained practitioner. Popular as a treatment instrument in sports medicine, the Electro-Acuscope is used to treat musculoskeletal injuries, such as lumbosacral sprains, shoulder strains, whiplash, trauma, temporomandibular joint pain, bursitis, carpal tunnel syndrome, and muscle spasms. It's also used for arthritis, bruises, herpes zoster infections, local skin infections and skin ulcerations, chronic fatigue syndrome, migraines, neuralgia, surgical incisions,

ELECTRO-ACUSCOPE

The Electro-Acuscope uses extremely low-frequency current to stimulate tissue repair. The device matches the current delivered to the resistance encountered in the damaged tissue, thereby working at a cellular level to regulate the repair process.

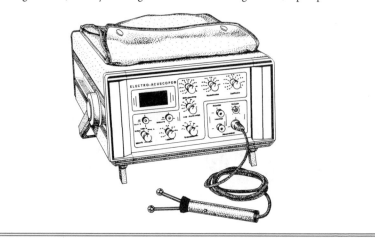

and palliative care of a ruptured disk in patients unwilling or unable to undergo surgery. (See *Electro-Acuscope*.)

Nogier auriculotherapy device

The Nogier auriculotherapy treatment device uses direct current (DC) or laser energy to treat acupoints on the ear. Similar to reflexology, in which treatment is administered through the foot, auriculotherapy operates on the concept that the entire body and all its organs can be identified at different points on the ear. Auriculotherapy can also be practiced with acupuncture needles, therapeutic magnets, and a glass rod technique for point massage.

While using the Nogier device to treat the patient, the practitioner takes a radial pulse. The increase or decrease in radial pulse amplitude, called the vascular autonomic signal, is used as an indicator for the progression of treatment.

Considerable training is required before using this device. Therapeutic applications include addictions, dyslexia, pain control (acute or chronic pain, back pain,

and pain from trauma), tinnitus, and Parkinsonian tremors. Its use is contraindicated for severe conditions, such as renal insufficiency and heart disease.

Other devices

Many bioelectrical acupuncture devices apply other frequencies from the low range of the electromagnetic spectrum. For example, a light beam generator has been used to direct photons of light to assist in restoring cells' normal energy state, thus promoting healing. Able to attain deep body penetration, it's described as effective for treating organ as well as skin problems.

Sound probes are reported to destroy parasites and anything not in resonance with the body, by emitting a tone of three alternating frequencies. Radiofrequency diathermy devices use radio waves to send penetrating heat deep into the tissues for improved blood flow, pain reduction, and healing.

Most bioelectrical acupuncture devices are used in similar ways. First, the practitioner uses the device to locate either traditional acupoints or a patient's trigger points of complaint. The practitioner searches for tissue impedance, which generates a pitched signal from the device. Then he uses the device to provide treatment consisting of low-level DC directed back into the identified points. Treatment lasts 30 minutes to 1 hour, and the patient may need to return for additional visits. Some patients can use the devices at home.

Hazards

Headache, nausea, and unpleasant sensations can occur with invasive or noninvasive bioelectrical acupuncture, requiring adjustment in the frequency and amperage of the device. Skin irritation and rash are also possible. If alterations in skin integrity occur, treatment may need to be postponed or treatment frequency reduced.

Clinical considerations

■ Bioelectrical acupuncture devices are contraindicated for pain of unknown cause and for severe conditions such as renal insufficiency and heart disease. These devices shouldn't be used for patients with demand-type cardiac pacemakers, or in transcerebral electrode placement (because of the remote risk of seizures) or electrode placement over the carotid sinus region (which regulates blood pressure).
■ Whether these devices may be used safely during pregnancy hasn't been established. However, in Europe TENS units have been used during labor and delivery to facilitate contractions.

Research summary

Controlled studies have demonstrated the benefits of bioelectrical acupuncture to treat postoperative pain, chemotherapy-induced illness, and renal colic and to induce contractions in post-term pregnancy. In research with rats, bioelectrical stimulation of acupuncture points has enhanced peripheral motor nerve regeneration and sensory nerve growth.

Biofeedback

Biofeedback teaches people how to exert conscious control over various autonomic functions with the help of physiologic feedback. Monitoring of physiologic function can be simple or quite complex with electronic machines. By observing the fluctuations of a particular body function — such as breathing, heart rate, or blood pressure — patients eventually learn how to adjust their reactions and other thoughts in order to alter that autonomic response. By learning to modify vital functions at will, patients develop the ability to control certain conditions such as high blood pressure without the use of medications or other conventional medical treatments.

The idea that people can control vital body processes voluntarily has been accepted in the West for only a few decades, but it has been practiced in the East, through meditation and yoga, for thousands of years. Today, biofeedback is widely used and approved by both conventional and alternative practitioners. It's popular with patients because it gives them a sense of control over their health problems and helps to lower health care costs; after 8 or 10 training sessions, the patient can usually learn to regulate the desired body process without the help of the monitoring device.

The most common forms of biofeedback are electromyographic (to measure muscle tension), thermal (to measure skin temperature), electrodermal (to measure the skin's electrical conductance), electroencephalographic (to measure brain wave activity), and respiration (to measure breathing rate). Increasingly sophisticated monitoring devices are continually expanding the applications for biofeedback. For example, sensors can now monitor the action of the internal and external rectal sphincters, allowing treatment of fecal incontinence; the activity of the bladder's detrusor muscle, allowing treatment of urinary incontinence; and esophageal motility and stomach acidity, providing information on ulcers and esophageal reflux.

The origins of biofeedback date back to the early 1960s, when Neil Miller, an experimental psychologist, suggested that the autonomic nervous system could be "trained." In a series of experiments, he showed that patients could learn how to control physiologic processes that were previously thought to be beyond voluntary control, such as heart rate, blood pressure, and GI function.

Biofeedback quickly began attracting widespread attention and in the late 1960s, researchers at the Menninger Foundation in Topeka, Kansas, discovered that elevating the temperature of the hands by biofeedback could alleviate migraine headaches. Since then, extensive research has led to numerous new applications for biofeedback as well as increasing acceptance by traditional health care providers, including medical doctors, physical therapists, psychiatrists, psychologists, and dentists.

TRAINING *Biofeedback practitioners need a firm grasp of both physiology and psychology. (In fact, many biofeedback therapists are trained psychologists.) Practicing biofeedback in the United States requires no license.*

Many private biofeedback schools throughout the United States train and certify clinicians. The Biofeedback Certification Institute of America in Wheat Ridge, Colorado, runs the major certification program for biofeedback practitioners and provides information about certified local practitioners.

Reported uses

Biofeedback has more than 150 applications for disease prevention and health restoration. It's used most often for stress-related disorders, such as insomnia, anxiety, headaches, hypertension, asthma, GI disorders (ulcers, irritable bowel syndrome), temporomandibular joint syndrome, and hyperactivity in children. The American Medical Association has even endorsed electromyelographic biofeedback for the treatment of muscle contraction headaches.

How the treatment is performed

Biofeedback machines are variations of common diagnostic monitoring systems that have been modified to produce a continuous flow of specific information to the patient. The equipment needed varies, depending on the targeted body function. For instance, a biofeedback machine geared toward helping the patient lower his heart rate might be a cardiac monitor with a light that flashes each time the heart beats. For biofeedback training involving muscle control or activity, a modified electromyelograph might be used. Relaxation and emotional stress can be monitored using a modified electroencephalograph.

Modified temperature probes are used in biofeedback training to treat migraines, hypertension, anxiety, and Raynaud's disease; lung volume measurements are used to train asthmatic patients to control their breathing; and modified sphygmomanometers are used to train patients to control hypertension. Some biofeedback machines require the use of special goggles to eliminate distractions, allowing the patient to focus on the feedback, which is projected on the inside of the goggle.

Electrodermal feedback (electrical conduction or resistance of the skin) allows an examiner to monitor changes in perspiration. Specialized motility sensors, which pick up movement of the GI tract, are used in the treatment of GI disorders. To treat curvature of the spine, a specialized biofeedback unit worn by the patient emits a soft beep if the patient slouches forward. If the patient doesn't straighten his posture, the device sounds a louder alarm.

In a typical session, electrodes are attached to the area of the body being monitored, such as the head (for brain wave activity), fingers (for pulse rate), or muscles (for muscle tension), according to the manufacturer's instructions. The electrodes feed information into a small monitoring box, which registers the results by a sound or light that varies in pitch or brightness as the body function fluctuates. A biofeedback practitioner interprets the signals and guides the patient in mental and physical exercises designed to help him achieve the desired result. The patient eventually trains himself to control his body's physiologic functions by altering thoughts, breathing, posture, or muscle tension.

Hazards

Biofeedback is contraindicated in patients with low blood pressure, psychiatric disorders (including severe depression), impaired attention or memory, or mental handicaps such as dementia. Patients may experience a local skin irritation from the electrodes used in the biofeedback monitoring.

Clinical considerations

■ Make sure that the patient continues to take prescribed medications, such as antihypertensives, while receiving biofeedback training.
■ Minimize distractions during the biofeedback session; they can prevent the patient from focusing and achieving optimum results.
■ Alternate electrode placement sites to reduce associated skin irritation.

 REIMBURSEMENT *Most insurance companies will reimburse only if a licensed practitioner prescribes and supervises the biofeedback technician.*

Research summary

According to the 1994 report *Alternative Medicine: Expanding Medical Horizons*, extensive research (including about 3,000 articles and 100 books) has demonstrated biofeedback's effectiveness in treating alcoholism, drug abuse, tension and migraine headaches, chronic pain syndromes, cardiac arrhythmias, essential hypertension, irritable bowel syndrome,

bronchial asthma, hyperactivity, attention deficit disorder, epilepsy, and hot flashes. Biofeedback is also effective in muscle reeducation and is the preferred treatment for Raynaud's disease and certain types of fecal and urinary incontinence.

Improvement has also been seen in patients with chronic pain, heart disease, difficulty swallowing, esophageal dysfunction, tinnitus, twitching of the eyelids, fatigue, and cerebral palsy. Biofeedback isn't recommended for severe structural problems, such as broken bones or herniated discs.

Biological dentistry

Holistic dentistry, whole body dentistry

Biological dentistry is the practice of dentistry with the realization that procedures done in the mouth can have profound impact on the patient. The biological dentist believes that many systemic symptoms and illnesses are, in fact, manifestations of problems in the mouth. Biological dentistry encompasses many facets. Major areas of interest to the biological dentist include: energetic wholeness; silver (mercury) fillings; root canals; cavitations; nutrition, supplementation, and homeopathics; fluoride; galvanic currents; and craniomandibular dysfunction.

Energetic wholeness

Biological dentists have developed a different mind-set from traditional dentists, one in which the body is viewed as an energetic whole. The concept dates to the 1930s when research by Cleveland dentist Dr. Weston Price demonstrated the systemic impact of tooth decay, malocclusion, and the poor processing of food. Other researchers of the day found similar connections.

In the 1950s and 1960s, Reinhold Voll, a German medical doctor, acupuncturist, and anatomy professor, developed an electroacupuncture device to measure skin resistance over acupuncture points. He found that changes in resistance reflected abnormalities in specific acupuncture meridians and, further, that each tooth and its surrounding bone structure related to specific organs, tissues, muscles, and vertebrae. He developed ways to determine cause and effect and used them to tell whether a certain tooth was having a negative impact on a specific organ (or visa versa) and to evaluate the effects of drugs, foods, herbs, and homeopathics on balancing the acupuncture or energy meridians. Many biological dentists today use instrumentation based on Voll's concepts, a form of testing known as electroacupuncture according to Voll (EAV), electrodermal screening, or meridian stress assessment.

Silver (mercury) fillings

Fillings that are usually called "silver" are actually 50% mercury; the remaining 50% is a combination of copper, tin, zinc, and silver. Biological dentists believe that the mercury contained in fillings causes many health problems for the following reasons:

- mercury leaches out of the fillings to all the tissues and organs
- the amount of mercury in the brain directly relates to the number of fillings in the mouth
- the amount of mercury in the brain of the fetus or newborn directly relates to the number of fillings in the mother
- mercury is extremely toxic, more so than lead or cadmium.

The view of traditional dentists is that the amount of mercury coming out of the fillings is too minute to be of concern; biological dentists believe that even a small amount of mercury is toxic.

Root canal

Dr. Price demonstrated, in almost 30 years of research, that when a tooth becomes nonvital, the bacteria within the dentinal tubules change from aerobic to nonaerobic and begin producing extremely potent toxins. Recent studies at the University of Kentucky by Haley and Pendergrass confirm the extreme virulence of these bacterial toxins. If allowed to pass beyond the confines of the tooth, these toxins can cause many systemic illnesses. Nonvital teeth also are believed to block energy flow along the meridians.

Cavitations

These holes in the bone usually occur in the mouth in an area where a tooth has been extracted. Cavitations can be a problem as they're believed to block energy flow along the meridians and act as a reservoir, holding high amounts of mercury and other extremely toxic compounds.

Nutrition, supplementation, homeopathics

Biological dentists stress the importance of nutrition and supplementation. Many biologic dentists use herbs and homeopathics as part of their treatment regimen.

Fluoride

Biological dentists don't believe in fluoridation of the public water supply.

Galvanic currents

Placement of dissimilar metals in the mouth creates galvanic currents that can be measured. Biological dentists observe that these can disrupt energy flow along acupuncture meridians and in general can act as an "interference field," causing various symptoms.

Craniomandibular dysfunction

Imbalance of the temporomandibular joint, the occlusion, or the cranial sutures can manifest as a multitude of systemic problems, especially musculoskeletal.

Reported Uses

Many holistic physicians realize the strategic role biological dentistry plays in health maintenance or restoration and regularly work in conjunction with biological dentists in treating systemic illnesses such as cancer, multiple sclerosis, hypothyroidism, chronic fatigue, and others.

How the treatment is performed
The dental procedures performed are similar to those used by the traditional dentist. In addition to X-rays, the biological dentist may use EAV or similar screening tests and diagnostic measurements to determine the patient's bioelectric and biochemical balance as well as his biophysical balance (the alignment of teeth, jaws, and temporomandibular joints). The biological dentist doesn't use mercury in the mouth, and tries to avoid using other metals whenever possible. When removing mercury fillings there are many steps taken prior to removal, during removal, and after removal to protect the patient. A biological dentist must be proficient in all aspects of traditional dental treatment.

Hazards
Complications and adverse effects of biological dentistry are similar to those that may occur with traditional dental procedures.

Research summary
Animal and human experiments show that the uptake, distribution in tissues, and elimination of amalgam mercury is significant. Research on the pathophysiologic effects of mercury centers on the immune system, renal system, oral and intestinal bacteria, reproductive system, and central nervous system.

birch

Betula lenta

Birch leaves contain tannin and gaultherine oil, which, when mixed with water, yields methyl salicylate. Other components of the leaves are triterpene alcohol, flavonoids (1.5%), proanthocyanidins,

and caffeic acid derivatives. These substances have a diuretic effect. Birch is available as dried leaves for tea, freshly pressed plant juices for internal use, and ointment and birch tar for topical use.

Reported uses
Birch is used as a gentle stimulant and astringent. A warm water infusion is used to stimulate diaphoresis, to flush out kidney stones, and to treat diarrhea, dysentery, cholera, and urinary tract infections.

Applied topically, birch may temporarily relieve rheumatic pain because of its methyl salicylate content. An infusion of birch is used to treat dandruff. Birch tar oil, or pix betulina, is used to treat scabies and skin infections.

Administration
- Dried herb: 2 to 3 g several times a day
- Infusion: three times a day or four times a day between meals
- Tea: Prepared from dried leaves or fresh plant juice and used orally as is or used to make an infusion, which is taken orally.

Hazards
Topical use of birch may cause irritation. There are no reported interactions.

Those who are dehydrated or allergic to birch trees should avoid use. Those with compromised cardiac or renal function should not use birch to treat edema.

Clinical considerations
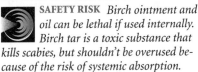 **SAFETY RISK** *Birch ointment and oil can be lethal if used internally. Birch tar is a toxic substance that kills scabies, but shouldn't be overused because of the risk of systemic absorption.*
- Make sure patient who's taking the herb orally drinks plenty of fluids because birch can cause dehydration.
- Advise patient not to exceed the recommended daily dose without consulting his health care provider.
- Advise patient to consult his health care provider if his condition doesn't improve in a few days.

- Instruct patient to discontinue use if his skin becomes irritated.
- Tell patient to remind prescriber and pharmacist of any herbal or dietary supplement that he's taking when obtaining a new prescription.
- Advise patient to consult his health care provider before using an herbal preparation because a treatment with proven efficacy may be available.

Research summary
The concepts behind the use of birch and the claims made regarding its effects have not yet been validated scientifically.

bistort

Adderwort, dragonwort, Easter giant, Easter mangiant, oderwort, osterick, patience dock, Persicaria bistorta, *sankeweed, sweet dock*

The leaves and rhizome of older bistort plants are cleaned, freed from green parts, cut up, and dried. Bistort contains 13% to 36% tannins, which give the herb the astringent effects that are helpful in treating diarrhea and sore or dry throat. Bistort powder is used to make an extract, infusion, ointment, or tincture for external use.

Reported uses
Bistort is used to treat digestive disorders, particularly diarrhea. It's also used as a gargle for mouth and throat infections and as an ointment for minor wounds.

Administration
- Tincture: 10 to 40 gtt diluted in a small amount of water and used as a gargle
- To treat minor mouth and throat irritations or infections: Infusion made with cold water and used as a gargle or a rinse.

Hazards
Bistort tincture contains alcohol and may precipitate a disulfiram or disulfiram-like

reaction, including flushing, dyspnea, vomiting, syncope, and confusion.
  There are no reported adverse effects with bistort.
  As a precaution, pregnant and breast-feeding patients should avoid use.

Clinical considerations
- Bistort is rarely used, and dosage information for internal use is sketchy.
- Because of the tannin content, overuse may increase mucous formation and irritate the intestines.
- If patient is pregnant or breast-feeding, advise her not to use bistort.
- Warn patient that herb is rarely used and that few dosage guidelines exist.
- Instruct patient to keep herb away from children.
- Tell patient to remind prescriber and pharmacist of any herbal or dietary supplement that he's taking when obtaining a new prescription.
- Advise patient to consult his health care provider before using an herbal preparation because a treatment with proven efficacy may be available.

Research summary
The concepts behind the use of bistort and the claims made regarding its effects have not yet been validated scientifically.

bitter melon

Art pumpkin, balsam apple, balsam pear, bitter cucumber, Carilla cundeamor, *cerasee,* Momordica charantia

The seeds of the bitter melon contain alpha-momorcharin and beta-momorcharin, which are abortifacients. The hypoglycemic effect of bitter melon is the result of the melon's charantin, polypeptide P, and vicine components. These substances reduce the blood glucose level and improve glucose tolerance.

Bitter melon may have antimicrobial effects and may inhibit viruses, including polio, herpes simplex 1, and human immunodeficiency virus. It may also have anti-inflammatory effects and relieve symptoms of GI ailments such as flatus, ulcers, constipation, and hemorrhoids. It's available as juice or as an extract in gel caps, and in products such as Bitter Melon Power.

Reported uses
Bitter melon is used to treat diabetes symptoms, and may help treat GI disorders.

Administration
■ To lower the blood glucose level: 2 oz of fresh juice or equivalent of 15 g of aqueous extract in gel cap form, every day.

Hazards
 SAFETY RISK *Bitter melon seeds contain vicine, which may cause an acute condition characterized by headache, fever, abdominal pain, and coma.*

Additional adverse effects associated with bitter melon include uterine bleeding, uterine contractions, abortion, hepatotoxicity, and hypoglycemia.

Bitter melon used in conjunction with insulin or oral antidiabetics may increase the hypoglycemic effect and cause a rapid drop in blood glucose level.

Bitter melon shouldn't be given to children because the red arils around the seeds may cause a toxic reaction. Also, pregnant women should avoid using it because it may cause uterine bleeding or miscarriage.

Clinical considerations
■ The juice of bitter melon has a bitter taste.
■ Bitter melon should be taken only in small doses and for no longer than 4 weeks.

■ The hypoglycemic effects of bitter melon are dose related, so dosage should be adjusted gradually.
■ If patient is pregnant or breast-feeding, advise her not to use bitter melon.
■ Inform diabetic patient that herb may cause hypoglycemia.
■ Instruct patient to immediately report headache, fever, and abdominal pain.
■ Tell patient to remind prescriber and pharmacist of any herbal or dietary supplement that he's taking when obtaining a new prescription.
■ Advise patient to consult his health care provider before using an herbal preparation because a treatment with proven efficacy may be available.

SAFETY RISK *Advise patient to store herb out of reach of children and pets because it can have toxic effects, including death.*

Research summary
Widely sold in Asian groceries as food, bitter melon is also a folk remedy for diabetes, cancer, and various infections. Preliminary studies appear to confirm the first of these folk uses, suggesting that bitter melon may improve blood sugar control in people with adult-onset (type 2) diabetes.

bitter orange

Bigarade orange, Citrus aurantium, *cortenza de naranja amarga, neroli, orange, pomeranzenschale, sour orange, zhi shi*

Bitter orange is an aromatic bitter with a spicy aroma and taste, derived from the dry outer peel of both ripe and unripe fruits of *Citrus aurantium,* minus the white, spongy parenchyma. It contains the flavanone glycosides naringin and neohesperidin, which are responsible for the bitter flavor. The volatile oils limonene, jasmone, linalyl acetate, geranyl acetate, and citronellyl acetate contribute to the aroma.

A bitter orange aqueous extract may have vasoactive effects. Topical bitter orange has antifungal effects and may be useful as an antiseptic. The plant that bitter orange comes from also contains synephrine and other sympathomimetics that cause central nervous system stimulation, insomnia, hypertension, and tachycardia; bitter orange may also have these effects. Bitter orange is available as a crude, dry orange peel for use in tea and traditional Chinese medicine, capsules, and tablets in weight-loss preparations, essential oil, and extracts for topical use.

Reported uses

Bitter orange is used to stimulate appetite, aid digestion, and relieve bloating. It's also used as an antifungal and as a gargle for sore throat, and may aid in weight loss.

Bitter orange is used to improve the taste and smell of herbal teas and is commonly added to sedative teas containing valerian or balm leaves.

In traditional Chinese medicine, bitter orange is used to treat prolapsed uterus, prolapsed anus or rectum, dysentery, abdominal pain, and other GI conditions.

Administration

- Herb: 4 to 6 g by mouth every day
- Extract: 1 to 2 g by mouth every day
- Tea: Prepared by steeping peel in 5 oz of boiling water for 10 to 15 minutes and then straining
- Tincture: 2 to 3 g by mouth every day.

Hazards

Bitter orange may be associated with erythema, blisters, pustules, dermatoses leading to scab formation, and pigment spots. It may decrease the effectiveness of antihypertensives, anxiolytics, and sedatives. There is an increased risk of photosensitivity reactions with sun exposure for patients taking bitter orange.

Pregnant and breast-feeding patients should avoid use because the effects are unknown. Patients with stomach or intestinal ulcers should avoid use because of bitter orange's toxic effect on the GI tract. Those with cardiovascular disease, anxiety, or insomnia should use bitter orange with caution. Bitter orange may be unsafe for use in children because large amounts can cause intestinal colic, seizures, and death.

Clinical considerations

- Frequent contact with the peel or oil, as through occupational exposure, can cause erythema, blisters, pustules, dermatoses leading to scab formation, and pigment spots.
- Warn patient not to delay seeking appropriate medical evaluation for indigestion, abdominal pain, or bloating because doing so may delay diagnosis of a potentially serious medical condition.
- If patient is pregnant or breast-feeding, is planning pregnancy, or suspects that she may be pregnant, advise her not to use bitter orange.
- Advise patient that use of bitter orange may be unsafe in children.
- Tell patient to remind prescriber and pharmacist of any herbal or dietary supplement that he's taking when obtaining a new prescription.
- Advise patient to consult his health care provider before using an herbal preparation because a treatment with proven efficacy may be available.

Research summary

Bitter orange may be effective when taken orally to stimulate appetite and for dyspeptic ailments. Currently there is insufficient scientific evidence evaluating its efficacy for other uses.

black catechu

Acacia catechu, *cutch, gambier, gambir*

Black catechu is the dried extract *Acacia catechu*, a tree native to Myanmar (Burma) and India. It's prepared by boiling the bark and sapwood of the tree and allowing the resulting decoction to evaporate into a syrup, which is then cooled in molds. Once solidified it's removed from the mold and broken into pieces. It contains 20% to 35% of catechutannic acid, 2% to 10% of acacatechin, quercetin, and red catechu.

The therapeutic properties of black catechu come from its tannic acid content. Tannic acid is an astringent with antisecretory properties. It acts locally by precipitating proteins such as damaged or necrotic tissue. Black catechu is available as dry powder, extract, lozenge, and tincture, in products such as Diarcalm, Elixir Bonjean, Enterodyne, and Spanish Tummy Mixture.

Reported uses

Black catechu is used to treat diarrhea and other GI disorders. As a gargle or lozenge, it's used for its astringent effects on mucous membranes and to treat sore throat.

Black catechu is also incorporated into ointments for topical use on furuncles, ulcers, and cutaneous eruptions. At one time, tannic acid was widely used to treat burns, but cases of fatal hepatotoxicity from systemic absorption ended this practice.

Administration

- Tincture: 0.3 to 2 g by mouth every day, divided into 0.5 g doses, three times a day, or 20 gtt in a glass of lukewarm water by mouth
- Topically: 20 gtt, undiluted, applied with a brush.

Hazards

SAFETY RISK *Ingestion of large amounts of tannic acid can cause nausea, vomiting, abdominal pain, and liver damage. Tannic acid barium enemas and tannic acid burn treatments may cause fatal hepatotoxicity from systemic absorption. The amount of black catechu needed to cause these reactions is unclear.*

Black catechu may be associated with nausea, vomiting, abdominal pain, and liver damage caused by tannin content.

The effectiveness of digoxin may be reduced when it's used with black catechu. The tincture contains alcohol; advise patient to avoid using black catechu with disulfiram, and metronidazole. Black catechu may interfere with iron absorption.

Pregnant and breast-feeding patients should avoid use because the effects are unknown. Patients with liver disease should also avoid use because of black catechu's tannin content. Those with a history of alcoholism should use black catechu with caution.

Clinical considerations

- Black catechu may exacerbate the intended therapeutic effects of conventional drugs.
- Warn patient not to delay seeking appropriate medical evaluation for symptoms of GI disorders because doing so may delay diagnosis of a potentially serious medical condition.
- If patient is pregnant or breast-feeding or is planning pregnancy, advise her not to use black catechu.
- Advise patient that safe oral dosing information is unknown.
- Many tinctures contain 15% to 90% alcohol and may be unsuitable for children, alcoholic patients, and patients with liver disease. Instruct patient with history of alcoholism or liver disease to check product label carefully for alcohol content.
- Advise patient not to apply black catechu to burned, damaged, or abraded skin.

- Tell patient to remind prescriber and pharmacist of any herbal or dietary supplement that he's taking when obtaining a new prescription.
- Advise patient to consult his health care provider before using an herbal preparation because a treatment with proven efficacy may be available.

Research summary
The concepts behind the use of black catechu and the claims made regarding its effects have not yet been validated scientifically.

black cohosh

Baneberry, black snake root, bugbane, bugwort, cimicifuga, Cimicifuga racemosa, *rattle root, rattleweed, richweed, squaw root*

Black cohosh is obtained from the fresh or dried rhizome and roots of *Cimicifuga racemosa*. Triterpene glycosides — including actein, cimigoside, and 27-deoxyactein — may produce the therapeutic effects. Black cohosh also contains salicylic acid.

Black cohosh may affect hormones such as estradiol, luteinizing hormone, follicle stimulating hormone, and prolactin. However, the precise mechanism of action is presently unknown.

Black cohosh is available as capsules, liquid extract, powder, tablets, and tincture, in products such as NuVeg Black Cohosh Root, Remifemin, and Wild Countryside Black Cohosh.

Reported uses
Black cohosh is effective for treating somatic and psychological symptoms of menopause, including hot flashes, diaphoresis, sleep disturbance, and anxiety. It doesn't affect vaginal epithelium and may be ineffective for treating menopausal vaginal dryness. German Commission E has approved black cohosh for premenstrual discomfort, dysmenorrhea, and menopausal symptoms of the autonomic nervous system. It may be safe for women with a history of breast cancer and other estrogen-sensitive cancers.

Administration
- Liquid extract (1:1 in 90% alcohol): 0.3 to 2.0 ml by mouth
- Tincture (1:10 in 60% alcohol): 2 to 4 ml by mouth
- Remifemin: 20 mg by mouth two times a day.

Hazards
Black cohosh may be associated with GI discomfort.

Tinctures contain alcohol and may cause a disulfiram or disulfiram-like reaction. Advise patient to avoid using with disulfiram and metronidazole.

Pregnant patients should avoid use because large doses may cause miscarriage or premature birth. Breast-feeding patients should avoid use because the effects aren't known.

Patients who are salicylate sensitive — including those with asthma, gout, peripheral vascular disease, diabetes, hemophilia, and kidney and liver disease — should use with caution.

Clinical considerations
 SAFETY RISK *Don't confuse black cohosh with blue or white cohosh.*
- Effective doses are equivalent to 40 mg per day of crude drug.
- The adverse reactions of and precautions for salicylates may apply to black cohosh.
- Black cohosh has no known benefits for osteoporosis or cardiovascular disease.
- Tincture may contain up to 90% alcohol and so may be unsuitable for children, alcoholic patients, and those with liver disease.
- Black cohosh isn't recommended for use for longer than 6 months.
- Signs and symptoms of overdose include nausea, vomiting, dizziness, ner-

vous system and visual disturbances, reduced pulse rate, and increased perspiration.
- If patient is pregnant or breast-feeding or is planning pregnancy, advise her not to use this herb.
- Encourage patient to have a proper medical evaluation before treating symptoms of menopause.
- Advise patient to keep black cohosh away from children and pets.
- Tell patient to remind prescriber and pharmacist of any herbal or dietary supplement that she's taking when obtaining a new prescription.
- Advise patient to consult her health care provider before using an herbal preparation because a treatment with proven efficacy may be available.

Research summary
The best evidence for black cohosh as a treatment for menopause comes from a double-blind study that followed 80 women for 12 weeks, comparing the benefits of black cohosh, conjugated estrogens (0.625 mg), and placebo. According to the reported results, black cohosh was actually more effective than estrogen, both in relieving symptoms and in normalizing the appearance of vaginal cells under microscopic evaluation.

black haw

American sloe, cramp bark,
dog rowan tree, European cranberry,
guelder rose, high cranberry,
king's crown, May rose, red elder,
rose elder, silver bells, snowball tree,
stagbush, viburnum,
Viburnum prunifolium, *water elder,*
Whitsun bosses, Whitsun rose,
wild guelder rose

Black haw is obtained from the root and stem bark of the plant, which contain scopoletin, tannins, oxalic acid, salicin, and salicylic acid. Scopoletin may be a uterine relaxant. It's available as dried bark and tincture.

Reported uses
Black haw is used to relieve menstrual cramps, and as an antidiarrheal, diuretic, antispasmodic, and anti-asthmatic. It's also used to prevent miscarriage.

Administration
- Tea: 2 teaspoons of dried bark boiled and simmered in 1 cup of water for 10 minutes, and then strained
- Tincture: 5 to 10 ml by mouth three times a day.

Hazards
Black haw may enhance the effects of anticoagulants, such as heparin and low-molecular-weight heparin and warfarin. It may also enhance the effects of antiplatelets, such as aspirin, clopidogrel, dipyridamole, nonsteroidal anti-inflammatory drugs, and ticlopidine. Black haw may also have antiplatelet effects, which may interact with anticoagulant or antiplatelet herbs and produce increased bleeding tendencies. Advise patient to use with caution with feverfew, garlic, ginger, ginkgo, and ginseng. The tincture contains alcohol and may cause a disulfiram or disulfiram-like reaction.

Pregnant patients shouldn't use black haw without the consent of an obstetrician. Breast-feeding patients should avoid use because the effects aren't known. Those with history of kidney stones should use with caution because black haw contains oxalic acid.

Clinical considerations
- Tincture may contain up to 90% alcohol and so may be unsuitable for children, alcoholic patients, and those with liver disease. Advise against use in these patients.
- Because black haw may have antiplatelet effects, monitor patient for bleeding and caution him to report unusual bleeding or bruising without delay.

- Warn patient not to delay seeking appropriate medical evaluation because doing so may delay diagnosis of a potentially serious medical condition.
- If patient has a history of kidney stones, advise him to consult his health care provider before using black haw.
- If patient is pregnant or breast-feeding, advise her to avoid use of black haw unless she has her health care provider's approval.
- Instruct patient to keep herb away from children and pets.
- Tell patient to remind prescriber and pharmacist of any herbal or dietary supplement that he's taking when obtaining a new prescription.
- Advise patient to consult his health care provider before using an herbal preparation because a treatment with proven efficacy may be available.

Research summary
The concepts behind the use of black haw and the claims made regarding its effects have not yet been validated scientifically.

black root

Beaumont root, Bowman's root,
Culveris root, hini, Leptandra virginica,
oxadoddy, physic root, tall speedwell,
tall veronica, whorlywort

Black root is derived from the whole root or root bark, which contains tannic acid, volatile oils, gum, resin, a crystalline principle, a saccharine principle resembling mannite, and a glucoside-resembling senegin. Its tannic acid content has astringent and antisecretory properties. Black root is available as dried root, powdered root bark, and tincture.

Reported uses
Fresh black root is used as an emetic. The dried root has a gentler action and is used to treat constipation and liver and gallbladder disease, and to increase bile flow. Historically, black root was used to treat bilious fever.

Administration
- Powdered root bark: 1 to 4 g by mouth
- Tea: ⅓ cup before each meal, not to exceed 1 cup of tea per day; prepared by steeping 1 teaspoon of black root in 1 cup boiling water for 30 minutes, then straining
- Tincture: 2 to 4 gtt by mouth in water.

Hazards

SAFETY RISK *Ingesting black root in large amounts can cause nausea, vomiting, abdominal pain, and liver damage because of its tannic acid content. The amount of black root required to cause these symptoms is unclear.*

Black root may reduce the effectiveness of digoxin. It decreases the absorption of iron. Laxatives and herbs with laxative effects — such as aloe, blue flag rhizome, butternut, cascara sagrada bark, castor oil, colocynth fruit, manna bark exudate, podophyllum root, rhubarb, senna, wild cumber fruit, and yellow dock root — may increase the cathartic effects of black root. Additive effects occur when black root is used with herbs that have potassium-wasting effects, such as gossypol, horsetail, and licorice.

Patients with gallstones or bile duct obstruction should avoid using black root. Those with a GI disease like colitis or irritable bowel syndrome that may be aggravated by the cathartic effects of black root should use it with caution.

Pregnant patients shouldn't use the herb because the fresh root has abortifacient and teratogenic effects. Also, breast-feeding patients should avoid use because the effects are unknown.

Clinical considerations
- Caution patient to use only the dry root, not the fresh root.
- Monitor patient for excessive diarrhea.
- Warn patient not to delay seeking appropriate medical evaluation because do-

ing so may delay diagnosis of a potentially serious medical condition.

- If patient is pregnant or breast-feeding or planning pregnancy, advise her not to use this herb.
- Advise patient not to drink more than 1 cup of black root tea per day.
- Advise patient to use caution when combining black root with other herbal, over-the-counter, or prescription laxatives.
- Tell patient to remind prescriber and pharmacist of any herbal or dietary supplement that he's taking when obtaining a new prescription.
- Advise patient to consult his health care provider before using an herbal preparation because a treatment with proven efficacy may be available.

Research summary
The concepts behind the use of black root and the claims made regarding its effects have not yet been validated scientifically.

blackthorn

Prunus spinosa, *sloe, wild plum flower*

Blackthorn is derived from the dried flowers and fresh or dried fruit of *Prunus spinosa*. The tannins in blackthorn berry have astringent effects, which help reduce mucous membrane inflammation. Blackthorn flower contains cyanogenic glycosides. Blackthorn is available as juice, marmalade, syrup, tea, and wine.

Reported uses
Blackthorn berry is added to mouth rinse and used to decrease mild inflammation of the oral and pharyngeal mucosa.

Blackthorn syrup and wine are used to purge the bowels and induce sweat, and blackthorn marmalade is used to relieve symptoms of dyspepsia.

Blackthorn flower is used orally to prevent gastric spasms and to treat common colds, respiratory tract disorders, bloat-

ing, general exhaustion, dyspepsia, rashes, skin impurities, and kidney and bladder ailments. It's also used for its laxative, diuretic, diaphoretic, and expectorant effects.

Blackthorn flower is also a component of teas that may help purify the blood.

Administration
- Oral berry: Mouth rinse up to two times a day; daily dose is 2 to 4 g
- Oral flower: 1 to 2 cups of tea by mouth during the day or 2 cups in the evening; prepared by steeping 1 to 2 g of blackthorn in 5 oz of water for 10 minutes, then straining.

Hazards
Blackthorn flower could be toxic because it contains cyanogenic glycosides.

There are no reported interactions with blackthorn.

Pregnant patients should avoid use because of blackthorn's teratogenic cyanogenic compounds. Breast-feeding patients should also avoid use.

Clinical considerations
- Blackthorn isn't recommended for long-term use. Warn patient that use should be short-term.
- If patient is pregnant or breast-feeding, advise her not to use blackthorn.
- Tell patient that although the safety and effectiveness of the herb are uncertain, its use as a coloring agent for tea is regarded as safe.
- Blackthorn may be stored for up to 1 year, away from light and moisture.
- Tell patient to remind prescriber and pharmacist of any herbal or dietary supplement that he's taking when obtaining a new prescription.
- Advise patient to consult his health care provider before using an herbal preparation because a treatment with proven efficacy may be available.

Research summary
The concepts behind the use of blackthorn and the claims made regarding its

effects have not yet been validated scientifically.

blessed thistle

Benediktenkraut, cardin,
Cnicus benedictus, *holy thistle,*
spotted thistle, St. Benedict thistle

Blessed thistle contains the sesquiterpene lactones cnicin and salonitenolide. Cnin, a glycoside, is responsible for the herb's bitterness, which stimulates the appetite and aids in digestion by encouraging the secretion of saliva and gastric juice. It may also act directly on the stomach and part of the small intestine.

Blessed thistle stimulates menstruation. It's characterized as a bitter tonic, astringent, diaphoretic, antibacterial, expectorant, antidiarrheal, antihemorrhagic, vulnerary, antipyretic, and galactagogue. The antibacterial properties come from the volatile oil and the cnicin component. It's available as capsules, decoction, dried herb, fluid extract, infusion, oil, tea, and tincture. The extract is a constituent in skin lotions, creams, and salves.

Reported uses
Blessed thistle is used orally to treat digestive problems such as liver and gallbladder diseases, loss of appetite, indigestion and heartburn, constipation, colic, diarrhea, dyspepsia, and flatulence. It may also improve memory, relieve menstrual complaints, control amenorrhea, regulate the menstrual cycle, increase perspiration, lower fever, enhance lactation, dissolve blood clots, control bleeding, and reduce rheumatic pain. It's also used as an expectorant and antibiotic.

Topically, blessed thistle poultice is used for furuncles, wounds, ulcers, and hemorrhage. Blessed thistle is added to alcoholic beverages during manufacturing as flavoring.

Administration
- Capsules: 2 capsules by mouth three times a day
- Decoction: 1 cup by mouth 30 minutes before meals; prepared by adding 1.5 to 2 g of finely chopped herb to 1 cup of water
- Liquid extract: (1:1 in 25% alcohol) 1.5 to 3 ml by mouth, three times a day
- Mean daily dose: 4 to 6 g of herb or equivalent preparations
- Tea: 3 cups by mouth every day; prepared by adding 2 g of dried herb to 1 cup of boiling water and steeping for 10 to 15 minutes
- Tincture: 1 to 2 ml by mouth three times a day.

Hazards
Adverse effects reportedly associated with blessed thistle include nausea, vomiting, diarrhea, and contact dermatitis.

Because blessed thistle increases stomach acidity, it may interact with antacids, H_2 antagonists, proton pump inhibitors, and sucralfate. Possible worsening of hypoglycemia may occur when blessed thistle is used with insulin and oral antidiabetics. Blessed thistle may potentiate the antibiotic activity of echinacea. There may be cross sensitivity with other herbs from the Compositae family such as mugwort and cornflower.

Pregnant and breast-feeding patients should avoid using blessed thistle because it may promote menstruation. Those with acute stomach inflammation, ulcers, or hyperacidity, should avoid using blessed thistle because it stimulates gastric juices. Those with a history of contact dermatitis, especially in relation to other members of the Compositae family — including ragweed, chrysanthemums, marigolds, and daisies — and those with diabetes, ulcers, acute stomach inflammation, and hyperacidity of the GI tract should used blessed thistle with caution.

Clinical considerations

 SAFETY RISK *Don't confuse blessed thistle with milk thistle* (Silybum marianum).

■ Infusions of more than 5 g per cup of tea may cause vomiting and stomach irritation.

■ Blessed thistle may cross-react with mugwort and cornflower.

■ If patient has diabetes, monitor his blood glucose level.

■ Warn patient not to delay seeking appropriate medical evaluation for indigestion, anorexia, or heartburn because doing so may delay diagnosis of a potentially serious medical condition.

■ If patient is pregnant or breast-feeding, advise her not to use blessed thistle.

■ If patient is taking a drug for diabetes, ulcers, or heartburn, instruct him to contact his health care provider before taking blessed thistle because his drug dosage may need to be adjusted.

■ If patient is collecting blessed thistle himself, advise him to wear protective clothes and glasses because the plant can cause inflammation of the skin, eyes, and mucous membranes.

■ Advise patient not to add milk or cream to blessed thistle tea; doing so may mute the gastric acid secretion.

■ Tell patient to remind prescriber and pharmacist of any herbal or dietary supplement that he's taking when obtaining a new prescription.

■ Advise patient to consult his health care provider before using an herbal preparation because a treatment with proven efficacy may be available.

Research summary
The concepts behind the use of blessed thistle and the claims made regarding its effects have not yet been validated scientifically.

bloodroot

Coon root, Indian plant, Indian red plant, paucon, pauson, red Indian paint, red puccoon, red root, Sanguinaria canadensis, snakebite, sweet slumber, tetterwort

Bloodroot contains isoquinolone alkaloid components, primarily sanguinarine, which have antimicrobial, antiseptic, anti-inflammatory, antihistamine, expectorant, antispasmodic, emetic, cathartic, pectoral, and cardiotonic effects.

Sanguinarine converted to a negatively charged iminium ion helps to inhibit plaque from settling on tooth enamel. Antibacterial properties of bloodroot fight organisms responsible for bad breath. Another alkaloid, cholerythrine, may have some anticarcinogenic effects.

Bloodroot is available for external use as decoction, extract, ointment, powder, and tincture, or for internal use as decoction and tincture. Extracts appear in commercial mouthwashes and toothpastes. Bloodroot is a constituent in products such as Lexat and Viadent.

Reported uses
Bloodroot is used as an emetic, cathartic, antispasmodic, decongestant, digestive stimulant, laxative, expectorant, dental analgesic, and general tonic. It's also used to treat bronchitis, asthma, croup, laryngitis, pharyngitis, congestion, deficient capillary circulation, nasal polyps, rheumatism, warts, ear and nose cancer (Fell technique), fever, sore throat, skin burns, and fungal infection.

Administration
■ Extract (1:1 in 60% alcohol): 0.06 to 0.3 ml (1 to 2 ml for emetic dose) by mouth three times a day
■ Rhizome: 0.06 to 0.5 g (1 to 2 g for emetic dose) by mouth three times a day
■ Tea: 1 cup by mouth several times a day; prepared by boiling 1 to 2 table-

spoon(s) of chopped rhizome in 17 oz of water for 15 minutes
- Tincture: (1:5 in 60% alcohol) 0.3 to 2 ml (2 to 8 ml for emetic dose) by mouth three times a day
- Wine: Prepared by steeping chopped bloodroot in brandy, then filtering.

Hazards

SAFETY RISK *Powdered rhizome or juice can destroy tissue. Large doses of the internal formulations can be poisonous. The FDA has classified bloodroot as unsafe.*

Adverse effects associated with bloodroot include headache, central nervous system (CNS) depression, ataxia, reduced activity, coma, hypotension, eye and mucous membrane irritation, glaucoma, contact dermatitis, nausea, vomiting, and shock.

Bloodroot may potentiate the action of antihypertensives, dopamine, and ganglionic or peripheral adrenergic blockers such as tubocurarine and norepinephrine. Use of bloodroot in conjunction with CNS depressants may have some additive effects. Bloodroot and corticotropin or corticosteroids may produce hypokalemia. Bloodroot may increase the antimicrobial activity of sanguinarine products containing zinc. It also may increase CNS effects if used with alcohol.

Pregnant and breast-feeding patients and those with infections or inflammatory GI conditions should avoid use. Those with GI irritation should use bloodroot with caution because it can irritate the GI tract; those with glaucoma, because it can affect glaucoma treatment.

Clinical considerations

- In most countries, bloodroot isn't used orally. Oral use can cause CNS depression and narcosis because of bloodroot's relaxant effect on smooth muscle.
- At higher doses, bloodroot produces interactions similar to diuretics and cathartics.

- If patient is taking an antihypertensive, monitor his blood pressure.
- Prolonged use of bloodroot may affect electrolyte levels, such as potassium, sodium, blood urea nitrogen, uric acid, and glucose.
- If overdose occurs or if patient ingests a large quantity of bloodroot, perform gastric lavage or induce vomiting and provide symptomatic treatment.
- Inform patient that bloodroot isn't recommended for oral use and that large doses can be poisonous. Tell him that toothpastes and mouthwashes containing bloodroot extracts are unlikely to cause harm if they aren't swallowed.
- If patient is pregnant, advise her not to use bloodroot.
- Advise patient to avoid contact with the eyes and mucous membranes because of bloodroot's irritant properties. Also advise him to take protective measures so he doesn't inhale the herb during crude herb processing.
- Tell patient to avoid alcohol while using bloodroot because of the risk of enhanced CNS depression.
- Warn patient that a component of the herb may cause cataracts.
- Tell patient to remind prescriber and pharmacist of any herbal or dietary supplement that he's taking when obtaining a new prescription.
- Advise patient to consult his health care provider before using an herbal preparation because a treatment with proven efficacy may be available.

Research summary
The concepts behind the use of bloodroot and the claims made regarding its effects have not yet been validated scientifically.

blue cohosh

Beechdrops, blueberry root, blue ginseng,
Caulophyllum thalictroides,
papoose root, squaw root, yellow ginseng

Blue cohosh is derived from the aerial parts of the plant, its roots, and its rhizomes. Pharmacologic effects are attributed to several glycosides and alkaloids, such as caulosaponin and methylcytisine. Caulosaponin is responsible for the herb's oxytocic effects and its effects on coronary vasculature as well as its ability to stimulate intestinal contractions. Methylcytisine produces nicotinic effects; for example, it elevates blood pressure and blood glucose level, stimulates respiration, and increases peristalsis. Blue cohosh is available as capsules, decoction, dried powder, liquid extract, tablets, tea, and tincture.

Reported uses

Blue cohosh is used to treat colic, sore throat, cramps, hiccups, epilepsy, urinary tract infections, inflammation of the uterus, asthma, memory problems, hypertension, muscle spasms, worm infestation, anxiety, restlessness and pain during pregnancy, and labor pains. It's used to stimulate uterine contractions and induce menstruation, and as an antispasmodic, antirheumatic, diaphoretic, expectorant, and laxative.

Blue cohosh may also have some antimicrobial activity. Low doses of the extract may inhibit ovulation. The roasted seeds of the herb are commonly used as a coffee substitute.

Administration

■ Dried rhizome or root: 0.3 to 1 g by mouth three times a day
■ Tea: 1 cup three times a day; prepared by steeping herb in 5 oz of boiling water, then straining
■ Liquid extract (1:1 in 70% alcohol): 0.5 to 1 ml by mouth three times a day.

Hazards

Adverse effects which are reportedly associated with blue cohosh include chest pain, vasoconstriction, hypotension, mucous membrane irritation, GI irritation, severe diarrhea, cramping, and hyperglycemia.

A *decreased* antidiabetic action of blue cohosh has been reported when it's used with acetazolamide, corticosteroids, dextrothyroxine, epinephrine, glucagon, oral contraceptives, phenothiazines, rifampin, thiazide diuretics, and thyroid-stimulating hormones.

An *increased* antidiabetic action of blue cohosh has been reported when it's used with allopurinol, anabolic steroids, chloramphenicol, clofibrate, fenfluramine, guanethidine, monoamine oxidase inhibitors, phenylbutazone, phenyramidol, probenecid, salicylates, sulfinpyrazone, sulfonamides, and tetracyclines.

Metabolism of blue cohosh may decrease when the herb is used with aminosalicylic acid, antihistamines, disulfiram, halothane, isoniazid, methylphenidate, phenothiazines, propoxyphene, sulfa drugs, and troleandomycin. Antacids and mineral oil may reduce anthelmintic effect of blue cohosh.

Blue cohosh may interact with antianginals and with nicotine replacement therapy. Diuretic activity of blue cohosh may potentiate the action of antihypertensives and peripheral adrenergic blockers. Barbiturates, diazoxide, loxapine, and vitamin B_6 may induce metabolism of blue cohosh. Clindamycin may enhance neuromuscular relaxing action of blue cohosh. Blue cohosh may increase metabolism of corticosteroids, digoxin, fluroxene, methadone, metyrapone, oral contraceptives, phenytoin, and tetracyclines. Blue cohosh may reduce the renal clearance of lithium, and may produce synergistic oxytocic activity when used with Sparteine. Severe hypertension may occur when blue cohosh is used with vasoconstrictors such as ephedrine, methoxamine, and phenylephrine. Alcohol may induce metabolism of blue cohosh, thus decreasing pharmacologic effects. Marijuana may cause a decreased antidiabetic action of blue cohosh.

 SAFETY RISK *Blue cohosh shouldn't be used during labor. Several adverse effects have been reported to the FDA, including fetal toxicity, neonatal stroke, and aplastic anemia after maternal use of herb during labor, and neonatal acute myocardial infarction associated with heart failure and shock.*

Pregnant patients should avoid use of blue cohosh because it may stimulate menstruation. Patients with cardiovascular disease and those with GI conditions should also avoid its use. Those with hypertension or diabetes should use blue cohosh with caution.

Clinical considerations
■ In the past blue cohosh has been listed as a drug in the USP and the National Formulary; however, because of serious safety concerns, its use isn't recommended.

■ The root of this herb can be toxic, and the danger associated with its use seems to outweigh the reported medicinal benefits.

SAFETY RISK *Raw blue cohosh berries are poisonous to children.*
■ Don't confuse blue cohosh with black cohosh.

■ Monitor patient's blood pressure and blood glucose, blood urea nitrogen, uric acid, and protein-bound iodine levels.

■ Monitor patient for signs and symptoms of overdose, which resemble those of nicotine toxicity. If overdose occurs, perform gastric lavage or induce vomiting, if needed.

■ Warn patient to avoid using blue cohosh during pregnancy, labor, and breast-feeding.

■ Tell patient to remind prescriber and pharmacist of any herbal or dietary supplement that he's taking when obtaining a new prescription.

■ Advise patient to consult his health care provider before using an herbal preparation because a treatment with proven efficacy may be available.

Research summary
There is virtually no credible evidence that blue cohosh is effective for any of the conditions for which it has been used. Several published reports cite cases of serious adverse effects in infants, apparently caused by blue cohosh.

blue flag

Dagger flower, daggers, dragon flower, flaggon, flag lily, fleur-de-lis, fliggers, flower-de-luce, gladyne, iris, irisin, Iris caroliniana, I. versicolor, *Jacob's sword, liver lily, myrtle flower, poison flag, segg, sheggs, snake lily, sweet flag, water flag, white flag root, wild iris, yellow flag, yellow iris*

Blue flag preparations are obtained from the rhizome portion of the plant. The primary useful ingredients are iridin and oleoresin. Blue flag may stimulate the flow of bile from the gallbladder to the duodenum. It's used as an anti-inflammatory, diuretic, laxative, and sialagogue, as well as a hepatic and dermatologic herb.

Reported uses
Blue flag is used to purify blood and free it from toxins. It's used to treat heartburn, belching, nausea, and headaches resulting from digestive disorders as well as disorders of the respiratory tract and thyroid gland. It's also used for its cathartic, emetic, and diuretic effects.

Blue flag is applied externally on sores and bruises to decrease inflammation.

Administration
■ Decoction: 1 cup of preparation by mouth three times a day; prepared by placing ½ to 1 teaspoon of dried herb in 1

cup of boiling water and simmering for 10 to 15 minutes
■ Solid extracts, powdered root: 10 to 20 grains by mouth
■ Tincture: 2 to 4 ml by mouth three times a day
■ Dried rhizome: 0.6 to 2 g three times a day
■ Liquid extract: 1 to 2 ml three times a day.

Hazards

 SAFETY RISK *The fresh root of blue flag is poisonous. Iridin poisoning in humans and animals and severe nausea and vomiting after consumption of fresh root have been reported. A patient who chooses to use the herb should use only small doses of the dried root.*

Reported adverse effects with the use of blue flag include headache, lacrimation, eye inflammation, throat irritation, and mucous membrane and skin irritation from the herb's furfural component.

Blue flag may potentiate the effects of anticoagulants by reducing absorption of vitamin K from the gut. It may also potentiate the action of antihypertensives, ganglionic, or peripheral adrenergics. Beta blockers such as meprobamate, phenobarbital, propranolol, and other sedative hypnotics such as chloral hydrate may decrease blue flag's anti-inflammatory effects.

Blue flag may cause hypokalemia when used in conjunction with corticosteroids and corticotropin. It may reduce the renal clearance of lithium. Blue flag may increase depletion of potassium when used with stimulant laxative herbs such as aloe, buckthorn fruit and bark, butternut, cascara sagrada bark, castor oil, colocynth fruit pulp, gamboge bark exudate, podophyllum root, rhubarb root, senna leaves and pods, yellow dock root, potassium-wasting herbs such as horsetail plant and licorice rhizome, and wild cucumber fruit.

Pregnant and breast-feeding patients and patients with infectious or inflammatory GI conditions should avoid use.

Clinical considerations
■ If patient is also taking digoxin, monitor his blood digoxin levels.
■ Monitor blood pressure and blood glucose, serum electrolyte, and uric acid levels.
■ If patient is also taking an anticoagulant, monitor International Normalized Ratio.
■ Warn patient not to take blue flag internally.
■ If patient is pregnant or breast-feeding, advise her not to use blue flag.
■ Caution patient that blue flag can cause severe irritation if it comes in direct contact with eyes, ears, nose, or mouth.
■ Tell patient to remind prescriber and pharmacist of any herbal or dietary supplement that he's taking when obtaining a new prescription.
■ Advise patient to consult his health care provider before using an herbal preparation because a treatment with proven efficacy may be available.

Research summary
Safety studies of blue flag have not been performed, and related species have been found to be toxic.

bogbean

Bean trefoil, bog hop, bog myrtle, bog nut, brook bean, buck bean, marsh clover, marsh trefoil, Menyanthes trifoliata, *moon flower, trefoil, water shamrock, water trefoil*

Bogbean is obtained from the dried rhizome of *Menyanthes trifoliata.* The useful components are a small quantity of volatile oil and the glucoside menyanthin, which is reported to stimulate saliva production and gastric secretion. Bogbean is available as a fluid extract, tablet, powder, and whole leaf.

Reported uses
Bogbean is used to treat loss of appetite, dyspepsia, gout, rheumatoid arthritis, osteoarthritis, rheumatism, and skin diseases. It's also used as a bitter to promote gastric secretion. In large doses, it's used as an emetic.

Administration
- Infusion: ½ cup by mouth, unsweetened, before each meal
- Tea: 1.5 to 3 g by mouth, daily; prepared by steeping 0.5 to 1 g of finely cut herb in boiling water (or cold water that's rapidly heated) for 5 to 10 minutes, then straining; 1 teaspoon equals 0.9 g of herb
- Tincture (1:5 in 45% alcohol): 1 to 3 ml by mouth three times a day
- Liquid extract (1:1 in 25% alcohol): 1 to 2 ml by mouth three times a day.

Hazards
Bogbean may be associated with GI irritation, and may increase the risk of bleeding if used with antiplatelet/anticoagulant drugs or herbs with anticoagulant or antiplatelet properties. It may negate the effects of antacids, H_2 antagonists, proton pump inhibitors, and sucralfate because it promotes gastric secretion. It may potentiate the effects of stimulant laxatives.

Bogbean isn't for use in patients with diarrhea, dysentery, or colitis. It's contraindicated in pregnant patients because it may stimulate menstruation and act as a stimulant laxative.

Clinical considerations
- Bogbean may alter the intended therapeutic effect of conventional drugs.
- Warn patient not to use bogbean to treat symptoms of anorexia, dyspepsia, or pain before seeking appropriate medical evaluation because doing so may delay diagnosis of a potentially serious medical condition.

- Educate patient on possible adverse effects that result from overdose, such as vomiting.
- Advise patient with diarrhea, dysentery, or colitis not to use the herb.
- Advise female patient to avoid use during pregnancy or breast-feeding.
- Tell patient to remind prescriber and pharmacist of any herbal or dietary supplement that he's taking when obtaining a new prescription.
- Advise patient to consult his health care provider before using an herbal preparation because a treatment with proven efficacy may be available.

Research summary
The concepts behind the use of bogbean and the claims made regarding its effects have not yet been validated scientifically.

boldo

Boldea, boldoa, boldu, boldus,
Peumus boldus

Boldo is derived from the dried leaves of *Peumus boldus*. It contains boldine, an isoquinoline alkaloid of the aporphine type, and a volatile oil that contains ascaridiole. Boldine may be effective as an antispasmodic, choleretic, and diuretic; it may also increase gastric secretions. The pharmacologic effects of the volatile oil are similar to those of boldine. Ascaridiole is an antihelminthic. Boldo is available as capsules, fluid extract, tablets, and tinctures of varying potencies.

Reported uses
Boldo is used to treat liver and gallbladder complaints, loss of appetite, dyspepsia, and mild spastic complaints. Boldo leaves, which are included in herbal teas for their diuretic and laxative effects, can cause significant diuresis. The oil is used to treat genitourinary inflammation, gout, and rheumatism.

Administration
- Boldo oil: 5 gtt by mouth
- Fluid extract (1:1 in 45% alcohol): 0.1 to 0.3 ml by mouth three times a day
- Pulverized herb for infusions: 4.5 g by mouth daily
- Tincture (1:10 in 60% alcohol): 0.5 to 2 ml by mouth three times a day.

Hazards

SAFETY RISK *In large doses, boldo stimulates the central nervous system, causing exaggerated reflexes, disturbed coordination, and seizures. In large doses, it may also paralyze motor and sensory nerves and muscle fibers, eventually causing death as a result of respiratory depression.*

Ascaridiole is a known toxin, and preparations of the volatile oil or distillates of the leaf should be avoided.

Adverse effects associated with boldo include exaggerated reflexes, disturbed coordination, seizures, paralysis of motor and sensory nerves and muscle fibers, and respiratory depression.

Boldo may have additive effects when used with diuretics.

Pregnant patients and patients with bile duct obstruction or severe liver diseases should avoid use.

Clinical considerations
- If patient has gallstones, advise him to consult his health care provider before using boldo.
- Caution patient that overdose may lead to neurologic symptoms, respiratory depression and, if severe enough, death.
- If female patient is pregnant, advise her not to use boldo.
- Advise patient to avoid preparations with the volatile oil of boldo or distillates of the leaf because of the toxic effects of ascaridiole. Inform patient that preparations with virtually no ascaridiole are available.
- Inform patient not to delay seeking appropriate medical intervention if symptoms persist after taking this herb.

- Tell patient to remind prescriber and pharmacist of any herbal or dietary supplement that he's taking when obtaining a new prescription.
- Advise patient to consult his health care provider before using an herbal preparation because a treatment with proven efficacy may be available.

Research summary
Boldo taken alone has not been well evaluated as a treatment for dyspepsia; however, a combination herbal treatment containing boldo (along with other herbs thought to stimulate the gallbladder) has been studied. In a double-blind trial, 60 individuals given either an artichoke leaf/boldo/celandine combination or placebo found improvements in symptoms of indigestion after 14 days of treatment. How this combination might be effective for treating dyspepsia is unclear.

boneset

Agueweed, crosswort, Eupatorium perfoliatum, *feverwort, Indian sage, sweating plant, teasal, thoroughwort, vegetable antimony, wood boneset*

Boneset is obtained from the complete aerial part of *Eupatorium perfoliatum*. It contains the components glucoside (eupatorin), volatile oil, resin, inulin, wax, sterols, triterpenes, and flavonoids. It also contains pyrrolizidine alkaloids, which cause hepatic impairment if consumed over a prolonged period, and tremetol, an unsaturated alcohol that lowers the blood glucose level.

Boneset acts as a diaphoretic, an antiphlogistic, and a bitter, which stimulates the appetite, aids digestion, and stimulates the body's immune system. Small doses of boneset may have diuretic and laxative effects, whereas large doses may result in vomiting and catharsis. Boneset is available as capsules, dried leaf or powder, fluid extract, and tablets in products such as Boneset Herb Organic Alcohol and Alvita Tea.

Reported uses

Boneset is used as a tonic to help restore systemic vitality and as a nutritional tonic to rejuvenate the body after a debilitating condition. It's also used to treat colds, catarrh, influenza, rheumatism, most fevers, and inflammation of the nose, throat, or tongue.

Administration

■ Fluid extract: 2 to 4 g of plant material by mouth
■ Infusion: Prepared by steeping 2 teaspoons to 2 tablespoons of crushed dried leaves and flowering tops in 8 to 16 oz of boiling water; administered three times a day
■ Tincture: 2 to 3 ml by mouth three times a day.

Hazards

SAFETY RISK *The herb contains pyrrolizidine alkaloids, which are hepatotoxic and hepatocarcinogenic, and may therefore cause hepatic dysfunction.*

Adverse effects associated with boneset include GI hemorrhage, fatty degeneration of the kidneys, fatty degeneration of the liver, hepatic dysfunction, hypoglycemia, and contact dermatitis.

There is an increased risk of hypoglycemia when boneset is used with insulin or oral antidiabetics.

Long-term use of boneset should be avoided. Those with liver disease and those who are pregnant or breast-feeding should avoid use.

Clinical considerations

SAFETY RISK *Symptoms of boneset overdose include weakness, nausea, lack of appetite, thirst, and constipation. Severe poisoning may result in muscle trembling and loss of motor control, progressing to paralysis and death.*
■ If patient is diabetic and is taking an oral antidiabetic, advise him to closely

monitor his blood glucose level because the tremetrol component of the herb may have a hypoglycemic effect.
■ Warn patient not to delay seeking appropriate medical evaluation because doing so may delay diagnosis of a potentially serious medical condition.
■ If patient is pregnant, advise her not to use boneset.
■ Tell patient to remind prescriber and pharmacist of any herbal or dietary supplement that he's taking when obtaining a new prescription.
■ Advise patient to consult his health care provider before using an herbal preparation because a treatment with proven efficacy may be available.

Research summary

The concepts behind the use of boneset and the claims made regarding its effects have not yet been validated scientifically.

borage

Beebread, Borago officinalis, *bugloss, burage, burrage, oxtongue, starflower*

Borage oil comes from the fatty oil of the seeds and flower of *Borago officinalis.* It may contain between 20% and 26% of the essential fatty acid gamma-linolenic acid (GLA). GLA has anti-inflammatory effects because of increased production of 15-hydroxy fatty acid and prostaglandin E_1, both metabolites of GLA, and astringent and sequestering effects.

Borage leaves are the dried leaves and flower clusters, which are harvested during the plant's flowering period and artificially dried at 104° F (40° C). They contain pyrrolizidine alkaloids, which are hepatotoxic and hepatocarcinogenic, and so may cause hepatic dysfunction. They also contain tannins, mucilage, malic acid, and potassium nitrate. In small amounts, borage may cause constipation because of its tannin content.

Borage's mucilage component may contribute to its expectorant effect; the malic acid and potassium nitrate components, to its mild diuretic effect. Borage is available as dried leaf or powder, fluid extract, oil, and tablets, in products such as Borage Bio-EFA, Borage Oil Softgels, Borage-Power, GLA-320 Borage Capsules, and Ultra GLA Capsules.

Reported uses
Borage is used externally as an astringent, a poultice for inflammation, and a treatment for eczema. The oil is used as treatment for neurodermatitis and as a GLA supplement.

Borage is used orally for its sequestering and mucilaginous effects in treating coughs and throat illnesses. It's used as an anti-inflammatory for kidney and bladder disorders, and for rheumatism. Borage is used as an analgesic, cardiotonic, sedative, and diaphoretic, and to treat phlebitis and menopausal complaints.

Administration
■ Oil: usually administered in vitamin capsules
■ For internal use: 1 oz dried leaves in 16 oz boiling water; 60 ml doses
■ Fluid extract: 2 to 4 ml by mouth.

Hazards
Gamma-linolenic acid can prolong bleeding time.

If used with anticonvulsants or phenothiazines, borage may lower the seizure threshold. Borage may increase the risk of bleeding if used with anticoagulants or antiplatelet agents.

Patients with liver disease or seizure disorders and those who are pregnant or breast-feeding should avoid use.

Clinical considerations
■ Borage leaves contain the potentially toxic pyrrolizidine alkaloids.
■ Liver function tests may be needed to help monitor patient for hepatotoxicity.
■ If patient has a history of seizures and is taking an anticonvulsant, monitor him for seizure activity because borage may lower the seizure threshold.

■ Borage leaves should be protected from light and moisture.
■ If patient is pregnant or breast-feeding, advise her not to use borage.
■ Warn patient of the potential for hepatic dysfunction and carcinogenic effects of borage plant preparations.
■ Advise patient that borage oil is usually safe and free from adverse effects when taken in therapeutic doses.
■ Advise patient not to delay seeking appropriate medical treatment if symptoms persist after taking borage.
■ Tell patient to remind prescriber and pharmacist of any herbal or dietary supplement that he's taking when obtaining a new prescription.
■ Advise patient to consult his health care provider before using an herbal preparation because a treatment with proven efficacy may be available.

Research summary
The concepts behind the use of borage and the claims made regarding its effects have not yet been validated scientifically.

broom

Basam, besenginsterkraut, besom, bizzom, breeam, broom top, broomtops, browme, brum, Cytisus scoparius, *ginsterkraut, green broom, hogweed, Irish broom top, Irish tops, sarothamni herb, Scotch broom, Scotch broom top*

Broom is derived from the dried and stripped flowers, the dried aerial parts, and the freshly picked flowers of *Cytisus scoparius*. The main alkaloid in broom is sparteine, a transparent, oily liquid, colorless when fresh, turning brown on exposure, with an aniline-like odor and a very bitter taste. It's slightly soluble in water, but readily soluble in alcohol and ether. Sparteine is a powerful oxytocic once used for inducing uterine contractions. It also has antiarrhythmic and bradycardic effects.

Scoparin, the other principal component, is a glucoside that occurs in pale yellow crystals, is tasteless, and is soluble in alcohol and hot water. It's responsible for broom's diuretic effect. Broom also contains flavonoids, biogenic amines, isoflavonoids, and other alkaloids. It's available as an aqueous essential oil extract, liquid extract, and tincture.

Reported uses

Aqueous essential oil extracts of broom are used internally to treat hypertension and cardiovascular and circulatory disorders as well as to stabilize circulation and elevate blood pressure. It's used as a cathartic and diuretic and, in large doses, as an emetic.

Broom is also used to treat pathologic edema, cardiac arrhythmia, nervous cardiac complaints, menorrhagia, hemorrhage after birth, hypotension, bleeding gums, hemophilia, gout, rheumatism, sciatica, gall and kidney stones, splenomegaly, jaundice, snake bites, and bronchial conditions, and to stimulate uterine contractions. Broom may be smoked like marijuana to produce euphoria and relaxation.

Administration

- Infusion: 1 cup fresh infusion by mouth three times a day
- Liquid extract (25% alcohol): 1 to 2 ml by mouth every day
- Tincture: 0.5 to 2 ml by mouth.

Hazards

 SAFETY RISK *The FDA has designated broom as an unsafe herb.*
Additive effects may occur if broom is used with antihypertensives. Herbal products prepared with alcohol may cause a disulfiram-like reaction. Broom may cause a hypertensive crisis if used with monoamine oxidase (MAO) inhibitors. Additive effects may occur if broom is used with quinidine. Additive effects may occur if broom is used with nicotine or smoking.

Those taking an MAO inhibitor, those with hypertension or atrioventricular block, and those who are pregnant should avoid use.

Broom may also cause headache.

Clinical considerations

- Advise patient that broom should be used only under a health care provider's supervision because it has the potential for abuse.
- Doses that contain more than 300 mg sparteine, or 30 g of drug, may cause dizziness, headache, palpitations, weakness, sweating, sleepiness, pupil dilation, and ocular palsy.
- If overdose occurs and patient doesn't vomit on his own, perform gastric lavage and administer activated charcoal. Treat spasms with chlorpromazine or diazepam. If patient becomes asphyxiated, intubation and oxygen respiration may be needed.
- Monitor blood pressure in patient who's using broom.
- Warn patient not to delay seeking appropriate medical evaluation for edema and cardiac complaints because doing so may delay diagnosis of a potentially serious medical condition.
- Advise patient who's taking an MAO inhibitor or is pregnant not to use broom.
- Tell patient to remind prescriber and pharmacist of any herbal or dietary supplement that he's taking when obtaining a new prescription.
- Advise patient to consult his health care provider before using an herbal preparation because a treatment with proven efficacy may be available.

Research summary

The concepts behind the use of broom and the claims made regarding its effects have not yet been validated scientifically.

buchu

Agathosma betulina, Barosma betulina,
B. crenulata, B. serratifolia, *bookoo,
bucco, bucku, buku, diosma*

Buchu consists of the dried leaves of
Barosma betulina, *B. crenulata*, and *B.
serratifolia*. It contains flavonoids, resin,
and mucilage. Buchu also contains a
volatile oil that's made up of more than
100 identified compounds, the principal
component of which is diosphenol,
which crystallizes at room temperature
(buchu camphor). Other major components of the oil include pulegone, limonene, and menthone.

Buchu is reported to have urinary
antiseptic, antibacterial, diuretic, anti-
inflammatory, and carminative properties. Diosphenol is thought to exert an
antibacterial effect, similar to that of
bearberry leaves. Like bearberry, this
phenol is excreted as a glucuronic acid
conjugate, which may account for similar
antibacterial properties. Volatile oil and
flavonoid components may be responsible for the anti-inflammatory effects.

Weak diuretic activity similar to coffee
or tea may come from the flavonoids
diosphenol and terpinen-4-ol present in
buchu leaf. Terpinen-4-ol increases
glomerular filtration rate and may irritate the kidneys. Pulegone is a hepatotox-
in and an abortifacient that stimulates
uterine contractions and may cause increased menstrual flow. Buchu is available as capsules, extract, herbal tea,
tablets, and tincture. It's also found in
commercial herbal blends used for diuresis.

Reported uses

Buchu has been used in Europe since the
16th century, and is still widely used by
advocates of herbs, particularly in South
Africa. However, German Commission E
lists buchu as an unapproved herb whose
effectiveness isn't documented.

Buchu is used to treat mild inflammation and infection of the kidneys and urinary tract in those with cystitis, urethri-
tis, prostatitis, and venereal disease. It's
also used to treat bladder irritation, gout,
stomachache, and constipation, and as a
mild diuretic, antiseptic, tonic, and stimulant. A douche prepared from an infusion of the leaves is used to treat yeast infections and leukorrhea.

Administration

- Fluid extract: 0.3 to 1.2 ml by mouth
three times a day
- For diuresis: Prepared by steeping 1 g
of herb in boiled water, covered, for 10
minutes, then straining; taken by mouth
several times a day
- Oral use: 1 to 2 g daily
- Tincture: 2 to 4 ml by mouth, up to
three times a day.

Hazards

Adverse effects that may be associated
with buchu include stomach or bowel irritation, kidney irritation, and increased
menstrual flow.

Buchu may enhance the effects of anticoagulants. Herbal products prepared
with alcohol may cause a disulfiram-like
reaction.

Pregnant patients and those planning
pregnancy should avoid use because of
buchu's abortifacient effects. Those with
liver disease should use buchu with caution because it may cause liver toxicity.
Those with kidney inflammation should
avoid use.

Clinical considerations

- Ingesting large amounts of buchu or
the oil can irritate the GI tract and kidneys.
- Buchu may alter the intended therapeutic effect of conventional drugs.
- If patient is taking an anticoagulant,
consider monitoring International Normalized Ratio, prothrombin time, partial
thromboplastin time, liver function, and
menstruation.

- Warn patient not to delay seeking appropriate medical evaluation because doing so may delay diagnosis of a potentially serious medical condition.
- If patient is pregnant or is planning pregnancy, advise her not to use buchu.
- Advise patient to alert her health care provider if after using buchu she experiences profuse menstrual flow or kidney, stomach, or bowel irritation.
- Tell patient to remind prescriber and pharmacist of any herbal or dietary supplement that he's taking when obtaining a new prescription.
- Advise patient to consult his health care provider before using an herbal preparation because a treatment with proven efficacy may be available.

Research summary
The concepts behind the use of buchu and the claims made regarding its effects have not yet been validated scientifically.

buckthorn

Alder buckthorn, alder dogwood, arrow wood, black alder bark, black dogwood, dogwood, frangula, frangula bark, glossy buckthorn, hartshorn, highwaythorn, ramsthorn, Rhamnus cathartica, R. frangula, *waythorn*

Dried buckthorn bark comes from the stems and branches of the *Rhamnus frangula* tree, which is imported from Russia, Yugoslavia, and Poland. It contains anthranoids and 3% to 9% anthraquinone glycosides, which include glucofrangulin A and B and frangulin A and B, which have a laxative effect.

The fresh bark contains reduced forms of anthrones and anthrone glycosides, which have an emetic component. Use of the untreated fresh herb can irritate the stomach mucosa, causing severe vomiting, colic, and bloody diarrhea.

Buckthorn's stimulant and irritant laxative effect on the large intestine is similar to, yet milder than, that of cascara sagrada. It has weaker antiabsorptive and hydragogic properties. The herb takes effect 6 to 8 hours after it's administered. Unlike bulk-forming laxatives, stimulant laxatives act directly on the intestinal mucosa and commonly result in gripping and loose stools.

Anthraquinones stimulate active chloride secretion and increase the amount of water and electrolytes discharged into the large intestine and passed in stool. The motility of the colon is increased as stationary and stimulating propulsive contractions are inhibited, thereby resulting in faster bowel movements. Buckthorn is available as capsules, fluid extract, liquid formulations, and tablets. It's also an ingredient in various teas.

Reported uses
Buckthorn is used as a laxative to treat constipation and to ease bowel evacuation in those who have anal fissures or hemorrhoids, and in those who have had rectal-anal surgery. It's also used orally to treat cancer. Buckthorn is also used as a tonic. Extracts of buckthorn bark are used topically in sunscreen products.

Administration
- Daily dose: Based on the quantity of its key component anthranoid, not on the quantity of dry herb; average daily dose based on hydroxyanthracine content is 20 to 180 mg; however, some sources list the daily dose as 20 to 30 mg of hydroxyanthracine derivative, calculated as glucofrangulin A
- Tea: Prepared by pouring boiling water over 2 g (1 teaspoon equals about 2.4 g; 1 scant teaspoon, 2 g) of finely ground herb and straining after 10 to 15 minutes
- Cold infusion: Prepared by letting the herb steep for 12 hours at room temperature.

Hazards
Overuse or abuse of buckthorn may interfere with the effects of antiarrhythmics because of potassium loss and may po-

tentiate the adverse effects of cardiac glycosides because of potassium loss. When buckthorn is used with corticosteroids or thiazide diuretics, there is an increased risk of hypokalemia, which may cause arrhythmias. The use of buckthorn and licorice may increase the risk of hypokalemia. The risk of hypokalemia is increased when buckthorn is used with potassium-wasting herbs such as horsetail herb or stimulant laxative herbs such as aloe, black root, blue flag rhizome, butternut bark, cascara sagrada bark, castor oil, colocynth fruit pulp, gamboge bark exudate, jalap root, manna bark exudate, podophyllum root, rhubarb root, senna leaves and pods, wild cumber fruit (*Ecballium elaterium*), and yellow dock root.

Buckthorn may be associated with GI cramping or gripping and dark yellow or red urine. Those with intestinal obstruction, abdominal pain of unknown origin, or acute inflammatory intestinal disease including appendicitis, colitis, Crohn's disease, and irritable bowel syndrome, should avoid using buckthorn. Pregnant and breast-feeding patients and children younger than age 12 should also avoid use. Those with fluid or electrolyte imbalances should use buckthorn with caution because long-term use or abuse can cause hypokalemia and loss of fluid.

Clinical considerations

■ If buckthorn is being used as a laxative, the dosage should be individualized to the smallest dose required to produce a soft stool.
■ Suggest that the patient try lifestyle changes — such as increasing dietary fiber and fluid intake and increasing exercise — to restore normal bowel function. Using a bulk laxative may also be preferable to using buckthorn.
■ Patient shouldn't use buckthorn for longer than 2 weeks without consulting his health care provider because overuse can cause intestinal sluggishness and loss of fluid and electrolytes, especially potassium. Consequences of chronic hypoka-

lemia include aggravated constipation, accelerated bone deterioration, nephropathies, albuminuria, hematuria, damage to the renal tubules, heart function disorders, and muscular weakness, especially when patient is also taking a cardiac glycoside or a diuretic.
■ Buckthorn takes effect 6 to 8 hours after it's administered, so it isn't suitable for rapid emptying of the bowels.
■ Patients with diarrhea or abdominal pain of unknown origin shouldn't use buckthorn.
■ If patient experiences adverse GI effects, advise him to reduce the dosage. If he experiences diarrhea or watery stools, he should stop using buckthorn.
■ It's unknown if the anthranoid level in buckthorn is high enough to cause diarrhea in breast-feeding infants.
■ Buckthorn may cause precancerous pigment changes in the intestinal mucosa.
■ Warn patient not to exceed the recommended dose. Signs and symptoms of overdose include vomiting and severe GI spasms.
■ Warn patient not to delay seeking appropriate medical evaluation because doing so may delay diagnosis of a potentially serious medical condition.
■ Advise patient who is pregnant or breast-feeding, or planning pregnancy, to avoid use.
■ Tell female patient to report planned or suspected pregnancy to her health care provider.
■ Inform patient that many so-called dieter's teas contain buckthorn.
■ Tell patient to remind prescriber and pharmacist of any herbal or dietary supplement that he's taking when obtaining a new prescription.
■ Advise patient to consult his health care provider before using an herbal preparation because a treatment with proven efficacy may be available.

Research summary
The concepts behind the use of buckthorn and the claims made regarding its

effects have not yet been validated scientifically.

bugleweed

Archangel, green ashangee, gypsy weed, gypsywort, Lycopus europaeus, L. virginicus, Paul's betony, sweet bugle, Virginia water horehound, water bugle, water hoarhound, wolf's foot, wolfstrappkraut

Bugleweed consists of the fresh or dried leaves and tops of *Lycopus europaeus* or *L. virginicus.* It contains flavonoids and hydrocinnamic and caffeic acid derivatives, including rosmaric acid, lithospermic acid, and their oligomerics, which are created through oxidation.

Bugleweed may have antithyrotropic activity — specifically, it may inhibit peripheral deiodination of thyroxine (T_4). Herb may also have hypoglycemic and antigonadotropic activity and may also decrease serum prolactin levels. Bugleweed is available as capsules, freshly pressed juice, powdered herb, tea, water-ethanol extract, and other galenic preparations for internal use, in products such as Bugleweed Herb Vcaps.

Reported uses
Bugleweed is used for mild hyperthyroidism, nervousness, insomnia, premenstrual syndrome, and breast pain. Tinctures and infusions were once used to decrease bleeding of menorrhagia and nosebleeds.

Administration
■ Teas: 1 to 2 g by mouth every day
■ Water-ethanol extracts: Equivalent of 20 mg of herb by mouth every day.

Hazards
Bugleweed may be associated with enlargement of the thyroid and increased prolactin secretion. Use of bugleweed with insulin or oral antidiabetics may increase the risk of hypoglycemia. It may interfere with iodine's metabolism, and may reduce the effectiveness of thyroid hormones, blocking peripheral conversion of thyroxine (T_4) to triiodothyronine (T_3). Bugleweed may produce additive effects if used with thyroid-suppressing herbs such as balm leaf and wild thyme plant.

Those with hypothyroidism or thyroid enlargement without functional disturbance and those receiving other thyroid treatments should avoid use. Pregnant and breast-feeding patients should also avoid use.

Clinical considerations
■ Because every patient's optimal level of thyroid hormone is different, the dosages provided are only rough estimates. Patient age and weight should be considered when determining dose.
■ Bugleweed may interfere with blood glucose control and may cause hypoglycemia. Monitor blood glucose level if patient has hypoglycemia or diabetes.
■ Bugleweed therapy shouldn't be stopped abruptly because sudden withdrawal can lead to increased prolactin secretion or exacerbation of the disorder being treated. Advise patient to discontinue bugleweed gradually unless a health care provider has directed otherwise.
■ Bugleweed may interfere with diagnostic procedures using radioisotopes.
■ Advise patient with hyperthyroidism to consult a health care provider for treatment. If patient is using other thyroid treatments, advise him not to use bugleweed.
■ If patient is pregnant or breast-feeding or is planning pregnancy, advise her not to use bugleweed, unless a health care provider who's an expert in the appropriate use of this herb has directed otherwise.
■ Tell patient to remind prescriber and pharmacist of any herbal or dietary supplement that he's taking when obtaining a new prescription.

■ Advise patient to consult his health care provider before using an herbal preparation because a treatment with proven efficacy may be available.

Research summary
Several very preliminary studies suggest that bugleweed may be helpful for treating mild hyperthyroidism.

burdock

Arctium lappa, A. minus, A. tomentosum, *Bardana, bardane root, beggar's buttons, burr seed, clot-bur, cocklebur, cockle buttons, edible burdock, fox's clote, great burr, happy major, hardock, hareburr, lappa, lappa root, love leaves, personata, philanthropium, thorny burr*

Burdock consists of the fresh or dried, first-year root of great burdock, *Arctium lappa*; common burdock, *A. minus*; or woolly burdock, *A. tomentosum*. The leaves and fruits may also be used. Burdock contains volatile oil, fatty oil, sucrose, resin, tannin, and large amounts of the carbohydrate inulin. Active constituents include podophyllin-type lignan derivatives and guanidinobutyric acid.

The fresh root and root extracts may have mild bacteriostatic and fungistatic activity and may also stimulate the flow of bile from the gallbladder to the duodenum. Polyacetylenes, specifically, arctiopiricin, may be responsible for the gram-positive and gram-negative antimicrobial properties.

Burdock may have antimutagenic, antitumorigenic, hypoglycemic, and uterine stimulant activity, and it may increase carbohydrate tolerance. The hypoglycemic and antimutagenic component may be a polyanionic, lignan-like compound. It's speculated that guanidinobutyric acid, a substance found in fruit extracts

derived from burdock, may be responsible for its hypoglycemic activity.

Burdock may also have antipyretic, diuretic, and diaphoretic properties. It may inhibit human immunodeficiency virus-1infection, antagonize platelet activating factor, prevent tumors, and affect the digestion of dietary fiber.

Burdock is available as capsules, liquid extract, fresh root, tinctures, and various topical formulations for cosmetic and toiletry products. It's available in products such as Arth Plus Capsules, Catarrh Mixture (oral liquid), Potter's G.B. Tablets, Gerard House Blue Flag Root Compound Tablets, Seven Seas Rheumatic Pain Tablets, Skin Eruptions Mixture (oral liquid), and Tabritis Tablets.

Reported uses
Burdock is used orally to treat cancers, renal or urinary calculi, GI tract disorders, constipation, catarrh, fever, infection, gout, arthritis, and fluid retention. It's also used as a blood purifier, diaphoretic, and aphrodisiac.

Burdock is used topically to promote healing and to treat skin conditions such as hair loss, dandruff, eczema, scaly skin, psoriasis, acne, and dry skin.

In traditional Chinese medicine, the burdock fruit is commonly combined with other herbs to treat colds, sore throat, tonsillitis, coughs, sores, and abscesses. In Asia, the root is considered a nutritious element of the daily diet.

Administration
■ Liquid extract (1:1 in 25% alcohol): 2 to 8 ml by mouth three times a day
■ Oral: 2 to 6 g of dried root by mouth three times a day
■ Tea: Prepared by placing 1 to 2.5 g (1 teaspoon equals 2 g) of finely chopped or coarsely powdered herb into 5 oz of boiling water for 10 to 15 minutes, then straining; consumed three times a day
■ Tincture (1:10 in 45% alcohol): 8 to 12 ml by mouth three times a day.

Hazards

SAFETY RISK *Burdock root closely resembles the toxic Atropa belladonna, commonly known as deadly nightshade root. For this reason, burdock should be used only when the fresh root or greens are collected by an expert with sufficient botanical knowledge. Advise patient to immediately report symptoms of belladonna toxicity: blurred vision, headache, drowsiness, slurred speech, loss of coordination, incoherent speech, restlessness, hallucinations, hyperactivity, seizures, disorientation, flushing, dry mouth and nose, rash, lack of sweating, and fever.*

Burdock may be associated with headache, drowsiness, slurred speech, loss of coordination, incoherent speech, restlessness, hallucinations, hyperactivity, seizures, disorientation, flushing, blurred vision, dryness of mouth and nose, rash, lack of sweating, allergic dermatitis (topical), and fever. It is possible, however, that these adverse effects — with the exception of allergic dermatitis — are actually associated with atropine contamination rather than with burdock itself.

Herbal products prepared with alcohol may cause a disulfiram-like reaction. Additive effects may occur when burdock is used with alcohol-containing products.

Burdock used in conjunction with insulin or oral antidiabetics may interfere with control of blood glucose level. Pregnant patients should avoid use because it may cause uterine contractions; breastfeeding patients, because it isn't known whether herb appears in breast milk.

Patients allergic to ragweed, chrysanthemums, marigolds, and daisies should use burdock with caution.

Clinical considerations

■ Monitor patient for signs of atropine toxicity as it's easy for an inexperienced herbalist to mistake burdock for the poisonous belladonna.

■ Liquid extract and tincture contain alcohol and may be inappropriate for alcoholic patients or those with liver disease.

■ Burdock may cause or exacerbate hypoglycemia. Dosage of insulin or antidiabetic may need to be adjusted. Instruct patient with diabetes or hypoglycemia to monitor his blood glucose level closely.

■ Warn patient not to delay seeking appropriate medical evaluation because doing so may delay treatment of a potentially serious medical condition.

■ If patient is pregnant or breast-feeding or is planning pregnancy, advise her not to use burdock.

■ Instruct patient to report any allergic symptoms to his health care provider.

■ Inform patient that some liquid formulations contain alcohol.

■ Tell patient to remind prescriber and pharmacist of any herbal or dietary supplement that he's taking when obtaining a new prescription.

■ Advise patient to consult his health care provider before using an herbal preparation because a treatment with proven efficacy may be available.

Research summary

German Commission E lists burdock as an unapproved herb and doesn't recommend its use because of a lack of data. None of the fresh herb's adverse properties have yet been proven to exist in the dried commercial product.

butcher's broom

Box holly, Jew's myrtle, knee holly, kneeholm, pettigree, Ruscus aculeatus, *sweet broom*

Butcher's broom consists of the dried rhizome and root of *Ruscus aculeatus,* an evergreen shrub native to the Mediterranean. It contains the steroid saponins ruscin, ruscoside, aglycones, neuruscogenin, and ruscogenin, and benzofuranes such as euparone and ruscodibenzofurane. Ruscogenin and neoruscogenin cause vasoconstriction by directly stimulating postjunctional alpha$_1$ and alpha$_2$

receptors of the smooth-muscle cells in the vascular wall. Two other steroid saponins may have cytostatic activity on a leukemic cell line.

Butcher's broom has diuretic, antipyretic, and anti-inflammatory properties. It may also be effective in treating venous disorders. Butcher's broom is available as capsules, extracts, ointments, and suppositories.

Reported uses
Butcher's broom is used extensively in Europe to treat circulatory disorders and has gained popularity in the United States. It's used orally to treat conditions of venous insufficiency such as pain, cramps, heaviness, and itching and swelling in the legs. It's also used to prevent atherosclerosis, to help mend broken bones, and as a laxative, diuretic, and anti-inflammatory.

Ointments and suppositories containing butcher's broom are used to relieve itching and burning from hemorrhoids. In early cultures, the asparagus-like shoots of butcher's broom were eaten as a food.

Administration
- Raw extract: 7 to 11 mg by mouth every day based on the total ruscogenin content (determined as the sum of neoruscogenin and ruscogenin components)
- Root powder: 100 to 3,000 mg by mouth every day.

Hazards
Butcher's broom may cause GI discomfort and nausea.

There are no known interactions with butcher's broom.

As a precaution, pregnant and breast-feeding patients should avoid use.

Clinical considerations
 SAFETY RISK *Don't confuse butcher's broom with Scotch broom or broom* (Cytisus scoparius L.) *or Spanish broom* (Spartium junceum L.).

- Warn patient not to delay seeking appropriate medical evaluation because doing so may delay treatment of a potentially serious medical condition.
- If patient is pregnant or breast-feeding, advise her to avoid use.
- Advise patient not to use butcher's broom in conjunction with other treatments for circulatory disorders without consulting his health care provider.
- Inform patient that although products containing butcher's broom may claim to be effective for treating circulatory problems of the legs, these products aren't FDA approved and may be ineffective for these conditions.
- Tell patient to remind prescriber and pharmacist of any herbal or dietary supplement that he's taking when obtaining a new prescription.
- Advise patient to consult his health care provider before using an herbal preparation because a treatment with proven efficacy may be available.

Research summary
Preliminary evidence from animal studies suggests that butcher's broom possesses anti-inflammatory properties and also constricts small veins. One small, double-blind study in 40 humans found improvements in vein function.

butterbur

Bladderdock, bog rhubarb, bogshorns, butter-dock, butterfly dock, capdockin, flapperdock, fuki, langwort, petasites, Petasites hybridus, *umbrella leaves*

Butterbur is derived from the rhizome, or rootstock, and leaves of the perennial shrub *Petasites hybridus.* It contains sesquiterpene lactones such as pestacins, angelicoyleneopetasol, fukione, and fukinolide. The antispasmodic and analgesic actions may result from the effects of pestacins on prostaglandin synthesis. Butterbur also contains volatile oils, pectin, mucilage, inulin flavonoids, and tannins.

Butterbur contains pyrrizolidine alkaloids, which are carcinogens and hepatotoxins. Butterbur is available as capsules, dried herb, and dried root in products such as Petadolex Standardized Extract.

Reported uses

Butterbur is used as an antispasmodic and analgesic. As an antispasmodic, it's used to treat urinary tract spasms, mild kidney stone disease, bile flow obstruction, dysmenorrhea, colic, bronchospasm, and cough. As an analgesic, it's used for backache, tension, and migraine headache.

Administration

- Capsules containing 50 mg of butterbur root extract — for example, Petadolex: 50 mg by mouth two times a day for migraine headache
- GI disorders: 5 to 7 g of dried herb by mouth every day.

Hazards

 SAFETY RISK *Butterbur's pyrrizolidine alkaloids are known hepatotoxins and carcinogens.*

Butterbur may be associated with sedation, hepatotoxicity, and cancer. It may have added anticholinergic adverse effects if used with antihistamines, atropine, phenothiazines, scopolamine, and tricyclic antidepressants.

If patient is pregnant or breast-feeding or has liver disease, butterbur is contraindicated because of its pyrrizolidine alkaloid content and antispasmodic effect.

Clinical considerations

- Because the pyrrizolidine alkaloids in butterbur are toxic, advise patient not to use herb for longer than 4 to 6 weeks annually.
- Monitor liver function, as indicated. Warn patient that many references discourage the use of oral butterbur because of liver toxicity associated with the primary component (pyrrizolidine alkaloid).
- Instruct patient to stop using butterbur immediately if he experiences skin discoloration, abdominal pain, nausea, or vomiting.
- Butterbur may be unsafe for children.
- If patient is pregnant or breast-feeding or is planning pregnancy, advise her not to use butterbur.
- Warn the patient not to delay treatment for an illness that doesn't resolve after taking butterbur.
- Tell patient to remind prescriber and pharmacist of any herbal or dietary supplement that he's taking when obtaining a new prescription.
- Advise patient to consult his health care provider before using an herbal preparation because a treatment with proven efficacy may be available.

Research summary

One German study showed a reduction in migraine severity and frequency after 4 weeks' treatment with butterbur. It suggests that patients with migraine may benefit from Petadolex prophylactic treatment.

cacao

Chocolate, cocoa, cocoa butter,
cocoa seed, cocoa seed coat,
Theobroma cacao

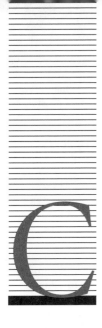

Cacao seed from the cacao tree is roasted, then pressed to extract cocoa butter,
also known as theobroma oil. The remaining cocoa cake is ground into cocoa
powder. Cacao contains 0.5% to 2.7%
theobromine, 0.25% caffeine, and other
methylxanthine alkaloids. Cocoa contains the antioxidant catechin. Unsweetened dark chocolate contains 47 mg of
caffeine and 450 mg of theobromine per
ounce. Milk chocolate contains about
6 mg caffeine and 45 mg of theobromine
per ounce. Theobromine has weaker
stimulant effects than caffeine but is a
more potent diuretic, cardiovascular
stimulant, and coronary dilator.

Reported uses
Cocoa powder and cocoa butter are
widely used in food products; cocoa butter is also used as a base for moisturizers,
cosmetics, and suppositories.
    Cocoa seed and cocoa seed coat are
used to treat intestinal conditions; diarrhea; liver, bladder and renal disease; diabetes; and others.

Administration
Dosage varies with the preparation.

Hazards
Adverse effects associated with cacao include central nervous system (CNS)
stimulation, tremor, insomnia, anxiety,

tachycardia, aggravation of GI ulcers, irritable bowel syndrome, and exacerbation of gastroesophageal reflux disease.

Interactions are possible between cacao and the following:

- acetaminophen, aspirin — increased analgesic effects due to caffeine in cacao
- alendronate — decreased alendronate bioavailability
- barbiturates — decreased caffeine effects because of increased metabolism and CNS depression
- beta agonists, such as albuterol, isoproterenol, or terbutaline — increased CNS and cardiovascular stimulation
- cimetidine, disulfiram, fluoroquinolones (such as ciprofloxacin, enoxacin, or norfloxacin), mexiletine, oral contraceptives — increased caffeine effects due to decreased metabolism
- clozapine — increased clozapine levels due to caffeine, increasing the risk of adverse reactions
- iron, zinc — decreased vitamin absorption
- lithium — increased lithium clearance
- monoamine oxidase (MAO) inhibitors, such as isocarboxazid, phenelzine, or tranylcypromine — possibly, hypertensive crisis with excessive caffeine intake
- phenylpropanolamine — increased caffeine effects due to additive sympathomimetic action (reports of manic psychosis with high doses of caffeine)
- terbinafine — increased caffeine effects due to decreased metabolism
- theophylline — decreased theophylline levels with excessive caffeine intake
- verapamil — increased caffeine effects due to decreased metabolism
- caffeine-containing herbs and herbal sympathomimetics, such as coffee, cola nut, ephedra, guarana, maté and tea, Ma huang — possibly, increased stimulant effects of cocoa products
- grapefruit juice — possibly, increased caffeine effects.

There are no known studies or reports regarding the effects of excessive chocolate consumption during pregnancy.

However, theobromine has been shown to be teratogenic in animals when given in doses dozens to hundreds of times the equivalent of normal human consumption of chocolate. High doses of caffeine —more than 300 mg per day—have been associated with lower birth weight and higher risk of spontaneous abortion in some studies. Caffeine appears in small amounts in breast milk.

Clinical considerations

- Caffeine may interfere with phenobarbital and serum uric acid assay.
- Because cacao may caused decreased absorption of vitamins such as iron or zinc, these supplements should be taken 2 hours either before or after cacao.
- Cocoa butter may be allergenic and comedogenic.
- A suggested link between cacao use and migraine and tension headache is controversial.
- Use of cacao may worsen symptoms of irritable bowel syndrome.
- Chocolate contains relatively low amounts of caffeine compared with other food sources.
- Advise pregnant or breast-feeding patient to avoid excessive chocolate consumption.
- Instruct patient to promptly report adverse effects.
- Inform patient not to delay treatment for an illness that doesn't resolve after taking cacao.
- Tell patient to remind prescriber and pharmacist of any herbal or dietary supplement that he's taking when obtaining a new prescription.
- Advise patient to consult his health care provider before using an herbal preparation because a treatment with proven efficacy may be available.

Research summary

The concepts behind the use of cacao for medicinal purposes and the claims made regarding its effects have not yet been validated scientifically. One recent study found no evidence of a relationship between the consumption of chocolate and coronary heart disease.

capsicum

African chilies, bird pepper, capsaicin, Capsicum annuum, C. frutescens, *cayenne, chili pepper, goat's pod, grains of Paradise, Mexican chilies, paprika, pimiento, red pepper, tabasco pepper, Zanzibar pepper*

The active component of capsicum, capsaicin, is isolated from the membrane and seeds of Capsicum peppers. Topically applied capsaicin depletes the neurotransmitter substance P from peripheral sensory neurons and blocks its synthesis and transport. Substance P is involved in transmitting pain and itch sensations from the periphery to the central nervous system and may have vasodilating effects. Capsaicin's effects may be similar to cutting or ligating a nerve.

Oral capsicum may inhibit gastric basal acid output and may inhibit platelet aggregation, but it doesn't alter prothrombin time or partial thromboplastin time. High-dose capsicum therapy may decrease coagulation (because of higher antithrombin III levels), lower plasma fibrinogen levels, and increase fibrinolytic activity. Capsaicin is highly irritating to mucous membranes and eyes.

Capsaicin is available for both oral and topical use in products such as cayenne pepper capsules, extract, and various topical preparations.

Reported uses

The FDA has approved topical capsaicin for temporary relief of pain from rheumatoid arthritis, osteoarthritis, postherpetic neuralgia (shingles), and diabetic neuropathy. It's being tested for treatment of psoriasis, intractable pruritus, vitiligo, phantom limb pain, mastectomy pain, Guillain-Barré syndrome, neurogenic bladder, vulvar vestibulitis,

apocrine chromhidrosis, and reflex sympathetic dystrophy. It's also used in personal defense sprays.

Oral capsicum is used for various GI complaints, including dyspepsia, flatulence, ulcers, and stomach cramps. It's used to treat hypertension and improve circulation. It's also used in some weight-loss and metabolic-enhancement products.

Administration

■ Oral: In some cultures, adults ingest up to 3 g by mouth every day of capsicum as a seasoning for various foods
■ Topical: For adults and children ages 2 years and older, capsicum is applied topically to affected area no more than three or four times a day. Hands should be washed immediately after capsicum application.

Hazards

Adverse effects associated with the use of capsicum include eye irritation, corneal abrasion, oral burning, diarrhea, gingival irritation, bleeding gums, cough, bronchospasm, respiratory irritation, burning sensation, stinging sensation, erythema, and contact dermatitis.

Risk of cough increases when capsicum is applied topically in patients who are on angiotensin-converting enzyme inhibitors. Capsicum may alter anticoagulant effects of anticoagulant and antiplatelet drugs. It may reduce bioavailability of aspirin and salicylic acid compounds. By increasing stomach acid, capsicum may also interfere with antacids, sucralfate, H_2 antagonists, or proton-pump inhibitors.

Herbal products prepared with alcohol may cause a disulfiram-like reaction. Absorption of theophylline may increase when the drug is administered with capsicum. Use of cayenne with anticoagulant or antiplatelet herbs (feverfew, garlic, ginger, ginkgo, and ginseng) may increase cayenne's anticoagulant effects, thus increasing bleeding tendencies.

Pregnant patients should avoid use because capsicum's effects on the fetus aren't known. Those who are breast-feeding and those with hypersensitivity to capsicum should also avoid use. Patients with irritable bowel syndrome should avoid use because of capsaicin's irritant and peristaltic effects.

 SAFETY RISK *Patients with asthma who use capsicum may experience bronchospasm.*

Clinical considerations

■ Alcoholic extracts may be unsuitable for children, alcoholic patients, patients with liver disease, and those taking disulfiram or metronidazole.

■ Topical capsaicin shouldn't be used on broken or irritated skin or covered with a tight bandage.

■ Adverse skin reactions to topical capsaicin are treated by washing the area thoroughly with soap and water. Soaking the area in vegetable oil after washing provides a slower onset but longer duration of relief than cold water. Vinegar water irrigation is moderately successful. Rubbing alcohol may also help. An emulsion of lidocaine and prilocaine provides pain relief in about 1 hour to skin that has been severely irritated by capsaicin.

 SAFETY RISK *Capsicum shouldn't be taken orally for longer than 2 days and then shouldn't be used again for 2 weeks.*

■ If patient is pregnant or breast-feeding or is planning pregnancy, advise her not to use this herb.

■ If patient is applying capsicum topically, inform him that it may take 1 to 2 weeks for him to experience maximum pain control.

■ Instruct patient to wash his hands before and immediately after applying topical capsaicin and to avoid contact with eyes and nose. Advise contact lens wearer to wash his hands and to use gloves or an applicator if handling his lenses after applying capsicum. If capsicum comes in contact with mucous membranes, advise flushing area with milk or water.

■ Inform patient not to delay treatment for an illness that doesn't resolve after taking capsicum. If he's applying it topically, advise him to contact his health care provider promptly if his condition worsens or if symptoms persist for 2 to 4 weeks.

■ Tell patient to store capsicum in a tightly sealed container, away from light.

■ Eating bananas may help with GI irritation from oral capsicum or cayenne pepper.

■ Tell patient to remind prescriber and pharmacist of any herbal or dietary supplement that he's taking when obtaining a new prescription.

■ Advise patient to consult his health care provider before using an herbal preparation because a treatment with proven efficacy may be available.

Research summary

Much clinical research has focused on the topical use of capsicum-containing products for temporary relief of pain. A recent study has shown that capsicum nasal drops may be beneficial in the treatment of cluster headaches. A few other studies have investigated topical capsicum for the treatment of psoriasis. All of these studies showed some positive results, but further investigation is warranted before recommending topical capsicum as an over-the-counter treatment.

caraway

Caraway seed, Carum carvi

Caraway contains a volatile oil that produces its characteristic taste and smell. It contains carvole and d-limonene (carvene), which may be active against GI discomfort. Caraway may also have weak antispasmodic activity. It's available as dried fruit and seed, alcohol-containing extract, and tincture.

Reported uses
Caraway is most commonly used as a spice. It's also used to treat GI upset, nausea, flatulence, bloating, menstrual discomfort, and incontinence; to promote lactation; and to stimulate appetite.

Caraway oil is used to make liqueurs, such as aquavit, and herbal mouthwashes.

Administration
- Dried fruit: 1.5 to 6.0 g/day, by mouth
- Extract: 3 or 4 gtt in liquid three to four times a day, by mouth
- Seeds: Chew 1 teaspoon three to four times a day
- Tea (prepared by adding 1 to 2 teaspoons of freshly crushed fruit to 5 oz of boiling water for 5 to 10 minutes): For adults, 1 cup two to four times a day by mouth, between meals; for children, 1 teaspoon
- Tincture: ½ to 1 teaspoon every day, up to three times a day, by mouth.

Hazards
Use of caraway may be associated with contact dermatitis. Herbal products prepared with alcohol may cause a disulfiram-like reaction.

Pregnant and breast-feeding patients should avoid using caraway, even in food, because of its antispasmodic effects.

Clinical considerations
- Many tinctures contain between 15% and 90% alcohol and may be unsuitable for children, alcoholic patients, patients with liver disease, and those taking disulfiram or metronidazole.
- Because the active component of caraway isn't water soluble, extracts and tinctures may be more effective than teas.
- If patient is pregnant, advise her not to use caraway.
- Inform patient not to delay treatment for an illness that doesn't resolve after taking caraway.
- Instruct patient to promptly report adverse reactions or new signs or symptoms.

- Tell patient to remind prescriber and pharmacist of any herbal or dietary supplement that he's taking when obtaining a new prescription.
- Advise patient to consult his health care provider before using an herbal preparation because a treatment with proven efficacy may be available.

Research summary
Both caraway seed and caraway oil have been approved by the German Commission E for use in mild dyspeptic conditions, flatulence, and GI fullness. A few German studies have shown clinically significant positive effects of a fixed caraway-peppermint oil preparation on gastroduodenal motility and non-ulcer dyspepsia.

cardamom
Elettaria cardamomum

Cardamom is obtained from the dried, almost ripened fruit of *Elettaria cardamomum*. Only the seeds of the fruit and the oils obtained from the seeds are used to prepare supplements. The active ingredients of cardamom are believed to be the seed's volatile oils, consisting primarily of cineol, alpha-terponyl acetate, and linalyl acetate. Cardamom may have antiviral properties. It's available as ground seeds and as a tincture.

Reported uses
Cardamom is used to soothe the stomach and treat dyspepsia. It's also used for its antispasmodic, antiflatulent, and motility-enhancing effects, making it potentially useful in other GI conditions.

Administration
- Ground seeds: Average daily dose is 1.5 g by mouth
- Tincture: 1 fluid dram per day, by mouth.

Hazards

Use of cardamom may be associated with gallstone colic. Herbal products prepared with alcohol may cause a disulfiram-like reaction.

Patients with gallstones should avoid use. Pregnant and breast-feeding patients should avoid use.

Clinical considerations

■ Tinctures may contain a significant amount of alcohol, making them unsuitable for children, alcoholic patients, and patients with liver disease.

■ Warn patient not to treat symptoms of gastric distress with cardamom before seeking appropriate medical evaluation because doing so may delay diagnosis of a potentially serious medical condition.

■ Instruct patient to promptly report adverse reactions and new signs or symptoms.

■ Tell patient to remind prescriber and pharmacist of any herbal or dietary supplement that he's taking when obtaining a new prescription.

■ Advise patient to consult his health care provider before using an herbal preparation because a treatment with proven efficacy may be available.

Research summary

The concepts behind the use of cardamom for medicinal purposes and the claims made regarding its effects have not yet been validated scientifically.

carline thistle

Carlina acaulis, *dwarf carline, ground thistle, southernwood root*

Carline thistle is obtained from the dried root of the *Carlina acaulis* plant. The root is used to prepare tea, wine, and tinctures that may be used internally or externally. The acetone extract and the essential oils found in the root of carline thistle are believed to possess antibacterial properties that seem to hinder the growth of *Staphylococcus aureus*.

Reported uses

Carline thistle is used orally to treat gallbladder disease, digestive problems, and alimentary tract spasms. It may also act as a mild diuretic and cause diaphoresis.

Externally, carline thistle has been used to treat dermatosis, rinse wounds and ulcers and, when used as a gargle, to alleviate symptoms associated with cancer of the tongue.

Administration

■ Tea: 3 cups every day; prepared by steeping 3 g of finely cut dried root in 5 oz of boiling water for 5 to 10 minutes

■ Tincture: 40 to 50 gtt 4 to 5 times every day, by mouth; prepared by steeping 20 g of chopped root in 80 g of 60% ethanol for 10 days

■ Topical preparation: Prepared by adding 30 g of dried root to 1 quart of boiling water, boiling for 5 to 10 minutes, then straining

■ Wine: 1 small glass before meals; prepared by steeping 50 g of the dried root in 1 quart of white wine for a minimum of 12 days.

Hazards

Adverse effects associated with carline thistle include allergic reactions. Herbal products prepared with alcohol may cause a disulfiram-like reaction.

Pregnant and breast-feeding patients should avoid use.

Clinical considerations

■ Patients with a history of seasonal allergies may be more likely to experience a hypersensitivity reaction.

■ Advise patient to seek medical attention immediately if he suspects he's having an allergic reaction to the herb. Instruct him to promptly report other adverse reactions or new signs and symptoms.

■ Wine and tincture preparations contain significant amounts of alcohol, mak-

ing them unsuitable for children, alcoholic patients, and patients with liver disease.
■ Encourage patient to consider other treatment options because little information about the safety and efficacy of carline thistle exists.
■ Tell patient to remind prescriber and pharmacist of any herbal or dietary supplement that he's taking when obtaining a new prescription.
■ Advise patient to consult his health care provider before using an herbal preparation because a treatment with proven efficacy may be available.

Research summary

The concepts behind the use of carline thistle and the claims made regarding its effects have not yet been validated scientifically.

carob

Ceratonia siliqua, *locust bean, locust pods, St. John's bread, sugar pods*

The fruit and seeds of the *Ceratonia siliqua* are used to prepare dry carob extracts. Carob is believed to act as a dietary binding drug and antidiarrheal; the exact mechanism of action is unknown. It's rich in dietary fiber and polyphenols. Because carob increases the viscosity of GI contents, it may have hypoglycemic and hypolipidemic effects.

Reported uses

Carob is used orally to treat acute nutritional disorders, diarrhea, obesity, dyspepsia, enterocolitis, sprue, and celiac disease. It's also used for vomiting and gastroesophageal reflux in infants and during pregnancy.

Carob can be found in health food products for weight loss and energy and as a chocolate substitute. Carob flour and extracts are used as flavoring agents in foods and beverages.

Administration

Oral use: 20 to 30 g of carob added to water, tea, or milk and consumed throughout the day.

Hazards

Inhaled carob powder can cause allergic rhinitis and asthma. There are no known interactions with carob.

Pregnant and breast-feeding patients should consult their health care provider before use.

Clinical considerations

 SAFETY RISK *Don't confuse this product with Carob tree,* Jacaranda procera, *or* Jacaranda caroba.
■ Warn patient not to treat a vomiting infant with carob before seeking appropriate medical evaluation because doing so may delay diagnosis of a potentially serious medical condition.
■ Discuss with patient other options for treating diarrhea or GI complaints.
■ Instruct patient to promptly report adverse reactions and new signs and symptoms.
■ Tell patient to remind prescriber and pharmacist of any herbal or dietary supplement that he's taking when obtaining a new prescription.
■ Advise patient to consult his health care provider before using an herbal preparation because a treatment with proven efficacy may be available.

Research summary

Carob has been studied as an ingredient in pediatric formula for the treatment of symptomatic gastroesophageal reflux with some positive results. One study demonstrated that a mixture of Gaviscon (aluminum hydroxide 80 mg and magnesium trisilicate 20 mg) plus a carob seed powder (Carobel) was more effective than the prescription medication cisapride. Another Swiss trial studied carob as a treatment for traveler's diarrhea and concluded that although carob treatment showed some positive results, they weren't clinically significant.

cascara sagrada

Bitter bark, buckthorn, chittem bark,
Frangula purshiana, *purshiana bark,*
Rhamni purshianae *cortex, sacred bark,*
yellow bark

Cascara sagrada is obtained from the dried bark of *Rhamni purshianae;* the bark must be aged 1 year or heat treated before use. Anthraglycosides, or anthraquinones, which consist primarily of cascarosides A and B, are the active ingredients.

Cascara is referred to as a stimulant laxative. When ingested, the herb causes the secretion of water and electrolytes into the small intestine. In the large intestine, the absorption of these products is inhibited, allowing the contents of the bowel to grow in volume. This increased volume then stimulates peristalsis and advances the bowel contents quickly through the large intestine for evacuation. Cascara may also have antileukemic properties. Historically, cascara has also been used for gallstones, liver ailments, and as a bitter tonic.

Cascara sagrada is available as cut bark, powder, and dry extract.

Reported uses

Cascara sagrada is used mainly as a stimulant laxative to treat constipation; the FDA has approved the herb for this use. It's also used to make teas, decoctions, elixirs, for cold maceration, and as a sunscreen in cosmetic products.

Administration

■ To treat constipation: 20 to 70 mg of hydroxyanthracene derivatives (calculated as cascaroside A) from the cut bark, powder, or dry extract, taken by mouth every day. Tea prepared by steeping 2 g of finely cut bark in 5 oz of boiling water for 5 to 10 minutes, then straining. Correct dose is the smallest necessary to maintain soft stools.

Hazards

SAFETY RISK *Prolonged use of cascara sagrada may lead to arrhythmias.*

Adverse effects of cascara sagrada include abdominal cramping, abdominal discomfort, vomiting, bloody diarrhea, albuminuria, hematuria, potassium deficiency, weight loss, and dermatitis. Colic and kidney irritation may result from intake of fresh rind.

Long-term use of cascara may lead to hypokalemia, which may enhance digoxin action. Concomitant use of cascara and laxatives increases the likelihood of diarrhea and fluid or electrolyte disturbances. There is an increased risk of potassium depletion if cascara is used with potassium-sparing diuretics and corticosteroids. There is an increased risk of potassium depletion if cascara is used with licorice root.

Those with intestinal obstruction, ulcerative colitis, appendicitis, abdominal pain of unknown origin, diarrhea, or acute intestinal inflammation, such as Crohn's disease, should avoid use of cascara sagrada. Children younger than age 12 and pregnant or breast-feeding patients should also avoid use.

Clinical considerations

■ Liquid and solid forms of cascara sagrada are for oral use only.
■ Effects are generally seen within 6 to 8 hours.
■ Tell patient not to begin using cascara if he's experiencing abdominal pain or diarrhea.
■ Advise patient that cascara isn't intended for long-term use and that he shouldn't use it for longer than 10 days without medical advice. Long-term use may cause hypokalemia that can lead to cardiac problems and muscle weakness. It may also cause lazy bowel, an inability to move bowels without a laxative.
■ *Pseudomelanosis coli,* a harmless pigmentation of the intestinal mucosa, may develop; it should reverse when patient stops taking the herb.

- Encourage patient to use milder methods of relieving constipation, including making dietary changes and using bulk-forming products, before using stimulant laxatives such as cascara.
- Herb may discolor urine, making diagnostic test interpretation more difficult.
- Overdose can cause diarrhea and fluid and electrolyte imbalance.
- Caution patient that children younger than age 12 and pregnant and breast-feeding patients shouldn't use cascara unless under the supervision of a health care provider.
- Advise patient not to use the fresh bark of the cascara plant because it can cause intestinal irritation, spasms, or cramping; bloody diarrhea; or severe vomiting.
- Tell patient to consult his health care provider if discomfort occurs. Discomfort may be resolved by lowering the dose or discontinuing the herb.
- Advise patient not to exceed the recommended dose and to discontinue use in the event of diarrhea or watery stools.
- Use only standardized anthraquinone-containing preparations. The effects of nonstandardized preparations are unpredictable.
- Tell patient to remind prescriber and pharmacist of any herbal or dietary supplement that he's taking when obtaining a new prescription.
- Advise patient to consult his health care provider before using an herbal preparation because a treatment with proven efficacy may be available.

Research summary
Cascara sagrada has been approved by the FDA as an over-the-counter laxative. A few recent studies have shown some antileukemic activity, but these are only in vitro and in mice. For humans, this and other uses of cascara sagrada have not yet been validated scientifically.

castor bean

African coffee tree, bofareira, castor, Mexico seed, Mexico weed, Palma Christi, Ricinus communis, *tangantangan oil plant, wonder tree*

Castor bean contains a constituent called ricin, a protoplasmic poison that causes cell death after binding to normal cells and disrupting deoxyribonucleic acid synthesis and protein metabolism. Ricin may have analgesic and antiviral properties. Castor bean is available as a paste for external use.

Reported uses
Castor bean is used externally as a paste to treat inflammatory skin conditions, boils, carbuncles, abscesses, inflammation of the middle ear, and migraines.

Administration
- Paste (made from ground seeds): Applied externally to affected areas two times a day for up to 15 days.

Hazards
 SAFETY RISK *Castor beans can be toxic when chewed and swallowed — 1 to 2 chewed seeds can be lethal for an adult. Plant leaves may also be poisonous.*

Adverse effects associated with castor bean include rash, toxic reaction, and allergic reaction. Potassium depletion from herb use can increase body's sensitivity to digoxin. Inhaled castor bean dust can cause allergic reaction.

Pregnant and breast-feeding patients should avoid use.

Clinical considerations
SAFETY RISK *Signs and symptoms of overdose or toxicity include severe stomach pain, nausea, hemoptysis, bloody diarrhea, and burning of the mouth. Seizures, hepatic and renal failure, and death can occur. If overdose occurs, provide supportive therapy.*

- Discourage oral use of castor bean.
- Advise patient not to use on broken or damaged skin and not to inhale castor bean dust.
- Advise patient to discontinue use if he develops a rash after use.
- Instruct patient to seek medical help immediately if he suspects he has taken an overdose.
- Warn patient to keep all herbal products away from children and pets.
- Tell patient to remind prescriber and pharmacist of any herbal or dietary supplement that he's taking when obtaining a new prescription.
- Advise patient to consult his health care provider before using an herbal preparation because a treatment with proven efficacy may be available.

Research summary
The concepts behind the use of castor bean and the claims made regarding its effects have not yet been validated scientifically.

catnip

Catmint, catnep, catswort, field balm,
Nepeta cataria

The leaves and flowering tops of *Nepeta cataria* are harvested between June and September for use in the preparation of catnip products. Iridoids, tannins, and the volatile oil nepetalactone are the major active ingredients. Catnip essential oil has sedative, carminative, and antispasmodic effects. It's a good source of iron, selenium, potassium, manganese, and chromium.

Catnip may also have diaphoretic and astringent effects. It may help relieve flatulence and colic. Catnip is available as capsules, dried leaf, tea, and tincture.

Reported uses
Catnip is used to treat colds, cough, fever, migraines, and hives. Dry leaves are smoked to treat bronchitis and asthma. It has also been used internally for menstrual cramps, dyspepsia, and colic because of its smooth muscle relaxant properties. Catnip has been used for insomnia, diuresis, and diaphoresis and for children with diarrhea. A topical poultice of catnip is used to relieve swelling.

Administration
- Decoction: 1 cup three times a day; prepared by steeping 1 to 2 teaspoons of tea in 6 to 8 oz of boiling water for 10 to 15 minutes, or boiling it in 6 to 8 oz of water, then simmering at low heat for 3 to 5 minutes
- Infusion: 1 cup three times a day; prepared by infusing 2 teaspoons of dried herb in 8 oz of boiling water for 10 to 15 minutes
- Tincture: 2 to 4 ml three times a day.

Hazards
 SAFETY RISK *Contraindicated in pregnant patients due to its uterine stimulant properties.*

Adverse effects associated with catnip include malaise, headache, sedation, abdominal discomfort, nausea, and vomiting. Benzodiazepines and catnip may cause additive central nervous system (CNS) depression. Herbal products prepared with alcohol may cause a disulfiram-like reaction.

Pregnant and breast-feeding patients should avoid use.

Clinical considerations
- Children and geriatric patients should start with weak preparations and increase the strength, as needed.
- Catnip abuse involves either smoking the dried leaves, similar to smoking marijuana, or making a volatile oil or extract of the herb, soaking tobacco in the extract, and then smoking the tobacco. If abuse is suspected, watch patient for signs of mood elevation, such as giddiness.
- If patient is pregnant or is planning pregnancy, advise her not to use catnip.

- Caution patient about potential sedative effects and impairment of cognitive ability. Instruct him to avoid activities requiring mental alertness (such as driving) until CNS effects are known.
- Extract may contain alcohol and may be unsuitable for children, patients with a history of alcohol abuse, or those with liver disease
- Instruct patient that liquid form needs to be shaken well before each use.
- Warn patient to keep all herbal products and drugs away from children and pets.
- Instruct patient not to drink alcohol when using catnip.
- Tell patient to remind prescriber and pharmacist of any herbal or dietary supplement that he's taking when obtaining a new prescription.
- Advise patient to consult his health care provider before using an herbal preparation because a treatment with proven efficacy may be available.

Research summary
The concepts behind the use of catnip and the claims made regarding its effects have not yet been validated scientifically.

cat's claw

Life-giving vine of Peru, samento, secondary root, una de gato, Uncaria tomentosa

---

The bark of the inner stalk, woody vine, or roots of *Uncaria tomentosa*, or cat's claw, are harvested for the plant's alkaloids, which are included in many pharmacologically active dietary supplements. Cat's claw inhibits urinary bladder contractions and has local anesthetic effects; its sterol components may have anti-inflammatory activity. Rhynchophylline may inhibit platelet aggregation.

Most cat's claw alkaloids have immunostimulant properties, which may stimulate phagocytosis. The major alkaloids dilate peripheral blood vessels, inhibit the sympathetic nervous system, and relax smooth muscles. Cat's claw may lower serum cholesterol levels and decrease heart rate.

Cat's claw is available as capsules, dried inner stalk bark or root for decoction, extract, powdered extract, and tea bags. Products include Cat's Claw Bark, Cat's Claw-Power, Devil's Claw, Devil's Claw Root, Garbato, Hausca, Paraguaya, Peruvian Cat's Claw Tincture, Toron, and Tambor.

Reported uses
Cat's claw is used to treat GI problems, including Crohn's disease, colitis, inflammatory bowel disease, and hemorrhoids. It's also used in cancer patients for its antimutagenic effects. Cat's claw has been combined with zidovudine to stimulate the immune system in patients with human immunodeficiency virus infection. It has been used to treat diverticulosis, ulcers, rheumatism, menstrual disorders, diabetes, prostate problems, gonorrhea, and cirrhosis, and to prevent pregnancy.

Topically, cat's claw is used to relieve pain from minor injuries and to treat acne.

Administration
- Capsules: 2 capsules (175 mg per capsule) by mouth every day or 3 capsules by mouth three times a day; dosage varies by manufacturer
- Extract (containing alcohol): 250 mg of cat's claw bark extract per milliliter, standardized to contain 3% of oxindole alkaloids
- Extract (alcohol free): 7 to 10 gtt three times a day; may increase to 15 gtt five times a day
- Powdered extract: 1 to 3 capsules (500 mg per capsule) by mouth two to four times a day
- Decoction: 2 to 3 cups per day; prepared by boiling 10 to 30 g inner stalk bark or root in 1 qt of water for 30 to 60 minutes

- Liquid or alcohol extract: 10 to 15 gtt two to three times a day, to 1 to 3 ml three times a day.

Hazards

Hypotension has been reported with use of cat's claw. Cat's claw may potentiate hypotensive effects of conventional anti-hypertensives. Its immunostimulant properties may counteract the therapeutic effects of immunosuppressants. Food enhances the absorption of cat's claw. Cat's claw may inhibit platelet aggregation and prolong bleeding when used with antiplatelets or anticoagulants.

Cat's claw is contraindicated in pregnant and breast-feeding patients, patients who've had transplant surgery, and patients who have autoimmune disease, multiple sclerosis, or tuberculosis. Those with a history of peptic ulcer disease or gallstones should use caution when taking this herb because it stimulates stomach acid secretion.

Clinical considerations

- Some liquid extracts contain alcohol and may be unsuitable for children, patients with a history of alcohol abuse, or patients with liver disease.
- This herb and its contents vary from manufacturer to manufacturer, and the alkaloid concentration varies from season to season; advise patient to purchase herb from the same reputable source each time.
- This product and its contents may vary among different manufacturers and demonstrates great seasonal variation in alkaloid concentration.
- Inform patient that herb should be used for no more than 8 weeks without a 2-week to 3-week rest period from the herb.
- Instruct patient to promptly report adverse reactions and new signs or symptoms.
- Instruct patient to keep herbs and drugs out of children's reach.
- Tell patient to remind prescriber and pharmacist of any herbal or dietary supplement that he's taking when obtaining a new prescription.
- Advise patient to consult his health care provider before using an herbal preparation because a treatment with proven efficacy may be available.

Research summary

Scientific studies of cat's claw have been conducted in Peru, Italy, Austria, and Germany, but as yet have yielded no conclusive proof of any healing benefit.

cat's foot

Antennariae dioica, *cat's ear flower, catsfoot, life everlasting, mountain everlasting*

Cat's foot flower consists of the fresh or dried flowers of *Antennariae dioica*. It contains anthracene derivatives, flavonoids, saponins, mucilages, and tannins. Cat's foot stimulates the flow of gastric and pancreatic secretions. It may raise blood pressure, and it may have spasmolytic, choleric, discutient, and astringent effects. Cat's foot is available as bulk dried herb.

Reported uses

Cat's foot is used to stimulate the flow of bile from the gallbladder to the duodenum, and to treat dysentery. It has also been used as a diuretic. In Europe, cat's foot is used to cure quinsy (peritonsillar abscess) and mumps and to treat bites of poisonous reptiles.

Administration

- Infusion: ½ to 1 cup by mouth every day; prepared by steeping 1 teaspoon fresh or dried flowering herb in ½ cup (120 ml) of boiling water for 10 minutes.

Hazards

There are no known adverse effects with the use of cat's foot; however, the tannin component of the plant may cause nausea, vomiting, constipation, or abdominal pain if ingested in large quantities. Hepatic damage may also occur with the use of large amounts.

Cat's foot may interfere with the intended therapeutic effect of antihypertensives. Tannins may also interfere with digoxin, iron-containing compounds, and alkaloids.

Pregnant and breast-feeding patients and patients with preexisting liver damage should not use cat's foot.

Clinical considerations

- Therapeutic use of cat's foot isn't recommended.
- If patient is using cat's foot, monitor his blood pressure at outset and regularly thereafter.
- Instruct patient to promptly report adverse reactions and new signs or symptoms.
- Tell patient to remind prescriber and pharmacist of any herbal or dietary supplement that he's taking when obtaining a new prescription.
- Advise patient to consult his health care provider before using an herbal preparation because a treatment with proven efficacy may be available.

Research summary

The concepts behind the use of cat's foot and the claims made regarding its effects have not yet been validated scientifically.

celandine

Chelidonii herba, Chelidonium majus, *greater celandine, jewel weed, pilewort, quick-in-the-hand, schöllkraut, slipperweed, swallow-wort, tetterwort, touch-me-not*

Celandine alkaloids are obtained from the flowering tops and roots of *Chelidonium majus*. When used topically, celandine has analgesic, antiseptic, and caustic effects.

When taken orally, the herb may have cytostatic activity with nonspecific immune stimulation and may facilitate bile flow in the GI system. It may also have antispasmodic and diuretic effects. Celandine is available as dry plant, dry root, liquid extract, ointment, tinctures, and in various multi-ingredient products.

Reported uses

Celandine is used orally to treat nonobstructive cholecystitis, jaundice, cholelithiasis, hypercholesterolemia, angina pectoris, asthma, breast lumps, constipation, diffuse latent liver complaints, stomach cancer, and gout. It may also help manage blood pressure, but such use isn't well documented.

Celandine is used topically as an analgesic, antiseptic, and caustic agent for eczema, blister rashes, scabies, scrofulous diseases, insect bites, warts, and hemorrhoids.

Administration

- Liquid extract: 1 to 2 ml by mouth three times a day
- Tincture: 10 to 15 gtt sublingually three times a day
- Herb decoction, infusion: 2 to 4 g powdered herb (not root) in 1 cup of boiling water three times a day
- Ointment: Applied to affected area three times a day, as needed
- Root decoction or infusion: 1½ cups of cold liquid every day; prepared by steeping 1 level teaspoon (about 0.5 g) of rootstock in 1 cup of boiling water for 30 minutes
- Topical juice: Mixed with vinegar and dabbed on no more than two or three warts at a time, two to three times a day.

Hazards

 SAFETY RISK *Overdoses of stem juice may cause paralysis and death.*

Adverse effects associated with the use of celandine include stupor, seizures, drowsiness, burning in the mouth, abdominal discomfort, nausea, vomiting, bloody diarrhea, salivation, hematuria, jaundice, contact dermatitis, and allergic response.

Extracts or tinctures prepared with alcohol may cause a disulfiram-like reaction. Celandine may have blood pressure lowering effects and may contribute to the antihypertensive effects of such medications. Changes in electrocardiogram results may occur when celandine is used in conjunction with digoxin.

Efficacy may be reduced if celandine is used with morphine derivatives or sulfonamides. Celandine may cause hypoglycemia when used with sulfonylureas.

Patients with latex or celandine allergy, pregnant patients, breast-feeding patients, and patients with painful gallstones, acute bilious colic, obstructive jaundice, or acute viral hepatitis should avoid using celandine.

Clinical considerations
- Dried celandine is less active than the fresh herb.
- Patient should be cautioned about cross-sensitivity between latex allergy and oral use of celandine.
- Overdose, especially of stem juice, could be toxic and life-threatening.
- Caution patient to use celandine only under a health care provider's supervision.
- Tell patient to alert his health care provider if he's allergic to latex or herbs before he starts using celandine.
- If patient is pregnant or is planning pregnancy, advise her not to use celandine.
- Warn patient not to exceed the recommended dosage.
- Advise patient to notify his health care provider and immediately seek medical attention if herb causes allergic reaction or yellowing of the skin or sclera.
- Inform patient that herb is not recommended for long-term use.
- Tell patient to remind prescriber and pharmacist of any herbal or dietary supplement that he's taking when obtaining a new prescription.
- Advise patient to consult his health care provider before using an herbal preparation because a treatment with proven efficacy may be available.

Research summary
The concepts behind the use of celandine and the claims made regarding its effects have not yet been validated scientifically.

celery

Apium graveolens, *smallage*

Celery is high in minerals, including sodium and chlorine, but is a poor source of vitamins. It may have antirheumatic, anti-inflammatory, diuretic, sedative, anticonvulsive, fungicidal, and anticarcinogenic effects. Celery juice has antihypertensive effects, and the oil may cause hypoglycemia.

Celery is available as capsules, dried fruits, dried seeds, liquid extract, tincture, and in multi-ingredient preparations for internal use.

Reported uses
Celery is used to relieve GI gas and colic and to treat bladder and kidney disorders, rheumatic arthritis, gout, and calculosis. Dieters use celery because of its high fiber content.

Celery oil is used as a spasmolytic and sedative for nervousness and hysteria and as an antiflatulent. It's also used to manage hypertension and blood glucose levels and to promote menses. Oil extract from the root is used to restore sexual potency impaired by illness.

Celery seeds are used to treat bronchitis and rheumatism.

Administration
- Capsules: 2 to 3 capsules by mouth two to three times a day
- Liquid extract (1:1 in 50% alcohol): 0.3 to 1.2 ml three times a day

- Decoction: Three times a day; prepared by boiling ½ teaspoon of seeds in 1½ cups of water briefly, then straining
- Dried fruits: 0.5 to 2 g or by prepared liquid substance 1:5 two to three times a day
- Infusion: Three times a day; prepared by steeping 1 to 2 teaspoons of freshly crushed seeds in 1 cup of water for 10 to 15 minutes
- Juice: 1 tablespoon two to three times a day before meals
- Oil: 6 to 8 gtt in water two times a day
- Tincture: 1 to 5 ml three times a day.

Hazards
Adverse effects associated with celery include sedation, respiratory difficulty, dermatitis, urticaria, depigmentation, hyperpigmentation, angioedema, and allergic reaction, including anaphylactic shock.

Celery has possible additive hypotensive effects when used with diuretics and antihypertensives. It has possible additive hypoglycemic effects when used with insulin and oral antidiabetics. It carries an increased risk of photosensitivity reactions with sun exposure.

Pregnant patients shouldn't use celery seed and shouldn't use more than a moderate amount of other parts of the plant. Patients with renal infection or renal insufficiency should avoid use.

Clinical considerations
- Ingestion of large amounts of celery oil may cause toxic reaction.
- If patient has diabetes and is using celery, instruct him to monitor his blood glucose level very carefully because celery may cause hypoglycemia.
- If patient is also taking a diuretic or an antihypertensive, monitor his blood pressure regularly.
- Instruct patient to promptly report adverse reactions and new signs or symptoms.
- If patient has a kidney infection or kidney disease, advise him not to use celery medicinally because the volatile oils can irritate the renal system.

- If patient is pregnant or is planning pregnancy, advise her not to use celery seed and to be extremely cautious if using celery in other forms for its therapeutic effects.
- Tell patient that storing the plant for extended periods of time may lead to an increased risk of phototoxicosis.
- Tell patient to remind prescriber and pharmacist of any herbal or dietary supplement that he's taking when obtaining a new prescription.
- Advise patient to consult his health care provider before using an herbal preparation because a treatment with proven efficacy may be available.

Research summary
The concepts behind the use of celery and the claims made regarding its effects have not yet been validated scientifically.

Cell therapy

Live cell proteins, live cell therapy, live protein therapy, live tissue extracts, liver growth factors

In cell therapy, live whole cells or extracts derived from living cells are administered in their natural, undenatured form either sublingually or by injection to improve or rejuvenate the function of targeted organs. Live cell therapy is promoted as a treatment for a wide range of specific conditions and also as a panacea to slow the effects of aging and degeneration.

Proponents of live cell therapy claim that the idea goes back thousands of years, referring to similar therapies found in the Kama Sutra, the Papyrus of Eber, and the writings of Hippocrates. The modern introduction of this therapy is credited to Paul Niehans, a Swiss endocrinologist. In 1931, Dr. Niehans was called in to care for a patient whose parathyroid gland had been inadvertently removed during goiter surgery. Hoping to provide temporary relief from the resulting convulsions, he administered a preparation of freshly macerated oxen parathyroid gland with the intention of providing some hormonal effect. This impromptu preparation provided more than temporary relief; the patient made a rapid and complete recovery.

Dr. Niehans' results were based on those seen in the work of Nobel laureate biologist Alexis Carrel. Starting in 1912, Dr. Carrel had performed experiments showing that spleen cells from young, healthy sheep placed in close proximity to old senescent cells would revitalize the older cells. Dr. Niehans believed that his injection of live parathyroid cells rejuvenated the remaining injured parathyroid cells, thereby restoring their function. He went on to administer over 45,000 live cell therapy injections over the next 42 years from his clinic in Switzerland. Similar treatments, using substances extracted from pituitary, adrenal, ovary, testes, or other glands, were common in the United States during the same period.

Reliance on live tissue extracts diminished with the availability of synthetic hormones and vitamin isolates. Use of live cell therapies further diminished as new research suggested that the benefits of these treatments resulted from their high vitamin, mineral, or hormonal content. However, effects such as the disappearance of chronic conditions remain unexplained. A therapy very similar to live cell therapy, called protomorphogen therapy, in which oral medications made from dried glandular or tissue extracts are administered orally, is still in widespread use among practitioners of nutritional medicine.

Early live cell therapy was based on the simple theory that administering an extract of a specific organ will improve that organ's function. Some products have a general effect; for example, mesenchyme extracts, derived from undifferentiated bovine embryonic connective tissue, are used for any condition involving tissues derived from mesenchyme cells — that is, bone, tendons, connective tissue, and the central nervous system. Dr. Niehans theorized that once ingested, these extract cells migrate to the area of greatest injury in the body, line up with the damaged cells, then start replicating to replace and rejuvenate damaged tissue.

Proprietary products currently on the market no longer contain live cells. Rather, they contain protein extracts from living cells that have been carefully extracted, purified, and preserved. These undenatured, or "live," proteins contain an array of still undefined growth factors and other cellular products that apparently stimulate the cells in similar tissue.

The product to be used is chosen according to the traditional model of Dr. Niehans' live cell therapy. Thymus extracts are used to increase and balance immune system activity. Mesenchyme extracts are used to stimulate repair and improve function in all mesenchyme-derived tissues. Adrenal extracts are given to improve adrenal function, liver extracts to improve liver function.

The number of live cell products currently sold is limited, but if current trends are predictive, their availability and variety will grow. Current products include thymus, mesenchyme, adrenal, pancreas, liver, brain, and shark cartilage.

Reported uses

Live cell therapy is recommended for a wide range of diseases and injuries. Products are frequently used in combination. For example, liver cirrhosis due to hepatitis C might be treated by using a combination of three products: thymus is used to rebalance immune function and decrease the damage the immune system causes the liver; liver extracts are used to increase liver function; and mesenchyme is used to repair liver damage.

How the treatment is performed

Live cell products are typically dispensed in 7 ml vials shipped frozen from the distributor and thawed one at a time just prior to use. A pretreatment test injection screens for allergic reaction. The extracts are administered either by I.M. injection or sublingually. Typical dosing protocols call for the administration of two vials per week during acute treatment and as few as one vial per month for long-term maintenance.

Hazards

Care must be taken regarding the source, transport, and storage. The Canadian facility, Aeterna, which manufactures the NatCell and Car T Cell lines, complies with Canadian pharmaceutical guidelines. Obvious concern for sanitary practice and contamination-free products exists. No adverse effects have been reported.

Cell therapy is not recommended for those with severe kidney disease, liver failure, or acute infections and inflammatory diseases. Patients who show an allergic reaction to the test injection should not receive the treatment.

Clinical considerations

There is still limited clinical experience with these products. Several possible contraindications go back to Dr. Niehans' work. In his Swiss clinic, Dr. Niehans wouldn't treat anyone who suffered from any infections, including dental problems, tonsillitis, or appendicitis, as he believed they led to failure of therapy. He also believed that sedatives or similar drugs weakened the effects of therapy. He wouldn't treat anyone until at least 6 to 8 weeks after a vaccination.

Research summary

Recently published studies suggest that live cell products are useful in treating liver disease, multiple sclerosis, chronic fatigue syndrome, and a range of other problems. However, these articles were often sponsored by the manufacturer and were peer reviewed.

RESEARCH *Berbari, et al. (1999) reported on the antiangiogenic effects of shark cartilage extract. Oral administration of the extract decreased wound angiogenesis. This is signifi-cant, as it's the first report published demonstrating this phenomenon. Antiangiogenic effect would be valuable in treating a number of disease processes, including metastatic progression of tumors, age-related macular degeneration, rheumatoid arthritis, and skin disorders such as psoriasis, hypertrophic scarring, and keloids.*

Cell-specific cancer therapy

The Center for Cell-Specific Cancer Therapy, located in Santo Domingo, Dominican Republic, and staffed by a nuclear engineer and a medical doctor, uses pulsed electromagnetic field therapy to treat a variety of cancers. According to the center, cancer cells emit an excessive amount of positively charged ions, making them a logical target for the center's bioelectromagnetic therapy called cell-specific cancer therapy (CSCT). No other cells in the body produce such an energy signature, and different cancers have distinctively different ionic signatures.

The goal of the center's therapy is to detect cancer cells by their signatures and destroy them by means of a pulsed electromagnetic field. This field reportedly alters the cancer cells' metabolism without harming surrounding healthy cells. Since opening in August, 1996, the center has treated 150 clients and claims a success rate of 50%. However, its claims haven't been verified independently.

Reported uses

The center claims that CSCT is most effective at detecting actively growing cancers. It reports having successfully treated even stage IV cancers.

How the treatment is performed

CSCT treatment consists of scanning the body and then marking the cancerous sites on a body map and on the patient. Using a proprietary electromagnetic device, called the CSCT-200, which is described as producing a pulsed electromagnetic field, the sound frequency of the cancer cells is identified and matched. The signal is then sent back into the cells, causing them to vibrate, rupture, and die. Treatment sessions generally last for 30 minutes, and are given twice a day for up to 3 weeks. The center considers the treatment successful when the CSCT-200 can no longer detect the cancer signals, and when conventional laboratory tests no longer detect cancer markers.

Currently, the Center for Cell-Specific Cancer Therapy focuses only on the scanner treatment without attention to other factors related to achieving long-term remission, such as nutrition, diet therapy, detoxification, dental work, and counseling.

Hazards
The center doesn't accept patients who have received conventional chemotherapy and radiation therapy because it maintains that such therapies can hinder the effectiveness of the CSCT treatment. The scanner reportedly can't perceive previously treated cancer cells that have received high doses of chemotherapy or radiation and yet survived. This is presumably because their metabolism has slowed and their ionic pattern is undetectable. These undetectable cells could recover to multiply again. However, by delaying conventional treatment, the patient risks cancer progression if CSCT fails.

CSCT scanning carries the potential risk of cumulative electromagnetic exposure.

Clinical considerations
Because the center maintains that conventional treatment can inhibit CSCT, a patient may reject or postpone conventional treatment in favor of this alternative treatment, potentially risking his life if the CSCT treatment is unsuccessful.

Research summary
CSCT bases its efficacy claims on operating principles that are grounded in current scientific knowledge of cancer. Although CSCT is considered noninvasive and nondestructive of healthy tissue, precise and objective research is needed to verify its effectiveness.

The use of pulsed magnetic fields for cancer therapy has been questioned on the grounds that such fields may stimulate cancer growth while simultaneously stimulating the immune system through a stress response. At the onset of treatment, it appears that the immune system wins out and the cancer subsides. However, when the stress response declines, the cancer may resume its replication.

centaury

Bitter bloom, bitter clover, bitter herb, canchalagua, Centaurii herba, Centaurium minus, C. umbellatum, *Centaury gentian, centory, Christ's ladder,* Erythraea centaurium, *feverwort, filwort, red centaury, rose pink, taus-endgüldenkraut, wild succory*

Centaury is derived from the dried flowering tops of common centaury and *Erythraea centaurium.* It contains phenolic acids, alkaloids, monoterpenoids, triterpenoids, flavonoids, beta-coumaric, caffeic acids, xanthones, fatty acids, alkanes, and waxes. The major component, gentiopicroside, has antimalarial effects. Centaury may have antipyretic and stomachic effects. The compounds erythrocentaurin and erytaurin may be responsible for centaury's bitter tonic effects. The phenolic acids may have antipyretic activity. Centaury is available as liquid extract, powder, tea, and tincture.

Reported uses
Centaury is mainly used to treat anorexia and dyspepsia. Externally, it has been

used to treat wounds. In folk medicine, centaury has been used for fevers, worm infestation, and high blood pressure.

Administration
■ Liquid extract (1:1 in 25% alcohol): 2 to 4 ml by mouth up to three times a day
■ Powder: Sprinkled on a wafer with honey
■ Tea: Prepared by steeping 2 to 3 g in 5 oz (150 ml) of boiling water for 15 minutes, then straining
■ Tincture (27% alcohol): 2 gtt in water or under tongue, as needed.

Hazards
Centaury may antagonize the effect of anticoagulants. Herbal products prepared with alcohol may cause a disulfiram-like reaction. There are no reported adverse effects with centaury.

Those with hypersensitivity to centaury or any of its components and those with stomach or intestinal ulcers should avoid use. Pregnant and breast-feeding patients should also avoid use.

Clinical considerations
■ Excessive use of centaury should be avoided because information about safety and toxicity is limited.
■ Warn patient who is taking an anticoagulant not to use centaury.
■ Encourage patient to promptly report adverse reactions and new signs and symptoms.
■ If patient is taking disulfiram or metronidazole or if he has a history of alcoholism or cirrhosis, inform him that he should avoid centaury liquid extracts and tincture because of their alcohol content.
■ Tell patient to remind prescriber and pharmacist of any herbal or dietary supplement that he's taking when obtaining a new prescription.
■ Advise patient to consult his health care provider before using an herbal preparation because a treatment with proven efficacy may be available.

Research summary
The concepts behind the use of centaury and the claims made regarding its effects have not yet been validated scientifically.

chamomile

Anthemis nobilis, *azulon,* Chamaemelum nobile, *chamomilla,* Chamomilla recutita, Chamomillae anthodium, *ground apple, kamilenblüten,* Matricaria recutita, *pin heads, wild chamomile*

Chamomile is derived from the fresh or dried flowers of *Matricaria recutita* and *Chamaemelum nobile.* It contains a volatile oil that consists of up to 50% alpha-bisabolol, which reduces inflammation and is an antipyretic. Bisabolol also shortens the healing times of superficial burns and ulcers and inhibits development of ulcers.

Chamomile essential oil has antibacterial and slight antiviral effects. Chamazulene, a minor component of the oil, has anti-inflammatory and antioxidant effects. The flavonoids apigenin and luteolin also contribute to the anti-inflammatory effect. Apigenin is primarily responsible for the anxiolytic and slight sedative effect through action on the central nervous system benzodiazepine receptors; it produces no anticonvulsant effects.

Bisabolol, bisabolol oxides A and B, and the essential oil of chamomile are probably best known for their antispasmodic effects. Other compounds in chamomile that exert antispasmodic effects include apigenin, quercetin, luteolin, and the coumarins umbelliferone and herniarine. Chamomile is available as capsules, liquid extract, raw herb, tea, and topical cream.

Reported uses
Chamomile is used orally to treat diarrhea, anxiety, restlessness, stomatitis, he-

morrhagic cystitis, flatulence, and motion sickness. Teas are used mainly for sedation or relaxation.

Chamomile is used topically to stimulate skin metabolism, reduce inflammation, encourage the healing of wounds, and treat cutaneous burns. It's also used for its antibacterial and antiviral effects.

The German Commission E has approved chamomile flower for use as an inhalation in skin and mucus membrane inflammations, bacterial skin diseases (including those of the oral cavity and gums), and respiratory tract inflammation and irritation. It's also used in baths and irrigation for anogenital inflammation, and internally for GI spasms and inflammatory diseases.

Administration
Liquid extract:
- For adults: 1:1 or 1:1.5 in 10% to 70% alcohol, 1 to 4 ml three times a day
- For children ages 2 and older: 1:4 strength alcohol-free extract, ⅛ to ¼ teaspoon directly or in water or juice two to three times a day
- For children weighing 14 to 27 kg (31 to 60 lb): ¼ to ½ teaspoon directly or in water or juice two to three times a day
- For children weighing 27 to 41 kg (60 to 90 lb): ½ to 1 teaspoon directly or in water or juice two to three times a day
- For children weighing 41 to 54 kg (90 to 119 lb): 1 to 2 teaspoons directly or in water or juice two to three times a day.

Tea for GI upset: Prepared by steeping 1 tablespoon (3 g) of chamomile or 1 chamomile tea bag in 100 to 150 ml of boiling water for 5 to 10 minutes, then straining
- For adults and children older than age 6: Three to four times a day between meals
- For children ages 5 to 6: 100 to 120 ml once to four times a day
- For children ages 3 to 4: 50 to 80 ml once to four times a day
- For inflammation of mucous membranes in the mouth and throat, tea is used as a wash or gargle. For young children, tea should be diluted.
- Topical cream: Applied four times a day to affected areas in both adults and children
- As a bath soak: 50 g added to 10 liters of water
- For massage: Raw herb or flowers used in massage oils, as needed.

Hazards
SAFETY RISK *People sensitive to ragweed and chrysanthemums or related Compositae family members (arnica, yarrow, feverfew, tansy, artemisia) may be more susceptible to contact allergies and anaphylaxis. Individuals with hay fever or bronchial asthma caused by pollens are more susceptible to anaphylactic reactions.*

Adverse effects associated with chamomile include conjunctivitis, eyelid angioedema, nausea, vomiting, eczema, contact dermatitis, sedation, and anaphylaxis. The coumarin content of chamomile may antagonize or potentiate the effect of an anticoagulant. Increased sedation may occur when chamomile is used with benzodiazepines, central nervous system depressants, and alcohol.

Pregnant patients should avoid use because of emmenagogue and abortifacient effects. Chamomile shouldn't be used in teething babies or in children younger than age 2. Safety in breast-feeding patients and those with liver or kidney disorders has not been established, so these patients should avoid use.

Clinical considerations
- Advise patient that chamomile may cause an allergic reaction or make existing symptoms worse in susceptible individuals. Signs and symptoms of anaphylaxis include shortness of breath, swelling of the tongue, skin rash, tachycardia, and hypotension.
- Since chamomile has antispasmodic activity in the GI tract, it may delay or alter the absorption of prescription medications given at the same time. Separate

the administration of chamomile from other medications by 1 to 2 hours.

- If patient is taking an anticoagulant, advise him not to use chamomile because of possible enhanced anticoagulant effects.
- If patient is pregnant or is planning pregnancy, advise her not to use chamomile.
- Instruct parent not to give chamomile to a child before checking with a knowledgeable health care provider.
- Tell patient to remind prescriber and pharmacist of any herbal or dietary supplement that he's taking when obtaining a new prescription.
- Advise patient to consult his health care provider before using an herbal preparation because a treatment with proven efficacy may be available.

Research summary

Germany's Commission E authorizes the use of various topical chamomile preparations for a variety of diseases of the skin and mouth. Commission E has also authorized oral chamomile as a treatment for pain and inflammation in the stomach and intestines, and inhaled chamomile vapor for asthma and other lung problems.

 RESEARCH *One double-blind study of 161 individuals found chamomile cream equally effective as 0.25% hydrocortisone cream for the treatment of eczema (Aertgeerts, et al., 1985).*

chaparral

*Chaparro, creosote bush,
dwarf evergreen oak, el gobernadora,
falsa alcaparra, greasewood, gumis,
hediondilla, hideonodo, jarillo,
Larrea tridentate, shoegoi,
Sonora covillea, tasago,
ya-temp, zygophylacca*

Chaparral is derived from the flowers, leaves, and twigs of *Larrea tridentate*. Its major constituent is the lignin nordihydroguaiaretic acid (NDGA), which makes up 1.84% of the plant's active compounds. NDGA has potent anti-inflammatory activity because of its ability to block the enzyme lipoxygenase. Lipoxygenase is a precursor to many inflammatory prostaglandins; therefore, by blocking this enzyme, chaparral may help treat certain inflammatory conditions.

Besides inhibiting platelet aggregation in those taking aspirin, NDGA also has some antioxidant effects. Other components of chaparral that add to its antioxidant activity include flavonoids, saponins, and lignins. The lignins also have amoebicidal, antiparasitic, and fungicidal activity. NDGA has also been reported to have antimicrobial activity against certain species of *Penicillium*, streptococci, *Staphylococcus aureus*, *Bacillus subtilis*, and *Pseudomonas aeruginosa*. Chaparral is available as liquid extract, oil infusion, tablet, tea, tincture, bulk powder, and capsules.

Reported uses

Chaparral is used orally as supportive therapy for cancer, dyspepsia, venereal disease, tuberculosis, and parasitic infections. It's used as an oral rinse to help prevent tooth decay, halitosis, and gum disease.

Chaparral is used topically as supportive therapy for allergies, dysmenorrhea, intestinal cramping, rheumatoid arthritis, and wound healing.

Administration

- As an antimicrobial: Tea used as a mouthwash and expectorated; powder applied topically on minor abrasions; tea prepared by steeping 1 teaspoon of leaves and flowers in 1 cup hot water for 10 to 15 minutes
- To treat allergy symptoms: 1 to 3 cups of tea by mouth every day for several days or 20 gtt of tincture of liquid extract (68% to 75% alcohol) by mouth every day, once to three times a day

- To treat arthralgia: 1 to 3 cups of tea by mouth every day or 20 gtt of tincture or liquid extract once to three times a day; treatment limited to a few days
- To treat autoimmune disease: 20 gtt of tincture by mouth once to three times a day
- To treat dysmenorrhea or intestinal cramps: Infused oil applied topically to abdomen, as needed
- To treat premenstrual syndrome: 1 to 3 cups of tea by mouth every day or 20 gtt of tincture by mouth once to three times a day; treatment limited to a few days.

Hazards

 SAFETY RISK *Chaparral may not be safe to use because of risk of hepatotoxicity, dermatitis, and tumor growth. Hepatotoxicity appears as toxic or drug-induced cholestatic hepatitis.*

Adverse effects associated with the use of chaparral include fatigue, anorexia, abdominal pain, nausea, loose stools or diarrhea, dark urine, induction of cortical and medullary cysts in the kidney, hepatotoxicity, acute hepatitis, jaundice, elevated liver function test results, cirrhosis, acute fulminant liver failure, weight loss, pruritus, contact dermatitis, fever, and tumor growth.

NDGA may interfere with platelet adhesion and aggregation in patients taking aspirin. Herbal products prepared with alcohol may cause a disulfiram-like reaction. Excessive doses of chaparral may interfere with the activity of monoamine oxidase inhibitors.

Those with a history of liver disease, alcohol abuse, hepatitis, renal insufficiency, preexisting renal disease, or chronic renal failure should avoid use. Pregnant and breast-feeding patients should avoid using the herb.

Clinical considerations

SAFETY RISK *Dosages are for adults only. Because pediatric dosing information isn't available, chaparral should not be used in children.*

- Most patients find the taste of chaparral teas and tinctures disagreeable, which limits the amount they can tolerate before feeling nauseated.
- Monitor patient for signs or symptoms of hepatic failure. Caution him to stop using chaparral if he experiences nausea, fever, fatigue, dark urine, or jaundice.
- Gastric lavage may be performed within 60 minutes of a potentially fatal ingestion. Activated charcoal may also be used when administered within 1 hour of a potentially fatal ingestion.
- Warn patient not to delay seeking appropriate medical evaluation because doing so may delay diagnosis of a potentially serious medical condition.
- Tell patient to remind prescriber and pharmacist of any herbal or dietary supplement that he's taking when obtaining a new prescription.
- Advise patient to consult his health care provider before using an herbal preparation because a treatment with proven efficacy may be available.

Research summary
The concepts behind the use of chaparral and the claims made regarding its effects have not yet been validated scientifically.

chaste tree

Chasteberry, monk's pepper,
Vitex agnus-castus

Chaste tree is derived from the dried, ripened fruit of *Vitex agnus-castus*. It contains the two iridoid glycosides, agnuside and aucubin, as well as flavonoids, essential oils, and progestins. The berries exert a progesterogenic effect on women and an antiandrogenic effect on men. Progestin components include progesterone, testosterone, and androstenedione. Chaste tree is believed to act directly on the hypothalamic–pituitary axis. The herb is also contained in various multivitamin supplements for women and in combination products used to alleviate menopausal symptoms. By increasing the release of luteinizing hormone, which in turn increases progesterone production in the ovaries, chaste tree helps to regulate the menstrual cycle.

A component in chaste tree has been shown to bind to dopamine receptors, thereby inhibiting the release of prolactin. This is particularly useful in treating premenstrual breast pain associated with excess secretion of prolactin. It may also act as a diuretic to reduce water retention before menstruation. Chaste tree is available as capsules, elixir, liquid extract, tablets, tea, and tinctures, in products such as Vitex, Vitex Alfalfa Supreme, Vitex Extract, Vitex 40 Plus, and Vitex Vegicaps.

Reported uses

Chaste tree fruit is used to treat menstrual irregularities such as amenorrhea or excessive menstrual bleeding, premenstrual complaints, menopausal symptoms, and fibroids. It's also used to increase breast milk production and treat fibrocystic breast disease, infertility in women, and acne. Chaste tree has also been used to control libido, decrease appetite, reduce flatulence, and enhance sleep.

Administration

■ Capsules: 150 to 325 mg/capsule (standardized to contain 0.5% agnuside) taken by mouth one or two times a day
■ Tinctures, liquid extracts: German Commission E recommends aqueous-alcoholic extracts (50% to 70% alcohol) with 30 to 40 mg of the active herb.

Hazards

Adverse effects associated with the use of chaste tree include headaches, GI upset, increased menstrual flow, itching, and urticaria.

Chaste tree may have an antagonistic effect when used with antihypertensives; using chaste tree in conjunction with beta blockers may cause hypertensive crisis. Chaste tree has a dopaminergic effect,

and therefore may interact with dopaminergic/anti-dopaminergic medications. Chaste tree may alter female hormones; for this reason, it shouldn't be used in conjunction with hormone replacement therapy.

Men, pregnant patients, breast-feeding patients, adolescents, those with hypersensitivity to chaste tree or its components, those with active urticaria, those receiving hormone replacement therapy, and those taking oral contraceptives should avoid use.

Clinical considerations

■ Caution male patient against using this herb because of the antiandrogenic effects.
■ Oral use of chaste tree can cause rash, urticaria, and pruritus. If these symptoms occur, patient should discontinue use.
■ If patient is using chaste tree orally, monitor her for signs or symptoms of hypersensitivity, including shortness of breath and swelling of the tongue.
■ Chaste tree can be used for 4 to 6 months to treat premenstrual syndrome or to regulate the menstrual cycle.
■ Women with amenorrhea or infertility can use chaste tree for 12 to 18 months.
■ If patient is pregnant or breast-feeding, advise her not to use chaste tree.
■ If patient is taking an antihypertensive, especially a beta blocker, advise her not to use chaste tree because of the potential for hypertensive crisis.
■ Remind patient that the herb is not fast acting, therefore benefit may not be seen right away.
■ Advise patient to keep chaste tree away from children and pets.
■ Tell patient to remind prescriber and pharmacist of any herbal or dietary supplement that she's taking when obtaining a new prescription.
■ Advise patient to consult with her health care provider before using an herbal preparation because a treatment with proven efficacy may be available.

Research summary

The concepts behind the use of chaste tree and the claims made regarding its effects have not yet been validated scientifically.

chaulmoogra oil

Chaulmogra, chaulmugra, Hydnocarpus, *hydnocarpus oil, hynocardia oil, kalaw tree oil, leprosy oil,* taraktogenos kurzii

Topical chaulmoogra oil comes from the expressed oil of the seeds of the chaulmoogra tree. The active ingredient in the oil is chaulmoogric acid, also known as hydnocarpic acid. The oil may have antimicrobial activity, especially against *Mycobacterium leprae.*

Other compounds that have been isolated from the chaulmoogra tree include palmitic acid, glycerol, phytosterols, and a mixture of fatty acids. Chaulmoogra oil is available as an oil and an ointment.

Reported uses

Chaulmoogra oil is used to treat rheumatoid arthritis, sprains and bruises, tuberculosis, and eczema, psoriasis, and other inflammations of the skin. It's applied topically to open wounds and sores.

In the past, chaulmoogra oil was used as supportive treatment for leprosy for its antimicrobial effects. It has since been replaced with newer, more effective drugs.

Administration

▪ Oil: Applied topically to lesions, as needed.

Hazards

SAFETY RISK *Chaulmoogra oil should never be taken orally because the seeds are poisonous due to their cyanogenic glycoside content. If accidental ingestion occurs, patient will likely require emergency cardiac and respiratory treatment.*

Symptoms of poisoning include paralysis, coughing, dyspnea, laryngospasms, kidney damage, visual disorders, headache, and muscle pain. There are no known interactions with chaulmoogra oil. Topical application of chaulmoogra oil may cause skin irritation.

Those with hypersensitivity to chaulmoogra oil or any of its components, pregnant patients, breast-feeding patients, and children should avoid use.

Clinical considerations

▪ Oil may be painful to administer to open wounds because it's highly viscous.
▪ Encourage patient with leprotic wounds or ulcers to seek out professional medical treatment and to discuss with his health care provider the possibility of using chaulmoogra oil ointment as adjunct therapy. Inform the patient that data is limited regarding the oil's safety and efficacy.
▪ If patient is pregnant or breast-feeding, advise her against use.
▪ Advise parents not to use the oil on children.
▪ Tell patient to remind prescriber and pharmacist of any herbal or dietary supplement that he's taking when obtaining a new prescription.
▪ Advise patient to consult his health care provider before using an herbal preparation because a treatment with proven efficacy may be available.

Research summary

The concepts behind the use of chaulmoogra oil and the claims made regarding its effects have not yet been validated scientifically.

Chelation therapy

Chelation therapy is a chemical process that removes metallic or mineral toxins (such as lead, mercury, copper, iron, arsenic, aluminum, and calcium) from the body by binding them to the amino acid, ethylenediaminetetraacetic acid (EDTA).

Administered I.V. by a doctor, the EDTA bonds with specific metals and minerals in the body and transports them to the urine for excretion.

Although chelation therapy is an accepted treatment for lead poisoning and other heavy metal toxicities, practitioners of complementary and alternative medicineclaim that it can be used to treat other medical problems, especially coronary artery disease. The theory is that EDTA binds to the calcium in arterial plaque and the resulting compound is excreted in the urine. In this way, proponents claim, chelation therapy can reverse atherosclerosis and possibly prevent the need for angioplasty and bypass surgery.

EDTA may act as an antioxidant, protecting the blood vessels and body tissues from inflammation caused by free radical damage. As a result, it's believed that chelation therapy with EDTA can relieve the pain associated with chronic inflammatory diseases, such as arthritis, lupus, and scleroderma, and even slow the aging process.

TRAINING *The American College for Advancement in Medicine (ACAM) in Laguna Hills, California, has established standards of practice and guidelines for EDTA chelation therapy. Other allied organizations are the American Board of Chelation Therapy in Chicago and the American Holistic Medical Association in Raleigh, North Carolina.*

Reported uses
When combined with specialized nutritional supplements, exercise, weight normalization, and dietary changes, proponents claim that EDTA chelation therapy is an effective method of preventing or treating conditions related to atherosclerosis, such as coronary artery disease, myocardial infarction (MI), angina, cerebrovascular accident (CVA), and peripheral vascular disease, and that it may ultimately prevent associated conditions such as gangrene and senility.

In addition, this therapy is thought to promote revascularization of the brain

after CVA, of the heart after MI, and of the peripheral circulation in patients with peripheral vascular disease. Through all of its biochemical effects, EDTA may also improve metabolic function.

How the treatment is performed
Administration of chelation therapy requires the placement of a peripheral I.V. line. EDTA chelation therapy is administered on an outpatient basis by a licensed doctor as outlined in the protocols of ACAM. The dosage of EDTA is individualized for each patient according to age, sex, weight, and renal function. Vitamins and minerals are usually added to the EDTA solution.

Many studies have been performed to investigate the possibility of oral chelation therapy. However, to date, this administration form has been unsuccessful because only 5% to 10% of the EDTA is absorbed orally, whereas the I.V. absorption rate is 100%.

A typical course of treatment consists of 20 to 30 sessions given 1 to 3 times per week. Each session lasts about 3½ hours. Most doctors who administer chelation therapy for cardiovascular disease also recommend that patients undertake a whole-foods, low-fat diet and an exercise program.

Hazards
Adverse effects of EDTA chelation therapy may include hypotension, hypoglycemia, headache, rash, and thrombophlebitis. Reports of kidney and bone marrow damage, cardiac arrhythmias, I.V. site irritation, anemia, and death during the early days of EDTA chelation therapy are attributed to excessive dosages of EDTA. Proponents of the therapy believe that the lower dosages recommended by the ACAM today are safe.

Clinical considerations
■ EDTA chelation therapy should be instituted only after consultation with pa-

tient's health care provider to avoid interference with any preexisting conditions or interactions with current medications.
■ EDTA chelation therapy is not recommended in children, pregnant women, or patients with renal failure or severe heart failure.

Research summary
Proponents point to studies they say prove the treatment's effectiveness, while mainstream critics condemn the studies as anecdotal and unscientific. The Food and Drug Administration has not approved EDTA for use in anything other than heavy metal poisoning.

chickweed

Adder's mouth, mouse ear, passerina, satin flower, starweed, starwort, Stellaria media, *stitch-wort, tongue-grass, white bird's eye, winterweed*

The leaves of chickweed contain potassium, phosphorus, and nitrate salts. Chickweed also contains 150 to 550 mg of vitamin C per 100 g of herb and the flavonoid rutin, which may explain its topical effects in the treatment of rheumatism; rutin is a counterirritant or rubefacient. Chickweed is available as a dry herb, fluid extract, ointment, tea, and tincture.

Reported uses
Chickweed is used to treat respiratory problems such as bronchitis, asthma, cold, flu, cough, and tuberculosis. It's also used to treat constipation and blood disorders. As a food, chickweed is eaten in salads.

In homeopathic medicine, chickweed is used to treat rheumatism and psoriasis. It's most often used topically as a cream to treat eczema, rashes, itching, and inflammation.

Administration
■ Dried herb: 1 to 5 g three times a day
■ Fluid extract (1:1 in 25% alcohol): 1 to 5 ml three times a day
■ Ointment (1:5 in a lard or paraffin base): Applied topically in liberal amounts for eczema and psoriasis, three to four times a day
■ Tea: 1 to 2 teaspoons of dried herb in 6 oz. of water
■ Tincture (1:5 in 45% alcohol): 1 to 5 ml three times a day.

Hazards
Ingestion of large amounts of chickweed may cause paralysis; however, little data exists to support toxicities. Herbal products prepared with alcohol may cause a disulfiram-like reaction.

Those with hypersensitivity to chickweed or its components should avoid use. Because chickweed contains high amounts of potassium and phosphorus, patients with chronic renal failure shouldn't use it. Pregnant and breastfeeding women should avoid ingesting amounts larger than those found in food.

Clinical considerations
■ Consuming excessive amounts of chickweed may cause nitrate poisoning, evidenced by hypotension and headache.
■ Instruct patient to promptly report adverse reactions — especially hypersensitivity reaction — and new signs or symptoms.
■ If patient is also taking a cardiac drug, monitor his electrolyte levels.
■ Warn patient not to delay seeking appropriate medical evaluation because doing so may delay diagnosis of a potentially serious medical condition.
■ Tell patient to remind prescriber and pharmacist of any herbal or dietary supplement that he's taking when obtaining a new prescription.
■ Advise patient to consult his health care provider before using an herbal preparation because a treatment with proven efficacy may be available.

Research summary
The concepts behind the use of chickweed and the claims made regarding its effects have not yet been validated scientifically.

chicory

Blue sailor's succory, Chehorii herba, Cichorium intybus, *hendibeh, succory, wild chicory, wild succory*

Choriin, a 6,7 hydroxycoumarin derivative, is a pharmacologically active component of chicory. Lactucin, a bitter component, may be responsible for chicory's sedative effects and ability to counteract the effects of caffeine. Other bitter substances, such as intybin, fructose, and inulin, may be responsible for chicory's actions on the GI tract as a digestive tonic. Inulin also has quinidine-like effects. Chicory is available as fresh and dried leaves, stems, and roots as well as dry root stock.

Reported uses
Chicory is often eaten like celery or roasted and used with, or in place of, coffee. It's also used as a sedative, mild diuretic, laxative, and digestive agent to manage indigestion or dyspepsia. Chicory is used as a salad green. It's been used in the past to treat cardiac arrhythmias; however, no human trials support this.

Administration
- Comminuted drug: 3 to 5 g/day
- Decoction: 1 to 1½ cups by mouth every day; prepared by adding 1 teaspoon rootstock to ½ cup cold water, boiling, then straining
- Infusion, tea: Prepared by adding 2 to 4 g of whole herb to 7 oz (210 ml) of boiling water for 10 minutes.

Hazards

SAFETY RISK *Some commercially prepared chicory products may contain crushed cashew shells, which can cause an allergic reaction similar to poison ivy. Chicory may also be contaminated with a fungicide or bacteria.*

Potential adverse effects of chicory include sedation, lower heart rate (not proven in human trials), contact dermatitis, and toxic allergic reaction. There are no reported interactions with chicory; however, the herb may have cardioactive effects and may interact with drugs affecting heart rate, heart rhythm, or blood pressure, though this has never been demonstrated or reported over the many years of its use.

Those with hypersensitivity to chicory and those who are pregnant should avoid use. Those with sensitivity to ragweed, chrysanthemums, marigolds, or daisies should use cautiously.

Clinical considerations
- Chicory is generally recognized as safe. Monitor blood pressure and heart rate in patient who's using it for its therapeutic effects, and advise patient to immediately report any heart abnormalities to his health care provider.
- Handling chicory can cause contact dermatitis.
- Advise patient to watch for adverse reactions, especially sedation and contact dermatitis.
- Warn patient not to perform activities that require mental alertness until central nervous system effects are known.
- Tell patient to remind prescriber and pharmacist of any herbal or dietary supplement that he's taking when obtaining a new prescription.
- Advise patient to consult his health care provider before using an herbal preparation because a treatment with proven efficacy may be available.

Research summary
The concepts behind the use of chicory and the claims made regarding its effects have not yet been validated scientifically.

Chinese cucumber

Alpha-trichosanthin,
Chinese snake gourd, compound Q,
GLQ 223, gua-lau, gualoupi (fruit peel),
gualouzi (seed), snakegourd fruit,
tian-hua-fen (root),
Trichsanthies kirilowii

Chinese cucumber juice contains trichosanthin and karasurin, proteins which effectively induce abortions. The purified protein alpha-trichosanthin from the root of Chinese cucumber is cytotoxic to some macrophages infected with human immunodeficiency virus (HIV) and monocytes and may increase CD4 cell counts in patients with acquired immunodeficiency syndrome (AIDS). Trichosanthin may be useful in treating lymphomas and leukemias by helping to kill leukemia-lymphoma cells. The herb may have antitumorigenic effects. Chinese cucumber is available as dry ripe fruit, dry seeds, dry roots, fresh roots, dry fruit peel, and purified trichosanthin.

Reported uses
Chinese cucumber is used to treat invasive nevi. In traditional Chinese medicine, Chinese cucumber is used orally with other herbs to treat fever, dry and productive cough, mastitis, angina, constipation, lung abscess, diabetes, and appendicitis.

Administration
■ To treat fever, congestion, or constipation: 9 to 15 g of dried fruit by mouth.

Hazards

 SAFETY RISK *This herb is used by some HIV-positive patients as adjunctive treatment. However, the extracts can be extremely toxic when in-*

jected and should be used only under the direction of a knowledgeable practitioner.

Most adverse effects associated with Chinese cucumber are linked to parenteral administration and include cerebral edema, cerebral hemorrhage, seizures, myocardial damage, nausea, vomiting, blood cell damage, acute pulmonary edema, fatal anaphylactic reactions, and prolonged anaphylactic reactions, including fever, follicular atresia, ovulation changes, and decreased hormone levels. Additive hypoglycemic effects may occur when Chinese cucumber is used with antidiabetic agents.

Those with a hypersensitivity to Chinese cucumber should avoid use. Patients who are pregnant or who are planning pregnancy should also avoid use.

Clinical considerations
■ Warn patient that extracts of Chinese cucumber are extremely toxic when administered parenterally.
■ Advise patient never to ingest this product unless under the supervision of a qualified health care provider.
■ Instruct patient to immediately report any shortness of breath or severe headache.
■ Monitor patient closely for hypersensitivity reactions and mental status changes. Effects may occur more than a decade after a trichosanthin injection.
■ Monitor complete blood count closely at regular intervals.
■ If patient is receiving an antidiabetic or another herb that could cause hypoglycemic additive effects, caution him to closely monitor his blood glucose level.
■ If patient is pregnant, advise her to avoid all contact with Chinese cucumber.
■ Advise patient that he should follow up regularly with his health care provider to evaluate the effectiveness of therapy.
■ Tell patient to remind prescriber and pharmacist of any herbal or dietary supplement that he's taking when obtaining a new prescription.
■ Advise patient to consult his health care provider before using an herbal

preparation because a treatment with proven efficacy may be available.

Research summary

The concepts behind the use of Chinese cucumber and the claims made regarding its effects have not yet been validated scientifically. The herb is currently being studied as a possible treatment for AIDS-related infections.

Chinese rhubarb

Canton rhubarb, China rhubarb, chong-gi-huang, da-huang, daio, garden rhubarb, Himalayan rhubarb, Indian rhubarb, Japanese rhubarb, medicinal rhubarb, racine de rhubarbee, rhabarber, Rheum officinale, R. palmatum, R. tanguitcum, Russian rhubarb, Shenshi rhubarb, tai huang, Turkey rhubarb

Chinese rhubarb contains the anthraquinone rhein, so higher doses have a stimulant laxative effect similar to that of cascara and senna. In contrast, lower doses have antidiarrheal effects because tannins (5% and 10%) in the herb have astringent effects. Laxative effects generally occur 6 to 10 hours after ingestion.

Chinese rhubarb may increase cardiac contractility, with the polysaccharides inhibiting calcium influx in the myocardium, and it may slow the progression of diabetic nephropathy and chronic renal failure. It may lower proteinuria, heal bleeding GI ulcers, and have antiviral, antibacterial, antineoplastic, and diuretic effects. The anthraquinones rhein and emodin may inhibit growth of *Staphylococcus aureus*. Chinese rhubarb is available as dry roots, stem parts, bark, and powder, in products such as Phytoestrol N, Abdominolon, Certobil, Cholaflux, Colax, Dragees Laxatives, Enteroton, Fam-Lax, Herbalax, Neo-Cleanse, Plantago Complex, Tisana Arnaldi, and Vegebyl.

Reported uses

Chinese rhubarb is used orally to treat jaundice, kidney stones, gout, headache, toothache, and skin and mucous membrane inflammation. It's also used topically to heal skin sores and scabs.

German Commission E has approved Chinese rhubarb as a treatment for constipation; lower dosages are used to treat diarrhea. In Chinese medicine, it's used to treat delirium, edema, amenorrhea, and abdominal pain.

Administration

- To treat constipation: 20 to 30 mg of rhein (1.2 g of whole roots and stem of Chinese rhubarb) as a single daily dose for a maximum of 14 days; or 1 teaspoon (5 to 6 g) of powdered root boiled in 1 cup of water for 10 minutes, taken 1 tablespoon (15 ml) at a time, up to 1 cup every day; or ½ to 1 teaspoon of tincture every day
- To treat diarrhea: ¼ to ½ teaspoon (1 g) of powdered root boiled in 1 cup of water for 10 minutes, taken 1 tablespoon (15 ml) at a time, up to 1 cup every day; or ¼ teaspoon of tincture once a day
- To treat toothache: By cotton swab directly on the affected tooth.

Hazards

Adverse effects associated with Chinese rhubarb include abdominal cramping, diarrhea, nausea, vomiting, reduced gastric motility, kidney stones, hematuria, discolored urine, hypokalemia, electrolyte imbalance, weakness, dehydration, and pigmentation of the intestinal mucosa.

The oxalate in Chinese rhubarb may form an insoluble compound with calcium, which may cause kidney stones. Chinese rhubarb may increase the risk of hypokalemia when given with corticosteroids and potassium-wasting diuretics. It may increase the cardiac toxicity of digoxin or other antiarrhythmics as a result of potassium loss and effects on drug absorption. Chinese rhubarb may potentiate the effects of laxatives. It may also potentiate anticoagulant effect by reducing absorption of vitamin K.

Those with hypersensitivity to the herb or its components, pregnant patients, breast-feeding patients, and children under age 2 should avoid use. Those with intestinal obstruction or ileus, appendicitis or chronic intestinal inflammation such as gastric or duodenal ulcer, Crohn's disease, ulcerative colitis, abdominal pain of unknown origin, or a history of kidney stones should also avoid use. Limit duration of use to less than 2 weeks to avoid bowel tolerance.

Clinical considerations

■ Oral ingestion of Chinese rhubarb may cause hypokalemia due to excessive diarrhea. Monitor levels of potassium and other electrolytes carefully.

 SAFETY RISK *Caution patient against using the leaf of Chinese rhubarb because it's extremely toxic.*

■ If patient has a medical condition such as small bowel disease, a stomach ulcer, or heart disease, advise him not to use Chinese rhubarb.

■ If patient is taking digoxin, warfarin, a corticosteroid, or a diuretic, tell him to notify his health care provider before using Chinese rhubarb.

■ If patient is also taking digoxin or another antiarrhythmic, monitor electrocardiogram results for cardiac toxicity.

■ Although Chinese rhubarb has been used to treat constipation, instruct patient not to take it without medical advice and even then to use it only when needed, to help reduce likelihood of hypokalemia. Advise him to use the smallest possible dose to achieve therapeutic effect.

■ If patient is also taking digoxin or another antiarrhythmic, monitor electrocardiogram results for cardiac toxicity.

■ If patient is also taking an anticoagulant, watch his International Normalized Ratio closely.

■ Lazy bowel syndrome may develop with prolonged use. Warn patient about laxative dependency, and instruct him not to take Chinese rhubarb for more than 2 weeks.

■ Patient may experience red or bright yellow discoloration of urine.

■ Use of Chinese rhubarb may interfere with diagnostic urine tests.

■ Tell patient to remind prescriber and pharmacist of any herbal or dietary supplement that he's taking when obtaining a new prescription.

■ Advise patient to consult his health care provider before using an herbal preparation because a treatment with proven efficacy may be available.

Research summary

The concepts behind the use of Chinese rhubarb and the claims made regarding its effects have not yet been validated scientifically.

Chiropractic

With more than 50,000 practitioners, chiropractic is the fourth largest health profession (after doctors, dentists, and nurses) in the United States and may be the most commonly used alternative therapy today. Stemming from the Greek words for "done by hand," chiropractic is a therapeutic system based on the belief that most medical problems are caused by misalignments of the vertebrae and can be corrected by manipulating the spine.

Like osteopathy, chiropractic originated in the Midwest in the late 19th century as a reaction to medical orthodoxy. Daniel Palmer, its founder, was a grocer and self-educated healer from Iowa. His theory that the spine plays a major role in health was sparked by an encounter with a janitor who had been stooped and deaf for 17 years following a spinal injury. Palmer noticed a misaligned vertebra in the man's spine and manipulated it back into place. Subsequently, the man was able to stand up straight without pain, and his hearing was restored. The story illustrates the two primary benefits that practitioners ascribe to chiropractic: relief of musculoskeletal pain and disability and reestablishment of internal organ function.

Palmer, who later opened the first school of chiropractic, taught that the human body seeks to maintain a state of homeostasis and has an innate ability to heal itself. This "innate intelligence" regulates all body functions through the nervous system. Because the nerves originate in the spine, Palmer reasoned that displaced vertebrae could disrupt nerve transmissions, a condition he called *subluxation*. He taught that eliminating subluxations allowed the body to carry out its job of maintaining equilibrium unimpeded.

Palmer believed that almost every disease ultimately stemmed from subluxation and that spinal manipulation could treat them all — an idea that became known as "one cause-one cure." Although few chiropractors today still adhere to this theory, the core of the chiropractic profession remains the detection and correction of vertebral misalignment.

Recent advances in the understanding of neurophysiology may provide a theoretical basis for visceral organ responses to chiropractic adjustment.

 TRAINING *Chiropractors are licensed in all 50 states, after completing a 5-year course of study, and are regulated by state chiropractic boards.*

The American medical establishment has recently ceased its former condemnation of chiropractic. This resulted from a 1991 Supreme Court ruling that the American Medical Association (AMA) had conspired to contain and eliminate the competitive profession of chiropractic — an antitrust violation. The judgment required the AMA to reverse its ban on professional cooperation between chiropractors and medical doctors and to pay a substantial settlement. Much of the financial settlement is being used for chiropractic research.

REIMBURSEMENT *Chiropractic treatment is covered by Medicare and many other insurance providers. The American Chiropractic Association in Arlington, Virginia, provides information and referrals.*

Reported uses

Although back pain is the most common reason that people see a chiropractor, any musculoskeletal condition clearly related to spinal or vertebral malfunction is a likely candidate for a chiropractic consultation. Other common problems treated by chiropractors are neck and shoulder pain, headaches, sports injuries, and work-related injuries such as carpal tunnel syndrome.

How the treatment is performed

Spinal manipulative therapy is often delivered manually. Some chiropractors use a special treatment table that can be adjusted to numerous positions. Others may use various devices in order to control more precisely the force and direction of adjustments as well as to administer higher force adjustments if necessary.

Chiropractic emphasizes a holistic approach to the diagnosis and treatment of a specific problem, seeking to understand how, for instance, pain in the knee might actually stem from a lower back dysfunction that isn't currently causing pain in the back itself. Physical examination focuses on possible subluxations, muscle strength, and postural and structural problems to determine whether spinal manipulative therapy is appropriate, and it may include X-rays.

The most common manipulation technique is the *high-velocity, low-amplitude thrust* (also known as osseous adjustment). It's performed by moving a joint to the end point of its current normal range of motion and then imparting a swift, low-amplitude, specifically directed thrust. This generally painless maneuver moves the joint beyond its current normal range of motion, while keeping within the anatomic limits of its range. Other

SPINAL ADJUSTMENT

The chiropractor is manipulating the patient's right superior sacroiliac joint fixation. With one hand stabilizing the patient's shoulder, he thrusts his other hand against the affected ilium. Bracing his thigh against the patient's leg, the chiropractor institutes a quick thrust using his own body weight.

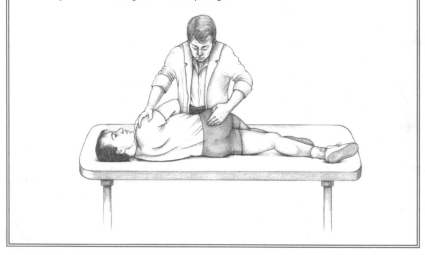

low-velocity adjustments are used when this standard adjustment isn't appropriate. In addition, some practitioners combine chiropractic with adjunctive therapies, such as joint mobilization, massage, nutrition therapy, heat or cold application, and ultrasound. (See *Spinal adjustment.*)

Hazards

Chiropractors claim that if performed by a trained professional, spinal manipulation should produce few if any complications. However, those who do not support chiropractic say manipulation of the lower spine can lead to such complications as leg weakness, bladder disturbance, and rectal and genital malfunction. They also note reports of life-threatening dissection of an artery during an adjustment.

Clinical considerations

Chiropractic manipulation is contraindicated in patients with conditions that might worsen as the result of a spinal ad-

justment, such as osteoporosis and advanced degenerative joint disease.

Research summary

Some chiropractors still claim they can cure any disease, from allergies and impotence to heart disease and cancer, with spinal manipulation. However, there is no supporting scientific evidence yet for most claims.

RESEARCH *In 1994, the Agency for Health Care Policy and Research (now the Agency for Health Care Quality) of the U.S. Department of Health and Human Services released "Acute Low Back Problems in Adults: Clinical Practice Guideline Number 14," a report developed by a panel of medical doctors, chiropractors, and other health professionals based on extensive research. This report endorsed spinal manipulation, either alone or in combination with nonsteroidal anti-inflammatory drugs, as an effective therapy for acute lower back pain, adding that it brought relief as well as*

functional improvement. The report rejected many standard medical treatments for
this condition, such as bed rest, traction,
and the use of painkillers. It also cautioned
against lumbar surgery, except in extreme
cases.

Similar research is currently being conducted to determine whether headaches,
particularly muscle tension headaches, respond better to chiropractic than to conventional medications.

chondroitin

CDS, chondroitin sulfate,
chondroitin sulfate A,
chondroitin sulfate C,
chondroitin sulfuric acid,
chonsurid, CSA,
galacosaminoglucuronoglycan sulfate

Chondroitin is a natural, biologic, high-
viscosity polymer found in the matrix
between joints. It helps maintain water
content and elasticity of the cartilage between joints, allowing for easy, painless
movement. Supplementation with chondroitin may enhance repair of degenerative injuries and inflammation. Chondroitin attracts fluid and nutrients into
the synovial space and thus may help
protect that area. Chondroitin is structurally similar to the low-molecular-
weight heparin derivative, danaparoid.

Chondroitin may help improve symptoms of osteoarthritis when used with
glucosamine and manganese ascorbate;
however, the American College of
Rheumatology doesn't recommend sub-
stituting chondroitin for traditional
treatment. Chondroitin is available as a
capsule containing bovine or shark cartilage, as a gel, or as a synthetic preparation in products such as ChondroFlex,
Cosamin DS, OsteoBiflex, and topical
Humatrix.

Reported uses

Chondroitin is used to decrease pain and
inflammation after extravasation with
ifosfamide, vindesine, doxorubicin, or
vincristine. It's also used to treat osteoarthritis.

Administration

- To treat osteoarthritis: 400 mg by
mouth two to three times a day, up to
1,200 mg per day.

Hazards

Adverse effects associated with the use of
chondroitin include epigastric pain, nausea, and allergic reaction. Chondroitin
may potentiate the effects of anticoagulant drugs.

Those with hypersensitivity to chondroitin or its components should avoid
use.

Clinical considerations

 SAFETY RISK Monitor patient for
allergic reactions, such as shortness
of breath or rash.

- To date, most chondroitin products are
of poor quality, not meeting labeled
amounts.
- Instruct patient not to discontinue
other arthritis treatment without discussing it with his health care provider.
- Little information exists about chondroitin's long-term effects.
- Tell patient to remind prescriber and
pharmacist of any herbal or dietary supplement that he's taking when obtaining
a new prescription.
- Advise patient to consult his health
care provider before using an herbal
preparation because a treatment with
proven efficacy may be available.

Research summary

Evidence suggests that chondroitin may
relieve symptoms of osteoarthritis more
effectively than placebo, and that results
endure for at least 1 year. Evidence that
chondroitin can alter the natural history
of osteoarthritis by slowing progressive
joint damage is weaker.

cinnamon

*Batavia cassia, cassia lignea,
Ceylon cinnamon, cinnamomon,
Cinnamomum verum, C. zeylanicum,
Saigon cassia, Saigon cinnamon*

The medicinal element of cinnamon is the oil extracted from the bark, particularly that of young trees, and the leaf. Cinnamaldehyde, an essential oil that accounts for 65% to 80% of the herb, possesses analgesic, antifungal, and antidiarrheal effects. Specifically, the essential oils from cinnamon bark are active against *Aspergillus parasiticus* growth. Cinnamon is available as a tea and tincture.

Reported uses

Cinnamon is used orally to treat loss of appetite, GI upset, bloating, flatulence, infections, fever, colds, and diarrhea. It's used topically as an astringent. In foods, it's used as a common spice and flavoring agent.

Administration

■ Tea: 1 cup of tea by mouth for a daily dosage of 2 to 4 g of bark; prepared by adding 0.5 to 1 g of bark to 7 oz (210 ml) of boiling water for 5 to 10 minutes and steeping

■ Tincture: 2 to 4 ml three times a day; prepared by moistening 200 parts cinnamon bark evenly with ethanol and percolate to produce 1,000 parts tincture.

Hazards

Adverse effects associated with cinnamon include sedation, sleepiness, depression, tachycardia, oral lesions, increased intestinal movement, tachypnea, allergic reactions to skin and mucosa, skin irritation, pruritus, and increased perspiration. There are no reported interactions with cinnamon.

Those with an allergy to cinnamon or Peruvian balsam should avoid use. Those who are pregnant or are planning pregnancy and those who have GI conditions, including ulcers, should avoid using cinnamon for therapeutic purposes because it may irritate the GI tract.

Clinical considerations

■ If patient is pregnant or is planning pregnancy, advise her not to use cinnamon medicinally.

■ Alert patient that cinnamon may cause an allergic skin reaction. Tell him to promptly report any adverse reactions and new signs or symptoms to his health care provider.

■ Advise patient to stop using cinnamon and to promptly contact his health care provider if he experiences stomach upset, diarrhea, or signs of bleeding.

■ Tell patient to remind prescriber and pharmacist of any herbal or dietary supplement that he's taking when obtaining a new prescription.

■ Advise patient to consult his health care provider before using an herbal preparation because a treatment with proven efficacy may be available.

Research summary

Germany's Commission E approves cinnamon for appetite loss and indigestion; however, these uses are backed by scant scientific evidence.

clary

*Clary sage, clear eye, muscatel sage,
Salvia sclarea*

The flowering tops and leaves of the *Salvia sclarea* yield an essential oil that's made up largely of alcohols and up to 75% linalyl acetate, linlol, pinene, myrcene, and phellandrene. Clary may have muscle relaxant, analgesic, anxiolytic, and some antiestrogenic effects. It's available as an oil and in products such as See Bright and Toute-Bonne.

Reported uses

Clary is used to treat mental fatigue, depression, anxiety, tension, and decreased libido. It's used as an astringent, anti-inflammatory, and antispasmodic, and to help restore hormonal balance and relieve symptoms of premenstrual syndrome or menopause.

The essential oil is used as a topical agent. In aromatherapy, it's used for baths, sprays, diffusers, and massages. Clary is also used as a flavoring agent in foods.

Administration

■ Atomizer: 8 gtt of the essential oil added to 1 oz (30 ml) of water in an atomizer
■ Bath: 8 gtt of the essential oil blended with 1 tablespoon of unscented bath oil or water and stirred well to disperse
■ Diffuser: 6 to 10 gtt of the essential oil added to 2 tablespoons water in diffuser bowl.

Hazards

Clary may cause drowsiness. Alcohol use with clary sage oil may result in enhanced sedation.

Women who are pregnant or are planning pregnancy should avoid use. Those who have breast cysts, uterine fibroids, or other estrogen-related disorders should avoid long-term use.

Clinical considerations

 SAFETY RISK *This essential oil is for external use only, primarily in aromatherapy.*

■ Warn patient not to treat migraine, depression, or anxiety with clary before seeking appropriate medical evaluation because doing so may delay diagnosis of a potentially serious medical condition.
■ If patient is pregnant or is planning pregnancy, advise her not to use the essential oil.
■ If patient is taking estrogen, instruct her to inform her health care provider.
■ Tell patient not to apply undiluted essential oils to skin.
■ Tell patient to remind prescriber and pharmacist of any herbal or dietary supplement that she's taking when obtaining a new prescription.
■ Advise patient to consult her health care provider before using an herbal preparation because a treatment with proven efficacy may be available.

Research summary

The concepts behind the use of clary and the claims made regarding its effects have not yet been validated scientifically.

clove oil

Caryophyllus, clove buds,
Syzygium aromaticum

Clove oil is derived from the dried, powdered flower buds of *Syzygium aromaticum.* The chief components of clove are the volatile oils eugenol (85%), eugenyl acetate, and beta-caryophyllene (5% to 8%). Clove oil is an analgesic and antiseptic. The eugenyl acetate component has antihistaminic and spasmolytic properties. Eugenol suppresses the pain pathways. Analgesic activity occurs by the inhibition of prostaglandin and leukotriene biosynthesis by inhibiting cyclooxygenase and lipoxygenase.

Clove oil inhibits gram-positive and gram-negative bacteria and may also have fungistatic, anthelmintic, and larvicidal effects. Clove oil is available for topical use or as a mouthwash.

Reported uses

Clove oil is used as a dental analgesic and antiseptic. It has also been studied for its potential to inhibit platelet aggregation.

Clove oil is used to relieve signs and symptoms of the common cold and to treat coughs, bronchitis, inflammation of the mouth and pharynx, and infections. It's also used as a spice and a flavoring for foods.

Administration

■ Mouthwashes: Aqueous solutions equal to 1% to 5% essential oil used as a rinse
■ Toothaches: Cotton dipped into undiluted oil, then applied topically to area of tooth pain.

Hazards

Adverse effects associated with the use of clove include hemoptysis, pulmonary toxicity, blood-tinged sputum (in clove cigarette smokers), depression, liver failure, altered electrolyte levels, irritation of skin and mucous membranes, toxic reaction, and disseminated intravascular coagulation. Theoretically, the herb may increase the effects of platelet aggregation inhibitors, although no interaction has been reported.

Clove oil isn't for use in children. Undiluted clove oil is unsafe for self-administration.

Clinical considerations

■ Allergic reactions to clove oil are rare.
■ Topical application of clove oil can be harmful to the teeth. Inspect patient's gums and mucous membranes for signs of local irritation.
■ Instruct patient to stop using clove oil if adverse reactions or local irritation occurs.
■ Tell patient to remind prescriber and pharmacist of any herbal or dietary supplement that he's taking when obtaining a new prescription.
■ Advise patient to consult his health care provider before using an herbal preparation because a treatment with proven efficacy may be available.

Research summary

The concepts behind the use of clove oil and the claims made regarding its effects have not yet been validated scientifically.

coenzyme Q10

Mitoquinon, ubidecarenone, ubiquinone

Coenzyme Q10 (CO Q10) is a lipid-soluble benzoquinone that's structurally related to vitamin K. It's found in every cell in the body, and acts as a free radical scavenger and membrane stabilizer. It's also an important cofactor in electron transport in the mitochondria. CO Q10 is available as capsules, softgels, and tablets, in products such as Maxi Cardio Co-Q10, Maxi-Sorb Co Q10, Mega Co Q10, and My Fav Coenzyme Q10.

Reported uses

Coenzyme Q10 is used to treat ischemic heart disease, hypertension, and heart failure. It's also used in the treatment of acquired immunodeficiency syndrome (AIDS), muscular dystrophy, and chronic fatigue syndrome. CO Q10 is used to protect against doxorubicin cardiotoxicity and to protect the myocardium during invasive cardiac surgery. It may also stimulate the production of blood cells. Low levels of CO Q10 have been found in patients with breast cancer, periodontal diseases, diabetes, and heart disease.

Administration

■ Oral use: 30 to 300 mg daily; dosages above 100 mg in divided doses, two to three times a day.

Hazards

Adverse effects associated with the use of CO Q10, though rare, include epigastric discomfort, loss of appetite, nausea, and diarrhea. Beta blockers may inhibit CO Q10-dependent enzymes. Hydroxymethylglutaryl coenzyme A (HMG-CoA) reductase inhibitors and gemfibrozil may decrease levels of CO Q10. CO Q10 may decrease insulin requirements in patients with type 1 diabetes mellitus. International Normalized Ratio may decrease when warfarin is used in conjunction with CO Q10. Oral hypoglycemics decrease serum CO Q10 levels, whereas food maximizes its absorption.

Those with a hypersensitivity to CO Q10, pregnant patients, and breast-feeding patients should avoid use.

Clinical considerations

■ Monitor vital signs and electrocardiogram results, as needed.
■ Warn patient not to treat signs and symptoms of heart failure — such as increasing shortness of breath, edema, or chest pain — with CO Q10 before seeking appropriate medical evaluation because doing so may delay diagnosis of a potentially serious medical condition.

SAFETY RISK *Advise patient with heart failure that CO Q10 shouldn't replace conventional drug therapy. Encourage him to discuss use of CO Q10 with his health care provider so treatment may be properly monitored.*

■ If patient is pregnant or breast-feeding, advise her not to use CO Q10.
■ If patient is diabetic, alert him to the signs and symptoms of hypoglycemia and hyperglycemia, and instruct him to monitor his blood glucose level.
■ Instruct patient to inform his health care provider if he's taking a cholesterol lowering or heart drug, an anticoagulant, or insulin.
■ Tell patient to remind prescriber and pharmacist of any herbal or dietary supplement that he's taking when obtaining a new prescription.
■ Advise patient to consult his health care provider before using an herbal preparation because a treatment with proven efficacy may be available.

Research summary

Patients with heart failure have significantly lower levels of CO Q10 in heart muscle cells than healthy people. This fact alone doesn't prove that CO Q10 supplements will help treat heart failure; however, it has prompted medical researchers to try using CO Q10 as a treatment for heart failure. Several double-blind studies have found that CO Q10

supplements, when taken along with conventional medication, can markedly improve symptoms and objective measurements of heart function.

coffee

*Arabian coffee, café, caffea,
Coffea arabica, espresso, java, mocha*

The medicinal components of coffee are derived from the seeds, or beans. Coffee seeds contain 1% to 2% caffeine, 0.25% trigonelline, 3% to 5% tannins, 15% glucose and dextrin, 10% to 13% fatty oil (trioleoyl glycerol and tripalmitoyl glycerol), and 10% to 13% proteins.

Caffeine, the active component of coffee, acts as a central nervous system stimulant. It has positive chronotropic effects on the heart, may increase gastric secretions, and may relax smooth muscles of the blood vessels and the bronchioles of the respiratory tract. Caffeine may increase low-density lipoproteins and total cholesterol levels in those consuming more than 5 cups of coffee per day. It also acts as a mild diuretic. Coffee is available as whole beans and as dried, freeze-dried, or ground beans. Spray-dried crystals are used for instant coffee.

Reported uses

Coffee is used most notably for its stimulant effects and for its ability to relieve malaise and weariness. It's also used for its diuretic and anti-inflammatory effects. In large doses, caffeine can be used to dilate the bronchioles during an asthma attack.

Administration

■ Maximum dose of caffeine: 1.5 g per day; less than 250 mg per day for non-pregnant adults; usually, 100 to 150 mg (1 cup brewed coffee) per day for pregnant adults.

Hazards

Adverse effects associated with coffee include insomnia, irritability, nervousness, dizziness, headache, hypertension, tachycardia, palpitations, irregular heart rate, ulcers, heartburn, vomiting, diarrhea, loss of appetite, abdominal spasms, stiffness, muscle spasms, tachypnea, increased total cholesterol and low-density lipoprotein (LDL) levels, hyperglycemia, and increased excretion of calcium. Reduced sedative effects are seen when coffee is used in conjunction with benzodiazepines. Slight increase in blood pressure may occur when coffee is used with beta blockers (metoprolol, propranolol). Coffee charcoal may interfere with the absorption of other drugs. Significant elevation in blood pressure and mania may occur when coffee is used with phenylpropanolamine. Increased stimulant effects and side effects may occur when used with other caffeine- or ephedrine-containing herbal or drug products. Coffee may potentiate the adverse effects of theophylline and increase jitteriness.

Caffeine is believed to increase the risk of late first and second trimester miscarriages. Caffeine consumed by a breast-feeding mother can cause sleep disorders in her infant. Patients who are pregnant, breast-feeding, or planning pregnancy should avoid use. Patients with ulcers or chronic digestive disorders and those with hypertension should also avoid use.

Clinical considerations

 SAFETY RISK *Although lethal overdose is unlikely, the first signs and symptoms of poisoning are vomiting and abdominal spasms.*

■ Sustained intake of coffee can lead to physical dependence. Withdrawal symptoms include headache and sleep disorders.
■ Advise patient with risk factors for heart disease, such as increased cholesterol level or hypertension, to discuss caffeine consumption with his health care provider.

■ Advise patient to inform his health care provider if he experiences difficulty sleeping or develops stomach upset or irritation. Discuss other potential adverse effects with patient and instruct him to promptly report signs and symptoms.
■ Advise patient who's pregnant, breast-feeding, or planning pregnancy to consider avoiding or limiting her caffeine intake.
■ Tell patient to remind prescriber and pharmacist of any herbal or dietary supplement that he's taking when obtaining a new prescription.
■ Advise patient to consult his health care provider before using an herbal preparation because a treatment with proven efficacy may be available.

Research summary

The concepts behind the use of coffee and the claims made regarding its effects have not yet been validated scientifically.

cola

Bissy nut, Cola acuminata, C. nitida, *cola nut, cola seeds, guru nut, kola nut, kola tree*

The medicinal components of cola are found in the seeds of *Cola acuminata* and *C. nitida*, trees of the cocoa family. The seed contains theobromine, theophylline, and 1.5% to 2.5% caffeine—all of which are central nervous system (CNS) stimulants.

Cola also has a diuretic effect, stimulates gastric acid production and gastric motility, and has mild chronotropic activity. It may contain potentially carcinogenic primary and secondary amines as well as tannins. Cola is available as liquid extract, cola nut, cola extract, tea, tincture, and wine, in products such as soft drinks, Starter, and Ultra Diet Pep.

Reported uses

Cola is used as a stimulant to counteract mental and physical fatigue and depression. Cola seeds are chewed to suppress hunger, thirst, morning sickness, and migraines. It's also used to flavor many popular carbonated soft drinks.

Administration

- Cola extract: 0.25 to 0.75 g per day
- Cola nut: 2 to 6 g every day in divided doses
- Fluid extract: 2.5 to 7.5 g per day
- Tea: 1 to 2 g of cola nut in 5 ounces of water three times a day
- Tincture: 10 to 30 ml per day
- Wine: 60 to 180 ml per day.

Hazards

Adverse effects associated with the use of cola include insomnia, restlessness, nervousness, excitability, tachycardia, palpitations, elevated blood pressure, and gastric irritation.

When cola is used in conjunction with beta agonists, such as albuterol, metaproterenol, salmeterol, and terbutalin, enhanced cardiac stimulation may occur. Enhanced cardiac and CNS stimulation may occur if cola is used with CNS stimulants, such as phenylpropanolamine or pseudoephedrine, or with decongestants. Cola may enhance the effect of diuretics. Abrupt caffeine withdrawal can increase the risk of lithium toxicity. Recommend consistent intake of caffeine-containing products during lithium therapy.

Hypertensive crisis can be precipitated if a person who's taking a monamine oxidase inhibitor consumes excessive amounts of caffeine. Using cola in conjunction with quinolone antibiotics can result in decreased caffeine clearance, leading to increased risk of adverse effects, such as increased blood pressure and heart rate and excessive CNS stimulation. Enhanced adverse effects may occur if cola is used with theophylline, or with other caffeine-containing products. Grapefruit juice may cause increased caffeine levels, leading to increased risk of adverse effects.

Those with underlying cardiac disease or renal insufficiency, geriatric patients, and those with a history of gastric or duodenal ulcers should avoid using cola. Pregnant and breast-feeding patients should limit use. Cola nut is contraindicated in those with chocolate allergy due to cross-sensitivity. Those with renal dysfunction should use cola cautiously.

Clinical considerations

- Monitor patient's heart rate and blood pressure.
- The diuretic effect of excessive cola may result in dehydration.
- Observe patient for signs of excess CNS stimulation. Before using a drug to treat symptoms of excitability such as insomnia, check to see if the patient should simply decrease his intake of cola.
- Because some cola preparations contain significant amounts of alcohol, children, alcoholic patients, patients with liver disease, patients receiving metronidazole or disulfiram, and pregnant and breast-feeding patients should avoid them.
- Stopping cola abruptly can sometimes lead to signs and symptoms of physical withdrawal, including headache, irritability, dizziness, and anxiety.
- Geriatric patients may be especially prone to adverse cardiac and CNS effects.
- Advise patient to limit his sources of caffeine, to avoid excessive cardiac and CNS stimulation.
- Advise patient who has hypertension or heart disease or is pregnant or breast-feeding to avoid cola preparations.
- Advise patient to consult his health care provider if he experiences palpitations or dyspepsia.
- Tell patient to inform all his health care providers about his use of cola.
- Instruct patient and family to avoid using alcohol preparations of cola in children, those with a history of alcohol abuse or liver disease, and those taking disulfiram or metronidazole.

- Advise patient that yellow staining of oral mucosa has been associated with chewing cola nuts.
- Tell patient to remind prescriber and pharmacist of any herbal or dietary supplement that he's taking when obtaining a new prescription.
- Advise patient to consult his health care provider before using an herbal preparation because a treatment with proven efficacy may be available.

Research summary
The concepts behind the use of cola and the claims made regarding its effects have not yet been validated scientifically.

Coley's toxins

Immunotherapy

Coley's toxins were first used by surgeon and cancer researcher William B. Coley at Memorial Hospital (now Memorial Sloan-Kettering Cancer Center) in New York. While reviewing over 100 cases of sarcoma, he became aware that patients who developed bacterial infections after surgery did better than those without postoperative infections. He began research on use of toxins in cancer patients and, in 1896, presented a paper to the Johns Hopkins Medical Society reporting regressions of sarcoma among 93 patients whom he had treated with the toxins. Dr. Coley chose bacteria that would cause a high fever and mobilize the patient's immune system to fight the cancer cells. Knowing that using live bacteria was dangerous, and because he determined that the immune reactions depended upon the toxins of the bacteria rather than the actual bacteria, he experimented with the toxins alone. He settled on a combination of heat-killed gram-positive *Streptococcus pyogenes* and non-pathogenic gram-negative *Serratia marcescens*. One of the biologically active ingredients in Coley's toxins is lipopolysaccharide (LPS), which causes hyper-

thermia. It causes a fever of 104° F to 105° F (40° C to 40.5° C) for 3 to 4 hours to enhance lymphocyte activity and boost the tumor necrosis factor (TNF).

The cell types most responsive to LPS are natural killer (NK) lymphocytes and macrophages. On detecting LPS, these cells release large amounts of inflammatory cytokines, one of which, TNF, is especially toxic to bacteria. Coley's toxins presumably involve activation of NK cells, and the products of these cells may combat the tumors.

Until 1930, Dr. Coley used these toxins to treat patients with a variety of cancers. Other physicians continued to use Coley's toxins through World War II. Many regressions of cancer were reported among patients treated, but the treatment fell into disuse with the advent of chemotherapy. The American Cancer Society for many years considered Coley's erysipelas toxins to be ineffective remedies. More recently, Coley's toxins have been cited as a promising treatment that may have been prematurely abandoned with the advent of modern radiotherapy and chemotherapy. Once considered unorthodox, such treatments for cancer might now be an adjunct to conventional surgery, chemotherapy, and radiation.

Reported uses
Coley's toxins are used outside the United States, in Mexico, Central America, Guatemala, Germany, and China. They've been used to treat renal, ovarian, breast, and testicular cancers; soft-tissue sarcomas; Hodgkin's disease; malignant melanoma; and cancers of the bone and connective tissue. Theoretically, joint treatment of bacterial toxins with radiation therapy might be beneficial for lesions that haven't metastasized or for controlling a symptomatic primary or secondary lesion in a patient with incurable metastases. Coley's toxins are used at some cancer clinics to "jump start" immune responses.

An adaptation of Coley's toxins, known as mixed bacterial vaccines, is administered to patients along with other immune-affecting agents at the Waisbren Clinic in Milwaukee, Wisconsin.

How the treatment is performed

The patient receives injections, either subcutaneous or I.V., every other week for 4 weeks and once a week thereafter. The dose schedule varies with the individual.

Coley's toxins are usually administered in a stepwise increasing dose, with the aim of maintaining a body temperature of 102.2° F (39° C) or higher. Patients must be monitored closely, and those who don't achieve this temperature receive higher doses.

Hazards

The most common side effects of the therapy include fever and nausea. Other less common side effects include headache, back pain, chills, angina, and occasionally herpes labialis. Overwhelming the immune system with Coley's toxins could result in serious infections in immune compromised patients.

Available evidence suggests that Coley's toxins aren't harmful or dangerous to humans suffering from various types of neoplasms, provided the toxins are administered properly as to dosage, site, and the usual aseptic precautions.

Clinical considerations

■ Coley's combined toxins are legal in the United States only if prepared and given within a physician's office. They may not be shipped.

■ One study cautioned that patients with severe hepatic insufficiency due to metastatic disease or other pathology, and patients who have had severe heart conditions, should not receive the toxins. It also indicated the need for prolonged toxin therapy, but found that toxins were not helpful if begun after massive radiation and chemotherapy had destroyed a patient's immune responsiveness.

Research summary

During the 1980s, Coley's toxins were tested in mice at Temple University, Philadelphia, and they compared favorably with other biological response modifiers because of their enhancing effects on the immune response and oncolytic properties at nontoxic levels.

A 1999 study (Richardson, et al.), funded by the National Institutes of Health, completed a cohort analysis of treatment with Coley's toxins. Using a retrospective cohort design with external controls, 128 patients treated with Coley's toxins in New York from 1890 to 1960 were compared with 1,675 control patients from the Surveillance Epidemiology End Result population-based cancer registry of patients who received the diagnosis in 1983. The study suggested that treatment with Coley's toxins is not associated with an increased risk of mortality. Given the tremendous advances in surgical techniques and medicine in general, any cohort of modern patients should have been expected to do better than patients treated 50 or more years ago, but no such statistical advantage for the modern group was observed in the study. In the absence of demonstrated harmful effects and some indication of positive effects, the study findings called for a reevaluation of this therapy.

Colonic irrigation

Colon hydrotherapy, colon therapy, colonic, colonic hydrotherapy, colonic therapy

Advocates of colonic irrigation believe that over time, pathogenic fungi, bacteria, mucus, and other debris accumulate in the colon leading to skin problems, constipation, and a lack of energy. Colonic therapy is a procedure designed to help improve the elimination of this toxic build-up by removing fecal matter from the colon walls and diluting the concentration of bacteria in the large intestine. This reduces proliferation of pathogenic bacteria and maintains proper levels of beneficial microflora. Once the colon is free of debris, the patient should notice changes in energy level, skin tone, weight, and stress level. In addition, a patient may no longer suffer from constipation or experience painful abdominal cramping or bloating. Enhanced absorption of vitamins and minerals is also noticed following a detoxification program using colonic therapy. The concept of colonic irrigation is based on the premise that intestinal waste products are a major contributor to disease and can poison the body if not removed.

Reported uses

One of the main uses for colonic irrigation is the treatment of chronic constipation. Inflammatory conditions of the colon can also be addressed using colonic therapy. Patients suffering from bloating, stomachache, or abdominal pain may also find relief using colonic therapy. Other conditions for which colonic therapy is used include acne, psoriasis, and eczema.

Patients with arthritis also seem to benefit from using colonic therapy. Some are thought to have increased bowel permeability, leading to a toxic condition in the GI tract in which toxins are continually reabsorbed into the blood. Once in the blood, these toxins attack the joints, leading to inflammation and stress.

Another major use for colonic therapy is in cancer patients. These patients tend to have deficient levels of various minerals, vitamins, and essential fatty acids. They may also suffer from constipation due to use of potent narcotic analgesics. Therefore, removing intestinal debris by colonic irrigation may lead to increased absorption of vitamins, minerals, and other key nutrients. Additionally, it may relieve constipation, allowing for enhanced elimination of toxins released from tumor cells.

RESEARCH *All studies but the 1997 study by Briel, et al., report on the potential adverse effects of colonic irrigation. In contrast, Briel and colleagues found significant results using colonic irrigation in patients with fecal soiling and fecal incontinence.*

How the treatment is performed

The day before the colonic irrigation is to take place, the patient is instructed to eat two salads. In the dinner salad, the patient adds 1 tablespoon of cooked corn in order to determine bowel transit time. The patient is also advised to avoid rice, pasta, and bread the day before and the day of the colonic irrigation and not to eat any food for at least 2 hours before the session.

With the patient lying on his side, a small plastic hose is gently inserted into the patient's rectum. This hose is connected to the colonic irrigation machine, which has controls for water temperature and volume. Water that has been filtered to remove bacteria, heavy metals, and chlorine begins to flow into the patient's rectum and throughout the colon. The volume of water, varied according to the patient's tolerance, induces peristaltic contractions of the colon, which expel the fecal matter into another hose leading back to the irrigation machine. This clear tube allows inspection of colon contents. The patient may experience a feeling of warmth during the session due to the presence of toxins in the fecal matter. During the irrigation, the therapist gently massages different areas of the abdomen to help dislodge and loosen areas of impaction. A session usually lasts 30 to 45 minutes. Most patients require a series of colonic irrigations to dislodge all of the fecal matter.

Hazards

If the therapist uses too much water, the treatment may be uncomfortable or painful. If the therapist uses too little water, the patient's bowel is forced to work harder to achieve peristalsis.

Overdistention of the colon during the procedure or an improperly inserted hose can cause perforation of the intestinal wall. A 1999 case report cited an incidence of perineal gangrene following a perforation of the bowel during colonic therapy.

An outbreak of amebiasis occurred in the early 1980s in a Colorado chiropractic clinic, most likely due to imcomplete cleaning of the irrigation machine between patients.

A cancer patient wishing to have a colonic irrigation performed should use caution. Administering a colonic irrigation to a patient who is weak may weaken him further. Close monitoring by an experienced health care provider is necessary.

Clinical considerations

 TRAINING *No certification is required to perform colon irrigation. Selecting an experienced physician or practitioner of alternative medicine to properly monitor the colonic therapy is important.*

Patients with diverticulitis, ulcerative colitis, Crohn's disease, severe hemorrhoids, tumors of the large intestine or rectum, excessive acidity in intestinal tract, and bowel perforation should not undergo colonic irrigation. No data exists regarding the safety of colonic irrigations in pediatric, maternal, and geriatric populations.

REIMBURSEMENT *Colonic irrigation is considered a legal medical practice in the United States. However, most third-party insurance payors do not reimburse patients for receiving colonic irrigations.*

Research summary

The literature contains several reports of colonic irrigation. However, most don't focus on validating the therapy in patients with bowel-related complications or diseases. Rather, they emphasize adverse effects and complications that can occur. A 1997 study showed positive results in patients with fecal soiling and fe-

cal incontinence, with the majority of patients in both groups claiming improvement in quality of life.

coltsfoot

Ass's foot, British tobacco, bullsfoot, coughwort, donnhove, fieldhove, flower velure, foal's-foot, foalswort, hallfoot, horse-foot, horsehoof, huflattichblatter, kuandong hua, Tussilago farfara

Coltsfoot contains 5% to 10% mucilage, which is believed to produce a soothing effect by physically coating the irritated mucosa of the mouth and throat. The plant's polysaccharides, flavonoids, and phenolic components may have anti-inflammatory and antibacterial activity. Also, the plant contains tussilagone, a sesquiterpene thought to have cardiovascular and respiratory stimulant properties, and a number of pyrrolizidine alkaloids, primarily senkirkine and senecionine, which are converted to toxic metabolites in the liver and have been associated with hepatotoxicity.

The dried leaf of coltsfoot is the part most commonly used for medicinal purposes. Although the flower also contains medicinal components, it's reported to have higher levels of pyrrolizidine alkaloids. Coltsfoot is available as tea, bulk leaf, capsules, leaf extract, and tincture.

Reported uses

Coltsfoot is used to soothe throat irritation and mild inflammations of the mouth and throat, to alleviate cough, and to treat symptoms of respiratory infections, acute and chronic bronchitis, laryngitis, asthma, colds, and emphysema. It's also used as a smoking mixture.

Administration

■ Leaf extract: 0.6 to 2 ml three times a day, not to exceed 1 mcg of pyrrolizidine alkaloids with a 1,2 necine structure

- Tincture: 2 to 8 ml three times a day
- Tea: Maximum of 6 g/day, or 10 mcg of pyrrolizidine alkaloids with a 1,2 necine structure; prepared by adding 1.5 to 2.5 g of cut leaf to boiling water.

Hazards

Adverse effects associated with the use of coltsfoot include lethargy, anorexia, abdominal pain (especially right upper quadrant pain) and swelling, nausea, vomiting, hepatotoxicity, liver changes and liver cancer, reversible hepatic veno-occlusive disease, jaundice, and allergic reaction.

Excessive consumption of coltsfoot may interfere with the effects of antihypertensives and cardiac drugs. Herbal products prepared with alcohol may cause a disulfiram-like reaction.

SAFETY RISK *Due to the risk of hepatotoxicity and liver cancer, coltsfoot isn't recommended for use by humans. Many countries have banned the internal use of other herbal products containing pyrrolizidine alkaloids because of the risk of liver toxicity.*

Clinical considerations

- Recommend alternative therapies that aren't associated with severe adverse effects — for example, over-the-counter lozenges or sprays.
- Some extracts may contain up to 45% alcohol, so children, alcoholic patients, those with liver disease, and those receiving metronidazole or disulfiram should avoid them.
- If patient has cancer or is undergoing chemotherapy, is pregnant or breast-feeding, or is planning pregnancy, advise against using coltsfoot.
- Some of coltsfoot's components may antagonize the effect of antihypertensives on blood pressure.
- Those with an allergy to plants in the Asteraceae family — such as ragweed, marigolds, daisies, and chrysanthemums — may experience hypersensitivity reactions to coltsfoot.

- The active ingredient, a mucilage, is destroyed when burned and smoked.
- Monitor blood pressure and liver function test results, and watch for signs and symptoms of hepatotoxicity, such as right upper quadrant pain, nausea, vomiting, abdominal distention, and jaundice. Instruct patient to report any of these signs at once.
- Warn patient that use in higher doses or for longer than recommended may increase the risk of liver toxicity and malignancy.
- Regardless of the preparation used, therapy should last no longer than 4 to 6 weeks per year, to prevent exposure to large amounts of pyrrolizidine alkaloids.
- Caution patient that manufacturers don't report the pyrrolizidine alkaloid content of their products, making it very difficult to determine the exact dose being ingested.
- Tell patient to remind prescriber and pharmacist of any herbal or dietary supplement that he's taking when obtaining a new prescription.
- Advise patient to consult his health care provider before using an herbal preparation because a treatment with proven efficacy may be available.

Research summary

The concepts behind the use of coltsfoot and the claims made regarding its effects have not yet been validated scientifically.

comfrey

Ass ear, black root, blackwort, boneset, bruisewort, consound, gum plant, healing herb, knitback, knitbone, salsify, slippery root, Symphytum officinale, *wallwort*

The medicinal components of comfrey are derived from the fresh or dried root and leaves of *Symphytum officinale*. Also used are the leaves and roots of Russian comfrey, also known as prickly comfrey, a hybrid of *S. officinale* and *S. asperum*.

Comfrey's medicinal effect may result from its allantoin content, which promotes cell proliferation and enhances wound healing. The roots contain more allantoin (0.6% to 0.7%) than the leaves (0.3%). Other components include rosmarinic acid—also believed to have anti-inflammatory properties—mucilage, and numerous pyrrolizidine alkaloids. Pyrrolizidine alkaloids are converted in the liver to toxic metabolites that have been linked to hepatotoxicity. The root contains a higher amount of pyrrolizidine alkaloids than the leaves.

Russian comfrey contains echimidine, which may be the most toxic pyrrolizidine alkaloid found in comfrey. Comfrey is available as alcohol-free root extract, compounded oil, cream, leaf extract, ointment, and root extract, in products such as Comfree.

Reported uses
Comfrey is used topically to treat bruises, sprains, joint inflammation, swelling, and ulcers. It's also used to help heal wounds.

Administration
■ Ointments and other external preparations containing 5% to 20% dried herb: Daily dose not to exceed 100 mcg of pyrrolizidine alkaloids with 1,2 unsaturated necine structure; applied topically to intact skin.

Hazards
Adverse effects associated with the internal use of comfrey include pancreatic islet cell tumors, urinary bladder tumors, hepatotoxicity, liver damage, veno-occlusive disease, and cancer. There are no reported interactions with the topical use.

Comfrey should not be consumed orally. Topical application should be limited to 10 days.

 SAFETY RISK *Several agencies, including the United States Pharmacopoeia's expert advisory panel and the American Herbal Products Associ-*ation, have identified comfrey preparations as potentially harmful because of reports of liver toxicity. Many countries have banned internal use of comfrey, so such use is highly discouraged.*

Clinical considerations
■ Advise patient that comfrey isn't recommended for internal use.
■ If patient has ingested comfrey, monitor for signs and symptoms of hepatotoxicity, including abdominal distention, nausea, right upper quadrant abdominal pain, and an elevated liver function test.
■ If patient is using comfrey to promote wound healing, monitor the wound being treated. Evaluate the possibility of an infectious cause of cellulitis or inflammation.
■ Inform patient that external preparations shouldn't be applied to broken or abraded skin.
■ Use of comfrey should be limited to 4 to 6 weeks per year, to prevent exposure to large amounts of pyrrolizidine alkaloids.
■ Tell patient to remind prescriber and pharmacist of any herbal or dietary supplement that he's taking when obtaining a new prescription.
■ Advise patient to consult his health care provider before using an herbal preparation because a treatment with proven efficacy may be available.

Research summary
The concepts behind the use of comfrey and the claims made regarding its effects have not yet been validated scientifically.

condurango

Condor-vine bark, condurango bark, condurango blanco, condurango cortex, eagle vine, Marsdenia condurango

The medicinal components of condurango are found in the bark of the branches and trunk of *Marsdenia condurango* and include numerous glycosides such as condurangin, which stimulates saliva and gastric juice secretion. Condurango can be found in many homeopathic preparations as a liquid extract, powdered bark, or tincture.

Reported uses
Condurango is used to stimulate appetite, alleviate dyspepsia, promote diuresis, and, in folk medicine, to treat stomach cancer. It may also be used to increase peripheral circulation. It's commonly used in South America as an alternative treatment for chronic syphilis.

Administration
- Aqueous extract: 0.2 to 0.5 g daily
- Bark: 2 to 4 g daily
- Liqueur, tea: 1 cup of liqueur or tea 30 minutes before each meal; liqueur prepared by steeping 50 to 100 g of bark in 1 qt (1 L) of wine for several days
- Tincture: 2 to 5 g for alcohol content (½ to 1 dram as needed).

Hazards
SAFETY RISK *There's a potential cross-sensitivity between condurango and natural rubber latex. Patients who have a severe allergy to latex and who use condurango may experience cutaneous reactions or respiratory compromise (shortness of breath, hypotension, tachycardia, or anaphylaxis).*

Adverse effects associated with condurango overdose include vertigo, visual changes, seizures, paralysis, and anaphylactic reaction. Herbal products prepared with alcohol may cause a disulfiram-like reaction. Tannins may bind iron and other drugs in the gut if taken simultaneously.

Pregnant and breast-feeding patients should avoid using condurango because it has an alkaloid component that resembles strychnine. Children and geriatric patients should also avoid use.

Clinical considerations
- If patient is taking condurango to alleviate dyspepsia, find out how serious his condition is and whether he has tried other therapies to treat it.
- If patient is taking condurango to stimulate his appetite, evaluate possible causes of his condition and whether he has also experienced significant weight loss because this may indicate a more serious condition.
- Patients who also report melena or hematemesis should be referred for further workup.

SAFETY RISK *Warn patient that overdose of condurango may produce dizziness, visual changes, seizures, and paralysis. Tell him to seek medical attention immediately if any adverse reactions occur.*

- If patient has a latex allergy, discourage use.
- If patient is pregnant or breast-feeding, advise her not to take the herb.
- If patient has a history of alcohol abuse or liver disease or is taking disulfiram or metronidazole, advise him to avoid taking preparations that contain alcohol.
- Warn patient to avoid using condurango with other drugs because information regarding interactions is lacking.
- Advise patient to report continued weight loss, GI bleeding, or worsening dyspepsia to his health care provider.
- Tell patient to remind prescriber and pharmacist of any herbal or dietary supplement that he's taking when obtaining a new prescription.
- Advise patient to consult his health care provider before using an herbal preparation because a treatment with proven efficacy may be available.

Research summary
The concepts behind the use of condurango and the claims made regarding its effects have not yet been validated scientifically.

coriander

Chinese parsley, cilantro,
Coriandrum sativum,
koriander, oriander

The medicinal elements of coriander are derived from the ripe, dried seed of *Coriandrum sativum*. It contains 0.5% to 1% essential oil. The volatile oil, which consists primarily of linalool, stimulates gastric acid secretion and has spasmolytic properties. It also provides vitamin C, calcium, magnesium, potassium, and iron. Coriander may have hypoglycemic, hypolipidemic, and antiseptic effects. It's available as capsules, pure coriander seed, essential oil, powder, and tea; it's also used in natural deodorant products and in curry powder.

Reported uses
Coriander is used to enhance appetite and treat dyspepsia, flatulence, diarrhea, and colic. It's also used to treat coughs, chest pains, fever, bladder ailments, halitosis, postpartum complications, colic, measles, dysentery, hemorrhoids, and toothaches.

In aromatherapy, the essential oil is used for its soothing effects and to improve blood circulation. Coriander is also used as a flavoring agent or spice in foods and as a fragrance in bath and beauty products. It can also be used to disguise the unpleasant taste of some medicines.

Administration
■ Dried seed: 3 g/day of crushed fruit
■ Tea: Between meals; prepared by pouring 7 oz of boiling water over 1 to 3 g of crushed coriander seed and steeping for 10 to 15 minutes
■ Tincture: 10 to 20 ml every day, after meals.

Hazards
SAFETY RISK *Breathing difficulty, airway tightness, and urticaria may occur in patients with severe* allergy to coriander. *Monitor patient for signs and symptoms of respiratory distress and vital signs closely.*

Adverse effects associated with coriander include allergic reaction and increased risk of photosensitivity reactions with sun exposure.

Patients with hypersensitivity to coriander or any of its components, pregnant patients, breast-feeding patients, and children should avoid use, as effects in these populations are unknown.

Clinical considerations
■ Some preparations may contain alcohol, so children, geriatric patients, those with a history of alcohol abuse or liver disease, and those taking disulfiram or metronidazole should avoid them.
■ Instruct patient not to take coriander if he is allergic to it or any of its components.
■ Assess patient's use of other therapies to manage GI complaints.
■ Evaluate patient for complications such as melena, hematemesis, and significant unintended weight loss.
■ Advise patient to seek emergency medical help immediately if he experiences adverse reactions, such as shortness of breath, rapid heart rate, or dizziness.
■ Advise patient to wear sunscreen and protective clothing outdoors and to avoid exposure to direct sunlight.
■ Tell patient to remind prescriber and pharmacist of any herbal or dietary supplement that he's taking when obtaining a new prescription.
■ Advise patient to consult his health care provider before using an herbal preparation because a treatment with proven efficacy may be available.

Research summary
The concepts behind the use of coriander and the claims made regarding its effects have not yet been validated scientifically.

corkwood

Corkwood tree, Duboisia myoporoides, *pituri*

Corkwood contains alkaloids, including hyoscyamine, hyoscine, scopolamine, atropine, and butropine. These components have potent anticholinergic properties and can be fatal in large doses. Corkwood is available as extract, leaves, and twigs.

Reported uses
Corkwood is used for its stimulant, euphoric, and hallucinogenic effects and may be used to treat motion sickness. Some patients chew the leaves and twigs. In homeopathy, corkwood is used to treat eye disorders.

Corkwood was used as a substitute for atropine and scopolamine before commercial sources were readily available.

Medicinal use of corkwood isn't currently recommended.

Administration
The use of corkwood is not well documented.

Hazards
Adverse effects associated with the use of corkwood include drowsiness, euphoria, excitation, hallucinations, other central nervous system (CNS) disturbances, altered heart rate, blurred vision, dry mucous membranes, paralyzed eye muscles, constipation, urine retention, and tachypnea.

Corkwood potentiates the anticholinergic effects of anticholinergics, such as atropine and tricyclic antidepressants. Corkwood may interfere with the efficacy of antiparkinsonians.

Patients with an allergy to corkwood or any of its components, atropine, or scopolamine should avoid use. Patients who are pregnant or breast-feeding and patients with glaucoma, intestinal disease

or obstruction, heart disease, or myasthenia gravis should avoid use.

Clinical considerations
 SAFETY RISK *Corkwood contains scopolamine, which is fatal in large doses.*

■ Inform patient that corkwood isn't recommended for medicinal use and can be dangerous or fatal in high doses.

■ Monitor patient for anticholinergic adverse effects and drug interactions, including rapid heart rate, decreased salivation, urine retention, constipation, and psychosis.

■ Tell patient that sgns and symptoms of overdose include tachycardia, tachypnea, constipation, urine retention, dry mouth, and CNS disturbances. Instruct him to promptly report adverse reactions and any new signs or symptoms.

■ If patient is pregnant or breast-feeding, advise her not to use corkwood.

■ Tell patient to remind prescriber and pharmacist of any herbal or dietary supplement that he's taking when obtaining a new prescription.

■ Advise patient to consult his health care provider before using an herbal preparation because a treatment with proven efficacy may be available.

Research summary
The concepts behind the use of corkwood and the claims made regarding its effects have not yet been validated scientifically.

cornflower

Bachelor's buttons, blue bonnet, bluebottle, bluebow, blue cap, blue centaury, Centaurea cyanus, *cyani flos, cyani-flowers, hurtsickle*

Cornflower is available as ray flowers, dried ray florets, and tubular florets of the cornflower plant. Several compounds—including anthocyans, flavonoids, and bitter principles — may be responsible for cornflower's activity. The flowers are generally considered to have tonic, stimulant effects and an ability to stimulate menstruation, with effects similar to blessed thistle.

Reported uses
Cornflower is used as a diuretic, an expectorant, a laxative, and as a stimulant for liver and gallbladder function. It's also used to treat cough, fever, menstrual disorders, vaginal candidiasis, and eczema of the scalp. It's used externally as an eye wash to treat eye inflammation and conjunctivitis.

Administration
The use of cornflower is not well documented.

Hazards
Allergic reaction may be associated with the use of cornflower. There are no reported interactions with cornflower.

Those with an allergy to cornflower or any of its components, geriatric patients, pregnant and breast-feeding patients, and children should avoid use.

Clinical considerations
■ Warn patient not to treat irregular menstrual periods with cornflower before seeking appropriate medical evaluation because doing so may delay diagnosis of an underlying medical condition. This herb should not be used to treat amenorrhea.
■ Tell patient to remind prescriber and pharmacist of any herbal or dietary supplement that he's taking when obtaining a new prescription.
■ Advise patient to consult his health care provider before using an herbal preparation because a treatment with proven efficacy may be available.

Research summary
The concepts behind the use of cornflower and the claims made regarding its effects have not yet been validated scientifically.

couch grass

Agropyron repens, *cutch, dog-grass, durfa grass,* Elymus repens, *Graminis rhizome, quack grass, quickgrass, quitch grass, Scotch quelch, triticum, twitch grass, wheat grass*

Couch grass contains the carbohydrate triticin, mucilages, sugar alcohols, soluble silicic acid, and volatile oils. The essential oil has an antimicrobial effect. Couch grass may also have a mild diuretic effect, probably a result of its sugar content. It increases urine volume when taken with water and prevents kidney stone formation. Dietary supplements of couch grass may use the rhizome, roots, and short stems of the plant. Couch grass is available as capsules, liquid extracts, tablets, and teas, in products such as Aqua-Rid, Arcocaps, and Diuplex.

Reported uses
German Commission E has approved couch grass to help treat urinary tract infections. Couch grass is also used to prevent kidney stones, as a diuretic, and to treat inflammatory diseases of the urinary tract and constipation as well as arthritis, bronchitis, the common cold, cough, fever, benign prostatic hyperplasia, and premenstrual syndrome.

Administration
■ Liquid extract (1:1): 4 to 8 ml, by mouth, three times a day
■ Tincture (1:5): 5 to 15 ml, by mouth, three times a day
■ Tea: 6 to 9 gm per day; prepared by adding 3 to 10 gm of herb to 1 cup boiling water.

Hazards
Electrolyte depletion and rash are associated with the use of couch grass. Herbal

products prepared with alcohol may cause a disulfiram-like reaction.

Patients with edema from cardiac or renal insufficiency should avoid use. Pregnant and breast-feeding patients should also avoid use.

Clinical considerations
- Liquid extracts may contain between 12% to 14% alcohol. If patient has a history of alcohol abuse or liver disease or takes metronidazole or disulfiram, advise him to avoid using this form of couch grass.
- If patient is pregnant or breast-feeding, advise her to avoid the use of couch grass.
- Discourage use of couch grass in geriatric patients and children because its safety and efficacy in these groups is unknown.
- Patients using couch grass for urinary tract irrigation should drink plenty of fluids.
- Warn patient not to delay seeking appropriate medical evaluation because doing so may delay diagnosis of a potentially serious medical condition.
- Tell patient to remind prescriber and pharmacist of any herbal or dietary supplement that he's taking when obtaining a new prescription.
- Advise patient to consult his health care provider before using an herbal preparation because a treatment with proven efficacy may be available.

Research summary
The concepts behind the use of couch grass and the claims made regarding its effects have not yet been validated scientifically.

cowslip

Artetyke, arthritica, buckles, butter rose, crewel, drelip, fairy caps, herb peterpaigle, key flower, key of heaven, may blob, mayflower, Our Lady's keys, paigle, palsywort, password, peagles, peggle, petty mulleins, plumrocks, Primula veris, P. officinalis

The medicinal parts of the cowslip are derived from the roots and flowers of *Primula veris*. Cowslip contains flavonoids, saponin glycosides, and volatile oil, which may be responsible for its ability to inhibit or dry secretions. It's available as dried flowers and roots, liquid extract, and tea.

Reported uses
Cowslip is used to treat asthma, cardiac insufficiency, dizziness, gout, headache, nervous diseases, neuralgia, tremors, and whooping cough and to inhibit or dry secretions. It's also used as an antispasmodic, diuretic, expectorant, hypnotic, and sedative.

Administration
Dosage of cowslip varies with the herb form.

Hazards
Adverse effects associated with the use of cowslip include heart dysfunction, nausea, vomiting, diarrhea, irritation of the digestive tract, destruction of red blood cells, liver damage, and allergic reaction.

Cowslip may potentiate the effects of antihypertensives and sedatives. It may potentiate electrolyte depletion when used with diuretics.

Patients with an allergy to cowslip or any other member of the primrose family, such as primrose, *Anagallis arvensis*, yellow loosestrife, moneywort, water violet, and cyclamen should avoid use. Pregnant and breast-feeding patients should also avoid use.

Clinical considerations

- Internal use isn't recommended because of cowslip's toxic effects.
- If patient is also taking a diuretic, monitor serum electrolyte levels.
- If patient is using cowslip externally, monitor for irritation to the skin and mucous membranes.
- If overdose occurs, perform gastric lavage, and then administer activated charcoal. Provide symptomatic and supportive measures.
- Warn patient not to delay seeking appropriate medical evaluation because doing so may delay diagnosis of a potentially serious medical condition.
- If patient is pregnant or breast-feeding or is taking a blood pressure drug or a diuretic, advise against using cowslip.
- Instruct patient to promptly report adverse reactions and new signs or symptoms.
- Tell patient to remind prescriber and pharmacist of any herbal or dietary supplement that he's taking when obtaining a new prescription.
- Advise patient to consult his health care provider before using an herbal preparation because a treatment with proven efficacy may be available.

Research summary

The concepts behind the use of cowslip and the claims made regarding its effects have not yet been validated scientifically.

cranberry

Bog cranberry, highbush cranberry, marsh apple, mountain cranberry, mooseberry, mossberry, trailing swamp cranberry, Vaccinium macrocarpon

The useful components of cranberry are obtained from the juice of the ripe cranberry fruit. It contains substances called proanthocyanidins that appear to prevent *Escherichia coli*, a common pathogen in urinary tract infections (UTIs), from adhering to the epithelial cells lining the bladder wall. Cranberry is available as capsules and tablets of concentrated extract, concentrated liquids, syrups, tinctures, juices, and sweetened juices, in products such as Cran-Actin, Cranberry-Plus, Emergen-C Cranberry, and Ultra Cranberry.

Reported uses

Cranberry is used to prevent UTIs, particularly in women prone to recurrent infection. It's also used to prevent kidney stones and to treat asthma, fever, and active UTI. It's used as a urine deodorizer in urinary incontinence. Cranberries are also eaten as a food.

Administration

- Capsules: 300 to 500 mg by mouth two to three times a day
- Cranberry juice, unsweetened: 8 to 16 oz (240 to 480 ml) a day to treat infection
- Cranberry tincture: 3 to 5 ml three times a day.

Hazards

Adverse effects associated with the use of cranberry include diarrhea and irritation if large quantities are ingested. Cranberry may decrease the effectiveness of weakly alkaline drugs, such as many antidepressants and prescription painkillers.

There are no reported precautions for the use of cranberry at this time.

Clinical considerations

- Tinctures may contain up to 45% alcohol. Patients with a history of alcohol abuse or liver disease or those taking metronidazole or disulfiram should be cautioned to avoid use of alcohol-containing preparations.
- Contrary to early investigations focusing on cranberry's ability to acidify the urine, its ability to prevent bacteria from adhering to the bladder wall seems to be more important in preventing UTIs.

Only the unsweetened, unprocessed form of cranberry juice is effective.

■ Cranberry is safe for use in pregnant and breast-feeding patients.

■ When consumed regularly, cranberry may be effective in reducing the frequency of bacteriuria with pyuria in women with recurrent UTIs.

■ Advise patient to notify the health care provider if signs or symptoms of a UTI appear. Explain that an appropriate antibiotic is usually needed to treat an active UTI.

■ If patient has diabetes, inform him that cranberry juice contains sugar but that sugar-free cranberry supplements and juices are available.

■ Tell patient to remind prescriber and pharmacist of any herbal or dietary supplement that he's taking when obtaining a new prescription.

■ Advise patient to consult his health care provider before using an herbal preparation because a treatment with proven efficacy may be available.

Research summary

Most of the research on cranberry to prevent UTIs has been conducted on commercial cranberry beverages, not dried cranberry powder.

Craniosacral therapy

An offshoot of chiropractic and osteopathy, craniosacral therapy is based on the theory that an unimpeded flow of cerebrospinal fluid (CSF) is the key to good health. CSF normally circulates from the cranium to the base of the spine. Practitioners believe that anything that impedes this flow or affects its rhythm can cause physical and mental problems.

Craniosacral therapy was developed in the early 1900s by William G. Sutherland, an American osteopathic doctor who believed that the bones of the skull move rhythmically throughout the day in response to the production of CSF in the ventricles. Craniosacral therapists claim

that they can actually palpate the flow of CSF by running their fingers over the skull or along the spine. According to their theory, any bumps or blows to the head can knock the skull bones out of alignment or cause them to become stationary or to move improperly. By gently manipulating these bones through massage or light pressure at the suture lines, they believe they can realign the bones, restore the free circulation of CSF, and remove strains and stresses built up in the meninges, allowing the entire body to function optimally.

TRAINING *Craniosacral therapy is most commonly practiced by osteopathic and chiropractic doctors who have been trained in the technique. The Upledger Institute in Palm Beach Gardens, Florida, provides information and referrals. The training consists of postgraduate instruction involving lecture, demonstration, and practice.*

Conventional medical practitioners say craniosacral therapy is based on theories that are inconsistent with the basic principles of anatomy taught in the West today. The current understanding of skeletal anatomy holds that the skull bones fuse together by age 2 and therefore can't be moved by manual pressure.

Reported uses

Proponents say craniosacral therapy can be used to treat chronic headaches, back or neck pain, sciatica, temporomandibular joint syndrome, depression, anxiety, and chronic fatigue in adults. However, they claim the most success in treating disorders in infants and children, including earaches, hyperactivity, and irritability, which they believe result from cranial injuries during the birthing process.

How the treatment is performed

Craniosacral therapy is usually performed with the patient lying prone and the therapist sitting behind the patient's head. The therapist begins by holding the patient's head and examining the placement and movement of the skull bones.

CRANIOSACRAL THERAPY TECHNIQUES

The following illustrations show some techniques used in craniosacral therapy.

The therapist attempts to relieve eyestrain and sinus pressure by decompressing the frontal bone and stretching the membrane beneath it.

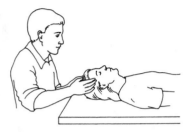

To relieve maxillary sinus conditions, the therapist applies pressure to the bones in the roof of the mouth, which balances the upper jaw.

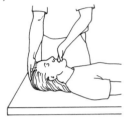

The jawbone is stretched to its limit to relieve temporomandibular joint syndrome.

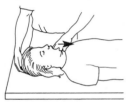

To help alleviate tinnitus, the therapist places his hands on the temporal bones and attempts to bring them back into alignment.

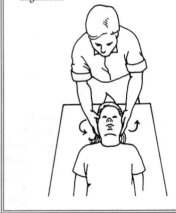

To relieve headache and stress, the therapist balances the large parietal bones on either side of the skull and stretches the membrane beneath them.

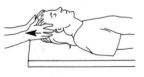

He then gently pulls, lifts, and stretches the bones into alignment. Patients report a feeling of deep relaxation during this process, which usually lasts from 30 minutes to 1 hour. Results of the therapy sometimes include relief of symptoms in distant parts of the body, such as leg pain. (See *Craniosacral therapy techniques.*)

Hazards
Some conventional medical doctors warn that craniosacral therapy should not be performed on infants or toddlers because their skull bones haven't become fused and manipulation of the delicate bone plates might be harmful.

Clinical considerations
This therapy may be an appropriate intervention for people who aren't comfortable with the physical intimacy of other manual healing techniques, such as Rolfing or massage.

Research summary

The mainstream scientific community has been unable to find evidence that the bones of the skull expand and contract in a rhythmic pattern that is palpable, as Sutherland claimed. As a result, even many osteopathic doctors have declined to embrace this therapy. However, the massage aspect may at least decrease stress and muscle tension and promote relaxation.

creatine

Creatine monohydrate

Creatine is a naturally occurring substance that can be obtained in red meat and other dietary sources. It may have an anti-inflammatory effect and may reduce levels of triglycerides in the blood. Creatine is available as pills, liquid, and powder, from many manufacturers in numerous combination products.

Reported uses

Creatine is used as a dietary supplement to increase strength and endurance, produce energy, enhance muscle size, improve stamina, and promote faster muscle recovery.

Administration

■ Athletes: 20 g taken by mouth every day for 3 days, then 5 g by mouth every day for the next 8 weeks, followed by 4 weeks with no supplementation, after which the cycle is repeated
■ Powder: Taken by mouth, mixed with 4 to 8 oz (120 to 240 ml) of orange or grape juice, up to four times a day.

Hazards

Adverse effects that may be associated with creatine include abdominal pain, bloating, diarrhea, dehydration, electrolyte imbalances, increased body weight, muscle cramps, and altered renal function. Because creatine is broken down and excreted by the kidneys as cre-

atinine, use of creatine affects renal function tests.

Cimetidine, probenecid, and trimethoprim may inhibit the tubular secretion of creatine, causing an increase in serum creatinine levels. Glucose may increase creatine storage in muscle. Nonsteroidal anti-inflammatory drugs (NSAIDs) may adversely affect renal function. Caffeine may reduce creatine's effects.

Those with a history of renal disease as well as pregnant and breast-feeding patients should avoid use.

Clinical considerations

■ Caution patient that creatine is useful only for intense exercise of short duration or when short bursts of strength are needed.
■ If muscle cramping occurs, patient should stop taking creatine and contact health care provider. A smaller dose may be needed.
■ Monitor patient's serum electrolyte levels and renal function, as needed.
■ If patient is taking cimetidine, probenecid, trimethoprim, or an NSAID, advise him to consult his health care provider before taking creatine.
■ If patient is a young athlete, discuss creatine's use and adverse effects with both the parents and the patient. Advise parents to monitor young athlete's use of creatine and to promptly report adverse effects to the health care provider.
■ Advise patient to drink plenty of fluids while taking creatine.
■ Tell patient to remind prescriber and pharmacist of any herbal or dietary supplement that he's taking when obtaining a new prescription.
■ Advise patient to consult his health care provider before using an herbal preparation because a treatment with proven efficacy may be available.

Research summary

Although the evidence for creatine is not definitive, of all sports supplements, it has the most evidence behind it. Numerous small double-blind studies suggest that it can increase athletic performance in sports that involve intense but short bursts of activity.

 RESEARCH *A double-blind study investigated creatine and swimming performance in 18 men and 14 women (Leenders, et al., 1999). Men taking the supplement had significant increases in speed during six 50-meter swims started at 3-minute intervals, as compared with men taking placebo. However, their speed did not improve when swimming ten 25-yard swims started at 1-minute intervals, perhaps due to the shorter rest time between laps.*

Interestingly, none of the women enrolled in the study showed any improvement with the creatine supplement. The authors of this study noted that women normally have more creatine in their muscle tissue than men do, so perhaps creatine supplementation (at least at this level) does not benefit women as it appears to benefit men. Further research is needed to fully understand this gender difference in response to creatine.

cucumber

Cowcumber, Cucumis sativus

Cucurbitin and fatty oil, contained in cucumber seeds, may have mild diuretic properties when ingested and a soothing effect when used topically. Cucumber flower may be a mild diuretic. Cucumber is high in potassium. It's available as emollient ointments and lotions.

Reported uses
Cucumber is used to treat high and low blood pressure, to cool and soothe irritated skin in patients with sunburn, and to provide fragrance in perfumes. It's also used as a cooling and beautifying agent.

Administration
Apply lotion or cream topically to affected areas, as needed. Wash with cucumber soaps and shower/bath gels as needed.

Hazards
Adverse effects associated with oral use of cucumber include fluid loss and electrolyte imbalances. Excessive use of cucumber may potentiate the effect of diuretics, leading to fluid and electrolyte disturbances.

Pregnant and breast-feeding patients should avoid medicinal use of cucumber.

Clinical considerations
■ Monitor patient for serum electrolyte imbalances. Monitor patient's fluid intake and output.
■ Warn patient not to treat swelling or edema with cucumber before seeking appropriate medical evaluation because doing so may delay diagnosis of a potentially serious medical condition.
■ If patient is pregnant or breast-feeding, advise her not to use cucumber medicinally.
■ Advise patient to promptly report adverse reactions to his health care provider.
■ Tell patient to remind prescriber and pharmacist of any herbal or dietary supplement that he's taking when obtaining a new prescription.
■ Advise patient to consult his health care provider before using an herbal preparation because a treatment with proven efficacy may be available.

Research summary
The concepts behind the use of cucumber and the claims made regarding its effects have not yet been validated scientifically.

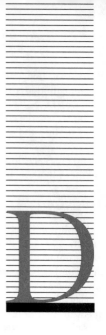

daffodil

Asphodel, daffy-down-dilly,
fleur de coucou, goose leek, Lent lily,
Narcissus pseudonarcissus

Daffodil contains alkaloids such as lycorine and galanthamine. In small doses,
lycorine may cause salivation, vomiting,
and diarrhea; in high doses, it causes
paralysis and collapse. Galanthamine is
an anticholinesterase that also exhibits
analgesic activity.

In resting bulbs, daffodil exhibits pilo-
carpine-like activity; in flowering bulbs,
it exhibits atropine-like activity. Daffodil
is available as a powder and an extract.

Reported uses
Daffodil is used as a topical astringent for
treating various wounds, burns, stiff
joints, and strained muscles.

Administration
■ Extract: 2 to 3 grains topically
■ Powder: 20 grains to 2 drachms topi-
cally.

Hazards

SAFETY RISK *Patients shouldn't
ingest any part of this herb orally
because the flowers and bulbs are
poisonous and can lead to rapid death.*

Adverse reactions associated with daffodil include central nervous system
(CNS) disorders, paralysis, fainting
episodes, cardiovascular collapse, miosis,
vomiting, salivation, diarrhea, respiratory
collapse, dermatitis, chills, and irritation

and swelling of the mouth, tongue, and throat. There are no known interactions with daffodil.

Clinical considerations

■ Accidental poisoning could result if daffodil bulbs are mistaken for onions.
■ Daffodils may affect CNS, causing paralysis and possibly death.
■ Instruct patient not to ingest any part of a daffodil by mouth.
■ Instruct parents to keep the plant out of reach of children and pets.
■ Instruct patient to seek immediate emergency medical help if CNS symptoms, such as numbness of extremities or paralysis, occur.
■ Tell patient to remind pharmacist of any herbal or dietary supplement that he's taking when obtaining a new prescription.
■ Advise patient to consult his health care provider before using an herbal preparation because a treatment with proven efficacy may be available.

Research summary

The concepts behind the use of daffodil and the claims made regarding its effects haven't yet been validated scientifically.

daisy

Bairnwort, bruisewort, common daisy, Day's eye, field daisy, moon daisy, wild daisy

The medicinal part of the daisy is derived from the dried flowering herb. It may have anti-inflammatory and astringent properties. Daisy is available as dried herb, fresh herb, and oil.

Reported uses

Daisy is used to treat migraine, neuralgia, rheumatism, GI complaints such as bloating and anorexia, and liver inflammation. It's also used to curb fevers.

The oil is used internally for rheumatic complaints, joint pain, and dysmenorrhea; externally, for gout, bruises, sprains, and wounds. Daisy has been used as an ointment or salve, applied directly to the inflammation site.

Administration

■ Infusion (1 teaspoon of dried herb steeped in boiling water for 10 minutes): three times a day by mouth
■ Tincture: 2 to 4 ml three times a day by mouth.

Hazards

SAFETY RISK *Components of the volatile oil can vary with the variety of daisy from which the oil is derived. Those that have a high thujone content are particularly toxic. Internal use should be avoided.*

There are no reported adverse reactions or interactions with daisy. Pregnant and breast-feeding patients should avoid use.

Clinical considerations

■ Monitor inflammation site for improvement, change, or worsening of inflammation.
■ Advise patient that daisy has a bitter, pungent taste.
■ Instruct patient to promptly report adverse reactions and new signs and symptoms to his health care provider.
■ Discuss with patient other proven medical treatments for his condition.
■ Tell patient to remind pharmacist of any herbal or dietary supplement that he's taking when obtaining a new prescription.
■ Advise patient to consult his health care provider before using an herbal preparation because a treatment with proven efficacy may be available.

Research summary

The concepts behind the use of daisy and the claims made regarding its effects haven't yet been validated scientifically.

damiana

Herba de la pastora, Mexican damiana, old woman's broom,
Turnera aphrodisiaca, T. diffusa, T. microphylla

The leaf and the stem of the damiana plant are the most commonly used components. Damiana was first used by the Mayans in the treatment of giddiness and loss of balance. Its primary use in the last century has been as an aphrodisiac, a use that was described in the scientific literature as early as 100 years ago.

Ethanolic extracts have central nervous system (CNS) depressant activity, and the quinone arbutin may be responsible for antibacterial activities. Damiana is available as capsules, powder, tea, and tincture.

Reported uses

Damiana is used mainly for its aphrodisiac effects, for prophylaxis, and for treating sexual disturbances. It's also used to control bedwetting, depression, constipation, and nervous dyspepsia; to strengthen and stimulate during exertion; and to boost and maintain mental and physical capacity.

Damiana is boiled in water and the steam is inhaled to relieve headaches. There have been some reports of recreational use, with euphoric and hallucinogenic effects.

Administration

- Extract: 2 to 4 ml by mouth three times a day
- Capsules: 2 to 4 g by mouth three times a day
- Tea: 1 cup (2 to 4 g) in 5 oz (150 ml) boiling water, by mouth three times a day.

Hazards

Adverse reactions associated with damiana include insomnia, headache, hallucinations, urethral mucous membrane irritation, and liver injury. Damiana may interfere with the action of antidiabetics.

Pregnant and breast-feeding patients shouldn't use this herb because the effects on them are unknown.

Clinical considerations

 SAFETY RISK *When more than 7 oz (198 g) of extract is consumed, patient may display tetanus-like convulsions and paroxysms.*

- Diabetic patients should discuss the use of damiana with a health care provider before taking it with an antidiabetic.
- Monitor blood glucose level closely in diabetic patient taking both damiana and an antidiabetic. Advise diabetic patient to check blood glucose level regularly and to report alterations to health care provider.
- Monitor liver function tests, as needed.
- Evaluate for drug use any patient claiming to have had damiana-induced hallucinations.
- Advise pregnant patient, breast-feeding patient, and patient of childbearing age to avoid using this herb because of a lack of sufficient information about its safety.
- Advise patient to avoid performing activities that require mental alertness until the herb's CNS effects are known.
- Tell patient to promptly report adverse reactions or new signs and symptoms to a health care provider.
- Tell patient to remind pharmacist of any herbal or dietary supplement that he's taking when obtaining a new prescription.
- Advise patient to consult his health care provider before using an herbal preparation because a treatment with proven efficacy may be available.

Research summary

The concepts behind the use of damiana and the claims made regarding its effects haven't yet been validated scientifically.

Dance therapy

Dance therapy (also known as dance movement therapy) capitalizes on the direct relationship between body movement and the mind. The music, rhythm, and synchronous movement associated with dance are believed to promote healing by improving mood, reducing social isolation, awakening old memories and feelings, and enhancing overall well-being.

Used throughout history to celebrate major events and heal the sick, dance was first adopted as a medical therapy in the United States in 1942, when dance teacher Marian Chace was asked to work with psychiatric patients at a Washington, D.C., hospital. Psychiatrists found that her dance classes seemed to benefit patients who were considered too disturbed to join in other group activities. Chace's work paralleled the work of Trudi Schoop, a dancer and mime who worked with non-communicative patients in California.

Today, dance therapists typically work with people who have emotional, social, cognitive, or physical problems. Depending on the goal, dance therapy can be done alone, with partners, or in a group. Range-of-motion exercises set to music or formal dance routines may be used in individual dance therapy. Group dance, probably the most common form of dance therapy, allows people of different physical abilities to participate. By tapping their feet or patting their thighs in time to the music, patients can feel a part of the session. Dance routines range from simple clapping and swaying to intricate aerobic sessions.

Founded in 1956, the American Dance Therapy Association (ADTA) promotes research, monitors standards for professional practice, and develops guidelines for graduate education. It also publishes the *American Journal of Dance Therapy* and maintains a registry of therapists.

TRAINING *The ADTA offers a registered dance therapist certification to professionals who have a master's degree and complete a supervised clinical internship. After an extended period of supervised work, the therapist is awarded the Academy of Dance Therapists registered certification, which qualifies her to teach, supervise, and engage in private practice.*

Reported uses

Dance therapy has been shown to improve the condition of patients with emotional, cognitive, or physical problems, and to help elderly people suffering from impaired mobility and social isolation. For emotionally disturbed patients, dance can help reduce depression and anxiety, lead to greater self-awareness, and provide a means of expressing feelings and developing relationships. For cognitively impaired patients, including those with mental retardation, dance is used to motivate learning, increase body awareness, and develop social and communication skills. For physically disabled patients, dance improves movement and circulation, enhances self-esteem, and provides a creative outlet that's fun. For elderly patients, dance can help maintain or improve physical mobility; enhance flexibility, circulation, and respiratory function; improve vitality and self-esteem; reduce isolation; and assist with the expression of fear and grief. (See *Understanding dance therapy*, page 174.)

Dance therapy is also used to reduce stress in patients with cancer, AIDS, or Alzheimer's disease, and in their caregivers as well. Healthy people use dance therapy to help prevent disease and maintain well-being because it promotes flexibility, strengthens muscles, and improves cardiovascular and pulmonary function. As an added benefit, the interaction with others provides socialization, touch, and a sense of connectedness.

UNDERSTANDING DANCE THERAPY

In dance therapy, visible movement represents personality. Practitioners of this therapy believe that in changing the way a person moves, dance therapy changes the totality of the way the person functions. For instance, the outward, visible manifestation of a disorganized personality may be fragmented movement; therefore, working to develop integrated or graceful movements will also integrate and organize the personality.

The physical activity entailed in dance therapy increases levels of endorphins—naturally occurring proteins in the brain that inhibit the transmission of pain impulses. The result is a naturally induced state of well-being. Movement of the whole body stimulates the circulatory, respiratory, skeletal, and neuromuscular systems. Additionally, the activation of muscles and joints reduces body tension. Practitioners believe that these physical effects, together with the relationship between physical movement and personality, bring about dance therapy's therapeutic effects.

How the treatment is performed

Adequate space and music are the only types of "equipment" needed for dance therapy. The music should be appropriate to the population, both in its pace and aesthetic appeal. Faster music can be used to stimulate the group, slower music to provide a calming effect.

Enough space should be provided to accommodate free movement of the participants. Chairs should be arranged around the periphery of the dance area for those who need to remain seated, or those who become tired during the session.

Prior to starting a dance session, the participants should be assessed for risk factors. The presence of one or more risk factors doesn't preclude group members from participating but may influence the type of dance and the length of the session. Risk factors include poor cardiovascular status and a history of chronic obstructive pulmonary disease or degenerative musculoskeletal problems. Muscle atrophy or obesity and the participant's exercise history should also be considered, along with their use of tobacco or alcohol.

After the dance therapist chooses appropriate music and dance, the room is arranged and the participants are introduced. The purpose of the session is explained and everyone is encouraged to participate according to ability. The practitioner should circulate through the group during the dance, providing encouragement and motivation to those who are hesitant. All participants' efforts should be praised.

After the session, the type of activity and the group's response should be documented. The participants should be encouraged to discuss the feelings they experienced while dancing.

Hazards

Because dancing is an aerobic activity, patients may experience signs of cardiovascular compromise, such as dizziness, flushing, profuse sweating, and disorientation. Rapid motion may cause dizziness. Group members who exercise strenuously may experience muscle soreness or strain.

Clinical considerations

■ If your patient experiences signs of cardiovascular compromise, help him to a seated position and obtain his vital signs. Compare the readings to the patient's baseline, and notify the doctor of any changes.

■ If your patient experiences muscle soreness, immobilize the affected body part, notify the doctor, and apply cold or heat therapy as ordered.

Research summary
Multiple case studies evaluating the efficacy of dance therapy have reported positive psychological outcomes in a wide range of phenomena including decreased anxiety, changes in self-concept or body image, decreases in depression, improved social interaction, and improved cognitive processes.

dandelion

Blowball, cankerwort, lion's tooth, priest's crown, swine snout, Taraxacum officinale, *wild endive*

In Germany, the herb and root of the dandelion are used as an appetite stimulant, diuretic, bile stimulator, and treatment for dyspepsia. The herb without the root is used for loss of appetite and dyspepsia involving flatulence and feelings of fullness. The dried roots are used as a coffee substitute. Dandelion is also used in salads and wines.

Traditionally, dandelion was used to treat liver, gallbladder, and spleen ailments. It's used as a mild laxative and antidiabetic. Dandelion is available as fresh greens, capsules, extract, tablets, tea, and tincture.

Reported uses
Dandelion has a diuretic effect, probably owing to the sesquiterpenes in its composition and its high potassium content. It may help prevent and treat kidney stones because of its disinfectant and solvent actions on urinary calculi.

The enzyme taraxalisin is present in dandelion roots. The insulin component, with its hypoglycemic effects, may affect the blood glucose level. Dandelion may have some immune-modulating effects.

It may also stimulate nitric oxide production, which is involved with immune regulation and defense, and may induce tumor necrosis factor alpha secretion in peritoneal cells.

Administration
■ Herb, fluid extract (1 g/ml of 25% ethanol): 4 to 10 ml by mouth three times a day
■ Fresh herb: 4 to 10 g cut herb by mouth three times a day
■ Infusion: 4 to 10 g in 5 to 9 oz (150 to 270 ml) water by mouth three times a day
■ Succus: 5 to 10 ml pressed sap from fresh plant by mouth two times a day
■ Tincture (1 g/5 ml of 25% ethanol): 2 to 5 ml by mouth three times a day
■ Herb with root, fluid extract (1 g/ml of 25% ethanol): 3 to 4 ml by mouth three times a day
■ Infusion: 1 tablespoon cut roots and herb in 5 oz (150 ml) water
■ Tincture (1 g/5 ml of 25% ethanol): 10 to 15 gtt by mouth three times a day.

Hazards
Adverse reactions associated with dandelion include GI discomfort, GI or biliary tract blockage, gallbladder inflammation, gallstones, contact dermatitis, and allergic reactions.

When used with drugs such as anticoagulants, or with anti-platelet drugs such as aspirin, clopidogrel, heparin, ticlopidine, warfarin, and NSAIDs, there is an increased risk of bleeding. When dandelion is used with antidiabetics, there is a possibility for potentiated effects, leading to hypoglycemia. Additive effects are possible when used with antihypertensives. Dandelion can also decrease blood ciprofloxacin levels. It's rich in minerals such as magnesium, which are known binders of fluoroquinolone antibiotics.

Those allergic to dandelion, those with photosensitive dermatitis and allergies to other Compositae plants, and those with bile obstruction, empyema, or ileus should avoid use.

Clinical considerations

- All parts of the dandelion plant are edible. The stems, leaves, and flowers can be harvested alone, or the whole plant — including the roots — can be used.
- Tinctures may contain between 15% and 60% alcohol and may be unsuitable for children, alcoholic patients, those with liver disease, and those taking metronidazole or disulfiram.
- Sesquiterpene lactones are thought to be the allergenic components, but not all people with dandelion dermatitis react to sesquiterpene patch testing.
- The bitter substances contained in the leaves may cause gastric discomfort.
- If patient is also taking an antidiabetic, monitor blood glucose level closely.
- Advise patient not to harvest dandelions from grounds that may have been treated with weed killer or fertilizer.
- Warn patient not to substitute dandelion therapy for a prescribed diuretic.
- If patient is taking a fluoroquinolone antibiotic, advise him not to use dandelions because of a possible decrease in blood antibiotic level.
- Advise patient to immediately report any rashes or signs of bleeding to his health care provider.
- Instruct patient to contact his health care provider if symptoms don't resolve or if new symptoms develop.
- Tell patient to remind pharmacist of any herbal or dietary supplement that he's taking when obtaining a new prescription.
- Advise patient to consult his health care provider before using an herbal preparation because a treatment with proven efficacy may be available.

Research summary

The scientific basis for the use of dandelion is scanty. Preliminary studies suggest that dandelion root stimulates the flow of bile. Dandelion leaves have also been found to produce a mild diuretic effect.

Detoxification

Detoxification, or cleansing, is being used increasingly as a therapeutic modality to support and improve health. Our bodies are exposed to the vast array of toxic chemicals, called xenobiotics, that are ubiquitous in our environment. Xenobiotics are easily absorbed by the body through the skin, lungs, or the mucosal lining of the gastrointestinal tract. Chronic health problems can develop if detoxification doesn't take place and these toxins are allowed to circulate within the body. Excretion of toxins is a difficult process; however, the more water-soluble the toxin, the easier it is to remove.

The liver plays an important role in the removal of toxins because it transforms fat-soluble toxins into excretable, water-soluble metabolites. The enzymatic (Phase I) and conjugation (Phase II) reactions are liver processes responsible for detoxification. Phase I reactions activate the body's enzymes to enhance their accessibility to Phase II. Phase II facilitates conversion of toxins to a water-soluble form for excretion in urine or stool. The proper functioning of the bowel is also paramount to successful detoxification.

Reported uses

Chronic health problems can often be traced to compromised digestive and detoxification function. Exposure to toxins, intestinal permeability defects, and parasitic infections are common conditions associated with gastrointestinal dysfunction. The liver's capacity for detoxification can become impaired due to excessive exposure to toxins as well as deficiencies in nutrients. Common signs and symptoms of toxicity include weakness, headaches, neurological disturbances, multiple chemical sensitivities, immune dysfunction, abdominal pain, bloating, inflammatory bowel disorders, liver disorders, and chronic skin disorders.

How the treatment is performed

Treatment modalities generally include three categories of procedures: reducing exposures to toxins, enhancing gastrointestinal function, and supporting the detoxification process.

- Reduce exposure to toxins:
  - lifestyle changes
  - environmental changes
  - dietary changes
- Optimize gastrointestinal function:
  - improve digestion
  - remove intestinal toxins and pathogens
  - heal intestinal mucosa
  - reduce oxidative damage
  - reestablish normal intestinal flora
- Support detoxification:
  - provide nutritional support for Phase I and II detoxification pathways
  - follow dietary guidelines for detoxification.

Reducing toxin exposure decreases the body's overall burden of toxins both directly, by avoiding the addition of new toxins, and indirectly, by improving the body's ability to defend itself. Lifestyle, environment, and dietary factors are essential in creating the body's total toxic load. The use of alcohol, caffeine, and prescription drugs is a lifestyle factor that increases the toxic burden. Environmental factors include exposure to volatile organic compounds such as solvents and formaldehyde, which are found in products ranging from automotive fuel to household cleaners and building materials. Foods represent the most common source of exposure to toxins; approximately 3,000 chemicals are used by the food industry for various types of food processing. Another 12,000 chemicals are used in food packaging materials. Numerous studies have found pesticide residues in a significant percentage of food samples. Organically grown and unprocessed or minimally processed foods may be an option to reduce toxin exposure. Avoiding exposure may necessitate significant changes in lifestyle and the environment.

Enhancing gastrointestinal function improves digestion and, consequently, increases absorption of nutrients. Gastrointestinal function is inadequate if the proper digestive enzymes and pH are unbalanced. Enzymes such as lipase, amylase, pancreatin, pepsin, and protease may be inactive in those patients with gastric or pancreatic hypofunction. This will lead to malabsorption of nutrients, food intolerance, and food allergy. Foods that aren't completely digested can putrefy in the intestine, producing toxins. Using plant enzymes can assist in promoting digestion and absorption of nutrients in those individuals with imbalances of gastrointestinal pH.

Lifestyle factors also influence digestive function. Thorough chewing of food is imperative to adequate digestion because it provides mechanical breakdown of foods and the necessary surface area for enzymatic activity to take place. Normal digestive secretions and motility may be impaired by depression and anxiety. Raw foods promote digestion because of their naturally occurring enzymes.

Fiber is essential for the maintenance of normal gastrointestinal function. Soluble fiber is fermented by colonic microflora, resulting in the production of short chain fatty acids such as butyric acid, which is essential for normal colonic functioning. Dietary fiber helps to bind to toxins and aids with elimination through the bowel. Oral use of bentonite clay has also been shown to help bind toxins and prevent their systemic absorption.

The gastrointestinal tract is considered one of the largest immune systems of the body. Faulty bowel mucosa compromises not only digestive and absorptive functions, but also vital immune functions. Defects of permeability can be caused by intestinal parasites, dysbiosis, impaired digestion, pancreatic insufficiency, food allergies, and the use of alcohol or NSAIDS.

Normal bowel flora help to prevent the establishment of intestinal pathogens through competitive inhibition. Probiotics such as *Lactobacillus* and *Bifidobacteria* species contribute to a healthy intestinal environment by maintaining optimum pH and producing important nutrients and enzymes. Elimination of intestinal pathogens is necessary for a healthy intestinal tract because they are often responsible for production of toxins, thereby placing an additional burden on the system. Preparations to restore balance to the intestinal flora include formulas containing plant extracts from *Artemisia annua*, allicin, berberine, *Hydrastis canadensis*, and *Allium sativa*. Enemas or colonic irrigations may be advised to facilitate toxin removal.

Glutathione, superoxide dismutase, catalase, beta carotene, vitamin E, selenium, and N-acetylcysteine are substances essential to detoxification. Vitamin and mineral co-factors required for cytochrome P-450 reactions include riboflavin, niacin, magnesium, iron, and several trace minerals. Cruciferous vegetables and quercetin have also been shown to support Phase I detoxification. Phase II detoxification is promoted by usage of calcium d-glucarate, which is a natural ingredient in certain fruits and vegetables and results in increased elimination of toxins. Other helpful agents include amino acids such as glycine, cysteine, glutamine, methionine, taurine, glutamic acid, and aspartic acid. Dietary supplementation may help to replace depleted supplies of nutrients needed for detoxification.

Dietary support to encourage hepatic detoxification includes emphasis on freshly prepared natural, organic, unrefined, and unprocessed foods containing a minimum of additives and chemical residues. Fresh vegetables and fruits, whole grains, and unrefined starches should constitute a significant portion of the diet. Red meats, animal fats, sugar and other simple and refined carbohydrates, salt, alcohol and caffeine should be consumed in moderation or, preferably, avoided. Elimination of allergenic foods can facilitate mucosal healing and decrease the body's total load of toxins.

The total body burden of toxins and resulting tissue damage tends to accumulate over time, leading to a cascade of illnesses. A comprehensive approach is needed to address reduction of toxin exposure, healing of the gastrointestinal tract, and support of the hepatic detoxification process.

Hazards

As the toxin load of the body decreases, there may be symptoms of headaches, fatigue, irritability, body aches, and strong cravings for foods removed from the diet.

Clinical considerations

- Patients with serious medical concerns should consult with a medical practitioner before making any dietary, lifestyle, or prescription changes.
- Caution patient that detoxification should be carried out only under the guidance of a qualified medical practitioner.

TRAINING *Resources for special training, which is advisable to facilitate optimal outcome, can be found through HealthComm International, Inc., Clinical Research Center, P.O. Box 1729, 5800 Soundview Drive, Gig Harbor, Washington 98335; Attn: Jeffrey S. Bland, PhD; or through Great Smokies Diagnostic Laboratories, Ashville, NC (www.gsdl.com).*

Research summary

Toxicity overload is becoming epidemic and is responsible for a host of chronic degenerative diseases. Reducing exposure to toxins, improving digestion, replacing intestinal pathogens with healthy bacteria, and support of detoxification with appropriate methods all contribute to lessening the toxic burden and promoting healing and optimal health.

devil's claw

Grapple plant, Harpagophytum procumbens, *wood spider*

Devil's claw has been used by native Africans as a folk remedy for diseases ranging from liver and kidney disorders to allergies, headaches, and rheumatism. It's marketed in Canada and Europe as a home remedy for the relief of arthritic disease. Devil's claw is available as capsules, fresh herb, and tincture.

Reported uses

Devil's claw is used for its anti-inflammatory and analgesic effects. It's also used to treat allergies, atherosclerosis, GI disturbances and heartburn, menstrual difficulties, menopausal symptoms, nicotine poisoning, neuralgia, and liver, kidney, and bladder diseases. In Germany, devil's claw is approved for use as an appetite stimulant and digestive aid.

Administration

- Decoction: 0.5 g in 150 ml water by mouth three times a day for loss of appetite; 1.5 g in 150 ml water by mouth three times a day for other conditions
- Fluid extract (1 g/ml): 0.5 ml taken by mouth three times a day for loss of appetite; 1.5 ml by mouth three times a day for other conditions
- Fresh cut tuber: 1.5 g by mouth every day
- Dried tuber/root: 6 g by mouth every day
- Infusion (4.5 g of herb in 300 ml, steeped in boiling water for 8 hours): three portions by mouth every day
- Standardized extracts: 600 to 800 mg by mouth three times a day; standardized to 2% to 3% iridoid glycosides or 1% to 2% harpagoside.

Hazards

Adverse reactions associated with devil's claw include headache, tinnitus, anorexia, and allergic reaction. Devil's claw may decrease blood glucose levels and have an additive effect when used concomitantly with antidiabetic agents. Herbal products prepared with alcohol may cause a disulfiram-like reaction.

Oral use of devil's claw should be avoided in pregnancy and lactation due to its oxytocic effects. Patients with gastric or duodenal ulcers should avoid use because devil's claw increases production of stomach acid. Patients taking a beta blocker, calcium channel blocker, antihypertensive, or antiarrhythmic should use cautiously because herb may have hypotensive, bradycardic, and antiarrhythmic effects. Patients with heart failure should use cautiously because herb may have negative inotropic effects at high doses.

Clinical considerations

- Devil's claw may increase the intended therapeutic effect of conventional drugs.
- Tinctures may contain between 15% and 60% alcohol and may be unsuitable for children, alcoholic patients, those with liver disease, and those taking metronidazole or disulfiram.
- Warn patient to seek appropriate medical evaluation right away, to avoid delaying diagnosis of a potentially serious medical condition.
- Advise patients taking a heart drug or a blood pressure drug to promptly report any light-headedness, dizziness, abnormal heartbeats, or swelling.
- Instruct patient to seek medical attention if symptoms don't resolve.
- Tell patient to remind pharmacist of any herbal or dietary supplement that he's taking when obtaining a new prescription.
- Advise patient to consult his health care provider before using an herbal preparation because a treatment with proven efficacy may be available.

Research summary

Devil's claw extracts contain chemicals that possess anti-inflammatory activity, the ability to reduce blood pressure, decrease heart rate, and slow anti-arrhythmic activities in animal studies. The literature states that these extracts appear to be free of significant toxicities when given for short periods of time; however, the long-term toxicity or potential interactions isn't known. The concepts behind the use of devil's claw and claims made regarding its effects must be studied further and validated scientifically.

RESEARCH *One double-blind study followed 89 individuals with rheumatoid arthritis for a 2-month period. The group given devil's claw showed a significant decrease in pain intensity and improved mobility (Lecomte et al., 1992). Another double-blind study of 50 people with various types of arthritis found that 10 days of treatment with devil's claw provided significant pain relief (European Scientific Cooperative on Phytotherapy, 1996-1997).*

dehydroepiandrosterone

DHEA

Dehydroepiandrosterone (DHEA) is a precursor of both estrogen and testosterone. It's secreted mainly by the adrenal glands. Both DHEA and its sulfate conjugate, DHEA-S, are converted in the periphery to androgens. Circulating levels of DHEA increase during childhood into early adulthood, but begin to drop with age — by age 60, levels are only 5% to 15% of what they are at age 20. Those with autoimmune and cardiovascular disease also have lower DHEA levels.

Responses to DHEA appear to be gender-specific. In women, supplementation increases both serum DHEA and testosterone levels; in men, it may have no effect on serum testosterone or estrogen levels. DHEA may be useful as treatment for depression and as an anti-aging supplement to restore neuroendocrine function, thus improving mood and increasing feelings of well-being. It may also be useful in treating systemic lupus erythematosus (SLE) and adrenal insufficiency.

Related compounds include androstenedione (metabolite of DHEA), and pregnenolone (precursor to DHEA). DHEA is available as tablets, capsules, sustained-release tablets, micronized tablets, chewing gum, liquid, sublingual drops, herbal tea, and cream. Common trade names include DHEA Fuel, DHEA Power; combination products include Andro-Stack 850, EAS Andro-6, Twinlab Growth Fuel, Twinlab 7-Ketofuel, and Twinlab Tribulus Fuel Stack.

Reported uses

DHEA is used to treat osteoporosis, depression, Alzheimer's dementia, Tourette syndrome, chronic fatigue syndrome, AIDS, migraines, erectile dysfunction, epilepsy, and cancer. It's also used to increase feelings of well-being, slow or reverse the aging process, increase sex drive, increase lean body mass, and decrease fat mass.

Administration

- Oral use: 25 to 200 mg by mouth every day
- Creams (10%): 3 to 5 g applied topically to skin every day.

Hazards

Adverse reactions associated with DHEA may include severe manic episodes, cardiac arrhythmias, and acne; androgenic or masculinizing effects, including hirsutism, in women; estrogenic effects, including gynecomastia, in men; and male-pattern baldness. DHEA may interact with medications that are eliminated by the CYP4503A4 route.

Those with cancers that are stimulated by estrogen, such as breast cancer, or by testosterone, such as prostate cancer, and those at risk for heart disease, should avoid taking DHEA. Pregnant patients should also avoid use because DHEA may have androgenic effects on female fetuses, may induce spontaneous abortion, or may inhibit fetal development.

Clinical considerations

■ DHEA isn't a natural supplement. It's a hormone, synthetically manufactured from soybeans or wild yams. Contrary to advertising claims, wild yams don't contain DHEA. They contain diosgenin, a precursor of DHEA, which may not be converted to DHEA in the body.

■ DHEA isn't intended for any patient younger than age 40 unless circulating levels of DHEA are less than 130 mg/dL if the patient is a woman, or less than 180 mg/dL if the patient is a man.

■ DHEA has orphan drug status for the treatment of corticosteroid-dependent SLE and for the treatment of severe burns in those who require skin grafting.

■ The typical dosage range is 50 to 200 ml daily, depending on the intended use and individual's response.

■ DHEA may increase levels of insulin-like growth factor, which may represent a risk for those with prostate cancer.

■ Monitor patient for adverse hormonal effects.

■ Long-term safety of DHEA supplementation is unknown.

■ Discuss with patient his reasons for taking DHEA.

■ Advise female patient to inform her health care provider if she becomes pregnant or plans to become pregnant in the near future.

■ Instruct female patient to report any weight gain, hair loss, growth of facial hair, or other masculinizing effects to her health care provider.

■ Instruct male patient to report any signs of breast growth and development to his health care provider.

■ Tell patient to remind pharmacist of any herbal or dietary supplement that he's taking when obtaining a new prescription.

■ Advise patient to consult his health care provider before using an herbal preparation because a treatment with proven efficacy may be available.

Research summary

Further studies are needed to confirm DHEA's potential to slow the aging process, improve mood, and aid in weight loss.

RESEARCH *A double-blind placebo-controlled trial of 280 men and women ranging in age from 60 to 79 years evaluated the effects of 50 mg of DHEA daily for 1 year (Baulieu et al., 2000). The results suggest that DHEA can slow the development of osteoporosis in women over 70. However, neither men nor younger women responded. A double-blind placebo-controlled study enrolled 40 men with difficulty achieving or maintaining an erection, who also had low measured levels of DHEA. (Reiter et al., 1999) The results showed that DHEA at a dose of 50 mg daily significantly improved sexual performance.*

dill

Anethum graveolens

Dill is available as fresh greens, dried greens, or dried seeds. The dried seeds contain an essential oil, carvone, that may have an effect on smooth and skeletal muscle response.

Reported uses

Dill is used to prevent and treat diseases affecting the GI and urinary tracts as well as the kidneys, and to treat sleep disorders and spasms. The seed is used as an antispasmodic and bacteriostatic. It's also used to treat dyspepsia. The upper stem and seeds of the plant are used, fresh or dried, as a flavoring agent and a garnish.

Administration

■ Oil of dill: 0.1 to 0.3 g, or 2 to 6 gtt, three times a day
■ Tea (2 teaspoons of mashed seeds steeped in 1 cup of boiling water for 10 minutes): 3 cups by mouth every day
■ Tincture: ½ to 1 teaspoon, up to three times a day.

Hazards

Herbal products prepared with alcohol may cause a disulfiram reaction. Contact with the juice from the fresh dill plant may cause skin to react badly when exposed to sunlight.

Those allergic to dill should avoid use.

Clinical considerations

 SAFETY RISK *Dill weed is high in sodium. Discourage excessive use in those with conditions that require sodium restriction, such as heart failure or renal failure.*

- Tinctures may contain between 15% and 60% alcohol and may be unsuitable for children, alcoholic patients, those with liver disease, and those taking metronidazole or disulfiram.
- Monitor patient's response to therapy, including improvement of symptoms and adverse reactions.
- Advise any patient with an allergy to dill to avoid use.
- Warn patient to seek appropriate medical evaluation right away, to avoid delaying diagnosis of a potentially serious medical condition.
- Instruct patient to promptly report adverse reactions and new signs or symptoms.
- Tell patient to remind pharmacist of any herbal or dietary supplement that he's taking when obtaining a new prescription.
- Advise patient to consult his health care provider before using an herbal preparation because a treatment with proven efficacy may be available.

Research summary

The concepts behind the use of dill and the claims made regarding its effects haven't yet been validated scientifically.

dong quai

Angelica polymorpha sinensis, A. sinensis, *Chinese angelica, dang-gui, tang-kuei*

Dong quai dietary supplements are obtained from the roots of *Angelica polymorpha*. Dong quai extracts contain at least 6 coumarin derivatives — including bergapten, osthol, oxy-peucedanin, and psoralen — and two furocoumarin derivatives, sen-byak-angelicole and 7-demrthylsuberosin. Coumarin derivatives have anticoagulant, vasodilating, and antispasmodic activity. Also, osthol may have central nervous system stimulant activity.

Other components found in the essential oil include *n*-butyl-pthalide, cadinene, isosafrole, and safrole. Safrole may be carcinogenic, so ingestion should be avoided. Root extracts may contain various lactones and vitamins A, E, and B_{12}. Dong quai extracts may have a modulatory effect on endogenous estrogens. Common trade names include Women's Ginseng, and combination products such as Menopausal Formula, Nature's Fingerprint, PMS Formula, and Rejuvex.

Reported uses

Dong quai is widely used in traditional Chinese medicine and continues to be popular in China and elsewhere. It's used to treat menstrual disorders, as an analgesic in rheumatism, and to suppress allergy symptoms.

Dong quai is used to treat anemia, hepatitis, hypertension, migraines, neuralgias, rhinitis, and gynecologic disorders including irregular menstruation, dysmenorrhea, premenstrual syndrome, and menopausal symptoms.

Administration

Capsules: 500 mg by mouth, or 1 to 2 capsules three times a day
Liquid extract: 1 to 2 gtt three times a day.

Hazards

Dong quai may cause bleeding gums, diarrhea, blood in the stool, hematuria, photodermatitis, bleeding, fever, or cancer. When used with warfarin, dong quai can potentiate anticoagulant effects. Similar effects are possible with other anticoagulants. There is also an increased risk of photosensitivity reactions with dong quai.

Patients taking an anticoagulant should avoid use. Because of potential effects on uterine contractions and unknown direct effects on the developing fetus, pregnant and breast-feeding patients shouldn't use dong quai.

Clinical considerations

- Monitor patient for signs of easy bruising or bleeding.
- If dong quai must be used with another anticoagulant, closely monitor PT and International Normalized Ratio.
- Monitor patient for photosensitivity reactions.
- If patient is pregnant or breast-feeding, advise her not to use dong quai.
- Advise patient to keep this and other herbal products out of reach of children.
- Tell patient to remind pharmacist of any herbal or dietary supplement that he's taking when obtaining a new prescription.
- Advise patient to consult his health care provider before using an herbal preparation because a treatment with proven efficacy may be available.

Research summary

The concepts behind the use of dong quai and the claims made regarding its effects haven't yet been validated scientifically.

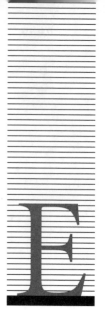

echinacea

American coneflower, black sampson,
black susans, cockup hat, comb flower,
Echinacea angustifolia, E. pallida,
E. purpurea, *hedgehog, Indian head,*
Missouri snakeroot, purple coneflower,
purple Kansas coneflower, red sunflower,
rudbeckia, scurvy root, snakeroot

Echinacea is obtained from the dried rhizomes and roots of *Echinacea angustifolia* and *E. pallida*, and the roots or aerial parts of *E. purpurea*. It may enhance immune system function, with the lipophilic fraction in the roots and leaves producing the most effective immunostimulation. When taken internally, echinacea may increase the number of circulating leukocytes, enhance phagocytosis, stimulate cytokine production, and trigger the alternate complement pathway. In vitro, some components are directly bacteriostatic and exhibit antiviral activity. Applied topically, echinacea can exert local anesthetic activity, antimicrobial activity, and anti-inflammatory activity, and it can stimulate fibroblasts.

Echinacea is available as capsules, glycerite, expressed juice, hydroalcoholic extract, lozenges, tablets, tea, tinctures (1:5, 15% to 90% alcohol), and whole dried root. Common trade names include EchinaCare Liquid, Echinacea Glycerite, Echinacea Herbal Comfort, Echinacea Xtra, Echina Fresh, Echinagel, EchinaGuard Liquid, EchinaGuard Pro, and Echinex.

Reported uses

Echinacea is used primarily for treating and preventing upper respiratory tract infections. It's also used to stimulate the immune system and heal wounds, including abscesses, burns, eczema, and skin ulcers. Echinacea may be used as an adjunct to a conventional antineoplastic therapy and may provide prophylaxis against upper respiratory tract infections and the common cold. In addition, it may be used for treatment of urinary tract and yeast infections (recurring vaginal candidiasis). Intravenous and intramuscular use has been reported in some studies to prolong survival time of patients with hepatocellular carcinoma.

Administration

- Capsules containing powdered *E. pallida* root extract: Equivalent to 300 mg by mouth three times a day
- Expressed juice of *E. purpurea* (2.5:1, 22% alcohol): 6 to 9 ml by mouth every day, not to exceed 8 weeks
- Hydroalcoholic tincture (15% to 90% alcohol): 3 to 4 ml by mouth three times a day
- Tea (simmer ½ tsp of coarsely powdered herb in 1 cup of boiling water for 10 minutes): 1 cup of freshly made tea taken several times daily for colds
- Whole dried root: 1 to 2 g by mouth three times a day.

Hazards

Echinacea has been associated with unpleasant taste, nausea, vomiting, minor GI symptoms, diuresis, allergic reaction, fever, and tachyphylaxis. The intravenous use of echinacea may lead to shivering, muscle weakness, and pain at injection site. Herbal products that contain alcohol may precipitate a disulfiram-like reaction when used with disulfiram or metronidazole. Decreased effectiveness may be observed when used with immunosuppressants such as cyclosporine. Preliminary evidence shows that echinacea can inhibit cytochrome P450 3A4 enzyme, affecting drugs metabolized by this system.

Echinacea preparations containing alcohol may enhance CNS depression when used with alcohol.

Patients with HIV infection, AIDS, tuberculosis, collagen disease, multiple sclerosis, or autoimmune disease should avoid use. Pregnant and breast-feeding patients should also avoid use.

Clinical considerations

- Daily dose depends on the preparation and potency but use shouldn't continue for more than 8 weeks. Consult specific manufacturer's instructions for parenteral administration, if applicable.
- Echinacea is considered supportive treatment for infection; it shouldn't be used in place of antibiotic therapy.
- Some active components may be water-insoluble.
- Echinacea is usually taken at the first sign of illness and continued for up to 14 days. Regular prophylactic use isn't recommended.
- Herbalists recommend using liquid preparations because it is believed that echinacea functions in the mouth and should have direct contact with the lymph tissues at the back of the throat.
- Some tinctures contain between 15% and 90% alcohol, which may be unsuitable for children and adolescents, alcoholics, and patients with hepatic disease.
- Advise patient not to delay seeking appropriate medical evaluation for a prolonged illness.
- Advise patient that prolonged use may result in overstimulation of the immune system and possible immune suppression. Echinacea shouldn't be used for more than 14 days for supportive treatment of infection.
- The herb should be stored away from direct light.
- Advise patient to keep this and other herbal products out of reach of children.
- Tell patient to remind pharmacist of any herbal or dietary supplement that he's taking when obtaining a new prescription.

- Advise patient to consult his health care provider before using an herbal preparation because a treatment with proven efficacy may be available.

Research summary

Approximately 15 double-blind, placebo-controlled studies provided evidence strongly suggesting that various echinacea species can significantly reduce the duration and severity of illness. However, regular prophylactic use of echinacea has not been found to significantly reduce the incidence of infections.

elderberry

Black elder, black-berried elder, blood elder, blood hilder, boor tree, common elder, danewort, dwarf elder, elder, ellanwood, ellhorn, European elder, S. ebulus, S. nigra

Elder flowers and berries have been used in traditional medicine and as flavorings for centuries. In folk medicine, the flowers have been used for their diuretic and laxative properties and as an astringent. Various parts of the elder have been used to treat cancer and a host of other unrelated disorders. Elderberry is available as an aqueous solution, berries, extract, flowers, oil, and wine.

Reported uses

Elderberry extracts are used to treat asthma, bronchitis, cough, epilepsy, fever, fungal infections, gout, headache, hepatic dysfunction, neuralgia, rheumatic diseases, and toothache. They are also used as diuretics, insect repellents, and laxatives.

Native Americans used tea made from elderberry flowers to treat respiratory infections. They also used the leaves and flowers in poultices applied to wounds, and the bark, suitably aged, as a laxative. The berries are frequently made into beverages, pies, and preserves, but they have also been used to treat arthritis.

Administration

- Infusion (add 3 to 4 g of elderberry flowers to 5 oz of simmering water): 1 to 2 cups by mouth several times daily
- Elderberry juice-containing syrup: Adults, 4 tablespoons daily for three days; children, 2 tablespoons daily for three days.

Hazards

Adverse reactions associated with elderberry include diarrhea, nausea, and vomiting. There are no known interactions with elderberry.

Pregnant and breast-feeding patients should avoid use.

SAFETY RISK *Elderberry has been associated with cyanide-like poisoning. Patients should avoid consumption of berries from the dwarf elder (S. ebulus) because it can contain an especially high content of cyanide-like compounds.*

Clinical considerations

- Don't confuse elderberry with American elder (*Sambucus canadensis*).
- Leaves and stems shouldn't be crushed when making elderberry juice because of potential for cyanide toxicity.
- Elderberry may interfere with the intended therapeutic effect of conventional drugs.
- Elderberry (especially *S. ebulus*) can cause cyanide-like poisoning — characterized by diarrhea, vomiting, vertigo, numbness, and stupor — particularly if uncooked portions are consumed. It can also cause toxic reaction in children if they use elderberry stems for peashooters.
- Uncooked elderberries are more likely to cause nausea.
- Monitor patients for nausea and vomiting.
- Warn patient not to treat symptoms of asthma, infection, or hepatic disease with elderberry before seeking appropriate

medical evaluation because doing so may delay diagnosis of a potentially serious medical condition.

■ Inform patient of the toxic potential of certain varieties of elderberry.

■ Advise patient to keep this and other herbal products out of children's reach.

■ Tell patient to remind pharmacist of any herbal or dietary supplement that he's taking when obtaining a new prescription.

■ Advise patient to consult his health care provider before using an herbal preparation because a treatment with proven efficacy may be available.

Research summary

The concepts behind the use of elderberry and the claims made regarding its effects haven't yet been validated scientifically.

elecampane

Elfdock, elfwort, horse-elder, horseheal, Inula helenium, *scabwort, velvet dock, wild sunflower*

Elecampane is obtained from the dried cut root and rhizomes of *Inula helenium*. Extracts generally contain a volatile oil whose chief components are alantolactone; isoalantolactone; 11,13-dihydro-isoalantolactone; 11,13-dihydroalan-lantolactone; and other sesquiterpen-lactones. These compounds may exhibit variable antiseptic, antibacterial, antifungal, diuretic, expectorant, and hypotensive activities. Elecampane is available as fluid extract, in powdered root preparations, and topical products.

Reported uses

Elecampane is used to treat diabetes, hypertension, diseases of the respiratory tract such as bronchitis, asthma, and cough, diseases of the GI tract, and diseases of the kidney and lower urinary tract. It's also used to stimulate appetite

and bile production, to treat dyspepsia and menstrual complaints, and to promote diuresis.

Administration

■ Dried root: 2 to 3 g by mouth three times a day

■ Fresh root: 1 to 2 tablespoons by mouth three times a day

■ Extract: 3 g dried root in 20 ml alcohol and 10 ml water by mouth three times a day

■ Tea (steep 1 g of ground herb in boiling water for 10 to 15 minutes): 1 cup every 4 hours up to three times a day as an expectorant.

Hazards

Adverse reactions associated with elecampane include mucous membrane irritation, allergic contact dermatitis and, with larger doses, nausea, vomiting, diarrhea, and cramps. There is a theoretical interaction with herbs with sedative properties and with hypoglycemic drugs, sedatives, and antihypertensives.

Those with a history of hypersensitivity or contact dermatitis should avoid use. Pregnant and breast-feeding patients should also avoid use.

 SAFETY RISK *Large doses of elecampane could cause signs of paralysis.*

Clinical considerations

■ Elecampane may interfere with the intended therapeutic effect of conventional drugs.

■ Monitor patient for signs of allergic reaction, especially dermatologic reactions.

■ The alantolactone component can irritate mucous membranes.

■ If overdose occurs, treat with gastric lavage, intestinal emptying, and activated charcoal.

■ Instruct patient to keep this and other herbal products out of children's reach.

■ Instruct patient not to store the herb in a plastic container.

■ Tell patient to remind pharmacist of any herbal or dietary supplement that he's taking when obtaining a new pre-scription.

■ Advise patient to consult his health care provider before using an herbal preparation because a treatment with proven efficacy may be available.

 SAFETY RISK *Advise patient that little evidence exists supporting therapeutic use of elecampane and that the herb can cause an allergic reaction.*

Research summary

The concepts behind the use of elecam-pane and the claims made regarding its effects haven't yet been validated scientif-ically.

Energy medicine

Vibrational healing, vibrational medicine

The human body is an electromagnetic unit. Electricity makes the heart beat and muscles expand and contract, and fires impulses across tiny fibers in the nervous system to make possible our every thought, mood, and physical reaction. Energy medicine, or vibrational medi-cine, is a form of therapy in which the patient's own electromagnetic, or energy, field is used to promote wellness or heal-ing. Energy medicine consists of a variety of therapeutic modalities, each of which has its own healing frequency, or ener-getic waveband.

Throughout history, the peoples of many nations have used various forms of vibrational energy for healing. Most tra-ditional cultures identify some form of a basic life force flowing from a universal creator. In China it's called *chi*; in ancient Greece, *pneuma*; in India, *prana*; in Japan, *qi*. To the native peoples of the North American continent, this force is known as the *flow of spirit*. To all these peoples, the life force is the basis of phys-ical, psychological, and spiritual health. These subtle, unseen energies are incor-porated in the therapeutic vibrational methods of the different modalities, as healers work to enhance or rebalance this life force, strengthening it where it's weak, and modulating it where it's exces-sive.

One popular form of energy medicine works with the patient's aura. The aura, or auric field, reflects how one's life is be-ing lived at the moment of observance. The vibration, color, and sound of the aura are all interrelated and represent a means of determining the frequency of energy in the auric field. A healer chan-neling energy to a client will often expe-rience reactions in his own body; for ex-ample, he may feel a vibration, "see" the color of the energy, or "hear" a sound he associates with a particular color or feel-ing (a phenomenon known as clairaudi-ence). There are seven layers of the auric field.

■ The etheric body or layer is joined di-rectly to the physical body, from which it extends outward 2 to 6 inches; it is re-ferred to as "etheric double" because it contains a blueprint as well as replica-tions of all the organs in the physical form.

■ The emotional body is the wellspring from which all our emotions, desires, joys, pains, sufferings, and passions emerge. Beliefs, perceptions, attitudes, and emotions — particularly fear — affect the body through the nervous, en-docrine, muscular, and immune systems; they can change the field or cause it to shut down.

■ The mental body is responsible for ra-tional, clear, and intellectual functions. It's responsible for the conscious (that which we are aware of) and the uncon-scious (that which has been repressed or forgotten and exists just beneath the sur-face of consciousness) mind, as well as memories.

■ The astral body bridges dimensions of matter and spirit and is transitional be-tween the first and last auric bodies. The astral body contains the entire personali-ty and contains all the extraordinary abilities — intuition, extrasensory perception, image projection, spiritual sight, and clairvoyance — as well as compassion for others.

■ The causal, or second etheric, body is the first layer of the spiritual realm, which contains the knowledge of the individual's purpose in life, his talents, and the lessons he must learn during the course of his lifetime.

■ The celestial body is the site of clear vision, in the spiritual sense of individual future, and is believed to contain a love that surpasses human love. It influences sight and other manifestations of visualization — insight, foresight, inspiration, clairvoyance, and physical manifestation. It's sometimes erroneously called the third eye.

■ The spiritual and cosmic consciousness, also called the ketheric layer or body, is said to be in direct contact with the divine universe; it's the body's energetic blueprint. It is also a center of knowing without thought or reason. Our spiritual life resides here.

The auric fields are created and controlled by the chakras. *Chakra* is a Sanskrit word meaning "wheel" or "circle of movement." The chakras are spirals of concentrated life force or vortices of energy. They're arrayed in a straight line at the center of the body, with the energy vortices of the second through the sixth extending out the front and back. The root chakra points downward, and the crown chakra points upward. In the northern hemisphere, healthy chakras spin in a clockwise direction, facing the front of a person. South of the equator, chakras spin in a counterclockwise direction. The direction of radiation, shape and diameter of a chakra indicate the state of its energy and the health of the corresponding or adjacent physical organs. (See *Characteristics of the seven primary chakras,* page 190.)

Six secondary chakras are located in the palms of the hands, backs of the knees, and soles of the feet near the arches. There are twenty smaller tertiary

chakras located on the tips of the fingers and toes. The second and third chakras in the hands are used to direct energy during healing practices; the second and third chakras in the feet are used to ground the healer while performing healing activities. Additionally, minor chakras are designated anteriorly over both hip joints, tips of the shoulder, and elbows.

Another type of energy medicine is non-local healing, in which the practitioner may be at some distance from the person to be healed. Non-local healing includes prayer, empathetic concern, and distant intentionality, in which healing thoughts and vibrations are sent to the person in need.

Reported uses
Energy medicine may be used in conjunction with a more traditional regimen to facilitate treatment of anemias, cancer, arthritis, colitis, Alzheimer's, inflammatory diseases, hypertension and heart disease, cellular diseases, viral diseases, overdoses, and fractures. Energy therapy isn't effective with genetic diseases.

How the treatment is performed
The healing practitioner begins by "centering" — that is, focusing his creative or healing intention by directing it inward — to ready himself for assessing and treating the patient. The practitioner draws energy into himself through his crown chakra and sends it to his own heart (to ensure that no harm is done), then out through his hands to the client. The energy may go through both hands, or through only the left hand, with the right hand drawing negative energy away from the client. The practitioner may envision a desire and commitment to creating a specific outcome for the patient; for example, fulfilling a personal goal or aspiration, or he may simply facilitate the energy to be used for the client's best interest. This creative, healing intention aligns the conscious, subconscious, and super conscious aspects of the mind; sets energy forces in motion; and may create

CHARACTERISTICS OF THE SEVEN PRIMARY CHAKRAS

Chakra	Location	Glands	Color	Issues
7. Crown	Slightly above the top of the head; 2 to 3 inches in diameter	Pituitary, pineal	Violet	Worthiness, trusting God
6. Brow	Just above eyebrow line; 1½ to 2 inches in diameter	Pituitary, hypothalamus	Indigo	Seeing and admitting what is or has happened
5. Throat	Larynx, just above junction of collarbones; 1½ to 3 inches in diameter	Thyroid, parathyroids	Blue	Safety in speaking out
4. Heart	1 inch above where ribs meet on lower chest; 1½ to 4 inches in diameter	Thymus	Green	Trust and love
3. Solar plexus	Centered in pit of stomach, 2 inches below joining of ribs; 1½ to 4 inches in diameter	Pancreas	Yellow	Self-image, self-esteem
2. Sacral	Few inches below the navel and above the pubic bone; 2 to 4 inches in diameter	Adrenals	Orange	Power
1. Root	Perineum; 1 to 3 inches in diameter	Gonads	Red	Survival, safety, basic instincts, sexuality

instantaneous healings or other manifestations.

Hazards

No adverse effects arising from energy medicine have been identified. Some clients may express discomfort with the intensified energy; at that point the therapist may move to another location or end the treatment.

The use of vibrational toxins may impede the success of energy therapy. Such toxins include alcohol (loosens and misaligns the subtle anatomy), cigarette smoke (clouds and weakens the subtle anatomy), and caffeine (disturbs the flow of energy). These affect the acupuncture meridian system that affects the etheric body, which in turn causes energy leaks in the emotional and mental bodies.

Clinical considerations

The client should be consulted about cultural items or rituals that are important to him, and these should be incorporated into the healing session in the manner agreed upon.

Research summary

Numerous studies support the efficacy of vibrational or energy medicine. However, further study regarding its efficacy is necessary.

Environmental medicine

As the name implies, environmental medicine is concerned with the effects of the environment on human health. More and more health care providers —

including both conventional medical and alternative therapy practitioners—are recognizing that such substances as chemicals, dust, molds, and certain foods can cause allergic reactions that may result in or exacerbate a wide range of disorders in susceptible persons. These disorders may manifest as a complex assortment of chronic or cyclic signs and symptoms, usually involving more than one organ system and often mediated by the immune system.

Chemical sensitivity to foods, allergens, and other substances in the environment appears to be a growing problem among wide segments of the population and may help to explain many signs and symptoms that have been difficult to diagnose and treat. Many experts attribute this increased incidence of sensitivity to the growth of the petrochemical industry since the end of World War II. The amount of chemical products produced today is overwhelming. Many of these substances—for example, petroleum products, insecticides, and household cleaners—can't be properly broken down by the body. According to specialists in environmental medicine, toxins from these products accumulate in the body, eventually resulting in a host of disorders ranging from neurologic and GI disturbances to mental problems and cancer.

Food allergies are considered a form of environmental illness. In this type of allergy, a specific food triggers an adverse reaction of the immune system. Other potential environmental challenges include chemicals in food, water, and air; inhaled materials such as pollens, molds, and dust; electromagnetic fields; ionizing and non-ionizing radiation; medical and recreational drugs; noise pollution; and temperature and humidity.

Individual sensitivity to chemicals varies widely. For example, some people experience adverse effects following exposure to the small amounts of formaldehyde in the environment, such as that emitted by building and furnishing materials such as new carpet. Until recently, most practitioners thought these patients were hypochondriacs, with psychosomatic symptoms, because no one else seemed to be affected as they were.

Specialists in environmental medicine classify ecological illness into two categories: differentiated and undifferentiated disease. Differentiated disease includes recognized clinical diagnoses that can be attributed wholly or partly to an ecological cause, such as hay fever and other seasonal allergies, asthma, eczema, and anaphylactic food allergies. Undifferentiated disease includes symptoms (often seemingly unrelated) that don't fit a standard diagnosis and are often attributed to psychological causes, but may have an underlying ecological cause. Illnesses in this category may include arthritis, colitis, depression, general malaise, fatigue, headaches, and aches and pains with no ascertainable cause.

Primary care practitioners are commonly the first contact for persons suffering from environmental sensitivities, although a growing number of doctors in the United States, Canada, and Europe are entering this specialty field. Allergies have been studied since the 19th century, but only in the last 30 years has the field of environmental medicine become widely recognized. The pioneer in environmental medicine was Theron Randolph, a Chicago allergy specialist who believed that sensitivity to common foods such as wheat, milk, eggs, and so forth, could cause a wide range of medical problems for certain people. By withholding the suspect food for 4 days and then giving the patient a challenge dose, Randolph was able to identify foods that triggered assorted symptoms, including fatigue, headaches, skin conditions, arthritis, asthma, GI disorders, and depression. He later discovered that chemicals such as formaldehyde could also cause serious problems in susceptible people.

In attempting to understand how environmental substances can ultimately cause disease, environmental medicine has used Hans Selye's general adaptation syndrome model. His model describes how continued exposure to stressors, such as environmental toxins, can develop into a maladaptive response. However, each individual's reaction to a particular toxin or combination of toxins is also affected by other factors, including heredity, history, psychological stressors, and nutritional status. In addition, a particular environmental challenge may have a greater or lesser effect on an individual from day to day, depending on his physical and mental condition as well as the presence of other challenges in the environment.

Reported uses
Environmental medicine has been found effective in the treatment of mold and pollen allergies, food allergies, chemical sensitivity, and assorted disorders.

How the treatment is performed
Because the response to a particular environmental stressor varies greatly from person to person, identifying the cause of a patient's symptom pattern can be very difficult. The first step is to obtain a detailed chronological history targeting exposure to possible environmental stressors over time and relating exposures to the appearance of symptoms. The history should include any possible influences on the development or course of the patient's symptoms, including a detailed description of his home and work environments, and of the effects of the seasons or any specific activity. Laboratory tests and a physical examination are performed to identify nutritional problems, organ system dysfunction, or problems with the body's detoxification process. Treatment may include any combination of the following modalities:

- Patient education
- Therapeutic customized diets
- Nutritional supplements
- Immunotherapies
- Psychotherapies

- Detoxification therapies
- Environmental controls
- Pharmaceutics.

Allergy and hypersensitivity tests are an important element in the assessment process. These tests may include both traditional allergy tests, such as scratch tests for allergies to pollen, and the newer antigen tests, such as serial end-point titration, provocative neutralization, and bronchoprovocation. Complex symptom patterns may require inpatient hospitalization in an environmental control unit, which is free from all common chemical exposures. The patient consumes only water until all symptoms disappear, at which time he is challenged by foods and inhaled chemicals to assess his responses. Several hospitals in the United States and Canada have environmental control units.

For suspected food allergies, the doctor may propose an elimination diet in which the suspected food is eliminated from the patient's diet for at least 10 days to see whether his symptoms disappear. Among the most common food allergens are dairy products, wheat, corn, eggs, soy products, peanuts, potatoes, tomatoes, sugar, and shellfish.

Once the causative environmental toxin or food allergen has been identified, the primary treatment is avoiding exposure to it. For persons with multiple sensitivities, avoidance can be very problematic. For example, a person sensitive to perfumes would theoretically need to stay away from enclosed spaces where people are wearing perfumes. This could severely restrict the patient's social life as well as limit his ability to work in many work environments.

Patient education is essential. Patients must understand the factors that contribute to their illness to ensure long-term improvement. Environmental controls in the home and workplace to reduce exposure to the causative agents are essential. Immunotherapy may be used to reduce the patient's sensitivity to the offending substance.

Hazards

The major concern when trying to eliminate environmental toxins from the body is to remove them fully. Mobilizing them from tissue stores in fat or bone may temporarily increase their toxicity. Great care must be taken to maintain liver and kidney function, promote bowel elimination, and prevent recycling of toxins back into the body.

Clinical considerations

■ Keep abreast of the wide range of effects that environmental toxins can have on complex disease states to identify possible environmental influences on the patient's illness.

■ Warn the patient that trial-and-error testing may be necessary to determine the cause of his symptoms.

■ Show the patient how to keep an accurate diary of his symptoms (or a food diary) to aid in diagnosis.

■ If testing determines that the patient has a food allergy, make sure he understands that he will have to eliminate the food from his diet or undergo immunotherapy to decrease his sensitivity to it. Some environmental practitioners recommend eating only organic foods; if this is the case, recommend local sources the patient can use.

■ Teach the patient and his family, friends, and coworkers as much as possible about his illness, its cause (if known), and the need to avoid the causative food or substance.

TRAINING   *The American Academy of Environmental Medicine (AAEM) provides a comprehensive, ACCME-accredited continuing medical education program dedicated to training physicians in all aspects of environmental medicine.*

Research summary

Studies have supported an environmental link to numerous disorders, including arthritis, asthma, eczema, urticaria, migraines, colitis, fatigue, depression, hyperactivity, vascular problems, and psychological problems. Other studies have focused on the diagnostic techniques used in environmental medicine, including a 1993 study that supported the effectiveness of provocation-neutralization testing.

Enzyme therapy

Enzymes are protein molecules that act as catalysts or initiators for most of the biochemical reactions that occur in the body. Without these initiators, cells and tissues would be unable to perform all the biochemical reactions required to meet the body's needs. Enzymes are essential for digestion, tissue repair, and cellular energy. Digestive enzymes break down food for energy, while other enzymes convert this energy for use by the body. Still other types of enzymes may help coagulate blood, help the lungs expel carbon dioxide, and help convert nutrients to make new tissue for muscles, nerve cells, bones, and skin. Vitamins, minerals, and hormones could not do their work without enzymes.

The enzymes used for digestion are produced by the salivary glands, stomach, pancreas, and small intestine; at each step in the process, specific enzymes break down various types of food. The four main categories of digestive enzymes are amylase, protease, lipase, and cellulase. *Amylase* breaks down carbohydrates and is found in saliva and digestive and pancreatic juices. *Protease* helps digest protein and is found in pancreatic and stomach juices. *Lipase* aids in fat digestion and is found in stomach and pancreatic juices. *Cellulase* digests fiber and must be consumed from plants because the body is unable to manufacture it.

Reported uses

Practitioners of conventional medicine prescribe enzyme replacement therapy to treat specific enzyme deficiencies, such as lactase deficiency, and chronic diseases that affect the digestive process, such as cystic fibrosis. CAM practitioners use enzyme supplements to treat conditions that are unrelated to enzyme deficiencies, on the principle that taking enzyme supplements strengthens the digestive system and a properly functioning digestive system can help prevent and remedy a variety of acute and chronic health problems. Enzyme therapy makes use of both pancreatic and plant-derived enzymes.

Pancreatic enzyme supplements are used to treat viral disorders, for which they work by digesting the virus's protein coating, and cancer, for which they work by dissolving the cancer cells' outer coating, allowing white blood cells to destroy them. There are reports of improvement in patients with multiple sclerosis, and some athletes take pancreatic enzymes after an injury to promote inflammation and thus accelerate healing.

Plant enzymes are used to relieve digestive disorders, sore throats, hay fever, and candidiasis. Specific enzymes may also be prescribed to assist in protein, carbohydrate, or fat digestion, depending on an individual's health needs.

How the treatment is performed

To aid digestion, enzymes are given with meals. When used for other problems, however, they are given between meals so they won't be used to break down food. Enzyme therapy practitioners also encourage patients to eat a diet rich in whole foods, with large amounts of raw fruits and vegetables, because cooking can destroy plant enzymes.

Bromelain is a very common enzyme that's available over the counter. It's derived from pineapples and is used primarily as an anti-inflammatory agent for conditions such as muscle pain, bursitis, arthritis, tendonitis, and bursitis. The strength of bromelain is given in milk clotting units (mcu) or gelatin digesting units (gdu). Both units are essentially the same. The higher the number of units, the more potent the enzyme, which

means less bromelain is required. Therefore, taking 300 mg of one brand may not be the same as taking 300 mg of another brand. Always check the potency along with the amount per capsule. In general, 250 to 750 mg of bromelain at 1,800 mcu (or gdu), three times a day, is considered sufficient to relieve symptoms associated with inflammation and bruising.

Hazards

Enzyme therapy may cause adverse GI reactions, such as nausea, vomiting, diarrhea, or obstruction. Insufficient information is available regarding enzyme use in pregnancy and lactation. Unless the benefits outweigh potential risks, the use of enzymes is discouraged.

 SAFETY RISK *Enzymes shouldn't be used in patients susceptible to allergic reactions.*

Clinical considerations

- Patients with pancreatitis, acute exacerbation of chronic pancreatic disease, or a known hypersensitivity to pork protein should avoid pancreatic enzyme therapy.
- If the patient is considering taking enzyme supplements for a disorder unrelated to enzyme deficiency, advise him that there is no scientific support for such treatment.

TRAINING *The knowledge for general use of systemic enzyme therapy can be obtained by attending a several-day seminar on the subject. Specific training is necessary for intracorporeal administration.*

Research summary

There is no scientific evidence to support the use of enzyme supplements to treat serious diseases such as cancer or multiple sclerosis. Both consumer groups and the Food and Drug Administration have condemned companies that tout enzyme supplements as cures for such diseases.

ephedra

*Brigham tea, cao ma huang
(Chinese ephedra), desert herb,
desert tea, E. shennungiana, E. sinica,
ephedrine, epitonin, joint fir, ma-huang,
mahuuanggen (root), Mexican tea,
Mormon tea, muzei mu huang
(Mongolian ephedra), popotillo,
sea grape, squaw tea, teamster's tea,
yellow astringent, yellow horse,
zhong ma huang*

Ephedra, or ephedrine, is derived from the crude extracts of the root and aerial parts of *E. sinica* and *E. shennungiana*; other forms include *E. nevadensis, E. trifurca, E. equisetina,* and *E. distachya.* Ephedrine has been used medicinally as a stimulant and for the management of bronchial disorders. It is believed that the various members of this genus were used more than 5,000 years ago by the Chinese to treat asthma. Ephedra has been used in Asian medicine to treat colds and flu, fevers, chills, headaches, edema, lack of perspiration, nasal congestion, aching joints and bones, coughing and wheezing. Today, ephedra continues to find a place in herbal preparations designed to relieve cold symptoms and to improve respiratory function.

The primary active ingredient of ephedra extract is ephedrine, although extracts generally contain between 0.5% and 2.5% of alkaloids of the 2-amino-phenylpropane type, including ephedrine, methylephedrine, pseudoephedrine, norephedrine, and norpseudoephedrine. Similar to the structurally related drug amphetamine, ephedrine acts by directly stimulating the sympathomimetic system and the central nervous system (CNS, alpha and beta agonists), possibly increasing heart rate, myocardial contraction, peripheral vasoconstriction with associated elevations in blood pressure, bronchodilation, and mydriasis. Ephedrine is active when given orally, parenterally, or ophthalmically.

Other components in ephedra extracts include volatile oils, catechins, gallic acid, tannins, flavonoids, inulin, dextrin, starch, and pectin. Ephedra is available as capsules, tablets, teas, and tinctures, in combination products such as Chromemate, Escalation, Excel, Herbal Ecstasy, Herbal Fen-Phen, Herbalife, Metabolife, and Power Trim.

Reported uses

Ephedra is used to treat respiratory tract diseases with mild bronchospasm. Although it's been in use by conventional practitioners since the 1930s to treat asthma, it has become less popular as more specific beta agonists have become available. Ephedra is also used as a cardiovascular stimulant. Pseudoephedrine remains a common ingredient in many OTC cough and cold preparations. It's also used to treat other conditions, including chills, coughs, colds, flu, fever, headaches, edema, and nasal congestion, and as an appetite suppressant. The alkaloid-free North American species is used to treat venereal disease.

Ma huang was traditionally used by Chinese herbalists during the early stages of respiratory infections and also for the short-term treatment of certain kinds of asthma, eczema, hay fever, narcolepsy, and edema. However, ma huang was not supposed to be taken for an extended period of time, and people with less than robust constitutions were warned to use only low doses or to avoid ma huang altogether.

Administration

■ Oral use: Adults, 15 to 30 mg total alkaloid, calculated as ephedrine, every 6 to 8 hours for a total maximum daily dose of 300 mg/day; children older than age 6, 0.5 mg total alkaloid/kg; recommended daily dose, 2 mg

■ Extract: 1 to 3 ml by mouth three times a day

- Tea: 1 to 4 g by mouth three times a day
- Tincture (1:1): Medium single dose 5 g by mouth
- Tincture (1:4): 6 to 8 ml by mouth three times a day.

SAFETY RISK *The FDA prohibits the sale of ephedra in quantities of 8 mg or more per dose, and advises individuals to take less than 8 mg every 6 hours, and no more than 24 mg daily. They further advise that ephedra products not be used for more than 7 consecutive days.*

Hazards

Side effects associated with ephedra include anxiety, confusion, dependency, dizziness, headache, insomnia, irritability, mania, motor restlessness, nervousness, psychosis, seizure, arrhythmias, cardiac arrest, hypertension, hypotension, MI, palpitations, stroke, tachycardia, nausea, constipation, uterine contractions, urinary disorders, hyperglycemia, hypoglycemia, and dermatitis.

When used with beta blockers such as propranolol, ephedra may enhance sympathomimetic effects on vasculature from unopposed alpha-agonist effects, thus increasing risk of hypertensive effects. Concurrent use with cardiac glycosides or halothane may disturb heart rhythm. Additive pharmacodynamic effects may be seen when ephedra is used with CNS stimulants such as dextroamphetamine. An increased sympathomimetic effect may be observed with guanethidine. MAO inhibitors used with ephedra may pose risk of hypertensive crisis. Oxytocin and secale alkaloid derivatives can also increase blood pressure. Concurrent use with theophylline may increase risk of GI and CNS adverse effects. When ephedra is used with caffeine or yohimbe, an additive sympathomimetic and CNS stimulation may be noted.

Pregnant patients should avoid use because of the risk of inducing uterine contractions and the unknown effects of the herb on the fetus. Those with glaucoma,

pheochromocytoma, thyrotoxicosis, underlying CV disease, or a history of cerebrovascular disease should avoid use. Diabetic patients should avoid use because of potential hyperglycemic effects. Those with sleep, mood, anxiety, and psychotic disorders should use with caution.

SAFETY RISK *Pills containing ephedra have been combined with other stimulants like caffeine and sold as "natural" stimulants in weight-loss products. Deaths from overstimulation have been reported.*

Clinical considerations

- Compounds containing ephedra have been linked to several deaths and more than 800 adverse effects, many of which appear to be dose related.
- Monitor patient's pulse and blood pressure.
- Ephedra shouldn't be used for more than 7 consecutive days because of the risk of tachyphylaxis and dependence.
- Patients with eating disorders may abuse this herb.
- Signs and symptoms of toxic reaction include diaphoresis, dilated pupils, muscle spasms, fever, and cardiac and respiratory failure.
- If overdose occurs, perform gastric lavage and administer activated charcoal. Treat spasms with diazepam, replace electrolytes with I.V. fluids, and prevent acidosis with sodium bicarbonate infusions.
- Advise patient not to use this herb in place of getting the proper medical evaluation of a prolonged illness.
- Advise patient with thyroid disease, hypertension, CV disease, or diabetes to avoid using ephedra.
- Advise patient to watch for adverse reactions, particularly chest pain, shortness of breath, palpitations, dizziness, and fainting.
- Instruct patient to store ephedra away from direct light.
- Advise patient to keep this and other herbal products out of children's reach.
- Tell patient to remind pharmacist of any herbal or dietary supplement that

he's taking when obtaining a new prescription.

■ Advise patient to consult his health care provider before using an herbal preparation because a conventional treatment with proven efficacy may be available.

 SAFETY RISK *Dosages high enough to produce psychoactive or hallucinogenic effects are toxic to the heart and shouldn't be used.*

Research summary

Current research and studies have shown that ephedra is a powerful drug with the potential for dangerous side effects. The FDA has issued recommendations regarding dosage and administration of this herbal derivative.

eucalyptus

Blue gum tree, Eucalypti globulus, *eucalyptol, fever tree, gum tree, red gum, stringy bark tree*

Eucalyptus oil, also known as eucalyptol, is steam-distilled from the twigs and long leathery leaves of the eucalyptus tree. Eucalyptus folium contains the dried leaves of older *Eucalypti globulus* trees. The leaves are collected after the tree has been cut down and allowed to dry in the shade. The primary component of eucalyptus oil is the volatile substance 1,8-cineol (cineole). Oil preparations are standardized to contain 80% to 90% cineole.

The effectiveness of the herb as an expectorant is attributed to the local irritant action of the volatile oil. Eucalyptus is available as dried herb, eucalyptus leaf, essential oil, and tea bags.

Reported uses

Eucalyptus is used internally and externally as an expectorant, and to treat infections and fevers. It's also used topically to treat sore muscles and rheumatism. A topical combination of eucalyptus and peppermint shows promise as an analgesic.

Administration

■ Essential oil: Used in massage blends for sore muscles, in foot baths or saunas, steam inhalations, chest rubs, room sprays, bath blends, and air diffusions; for external use only

■ Leaf: Average daily dose is 4 to 16 g by mouth every 3 to 4 hours

■ Oil: For internal use, average dose is 0.3 to 0.6 g by mouth every day

■ Tea: For infusion, steep 6 oz of dried herb in boiling water for 2 to 3 minutes, and then strain; for decoction 6 to 8 oz of dried herb boiled for 3 to 5 minutes

■ Tincture: Take 3 to 4 g by mouth every day.

Hazards

Adverse reactions may include nausea, vomiting, diarrhea, and asthma-like attacks. Enhanced effects may be noted when administered with antidiabetics. Eucalyptus oil induces detoxification enzyme systems in the liver; therefore, the oil may affect any drug that the liver metabolizes. When given with other herbs that cause hypoglycemia (basil, glucomannan, Queen Anne's lace), decreased blood glucose levels may be observed.

Patients who have had an allergic reaction to eucalyptus or its vapors should avoid use. Those who are pregnant or breast-feeding, have liver disease, or have intestinal tract inflammation should avoid use.

 SAFETY RISK *Essential oil preparations shouldn't be applied to a child's face because of risk of severe bronchial spasm.*

Clinical considerations

■ Inform patient of potential adverse effects.

■ Monitor patient for allergic reaction.

■ In susceptible patients, particularly infants and children, the application of eucalyptus preparations to the face or the inhalation of vapors can exacerbate bronchospasm.

■ Monitor blood glucose level in diabetic patients taking eucalyptus.

■ Oral administration may cause nausea, vomiting, and diarrhea.

■ If poisoning or overdose occurs, don't induce vomiting. Vomiting may increase the risk of aspiration. Administer activated charcoal and treat symptomatically.

■ Advise the patient to stop taking eucalyptus immediately and to check with health care provider if difficulty breathing, hives, or skin rash occur.

■ Keep away from children and pets.

■ Tell patient to remind pharmacist of any herbal or dietary supplement that he's taking when obtaining a new prescription.

■ Advise patient to consult his health care provider before using an herbal preparation because a conventional treatment with proven efficacy may be available.

SAFETY RISK *The oil shouldn't be taken internally unless it has been diluted. As little as a few drops of oil for children and 4 to 5 ml of oil for adults can cause poisoning. Signs include hypotension, circulatory dysfunction, and cardiac and respiratory failure.*

Research summary
The concepts behind the use of eucalyptus and claims made regarding its effects haven't yet been validated scientifically.

evening primrose

*Fever plant, king's cure-all,
night willow-herb,* Oenothera biennis,
rock-rose, sand lily, scabish, sun-drop

Evening primrose oil is extracted from the seeds of *Oenothera biennis*. It contains the amino acid tryptophan and a high concentration of essential fatty acids, in particular *cis*-linoleic acid (CLA) and gamma-linoleic acid (GLA). The va-

riety of evening primrose grown for commercial purposes produces oil with 72% CLA and 9% GLA. These fatty acids are prostaglandin precursors.

Conversion of the prostaglandin precursors into prostaglandins is the basis for using this oil to stimulate cervical ripening, prevent heart disease, and reduce symptoms of rheumatoid arthritis. Its efficacy in other clinical conditions may result from its supply of fatty acids. Evening primrose is available as capsules, liquid, oil, and tablets (evening primrose complex), in products such as Mega Primrose Oil, Original Primrose for Women, and Royal Brittany Evening Primrose Oil.

Reported uses
Used by midwives to stimulate cervical ripening during pregnancy at or near term and to ease childbirth. Also used to manage cyclic mastitis, premenstrual syndrome, and neurodermatitis. Used as a dietary stimulant. Used to treat eczema and diabetic neuropathy in Europe, although recent evidence doesn't support its use for these conditions. Also used to treat hypercholesterolemia, rheumatoid arthritis, inflammatory bowel disease, Raynaud's disease, Sjögren's syndrome, chronic fatigue syndrome, endometriosis, obesity, prostate disease, hyperactivity in children, and asthma.

Administration
■ Oral use: Based on GLA content; typically, 1 to 2 capsules (0.5 to 1 g) three times a day

■ Cyclic mastitis: 3 g by mouth every day in 2 or 3 divided doses

■ Diabetic neuropathy: 4 to 6 g by mouth every day

■ Eczema in children: 2 to 4 g by mouth every day

■ Rheumatoid arthritis: 5 to 10 g every day.

Hazards
Adverse reactions may include headache, nausea, diarrhea, bloating, vomiting, flat-

ulence, and allergic reactions. When given with drugs that lower the seizure threshold such as tricyclic antidepressants, phenothiazines, and other epileptogenic drugs, there is an increased risk of seizures.

Those with an allergy to evening primrose oil and pregnant and breast-feeding patients should avoid use. Those with a history of epilepsy and those taking a tricyclic antidepressant, phenothiazine, or another drug that lowers the seizure threshold should also avoid use.

Clinical considerations
- Monitor patient for allergic reaction.
- The fatty oil, extracted from the seeds of the evening primrose plant by a cold extraction process, is available standardized for fatty acid content.
- Drug effects may be delayed: patients with cyclic mastitis and premenstrual syndrome may not see improvement for 4 to 6 weeks, with maximum benefit in 4 to 8 months; those with eczema may experience decreased pruritus in 3 to 4 months; and patients with diabetic neuropathy may see improvement in 3 to 6 months.
- Vitamin E may be given with evening primrose oil to prevent the formation of toxic metabolites.
- Tell patient to discontinue the herb if they have signs or symptoms of an allergic reaction, such as trouble breathing, hives, itchy or swollen skin, or rash.
- Advise patient to consult with her health care provider before using evening primrose oil during pregnancy or while breast-feeding.
- Advise patient to take herb with food to minimize adverse GI reactions.
- Tell patient to remind pharmacist of any herbal or dietary supplement that he's taking when obtaining a new prescription.
- Advise patient to consult his health care provider before using an herbal preparation because a conventional treatment with proven efficacy may be available.

SAFETY RISK *The oil may unmask previously undiagnosed epilepsy, especially when taken with a drug that treats depression or schizophrenia.*

Research summary
The concepts behind the use of evening primrose oil and the claims made regarding its effects haven't yet been validated scientifically.

eyebright
Euphrasia, Euphrasia officinalis

Eyebright has been used medicinally for centuries; Theophrastus (c. 372–287 B.C.) and Dioscorides (18th Century) prescribed infusions for topical application in the treatment of eye infections. The plant is used in homeopathic remedies to treat conjunctivitis and other ocular inflammations. Major components include a glycoside (aucuboside), a tannin (aucubin), caffeic and ferulic acids, sterols, choline, basic compounds, and a volatile oil. Eyebright also contains vitamins A and C. It's available in capsules.

Reported uses
Eyebright is used topically in the form of lotions, poultices, and eye baths for ophthalmic disorders, including treatment of blepharitis, conjunctivitis, sties, and eye fatigue. It's also used internally for coughs, hoarseness, and respiratory infections.

Administration
- Capsules, tablets: 1 to 2 capsules or tablets by mouth three times a day
- Liquid extract (alcohol free): 1 to 2 ml (28 to 56 gtt) by mouth three times a day
- Liquid extract (25% alcohol): 2 to 4 ml (40 to 80 gtt) by mouth three times a day
- Tea (for infusion, steep 1 to 2 teaspoons of finely cut herb in 6 oz of boiling water for 5 to 10 minutes; for decoction, boil 1 to 2 tsp of finely cut herb in 6

to 8 oz of boiling water for 3 to 5 minutes): Up to three times a day by mouth
■ Tincture (45% alcohol): 2 to 6 ml (½ to 1 tsp) by mouth three times a day.

Hazards
Side effects may include confusion, cephalgia, insomnia, weakness, sneezing, toothache, hoarseness, stomach upset, polyuria, cough, dyspnea, diaphoresis, yawning, and intense pressure in the eyes with tearing, itching, redness, swelling, photophobia, and changes in vision. Use with disulfiram or metronidazole may precipitate a disulfiram-like reaction. Use with alcohol may lead to enhanced central nervous system effects.

Pregnant and breast-feeding patients and children should avoid use. Patients with ophthalmic disease such as glaucoma should also avoid use.

 SAFETY RISK *Ophthalmic use of eyebright is strongly discouraged.*

Clinical considerations
■ Warn patient not to treat symptoms of ophthalmic disorders with eyebright before seeking appropriate medical evaluation because doing so may delay diagnosis of a potentially serious medical condition.
■ Advise patients with glaucoma to avoid use.
■ Many tinctures contain between 25% and 45% alcohol and thus shouldn't be used by alcoholic patients, those with liver disease, or those taking disulfiram, metronidazole, a benzodiazepine or a barbiturate.
■ Caution patient not to apply eyebright directly to his eye because the sterility of the products can't be guaranteed.
■ Tell patient that if he has trouble breathing or develops hives, or if his skin is itchy or swollen or breaks out in a rash, to stop taking this herb and contact his health care provider immediately.
■ Instruct patient to keep the herb away from children and pets.
■ Tell patient to remind pharmacist of any herbal or dietary supplement that

he's taking when obtaining a new prescription.
■ Advise patient to consult his health care provider before using an herbal preparation because a conventional treatment with proven efficacy may be available.

Research summary
Although many believe that eyebright has antibacterial and astringent properties, none of the chemical components has been associated with a significant therapeutic effect. The German Commission E recommends against the use of eyebright for therapeutic purposes.

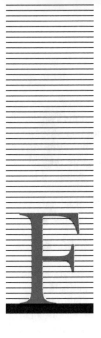

false unicorn

Blazing star, Chamaelirium luteum,
devil's bit, drooping starwort,
fairy-wand, helonias root, rattlesnake

False unicorn root, which is derived from
Chamaelirium luteum, contains the
steroid saponin mixture chamaelirin.
Other components that have been isolated from the root extract are oleic, linoleic, and stearic acids. Chamaelirin is believed to be responsible for the oxytocic,
diuretic, and anthelmintic effects of the
herb. The herb was first used by practitioners in the Eclectic medical movement
of the late 19th and 20th centuries. Its
chief use was for treating amenorrhea
and morning sickness. Although the root
probably has no effect on uterine tissue,
it may exert its effect by increasing human chorionic gonadotropin release.
False unicorn root is available as dried
root or rhizome, liquid extract, and tincture.

Reported uses
False unicorn is used to treat dysmenorrhea, amenorrhea, and morning sickness.
It's also used as an appetite stimulant,
anthelmintic, diuretic, emetic, and insecticide, and as a uterine tonic taken during pregnancy to prevent miscarriage.

Administration
- Tea: by mouth three times a day
- Liquid extract (45% alcohol): 1 to 2 ml
(20 to 40 gtt) by mouth three times a day

■ Tincture (45% alcohol): 2 to 5 ml (½ to 1 tsp) by mouth three times a day.

Hazards

Adverse reactions associated with false unicorn root include gastric upset and vomiting. When administered with estrogen and progesterone, false unicorn root may alter the action of hormones that affect the uterus.

The safety of false unicorn in pregnancy can't be guaranteed.

Clinical considerations

■ Many tinctures contain between 25% and 45% alcohol and shouldn't be used by alcoholic patients, those with liver disease, or those taking a drug such as disulfiram, metronidazole, a barbiturate, a benzodiazepine, or a cephalosporin.
■ High doses may cause stomach upset and vomiting.
■ Advise patient not to use false unicorn root without consulting her health care provider, especially if she's pregnant or breast-feeding.
■ Warn patient not to delay seeking appropriate medical evaluation because doing so may delay diagnosis of a potentially serious medical condition.
■ Instruct patient to stop taking this herb and to contact a health care provider immediately if he experiences difficulty breathing, hives, itchy or swollen skin, or a rash.
■ Tell patient to remind pharmacist of any herbal or dietary supplement that he's taking when obtaining a new prescription.
■ Advise patient to consult his health care provider before using an herbal preparation because a conventional treatment with proven efficacy may be available.

Research summary

The concepts behind the use of false unicorn root and the claims made regarding its effects haven't yet been validated scientifically.

Fasting

Fasting—the restriction of dietary intake to liquids—may allow the body to rid itself of toxins while promoting healing. Because the body expends a great deal of energy breaking down foods, a fast, which usually last from 2 to 5 days, may provide a resting period for the body. While the digestive system rests, the excretion of toxins continues and no new toxins are being introduced into the body. In addition to its physical healing effects, fasting may promote mental and spiritual well-being.

Fasting has been practiced for centuries in many cultures. Ancient cultures used fasts not for weight loss or detoxification, but as a means of self-deprivation for religious purposes. Today, Islam and Judaism still require fasting on certain holidays.

All fasting regimens allow fluids—either water, juices, or herbal teas. Many naturopathic doctors recommend fasting, usually twice a year for 5 days, as part of a regular health maintenance program. Some recommend a vegetable juice fast, while others consider juice a food and recommend water only.

Reported uses

Fasting is believed to enable the body to cleanse the liver, kidneys, and colon, flush out toxins, and purify the blood. The energy the body saves during a fast can be redirected to other functions, such as revitalizing the immune system. Some of the conditions that may benefit from fasting include hypertension, arthritis, food allergies (identification and elimination), inflammatory diseases, and headaches.

How the treatment is performed

Therapeutic fasting regimens vary according to the philosophy of the practitioner and the purpose of the fast. The patient usually must undergo some form of preparation before beginning the fast, such as eating raw fruits and vegetables or drinking certain fluids for a prescribed amount of time. For example, he may be instructed to drink a specified amount of water along with pure juices and two to three cups of herbal tea each day. The practitioner will determine the duration and type of fast (water or juice) that is appropriate for the patient. Most practitioners suggest a 2- to 3-day fast, although longer fasts are sometimes recommended.

When a water fast is used, it's recommended that the patient drink at least three glasses of distilled or spring water daily. Some practitioners believe that a juice fast is less stressful on the body because juice provides necessary nutrients and can prevent low blood glucose levels. In addition, water fasting may cause the body to release toxins too quickly, resulting in headaches. Vegetable juices are preferable to fruit juices, which contain large amounts of sugar.

A patient who is ending a fast shouldn't resume eating with a single large meal because the GI system needs time to replenish digestive juices. Rather, he should eat several small meals spaced several hours apart to allow his body time to readjust to solid food. The patient should also avoid eating highly refined or spicy foods to prevent diarrhea, vomiting, or abdominal pain. The longer the fast, the more consideration and care is needed when reintroducing food. Water fasts are usually broken first with fruit or vegetable juices, with the reintroduction of solid foods taking place gradually. Juice fasts are usually followed by a 2-day diet of fresh raw fruits and vegetables.

Hazards

Some practitioners of conventional medicine claim that fasting may impair the immune system by depriving the body of essential nutrients. In addition, when blood glucose levels decline, the body starts breaking down muscle to provide energy. This muscle breakdown results in increased production of ammonia and nitrogen, leaving the patient weak, tired, and nauseated.

Other adverse effects may include dry skin or skin eruptions, headaches, dizziness, irritability, coated tongue, foul-smelling stools, body aches, and mucous discharge; however, fasting advocates say these symptoms are signs that toxins are leaving the body. More serious complications, such as cardiac arrhythmias (from electrolyte imbalances), anemia, hypotension, and bradycardia, have also been reported. The longer the fast, the more dangerous it becomes.

Fasting is contraindicated in pregnancy and breast-feeding.

Clinical considerations

■ Urge patients to consult a health care provider before beginning any type of fast. This is especially important for patients with health problems and those taking prescribed medications. Dosage requirements may change during a fast.
■ Fasting is contraindicated for patients with diabetes, eating disorders, epilepsy, kidney disease, severe bronchial asthma, stomach ulcers, ulcerative colitis, tuberculosis, or malnutrition. It's also not recommended for children, the elderly, or pregnant or lactating women.
■ If you are caring for a fasting patient, advise him to notify a health care provider if he experiences any adverse reactions, especially potentially life-threatening ones such as an irregular heartbeat.

 TRAINING *No formal training for practitioners who guide patients in fasting exists in the United States.*

Research summary
The concepts behind the use of fasting and the claims made regarding its effects haven't yet been validated scientifically.

Feldenkrais method

The Feldenkrais method takes a functional approach to reorganizing the body and behavior into new and more expanded motor patterns. The method is a form of somatic education that works by teaching patients to become more aware of the habitual neuromuscular patterns and rigidities of their bodies and by expanding their options for new ways of moving. It focuses on the patient's ability to regulate and coordinate movement by working through the nervous system.

Moshe Feldenkrais, a Russian-born Israeli physicist, mechanical engineer, and judo expert, developed his gentle method of bodywork in an attempt to rehabilitate his own knee, which he injured in an athletic accident. He studied anatomy, physiology, and psychology in the hope that he might be able to avoid surgery. The result of this search for a deeper understanding of the body and its functioning was the development of an entire philosophy of life that underlies the Feldenkrais method.

Feldenkrais came to believe that people practice a skill only until they achieve a desired goal. For instance, an infant sees adults and children moving around and doing things for themselves, and strives to do the same. Once he achieves that goal, he stops developing the skill that got him there. The same is true of such skills as speech and social interaction. Feldenkrais maintained that "settling for whatever technique helps achieve a goal" means that people tend to learn inefficient and unhealthful patterns of movement, speech, and emotional and social skills. As a result, most people learn to make do with 5% of their potential without realizing that their development has been stunted. In terms of movement, this means that people learn unconscious patterns of musculoskeletal behavior that limit their ability to function optimally.

Feldenkrais argued that habitual patterns of muscle movement underlie self-awareness and emotional actions and reactions. "We know what is happening within us as soon as the muscles of our face, heart, or breathing apparatus organize themselves into patterns, known to us as fear, anxiety, laughter, or any other

feeling," he wrote. Because of the key role of the muscular system in the development and ordering of mental, emotional, social, and physiologic systems, Feldenkrais believed that his exercises could not only increase flexibility, coordination, and range of motion, but also lead to enhanced functioning in other aspects of life.

TRAINING *Classes in the Feldenkrais method are taught in either group sessions or private one-on-one sessions. Practitioners must complete 800 to 1,000 hours of training over a 3-year to 4-year period. The Feldenkrais Guild of North America in Oregon sponsors training programs, provides information to the public, makes referrals, and maintains a Web site (www.feldenkrais.com).*

Reported uses

Feldenkrais considered his technique to be a training method to improve coordination, flexibility, range of motion, and function, rather than a medical therapy. The method can benefit anyone — young or old, physically fit or physically challenged — but is especially useful for people experiencing chronic or acute pain of the back, neck, shoulder, hips, legs, or knees. Practitioners also report success in dealing with central nervous system disorders (such as multiple sclerosis, cerebrovascular accident, and cerebral palsy).

How the treatment is performed

The group classes require no special equipment. The private sessions require a table or chair on which the student can lie down or sit; pillows, blankets, and other props may be used to facilitate certain movements.

The Feldenkrais method uses two trademarked approaches: Awareness Through Movement, which consists of group lessons, and Functional Integration, which offers private lessons tailored to the individual student. In the group classes (which last 30 to 60 minutes), the teacher verbally leads the students through a series of exercises designed to help them become more aware of their bodies and develop new patterns of movement. The exercises are performed in a slow, relaxed way, progressing from easy movements to movements of greater range and complexity. The emphasis is on enjoyment and avoiding pain. A variety of different lessons may be used, depending on the students' needs.

Functional Integration consists of gentle body work attuned to the individual student's needs. The student is fully clothed and may lie on a table or be in a sitting or standing position. Through touch, the teacher senses the student's patterns of neuromuscular "organization" and suggests more comfortable and functional patterns. The result ideally is more fluid movements and a decrease in "restrictive" patterns that create pain, tension, and stiffness. A typical session lasts 45 to 60 minutes.

Hazards
Because of its gentle technique, the Feldenkrais method is unlikely to cause any complications.

Clinical considerations
▪ The Feldenkrais method may be appropriate for patients with limitations caused by accidents. It can be incorporated into a rehabilitation program.
▪ Tell patient that it may take time to retrain himself to properly align his body.
▪ Patient must be able to follow verbal commands for the Awareness Through Movement part of the method.

Research summary
The concepts behind the use of the Feldenkrais method and the claims made regarding its effects haven't yet been validated scientifically.

fennel

Fenkel, Foeniculum vulgare,
*large fennel, sweet or bitter fennel,
wild fennel*

Fennel was known to the ancient Chinese, Indian, Egyptian, and Greek civilizations. It was in great demand during the Middle Ages. The plant was introduced to North America by Spanish priests and the English brought it to their settlements in Virginia. All parts of the plant have been used for flavorings. The oil has been used to protect stored fruits and vegetables against infection by pathogenic fungi. Fennel has been used for treatment of gastroenteritis and indigestion, to stimulate lactation, as an expectorant and emmenagogue and, reportedly, as an antidote to poisonous herbs, mushrooms and snakebites.

Fennel oil is obtained from the ripe or dried seeds of either sweet or bitter fennel. The composition of the oil varies slightly, depending on the source. Fennel oil extracted from bitter fennel is made up primarily of 50% to 75% trans-anetholes, 12% to 33% fenchone, and 2% to 5% estragole. Fennel oil extracted from sweet fennel is made up of 80% to 90% trans-anetholes, 1% to 10% fenchone, and 3% to 10% estragole. Additional components are present in smaller quantities. Fennel oil stimulates GI motility, and at high levels it has antispasmodic activity. The anethole and fenchone components have a secretolytic effect on the respiratory tract, probably a result of fennel's local irritant effects on the respiratory tract. Fennel is available as essential oil, honey syrup, seeds, and herbal tea.

Reported uses
Fennel is used as an expectorant to manage cough and bronchitis. Also used to treat mild, spastic disorders of the GI tract, feelings of fullness, and flatulence. Fennel syrup has been used to treat up-

per respiratory tract infections in children.

Administration

- Essential oil: 0.1 to 0.6 ml by mouth every day, up to 2 weeks
- Honey syrup with 0.5 g fennel oil/kg: 10 to 20 g by mouth every day, up to 2 weeks
- Seeds (crushed or ground, used for teas or other beverages): 5 to 7 g by mouth every day, up to 2 weeks.

Hazards

Adverse reactions associated with fennel oil include hallucinations, nausea, and vomiting, photodermatitis, contact dermatitis, and allergic reaction. There is an increased risk of seizures when given with drugs that lower the seizure threshold or anticonvulsants. There is also an increased risk of photosensitivity reaction with fennel use.

Those with sensitivity to fennel, celery, or similar foods and herbs should avoid use. Pregnant patients, small children, and those with a history of seizures should also avoid use. Diabetic patients should use the honey syrup cautiously because of the sugar content.

 SAFETY RISK *The use of fennel oil has been associated with seizures and pulmonary edema.*

Clinical considerations

- Ask patient whether he has an allergic response to celery, fennel, or similar spices and herbs.
- If patient has diabetes, warn him about the sugar content of the product.
- Tell patient to stop taking this herb and contact health care provider immediately if he experiences difficulty breathing, hives, or a rash.
- Tell patient to remind pharmacist of any herbal or dietary supplement that he's taking when obtaining a new prescription.
- Advise patient to consult his health care provider before using an herbal preparation because a conventional treatment with proven efficacy may be available.

SAFETY RISK *Advise patient that the maximum length of use shouldn't exceed 2 weeks. Don't mistake poison hemlock for fennel. Hemlock can cause vomiting, paralysis, and death. Know the source of preparation before administering fennel.*

Research summary

The concepts behind the use of fennel and the claims made regarding its effects haven't yet been validated scientifically.

fenugreek

Bird's foot, bockshornsamen,
Foeniculum vulgare, *Greek hay seed,*
Trigonella foenum-graecum

Fenugreek has been used for millennia both as a medicine and as a spice in Egypt, India, and the Middle East. Traditional medicinal uses include the treatment of wounds, bronchitis, digestive problems, arthritis, kidney problems, male reproductive conditions, boils, diabetes, cellulitis, tuberculosis, and GI problems. Investigations in animals have found the seeds to reduce serum cholesterol and glucose levels.

Active components in fenugreek include mucilages, proteins, steroid saponins, flavonoids, and volatile oils. Trigonelline, an alkaloid found in fenugreek, is degraded to nicotinic acid (niacin), which may partially explain its ability to lower serum cholesterol levels. Steroid saponins may also lower blood glucose and plasma glucagon levels and enhance food consumption and appetite. The seeds contain up to 50% mucilaginous fiber that, because of their ability to absorb and expand, are commonly used to treat diarrhea and constipation. The seeds also contain coumarin compounds. Fenugreek is available as capsules, paste, powder, ripe seeds, dried seeds, and as a spice.

Reported uses

Fenugreek is used to treat GI complaints and to relieve upper respiratory tract congestion and allergies. It's also used to lower cholesterol, blood glucose, insulin, and hemoglobin A1C levels, to improve glucose tolerance, and as an appetite stimulant.

Topically, a preparation of fenugreek is applied to treat skin inflammation, muscle pain, and gout, and to aid in the healing of wounds or skin ulcers.

Administration

- External: A poultice is prepared by mixing 50 g of powdered fenugreek with 1 qt (1 L) of water, and applied topically to the affected area, as needed
- Internal: An infusion is prepared by steeping 0.5 g of fenugreek in cold water for 3 hours, and then straining. Honey may be used to sweeten the infusion. The dosage is 6 g by mouth, or a cup of tea taken several times a day.

Hazards

Adverse reactions to fenugreek include maple-syrup odor to urine, hepatotoxicity, jaundice, nausea, vomiting, increased bilirubin level, hypoglycemia, contact dermatitis (with external use), flushing, wheezing, watery eyes, numbness, rash, and angioedema (after inhalation, ingestion, or topical anesthesia).

When taken with adrenergic blockers, there is an additive vasodilating effect that may lead to hypotension. There is risk of increased prothrombin time (PT) and International Normalized Ratio (INR), and potential risk of abnormal bleeding, when fenugreek is taken with anticoagulants such as aspirin, NSAIDS, heparin, low-molecular-weight heparins, and warfarin. Fenugreek also has the potential to decrease blood glucose levels when administered to those taking hypoglycemics, including insulin. A decreased uricosuric effect is noted with probencid

and sulfinpyrazone. Because of the fibrous content in fenugreek seeds and its binding potential, absorption of drugs may be altered. Advise patient to avoid using fenugreek within 2 hours of other drugs.

Pregnant patients should avoid use because of the herb's potential abortifacient properties; alcohol and water extracts of the herb may stimulate uterine activity. Those with liver disease, peptic ulcers, or severe hypotension should avoid use because of the formation of nicotinic acid. Breast-feeding patients, and those who have had a previous allergic reaction to fenugreek or nicotinic acid, should also avoid use.

Clinical considerations

- If patient is taking an anticoagulant, monitor PTT, INR, and PT. Monitor the patient for abnormal bleeding.
- Appearance of rash or contact dermatitis may indicate sensitivity to fenugreek.
- Nausea, vomiting, jaundice, or elevated bilirubin level may indicate liver damage and hepatotoxicity from nicotinic acid. If patient develops these signs or symptoms, he should immediately stop using the herb.
- If patient is pregnant, planning to become pregnant, or breast-feeding, advise her not to use fenugreek.
- Caution patient that a rash or abnormal skin change may indicate an allergy to fenugreek and that nausea, vomiting, and skin color changes may indicate liver damage. Tell patient to discontinue use if such signs and symptoms appear.
- Remind patient not to take fenugreek at the same time as other drugs and to separate administration times by 2 hours.
- Tell patient to remind pharmacist of any herbal or dietary supplement that he's taking when obtaining a new prescription.
- Advise patient to consult his health care provider before using an herbal preparation because a conventional treat-

ment with proven efficacy may be available.

Research summary

Current studies continue to elucidate the mechanism of fenugreek's abilities to lower cholesterol and glucose levels. Recent studies also show the ability of the plant to decrease the quantity of calcium oxalate deposited in the kidneys.

feverfew

Altamisa, bachelor's button, chamomile grande, Chrysanthemum parthenium, *featherfew, featherfoil, feather-fully, febrifuge plant, flirtroot, midsummer daisy, mutterkraut, nose bleed, Santa Maria, tanacetum,* Tanacetum parthenium, *vetter-voo, wild chamomile, wild quinine*

Feverfew has a long history of use in traditional medicine, especially among early European herbalists. Recently, it has become a popular remedy for migraine headaches, menstrual pain, asthma, dermatitis, arthritis, and as an antipyretic. It's been used as an insect repellant and balm for insect bites, as well as an antidote for overindulgence in opium.

Feverfew has more than 35 chemical components, of which parthenolide, a germacranolide, is the primary constituent. Sesquiterpene lactones are the most well-known and studied constituent of feverfew. Monoterpenes, such as camphor; flavonoids, such as luteolin and apigenin; and volatile oils, including angelate, costic acid, and pinene are also found in feverfew. Traces of melatonin appear in pure leaves and commercial preparations of the herb.

Parthenolide is thought to be the major component responsible for the pharmacologic effects of feverfew. It inhibits prostaglandin synthesis, platelet aggregation, serotonin release from platelets, release of granules from polymorphonu-

clear leukocytes, histamine release from mast cells, and phagocytosis. Parthenolide may have thrombolytic, cytotoxic, and antibacterial activity and may cause contraction and relaxation of vascular smooth muscle.

Monoterpenes, and possibly melatonin, may be responsible for feverfew's sedative and mild tranquilizing effects. Feverfew is available as capsules, dried leaves, liquid, powder, seeds, and tablets, in products such as Feverfew Extract Complex, Feverfew LF and FL-GBE, Feverfew Power, Migracare Feverfew Extract, Migracin, MigraSpray, MygraFew, Partenelle, and Tanacet.

Reported uses

Feverfew is used most commonly to prevent or treat migraine headaches and to treat rheumatoid arthritis. It's also used to treat asthma, psoriasis, menstrual cramps, digestion problems, and intestinal parasites; to debride wounds; and to promote menstrual flow. Feverfew is used as a mouthwash after tooth extraction, a tranquilizer, an abortifacient, and an external antiseptic and insecticide.

Administration

- Infusion (steep 2 tsp of feverfew in a cup of water for 15 minutes, or double the amount of feverfew and allow it to steep for 25 minutes): Dosage is 1 cup of the mild infusion three times a day; stronger infusion is for topical use
- Powder: Recommended daily dose is 50 mg to 1.2 g
- Migraines: Dosage is 125 mg of dried leaf preparation every day; *T. parthenium* content should be standardized to contain at least 0.2% parthenolide, equivalent to 250 mcg of feverfew.

Hazards

Adverse reactions to feverfew include dizziness, tachycardia, mouth ulcerations, GI upset, and contact dermatitis. Feverfew inhibits prostaglandin synthesis and platelet aggregation. Monitor patients taking anticoagulants, antiplatelet drugs including aspirin, and thrombolytics for increased bleeding tendency.

Pregnant women should avoid use because of its potential abortifacient properties. Breast-feeding patients should also avoid use. Patients allergic to members of the daisy, or *Asteraceae*, family — including yarrow, southernwood, wormwood, chamomile, marigold, goldenrod, coltsfoot, and dandelion, should avoid use. Patients who have had previous reactions to feverfew shouldn't take it internally. Feverfew shouldn't be used in children younger than age 2.

Clinical considerations

- Educate patient about the potential risk of abnormal bleeding when combining herb with an anticoagulant, such as warfarin or heparin, or an antiplatelet, such as aspirin or another NSAID.
- If patient is taking an anticoagulant, monitor INR, PTT, and PT. Monitor patient for abnormal bleeding.
- Advise patient to discontinue use immediately if he experiences rash or contact dermatitis because these may indicate sensitivity to feverfew.
- Abruptly stopping the herb may cause "post-feverfew syndrome," involving tension headaches, insomnia, joint stiffness and pain, and lethargy.
- If patient is pregnant, planning to become pregnant, or breast-feeding, advise her not to use feverfew.
- Tell patient to remind pharmacist of any herbal or dietary supplement that he's taking when obtaining a new prescription.
- Advise patient to consult his health care provider before using an herbal preparation because a conventional treatment with proven efficacy may be available.

Research summary

Studies comparing feverfew's efficacy in controlling migraines to placebo have generally found a significant clinical benefit from the use of feverfew. Preliminary safety data from clinical trials suggest that the plant is relatively safe, although the incidence of mouth ulcers has been high in some trials. The plant does not appear to be mutagenic, and shouldn't be used by pregnant women.

figwort

Carpenter's square,
heal-all scrofula plant, kernelwort,
rosenoble, Scrophularia nodosa,
throatwort

The useful constituents of figwort are derived from the dried flowers and leaves of *Scrophularia nodosa*. It contains iridoids, flavonoids, tannins, and phenolic acids. Iridoid and phenylethanoid glycosides have also been isolated from the aerial parts of the plant. Two of these glycosides, harpagoside and harpagide, may have heart-strengthening and anti-inflammatory properties. It's available as dried herb and root, liquid extract, and tincture.

Reported uses

Figwort is used externally to treat skin conditions, such as eczema and psoriasis. It may also help heal wounds, ulcers, burns, and hemorrhoids. In homeopathic medicine, figwort is used to treat decreased resistance, tonsillitis, and lymph edema. It's used internally for its mild laxative effect and its mild diuretic and heart-strengthening properties.

Administration

- Liquid extract (1:1 preparation in 25% alcohol USP): 2 to 8 ml by mouth three times a day
- Tea (steep 2 to 8 g of dried leaves and stems in 5 oz of boiling water for 5 to 10 minutes: three times a day
- Tincture (1:10 preparation in 45% alcohol USP): 2 to 4 ml by mouth three times a day.

Hazards

Figwort may contain cardiac glycosides; potential interactions may occur when given with antiarrhythmics or digoxin. Figwort may increase blood glucose level and therefore may decrease the effectiveness of hypoglycemics, such as insulin, metformin, or sulfonylureas. Administration with other cardiac glycoside-containing herbs such as black hellebore, digitalis leaf, lily-of-the-valley, motherwort, oleander leaf, pheasant's eye, pleurisy root, or uzara could lead to increased cardiac effects.

Those with preexisting cardiac abnormalities including arrhythmias and conduction disturbances should avoid use. Pregnant and breast-feeding patients should also avoid use.

Clinical considerations

▪ Figwort may interfere with the intended therapeutic effect of conventional drugs.

▪ Monitor patient for cardiac abnormalities. Inform patient about the potential for cardiac abnormalities. If patient experiences any cardiac disturbances while taking figwort, instruct him to discontinue the herb and to immediately report symptoms to his health care provider.

▪ If patient has diabetes, monitor him for fluctuations in blood glucose level because herb may cause hyperglycemia. Instruct diabetic patient to monitor blood glucose level frequently and to watch for abnormal fluctuations.

▪ If patient is pregnant, planning to become pregnant, or breast-feeding, advise her not to use figwort.

▪ Advise patient to keep the herb away from children and pets.

▪ Tell patient to remind pharmacist of any herbal or dietary supplement that he's taking when obtaining a new prescription.

▪ Advise patient to consult his health care provider before using an herbal preparation because a conventional treatment with proven efficacy may be available.

Research summary

The concepts behind the use of figwort and the claims made regarding its effects haven't yet been validated scientifically.

flavonoids

Anthocyanins, bioflavonoids, chalones, flavones, flavanols, flavonones, isoflavonoids

Plants contain compounds called flavonoids that give them their characteristic colors and hues. The term "flavonoid" is derived from the Latin word "flavus" which means "yellow," for one of the colors seen in some higher orders of plant species.

The presence of flavonoids was first detected in the 1930s by Albert Szent-Gyorgi, a Hungarian-born American biochemist. Szent-Gyorgi won a Nobel prize in medicine for his pioneering work on vitamin C. He originally named flavonoids "vitamin P." One of the first substances that Szent-Gyorgi found containing a flavonoid was in the rinds of citrus fruits, which he named "citrin." He found that combining citrin with vitamin C enhanced its absorption and strengthened vitamin C's antioxidant properties. He also discovered that this compound helped strengthen blood vessels, especially the capillaries, and aided in the prevention of capillary fragility. Although not considered essential in the same manner as vitamins, flavonoids play a major role in health maintenance.

Flavonoids are found in a wide range of foods, including citrus, soy, green tea, tomatoes, apples, and grapes. Over 4,000 flavonoids have been identified to date.

Reported uses

Flavonoids can be considered antioxidants, which are compounds that guard against the destructive forces produced by substances known as free radicals. Free radicals are molecules that lack electrons, which makes them unstable; such molecules try to stabilize themselves by stealing an electron from nearby molecules, thereby rendering stable molecules unstable and causing radical change to the cell. This mutation of the cell has now been linked to such conditions as cancer, arthritis, blood transport disorders, cardiovascular disease, and allergies. The bulk of the research has focused on the properties and efficacy of bilberry, green tea, oligomeric proanthocyanidins (OPCs), quercetin, and soy.

Bilberry

Bilberry (*Vaccinium myrtillus*), also known as European blueberry, contains potent flavonoids known as anthocyanosides. These compounds help to stabilize connective tissue by increasing the integrity of the collagen matrix and the production of collagen, and by preventing the destruction of collagen connective tissue around blood vessels. Collagen is a fibrous structural protein that can be found in all parts of the body. It's also dispersed in the vitreous liquid of the eye to form a gel that helps maintain the proper stiffness and shape of the eye. The antioxidant effects of bilberry can be seen when it's used in the treatment of ophthalmic disorders such as glaucoma and night blindness. In glaucoma, bilberry increases the tensile strength and integrity of the collagen, which may decrease intraocular pressure. Night blindness may also be helped by bilberry's anthocyanosides, which speed up the regeneration of the rods in the retina of the eye. The rods help with night vision and low light adaptation.

Green tea

Green tea contains flavonoids and antioxidants called polyphenols, which may guard against progression of certain cancers. It's suggested that green tea's antimutagenic and anticarcinogenic characteristic may be based on its action of blocking cell membrane receptors and suppressing nitrosamine production.

Green tea may also lower total cholesterol levels and LDL cholesterol oxidation. It may not be appropriate for certain patients because it contains caffeine.

Oligomeric proanthocyanidins

Oligomeric proanthocyanidins (OPCs) are potent antioxidants that can be found in red wines and grapeseed extracts. Originally discovered in the 1950s by the French scientist Jack Masquelier, OPCs may be the basis of the so-called "French Paradox" which refers to the fact that although French cooking contains more saturated fats and cholesterol producing foods, the French are 2.5 times less likely to die of coronary artery disease and its complications. Several studies have shown that red wine contains more of the OPCs than white wine and that the alcohol content is not related to the benefits.

Quercetin

Quercetin has one of the highest antioxidant effects of any flavonoid and is most widely used in the prevention and treatment of allergies and asthma. It acts by strengthening the mast cell wall and thus inhibiting the release of histamine. Quercetin also inhibits the production of cyclooxygenase and leukotrienes. These substances can cause vasoconstriction and bronchoconstriction. Quercetin does not cause the CNS depressant effects that are usually produced by prescription and OTC antihistamines. Some products also contain other flavonoids, such as hesperidin and rutin, along with quercetin; this combination may induce a synergistic affect. The pineapple stem enzyme may also be included. This aids in absorption and produces an anti-inflammatory effect.

Soy

Soy contains two widely studied isoflavonoids, daidzein and genistein. These compounds are also referred to as phytoestrogens. Phytoestrogens are 1/400 the strength of human estrogen and act as agonists and antagonists. If circulating estrogen is high, these compounds bind to receptor cells and reduce the hormone's action. Soy also acts to stimulate the receptor site if estrogen levels are low — as, for example, during menopause — and may, therefore, help control hot flashes. These isoflavonoids may also block the production of hormone-induced cancers such breast cancer, uterine cancer, and prostate cancer. Isoflavonoids may be obtained from eating soy products or by taking supplements. Sources of soy include tofu and soybeans.

Administration

- Bilberry: 80 to 160 mg three times a day
- Green tea: 6 to 10 cups, or 500 mg, a day
- OPCs: based on 2mg/kg of body weight
- Quercetin: 500 mg four times a day
- Soy: 50 to 100 mg of soy supplement a day.

Hazards

- Bilberry: Because the herb may inhibit platelet aggregation, it may be unsuitable for those with a bleeding disorder. In addition, bilberry may have additive effects when used with the drug warfarin.
- Green tea: Adverse effects include nervousness, insomnia, tachycardia, hyperacidity, GI irritation, decreased appetite, constipation, diarrhea, increased blood glucose and cholesterol levels, asthma, and allergic reactions. In addition, the caffeine in green tea may increase the stimulatory effects of ephedrine or any drug that acts as a stimulant. Administration with warfarin may lead to a decreased INR. Simultaneous use of green tea and iron supplementation reduce the absorption of iron. Green tea is contraindicated in breast-feeding patients, infants, and small children. Pregnant women should avoid or minimize use because of the caffeine. Patients with cardiovascular or renal disease, hyperthy-

roidism, spasms, and psychic disorders should use cautiously
- OPCs: No adverse effects are associated with OPCs.
- Quercetin: No adverse effects are associated with the use of quercetin. However, high doses may cause blood vessel dilation and blood thinning.
- Soy: Adverse effects include gastrointestinal effects, such as stomach pain, loose stool, and diarrhea, asthma, and allergic reaction. In addition, soy may cause decreased absorption of calcium, iron, and zinc supplements. It may reduce the effects of estrogen, raloxifene, and tamoxifen. Patients hypersensitive to soy or soy-containing products shouldn't use this product. High doses of soy protein may have harmful effects in women with breast cancer. Infants shouldn't be fed soy-based formulas because of high isoflavone content. Inhalation of soy dust led to an asthma outbreak in 26 workers exposed to soy powder when unloading the product.

Clinical considerations

Since they are water-soluble compounds, flavonoid supplements may be administered with food if a patient is experiencing any type of gastrointestinal problems.

Research summary

The concepts behind the use of flavonoids and the claims made regarding their effects haven't yet been validated scientifically.

flax

Flaxseed, leinsamen, lini semen, Linum usitatissimum, *linseed, lint bells, linum, winterlien*

Flax has been used for more than 10,000 years as a source of fiber for weaving or clothing. Linseed oil, derived from the flaxseed, has been used as a topical demulcent and emollient and as a laxative, particularly for animals. Flax contains mucilages, cyanogenic glycosides, 10% to 25% linoleic acid, oleic acid proteins (albumin), xylose, galactose, rhamnose, and galacturonic acid. Cyanogenic acids, with the activity of a certain enzyme, have the potential to release cyanide. Linolenic, linoleic, and oleic acids are classified as omega fatty acids.

The mucilaginous fiber absorbs and expands. The omega fatty acid component may decrease serum total cholesterol and low-density lipoprotein levels and may decrease platelet aggregation. Flax is available as capsules, flour, fresh flowering plant, oil, and whole seeds, in products such as Dakota Flax Gold, Flax Seed Oil, and Flax Seed Whole. Many cereals and pancake and muffin mixes contain flax.

Reported uses
Flax is used internally to treat diarrhea, constipation, diverticulitis, irritable bowel syndrome, gastritis, enteritis, bladder inflammation, and colons damaged by laxative abuse. In traditional medicine flax is used for removal of foreign bodies in eyes, and in the treatment of coughs and colds, constipation, and urinary tract infections. It's also used as a poultice for skin inflammation.

Administration
■ Gastritis, enteritis: Dosage is 1 tablespoon of the whole or bruised seed, not ground, mixed with 5 oz of liquid and taken two or three times a day. An alternative method involves soaking 5 to 10 g of whole seed in cold water for 30 minutes; the liquid is discarded, the seeds are ground, and 2 to 4 tablespoons are used as linseed gruel
■ Ophthalmic: A single moistened flaxseed is placed under the eyelid until the foreign object sticks to the mucous secretion from the seed
■ Topical: A hot poultice or compress is made from 30 to 50 g of the flour and applied as needed.

Hazards
Use of flax may result in intestinal blockage. Because of its fibrous content and binding potential, drug absorption may be altered or prevented. Advise patient to avoid using flax within 2 hours of a drug.

Those with an ileus, those with esophageal strictures, and those experiencing an acute inflammatory illness of the GI tract should avoid use. Pregnant and breast-feeding patients and those planning to become pregnant should also avoid use.

Clinical considerations
■ When flax is used internally, it should be taken with more than 5 oz of liquid per tablespoon of flaxseed.
■ Instruct patient to drink plenty of water when taking flaxseed.
■ Cyanogenic glycosides may release cyanide; however, the body only metabolizes these to a certain extent. At therapeutic doses, flax doesn't elevate cyanide ion level.
■ Even though flax may decrease a patient's cholesterol level or increase bleeding time, it's not necessary to monitor cholesterol level or platelet aggregation.
■ Warn patient not to treat chronic constipation, other GI disturbances, or ophthalmic injury with flax before seeking appropriate medical evaluation because doing so may delay diagnosis of a potentially serious medical condition.
■ If patient is pregnant, plans to become pregnant, or is breast-feeding, advise her not to use flax.
■ Instruct patient not to take any drug for at least 2 hours after taking flax.
■ Tell patient to remind pharmacist of any herbal or dietary supplement that he's taking when obtaining a new prescription.
■ Advise patient to consult his health care provider before using an herbal preparation because a conventional treatment with proven efficacy may be available.

Research summary
Preliminary evidence suggests that diets supplemented with ground flaxseed can improve the lipid profile of hypercholesterolemic patients, reducing certain atherogenic risk factors.

Flower remedies

Flower essences

Although many cultures have used flower remedies for healing purposes over the centuries, the practice didn't emerge in the West until the early 1920s with the research of Edward Bach, a pathologist, immunologist, and bacteriologist. Prepared from the flowers of wild plants, bushes, and trees, flower remedies are used to help stabilize emotional stresses that reflect the root cause of disease. Bach believed the basis of illness was found in disharmony between the spiritual and emotional aspects of human beings. This disharmony, found whenever conflicting moods produced fear, lassitude, uncertainty, loneliness, over-sensitivity, despair, excessive concern, and insecurity, lowered the body's vitality and resistance to disease. By assisting with the integration of emotional, spiritual, and physiological patterns, the remedies are used to produce a soothing, calming effect, thereby allowing the body to heal itself.

Bach discovered the works of Samuel Hahnemann, the founder of homeopathy, while working at London Homeopathic Hospital. When he considered Hahnemann's theories in light of the tranquility and inner harmony he experienced when outdoors in natural surroundings, he concluded that the solutions to disease-causing states could be found among plants, trees, and herbs. Bach searched the English countryside for curative plants and conducted research into their uses, often testing the remedies on himself prior to offering them to patients.

Bach opposed those aspects of modern medicine that address only the physical elements of illness. He believed that conventional treatments, such as pills, drugs, and surgery, were often counter-productive because, in many instances, the temporary relief they produced suggested a complete return to health while negative mental and emotional patterns continued unchecked. True healing was thereby postponed and the inevitable result was more serious illness at some later date. Bach's remedies were, therefore, intended to treat the mood and temperament of the patient rather than the physical illness.

Flower remedies are made by floating freshly picked blooms in bowls of spring water and leaving them in sunlight. In this way the "essence" of the flower is transferred to the water. More woody plants, or flowers that bloom when the sun is weak, are prepared by boiling for half an hour. The resulting solution is then fixed in proportions with brandy, which acts as a preservative, and stored in a dark glass bottle. Portions of that "mother" solution are then distributed in 1-ounce dropper bottles.

There are 38 flower remedies in all; 12 relate to what Bach saw as the key personality types, and 26 are used to bring relief from different kinds of emotional discomfort and distress. The most famous, Rescue Remedy, often used as first aid, is actually a combination of 5 flower remedies. The Bach Flower Remedies are included in the Supplement to the 8th edition of the Homeopathic Pharmacopoeia of the United States and are officially recognized as homeopathic drugs.

TRAINING *Today there are many varieties of flower remedies, or essences, as they are often called, and the preparation is essentially the same. In the mid-1970s, Richard Katz researched new flower essences and founded the Flower Essence Society. The Society now has a database of over 100 essences from different flowers in over 50 countries, has training programs available, and sponsors* and assists controlled scientific studies on flower essence therapy. It conducts seminars and certification programs for active flower essence practitioners and for the general public. The Practitioner Certification program is available to all participants who complete the Practitioner Intensive. This nine-month program involves classes and complete documentation of three in-depth case studies. In addition, practitioners using Bach's original 38 remedies can be certified by the Bach Foundation in Mt. Vernon, England, or at other sites throughout the world operated by Nelson Bach Ltd. The Practitioner Certification Training is a 6-month program, after which practitioners sign a Code of Practice that includes ethical standards and specifies that practitioners are not licensed to diagnose medical illness or otherwise practice medicine.

Reported uses

Flower remedies are simple to use alone or in combination with any of the other remedies, and are relatively inexpensive. They're available in both liquid concentrate and cream form and are used to treat a wide range of personal difficulties, such as everyday stress-related problems, periods of transition, and job-related tensions. Flower remedies are also used to treat hyperactivity in children, dieting and eating problems, learning difficulties, sleeping problems, mild depression, and the trauma of bereavement, separation, or divorce.

The cream helps to hasten the healing of abrasions and lacerations. Relief is often achieved when massaged into swollen and painful joints. Although not a substitute for emergency medical care, Rescue Remedy has been reported to significantly calm the sufferer who is experiencing fear and panic. Health practitioners such as chiropractors, dentists, psychiatrists, and massage therapists also use flower remedies as an adjunct to conventional therapy.

How the treatment is performed

For occasional negative moods, emotional difficulties, or an immediate stressful situation, drops may be placed under the tongue, or in a small glass of water or juice, four times daily. The client sips the remedy at intervals throughout the day until improvement is shown. In some circumstances, as with Rescue Remedy, it's safe to take every 10 to 15 minutes as needed. The concentrate can also be applied directly to the temples, wrists, or behind the ears, or in compresses or baths. In general, the strength of the remedy is determined by the frequency of the dosing, not by the number of drops taken at one time.

For long-term distress, the practitioner may determine the correct remedy by interviewing the client, or by having the client complete a questionnaire that will guide the practitioner's choice. Remedies are prepared by adding 2 to 4 drops of each flower essence chosen, with a teaspoon of brandy, apple cider vinegar, or vitamin C powder as a preservative, into an opaque 1-ounce bottle, which is then filled with spring or filtered water (distilled or carbonated water shouldn't be used). Four to six drops are taken under the tongue or in water four times a day.

The personal formula is continued until emotional difficulties are resolved, or there is a lifting of the negative emotional state, or a stabilizing of the over-reactive personality traits. Once symptoms have resolved, the remedies may be discontinued. New formulas can be made as needed. Because the remedies have a unique and personal effect on each person, the specific effects and duration of treatment can't be predicted. In general, most people experience improvement within 1 to 12 weeks; however, some take longer. Some change may be noticed within 1 to 3 weeks.

Hazards

Flower remedies are suitable for people of all ages. There are no known contraindications. Though rare, some may experience a minor reaction such as a rash, mild diarrhea, or an accentuation of the emotion for which they are taking the remedy. Since the remedies are nontoxic, these reactions may be part of the process of confronting feelings or a result of the process of detoxification. In some cases, adverse reactions may result from the patient's unconscious resistance to change.

Clinical considerations
■ Some patients may experiences a "peeling effect" — that is, as the initial emotional difficulty resolves, underlying emotions may surface and the need for additional remedies may arise.
■ Advise patient to discontinue use if an adverse reaction, such as rash or diarrhea, occurs, and to consult his health care practitioner.
■ Though the alcohol preservative volume is minuscule, if alcohol-sensitive the person may need to dilute the concentrate before taking.

Research summary
While numerous published anecdotal reports support the positive effects of flower remedies — including many from physicians and psychiatrists — the concepts behind their use haven't yet been validated scientifically. The Flower Essence Society, in an attempt to compile a foundation of research into the efficacy of flower remedies, compiles case studies and practitioner reports of the clinical use of essences. The studies include in-depth longitudinal cases backed by detailed practitioner documentation. In addition, the Flower Essence Society sponsors and assists controlled scientific studies on flower essence therapy.

 RESEARCH *Jeffrey Cram, a research and clinical psychologist with the Sierra Health Institute in Nevada City, California, has completed two double-blind, placebo-controlled studies of the effects of flower essences on stress. In the first he found muscular activity (EMG) at spinal locations corresponding to the heart and throat chakras had signifi-*

cantly reduced levels of reactivity after the use of the flower essences. In another study, those taking a flower essence formula showed far less reactivity to lights, as measured by the beta wave brain activity at nine sites clustered around the frontal lobes, and by muscle activity in the heart chakra area.

fumitory

Beggary, common fumitory, earth smoke, Fumaria officinalis, *wax dolls*

Fumitory has been known since antiquity and was described in herbals from the Middle Ages. The dried or fresh flowering plant — the above-ground part — is used medicinally. Active components include hydroxycinnamic acid derivatives, flavonoids such as rutin and fumaric acid, and isoquinoline alkaloids such as scoulerine, protopine, fumaricine, fumariline, and fumaritine.

Isoquinolone alkaloids may contribute to the herb's antispasmodic effects on the gallbladder, bile ducts, and GI tract. Cinnamic acid has a choleretic effect. Fumaric acid works as an antioxidant, a flavoring agent, and a chelating agent. Flavonoids and their derivatives may improve capillary function by decreasing abnormal leakage. Available as leaves, liquid extract, powder, and tincture.

Reported uses
In traditional medicine, fumitory is used to treat eczema and other dermatologic conditions. It's also used as a laxative and a diuretic, and to relieve liver, gallbladder, and GI complaints. Fumitory is used to treat cystitis, atherosclerosis, rheumatism, arthritis, hypoglycemia, and infections, and as a blood purifier.

Fumitory is also used topically to treat skin diseases such as chronic eczema and psoriasis.

Administration

- For gallbladder complaints: Infusion is prepared by pouring boiling water over 2 to 3 g of fumitory, and then straining after 20 minutes. Dosage is 1 cup warmed and taken before meals
- Internal use: Dosage is 6 g by mouth or 1 cup of tea several times a day
- Liquid extract (1:1 preparation in 25% alcohol USP): Dosage is 2 to 4 ml by mouth three times a day
- Tincture (1:5 preparation in 45% alcohol USP): Dosage is 1 to 4 ml by mouth three times a day.

Hazards

Fumitory may increase intraocular pressure and reverse the effects of anti-glaucoma drugs. Increased hypotension may be seen with antihypertensives. Tinctures and extracts contain significant levels of alcohol, increasing the risk for a disulfiram-like reaction. Fumaric acid is classified as a chelating agent; it may bind to other drugs and alter absorption. Increased CNS effects may be noted with alcohol use.

Patients with glaucoma or pregnant and breast-feeding women should avoid use. Because fumaric acid may cause renal failure, those with renal dysfunction should also avoid use.

 SAFETY RISK *Side effects associated with fumitory include hypotension, increased intraocular pressure, and acute renal failure.*

Clinical considerations

- Monitor patients for renal dysfunction — serum creatinine and BUN levels — because fumaric acid may cause renal failure.
- Because tinctures and extracts contain significant levels of alcohol, they may be unsuitable for children, alcoholics, those with a previous history of alcohol abuse, those with preexisting liver disease, and those taking disulfiram or metronidazole.
- If patient is pregnant or breast-feeding or is planning to become pregnant, advise her not to use fumitory.

- Inform patient of the potential for hypotension when using fumitory with an antihypertensive, and instruct him to report feelings of weakness, dizziness, or light-headedness to his health care provider.
- Remind patient not to take fumitory with any drug; instruct him to separate administration times by 2 hours.
- Caution patient not to use fumitory with alcohol.
- Instruct patient to report feelings of increased eye pressure or pain and to stop taking the herb immediately if he experiences such symptoms.
- Tell patient to remind pharmacist of any herbal or dietary supplement that he's taking when obtaining a new prescription.
- Advise patient to consult his health care provider before using an herbal preparation because a treatment with proven efficacy may be available.

Research summary

Fumitory has been investigated for its therapeutic potential in the management of cardiovascular and hepatobiliary disorders. Preliminary animal and human data suggest that the plant has pharmacologic activity, which requires further elucidation. Fumitory has not been associated with significant toxicity.

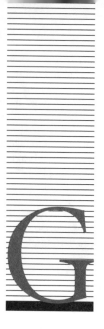

galangal

Alpinia officinarium, *catarrh root, China root, Chinese galangal, Chinese ginger, colic root, East India catarrh root, East India root, galanga, Gao Liang Jiang, gargaut, greater galangal, India root*

Alpinia officinarium rhizome contains a volatile oil, resin, flavonoids, galangol, kaempferide, galangin, and alpinin. The volatile oil may play a role in the herb's active medicinal properties such as calming the stomach. Galangal is available as dried powder, fluid extract, oil, rhizome, and tea.

Reported uses
Galangal is used to relieve flatulence, dyspepsia, nausea, vomiting, loss of appetite, and motion sickness. It's also used to treat fevers, colds, cough, sore throat, bronchitis, infection, rheumatism, and liver and gallbladder complaints. Used to inhibit prostaglandin synthesis. Used as an antibacterial and antispasmodic. Also used as a spice because of its pungent and spicy flavor and as a perfume. Used in homeopathic medicine as a stimulant.

Administration
■ Infusion (pour 150 ml boiling water over 0.5 to 1 g [1 teaspoon = 2 g] of herb, and then strain after 10 minutes): 1 cup 30 minutes before meals
■ Tincture: 2 to 4 ml by mouth every day (2 to 4 g)

- Rhizome: 2 to 4 g by mouth every day.

Hazards
High doses of essential oil may cause hallucinations. Acid-inhibiting drugs, such as antacids, sucralfate, H2 antagonists, and proton pump inhibitors, may interact with this herb due to alpinia's increase of stomach acid.

Pregnant and breast-feeding patients should avoid use.

Clinical considerations
- Galangal isn't widely used in the United States and may be difficult to obtain. Warn patient to use caution when obtaining products from unknown origins.
- This herb may interfere with the intended therapeutic effect of conventional drugs.
- Advise patient that dosing may be difficult if he's using galangal powder that's made for cooking. Tell him to consult a health care provider with a background in natural medicine before use.
- Warn patient that the essential oil may cause hallucinations.
- Tell patient to remind pharmacist of any herbal or dietary supplement that he's taking when obtaining a new prescription.
- Advise patient to consult his health care provider before using an herbal preparation because a conventional treatment with proven efficacy may be available.

Research summary
Decoctions of this herb are reported in the literature to show inhibitory effects in vitro against many pathogenic bacteria, including the anthrax bacillus, hemolytic *Streptococcus*, and various strains of *Staphylococcus*.

Dilute decoctions of this herb are also reported in the literature to have a stimulatory effect on guinea pig intestinal specimens of smooth muscle, while higher concentrations showed an inhibitory effect.

galanthamine

Galantamine,
galanthamine hydrobromide,
Galanthus nivalis, G. woronowii

Galanthamine is an alkaloid and a selective, long-acting acetylcholinesterase inhibitor derived from the plant *Galanthus nivalis* or *G. woronowii*. It antagonizes the muscle relaxation caused by nondepolarizing, curare-like muscle relaxants. Galanthamine may also modulate nicotinic cholinergic receptors and help improve daily functioning in patients with Alzheimer's disease. It's available in oral and I.V. solutions and tablets, in products such as Jilkon, Lycoremin, and Nivalin.

Reported uses
Galanthamine is used to treat symptoms of Alzheimer's disease, neuromuscular disorders, and mania. It's also used postoperatively to reverse the effects of neuromuscular blockers.

Administration
- Alzheimer's disease: Dosage is 20 to 50 mg by mouth every day, administered in 2 to 3 divided doses; the lowest possible dose should be used.
- Reversal of neuromuscular blockers: Dosage is 0.3 mg/kg I.V.

Hazards
Galanthamine may cause agitation, sleep disturbances, insomnia, light-headedness, bradycardia, nausea, vomiting, diarrhea, and anorexia. When used with other cholinergics (parasympathomimetics), there is the potential to increase adverse effects including bradycardia, hypotension, and respiratory distress.

Those with a known allergy or hypersensitivity to galanthamine should avoid use. Pregnant and breast-feeding patients, and those with gastrointestinal ulcer, Parkinson's disease, severe heart disease, bradycardia, bronchial asthma, epilepsy, hyperkinesia, ileus, or ureter occlusion should also avoid use.

Clinical considerations

- Galanthamine is considered an investigational drug in the treatment of Alzheimer's disease. More studies are being conducted to assess its efficacy. It may not be available for public use.
- Response to drug for Alzheimer's disease and mania may take 6 to 8 weeks.
- If patient is also taking an antiparkinsonian, monitor closely for symptom improvement or progression and adverse effects.
- Monitor patient for agitation, weight loss, and bradycardia.
- If patient is pregnant or breast-feeding, advise her not to use galanthamine.
- Tell patient to take with meals, if possible.
- Tell patient to remind pharmacist of any herbal or dietary supplement that he's taking when obtaining a new prescription.
- Advise patient to consult his health care provider before using an herbal preparation because a conventional treatment with proven efficacy may be available.

Research summary

The concepts behind the use of galanthamine and the claims made regarding its effects haven't yet been validated scientifically.

garlic

Allium sativum, *camphor of the poor, clove garlic, nectar of the gods, poor man's treacle, rustic treacle, stinking rose*

Garlic was valued as an exchange medium in ancient Egypt and its virtues were described in inscriptions on pyramids. The folk uses of garlic have ranged from the treatment of leprosy in humans to managing clotting disorders in horses.

Healers prescribed the herb during the Middle Ages to cure deafness, and the Native Americans used garlic as a remedy for earaches, flatulence, and scurvy.

Medicinal ingredients of garlic are obtained from the bulb of the *A. sativum* plant. The aroma, flavor, and medicinal properties of garlic are primarily the result of sulfur compounds including alliin, ajoen, and allicin. Also found in garlic are vitamins, minerals, and the trace elements germanium and selenium.

Garlic may act as an HMG-reductase inhibitor, thus moderately decreasing cholesterol and triglyceride levels. It can increase fibrinolytic activity and inhibit platelet aggregation, which is probably the work of allicin and ajoene. (Garlic oil used alone does not have this effect.) Garlic lowers blood pressure and may lower blood glucose level by increasing the body's circulating insulin and by increasing glycogen storage in the liver. It works as an antibacterial against both gram-positive and gram-negative organisms, including *Helicobacter pylori* (the causative organism in many peptic ulcers and in certain gastric cancers). It may also have antifungal, antiviral, and antitumorigenic effects. Garlic prevents endothelial cell depletion of glutathione, which is thought to be responsible for its antioxidant effects.

Garlic is available as aqueous extract (1:1), capsules, fresh cloves, garlic oil, powdered cloves, softgel capsules, solid garlic extract, tablets, cream (ajoene 0.4%), and gel (ajoene 0.6%). Common trade names include Garlicin, Garlic Powermax, Garlinase 4,000, GarliPure, Garlique, Garlitrin 4,000, Kwai, Kyolic Liquid, and Wellness Garlicell.

Reported uses

Garlic is used most commonly to decrease total cholesterol and triglyceride levels, and to increase HDL cholesterol level. It's also used to help prevent atherosclerosis because of its effect on blood pressure and platelet aggregation. Garlic is used to decrease the risk of cancer, especially cancer of the GI tract. In traditional medicine it's used to treat cough, colds, fevers, and sore throats. Garlic is also used orally and topically to fight infection through its antibacterial and antifungal effects.

Administration
Garlic is taken as 900 mg of dried powder, 2 to 5 mg of allicin, or 2 to 5 g of fresh clove. The average dose is 4 g of fresh garlic or 8 mg of garlic oil every day.

Hazards
Adverse reactions associated with garlic include headache, insomnia, fatigue, vertigo, tachycardia, orthostasis, halitosis, heartburn, flatulence, GI distress, nausea, vomiting, bloating, diarrhea, asthma, shortness of breath, contact dermatitis, burns, facial flushing, and body odor.

When taken with anticoagulants, NSAIDs, antiplatelet agents, or other herbs that exert anticoagulation effects such as feverfew and ginkgo, garlic may increase bleeding time, PT, and INR. Blood glucose level may be decreased with hypoglycemics and herbs that exert hypoglycemic effects, like glucomannan. Acetaminophen and other drugs metabolized by the cytochrome P450 enzymes 2E1, 2B1, and 2D6 may be altered by garlic. Garlic can lower serum cholesterol concentrations and test results.

Patients allergic to garlic should avoid use. Pregnant and breast-feeding patients should avoid use if consuming it in amounts greater than used in cooking. Should be used with caution in young children and in those with severe hepatic or renal disease.

 SAFETY RISK *Garlic has been associated with hypersensitivity reactions.*

Clinical considerations
- Therapeutic doses of garlic aren't recommended for patients with diabetes, insomnia, pemphigus, organ transplants, or rheumatoid arthritis, or for post-surgical patients.
- Monitor patient for signs and symptoms of bleeding.
- Garlic may lower blood glucose level. If patient is taking an antihyperglycemic, watch for signs and symptoms of hypoglycemia and monitor his serum glucose level.
- Advise patient not to delay seeking appropriate medical evaluation because doing so may delay diagnosis of a potentially serious medical condition.
- Advise patient to consume garlic in moderation, to minimize the risk of adverse reactions.
- Discourage heavy use of garlic before surgery.
- Advise patient that using garlic with anticoagulants or antiplatelet agents like NSAIDs may increase the risk of bleeding.
- Caution patient using garlic as a topical antiseptic to avoid prolonged exposure to the skin because burns can occur.
- Tell patient to remind pharmacist of any herbal or dietary supplement that he's taking when obtaining a new prescription.
- Advise patient to consult his health care provider before using an herbal preparation because a treatment with proven efficacy may be available.

 SAFETY RISK *Garlic oil shouldn't be used to treat inner ear infections in children.*

Research summary
Garlic and its extracts have a long history of folk use and recent research has indicated that the herb has significant pharmacologic activity when administered even in small doses. These include effects on blood sugar, cholesterol and lipid levels, and a distinct antithrombotic effect.

 RESEARCH *In one study, 432 individuals who had suffered a heart attack were given either garlic oil extract or no treatment over a period of 3 years. (Bordia, 1989) The results showed a significant reduction of second heart at-*

tacks and about a 50% reduction in death rate among those taking garlic.

Gem therapy

Crystal therapy

Since ancient times, people have believed that crystals have supernatural powers. Throughout history people have worn crystals in amulets, as love tokens, and for simple decoration in jewelry. Wearing crystals often brought a sense of peace to the wearer, and over time healers began to use crystals to affect healing of a variety of illnesses.

Renewed awareness of the various uses for crystals began in late 1970s, with the increasing use of crystals as tools to help people focus energy. Human problems are seen as a result of blockages, congestion, and depletion of energy. The universe is a field of energy with different levels that flow into one another. Crystals are used to detect and clear blockages in the body's energy flow, bringing it back into alignment and harmony with the universal energy flow.

Crystals increase the effects of other healing modalities; for example, acupuncture is 10% to 12% more successful when the needles are coated with quartz crystal. Crystals can enhance muscle testing and protect wearers from some radiation. It has been shown that simply wearing or putting a crystal in the home or workspace has positive effects. People occasionally experience feelings of discomfort when wearing a particular piece of jewelry without knowing why; it's believed that the feeling is caused by the energy level of the crystals in the jewelry.

In general, the colors of crystals correspond to the seven main colors of the visible spectrum and each, in turn, resonates with one of the seven primary chakras. (See *Gemstones and the seven primary chakras.*)

Reported uses

Crystalline structures can collect, focus, and emit electromagnetic energy; they transmit and receive radio waves, power quartz watches, set timers on computers, and release the sound recorded on records. Crystals are believed to affect the body by influencing the etheric layer, located 2 to 4 inches from the body and is just outside our visual range. Crystals are used as guides to help focus energies and get us in touch with the universal forces around us. Crystals are not forces themselves, but merely reflect energy, amplify it, and tune it for our use. Crystals are used as guides into the world of spiritual awareness.

Roeder (1994) lists 66 categories of disorders, with 2 to 16 combinations of three crystals to be used as treatment choices for each disorder. For example, allergies may be treated with blue lace agate, picture jasper, and rhodonite; blocks and resistances may respond to amethyst, aqua aura, and rainbow fluorite or sugilite, diamond, and bustamite; hyperthyroidism may be treated with rhyolite, emerald, and any brown stone. Crystals may also be used to obtain positive results; for example, a person seeking business success may use amber, azeztulite, turquoise, picture jasper, or topaz.

How the treatment is performed

Various crystals are used for different purposes. Amethysts are related to transformation and travel and may therefore be kept in the car to enhance safety. They're also used to treat addictions and other excesses; for example, it's believed that placing a small piece of amethyst under the tongue for 10 minutes will help in stopping smoking. Amethysts shouldn't be used by those with hyperactivity, schizophrenia, or mental retardation. Citrine is used for those most resistant to treatment; herkimer is useful to affect dreams; smoky quartz is a grounding tool that helps the wearer regain contact with reality; aquamarine is used for reconciliation, phobias, paralyzing fears,

GEMSTONES AND THE SEVEN PRIMARY CHAKRAS

Chakra	Color	Crystals
Root chakra	Red	Ruby and garnet
Sacral	Orange	Carnelian and orange jasper
Solar plexus	Yellow	Amber, citrine, yellow topaz
Heart	Green	Emerald and malachite
Throat	Blue	Sapphire and lapis lazuli
Brow	Violet	Amethyst and violet fluorite
Crown	Magenta	Rose quartz

and human relations in general; and red coral is used to promote the growth of bone cells. Crystals are typically programmed prior to use; that is, the crystal to be used is charged and empowered with the intended use. Fundamental laws for programming a crystal include:

- Compassion — the desire to relieve the client's suffering
- Non-attachment — objectivity regarding results, awareness of the client's responsibility to heal himself
- Intention — the end result or outcome.

With these feelings in mind, the practitioner holds the crystal cupped in his hands and gently breathes on it, thereby charging it with the intended purpose. A charged crystal may be used for up to 28 days.

Crystals are used in a variety of ways. Practitioners of Reiki, a Japanese method that uses the laying-on of hands to facilitate healing, may select nine different crystals of different colors and lay them on the seven main chakras, one between the feet, and one held in the practitioner's hand. People react very strongly to colors, both visually and through the chakras. Each chakra is stimulated and supported by the color energy of the crystals. Red garnet may be used to activate joy, orange amber to facilitate suc-

cess in life, and dark blue lapis lazuli to strengthen faith and peace. Alternatively, the practitioner may select seven crystals of the same type to stimulate the same aspect of all the chakras. Crystals may be placed directly on the chakra for 20 to 45 minutes.

A technique used by Ayurvedic and gemstone therapists in India for many years calls for gemstone powders to be ingested after being burned to ash. Crystals may also be ingested in the form of gem elixirs, which are prepared in a manner similar to flower essences — the gem is placed in a clear bowl of water, which sits in bright morning sunlight for several hours. It's believed that the magnetic influence of solar power energetically imprints some of the subtle energy pattern of the gem into the water. The resulting elixir is then placed, several drops at a time, under the tongue. Two unique gem elixirs are prepared from the magnetic materials of lodestone and magnetite. Lodestone is said to align our physical body's biomagnetic field with the earth's magnetic field. It is also a general tonic for the endocrine system and may also be valuable in stimulating tissue regeneration, balancing the acupuncture meridians and the opposing forces of yin and yang, and helping with detoxification from radiation exposures. The elixir of magnetite is said to enhance blood circulation, as well as energize and align the chakras, meridians, and subtle or spiritual bodies.

To protect the crystal, it should be wrapped in leather or 100% cotton, silk, wool, or linen fabric, which is always red in color. (It's believed that red has the slowest rate of absorption of luminous vibrations.) If the crystal is worn, it should be placed between the heart and solar plexus chakras, with the point down; if double pointed, both points should be left unwrapped.

Hazards
There are no adverse effects associated with the use of crystals.

Clinical considerations
Having a cleaned crystal in the office may enhance a healing environment. Using crystals for healing requires reading and training with a knowledgeable practitioner.

Research summary
The concepts behind the use of gem therapy and the claims made regarding its effects haven't yet been validated scientifically.

gentian

Bitter root, bittersweet, bitter wort, Gall weed, Gentiana, Gentiana lutea, *yellow gentian*

The gentians have been used for centuries as bitters to stimulate the appetite, improve digestion, and treat a variety of gastrointestinal complaints. The medicinal components are derived from the roots and rhizome of *G. lutea* species and include the following: amarogentin, gentiopicrin, gentiopicroside, swertiamarin, the alkaloids gentianine and gentialutine, xanthones, carbohydrates, pectin, tannins, triterpenes, and volatile oils.

Both gentian and stemless gentian are approved for food use. Stemless gentian usually is consumed as a tea, or in alcoholic extracts such as Angostura Bitters. Gentian extracts are used in a variety of foods, cosmetics, and some antismoking products. The plant has been used externally to treat wounds and internally to treat sore throat, arthritic inflammations, and jaundice. Gentian may stimulate gastric secretions. Because it's usually administered with alcohol, it's difficult to determine whether the gentian or the alcohol is having the gastric effects. It's available as bitter tonic, dried powder, dried root, extract, tincture, and tea.

Reported uses
Gentian is used to stimulate appetite and to aid in digestion by stimulating gastric juices. It's also used to treat flatulence and feelings of fullness. Gentian may have some anti-inflammatory effects.

Administration
■ Dried rhizome or root: 2 to 4 g by mouth every day
■ Liquid extract (1:1 g/ml): 2 to 4 g by mouth every day (1 to 2 ml, two to three times daily, 1 hour before meals)
■ Tea: Steep 1 to 2 g (½ teaspoon) of the herb in boiling water for 5 to 10 minutes
■ Tincture: (1:5 in 45% alcohol) 1 to 4 ml by mouth three times a day; average dose is 1 to 3 g every day.

Hazards
Adverse reactions associated with gentian include headache, GI upset, nausea, and vomiting. There may be an increased sedative effect when administered with barbiturates or benzodiazepines because of the alcohol content in the liquid preparations. The potential for disulfiram-like reactions exists with cephalosporins, disulfiram, and metronidazole because of the alcohol content in the liquid preparations. Theoretical interaction with acid-inhibiting drugs (antacids, sucralfate, H-2 antagonists, proton pump

inhibitors) is due to gentian's increase of stomach acid.

Patients with stomach or duodenal ulcers or excessive acid production (Zollinger-Ellison Syndrome) shouldn't use. Pregnant and breast-feeding patients should also avoid use. Patients with hypertension should use with caution.

Clinical considerations

- Tell patient to discontinue use if stomach upset occurs.
- Advise patient that the tincture form contains alcohol.
- Advise patient to keep product out of direct light.
- Tell patient to remind pharmacist of any herbal or dietary supplement that he's taking when obtaining a new prescription.
- Advise patient to consult his health care provider before using an herbal preparation because a conventional treatment with proven efficacy may be available.

SAFETY RISK *Don't confuse gentian with gentian violet, also known as crystal violet; they have different uses.*

Research summary

Gentian is a widely recognized plant that has been used as a bitter tonic for centuries. It is believed that a small amount of the extract (usually mixed with alcohol) can stimulate appetite and improve digestion. Aside from this, none of the other effects is well documented in humans. Therefore, the concepts behind the use of gentian and the claims made regarding its effects haven't yet been validated scientifically.

Gerson diet

The Gerson diet is one of a number of "metabolic" therapies that use a combination of diet, nutritional supplements, detoxification, and enzyme therapy to rebuild the immune system and fight dis-

ease. It's essentially a lacto-vegetarian regimen consisting of large quantities of fruits and vegetables in the form of freshly squeezed juice. In addition to the dietary guidelines, sodium intake is restricted, potassium and other assorted supplements are taken, and coffee enemas or colonic irrigation are used for detoxification.

Gerson began experimenting with diet in an attempt to relieve his own migraine headaches; after succeeding, he tried dietary changes to treat various diseases in his patients (including Albert Schweitzer). Gerson gained renown in Germany for successfully treating tuberculosis of the skin (lupus vulgaris) with a low-salt diet. He continued experimenting with different diet combinations for various diseases (including asthma, arthritis, and cancer); by the time he emigrated to the United States in 1936, he was concentrating on cancer.

Gerson came to believe that cancer was a degenerative disease stemming from impaired metabolism and that proper liver function was crucial to proper metabolic functioning. He also placed great importance on maintaining a proper balance of sodium and potassium, believing that an imbalance (excessive sodium levels) helped create an internal environment conducive to tumor growth. Gerson believed that his stringent treatment program reversed the conditions that were necessary to sustain such growth.

Reported uses

The Gerson Institute oversees a clinic in Tijuana, Mexico, that offers the Gerson treatment to about 600 patients a year. After an initial treatment period at the clinic, patients continue the regimen at home for 1 to 2 years or until their immune systems are considered sufficiently restored. The Institute claims success in treating certain types of cancer, heart disease, arthritis, and chronic fatigue syndrome.

How the treatment is performed
Gerson's program includes the following measures, among others:

■ A low-salt, low-fat, high-potassium diet consisting of three vegetarian meals daily prepared from organic foods
■ 8 oz (237 ml) of freshly prepared fruit or vegetable juice, prepared in a special press to reduce enzyme breakdown and enhanced with potassium, every hour for 13 hours each day (for the first 4 weeks) to bombard the body with nutrients and correct the sodium-potassium imbalance
■ Supplements of pepsin, potassium iodine (Lugol's solution), niacin, pancreatin (a digestive enzyme from bovine pancreas), and thyroid hormone
■ Coffee enemas daily to promote the release of toxins from the liver
■ Avoidance of all processed, canned, bottled, and frozen foods as well as foods cooked in aluminum pots
■ Limited dairy products and permanent avoidance of salt, berries, pineapple, pickles, nuts, mushrooms, soybeans, oil, coffee, chocolate, and refined sugar and flour.

Hazards
Excessive intake of potassium can result in renal failure, arrhythmias, and sudden death. Vitamin toxicity may also occur. Coffee enemas disrupt the GI system's natural balance of flora and can cause dehydration, fatigue, and malaise. Regular use of coffee enemas can result in nutritional deficiencies and have been linked to dangerous electrolyte imbalances.

Clinical considerations
■ Advise patient to have regular blood tests to check for potassium imbalance and vitamin toxicity.
■ Teach patient the signs and symptoms of dehydration, such as decreased urinary output, dark urine, and increased thirst and skin turgor.

 TRAINING *The training program is only open to licensed medical professionals. It consists of four*

phases, including a two-week internship, for accreditation by the Gerson Institute.

Research summary
In 1959, the NCI reviewed the 50 case histories presented in Gerson's book, *A Cancer Therapy: Results of 50 Cases,* and concluded that Gerson's data failed to meet the basic criteria for evaluating clinical benefit. A more recent study by Austrian researchers, which involved use of a modified Gerson plan as an adjunctive treatment for cancer, reported subjective benefits, including pain relief and less severe adverse effects from chemotherapy.

Although the fundamental aspects of Gerson's diet — increased intake of fruits and vegetables, decreased intake of sodium and fat — are consistent with accepted theories about reducing cancer risk, the medical establishment on the whole doesn't accept Gerson's theory that diet and detoxification can cause tumor regression.

ginger

Black ginger, gingembre, zingiber, Zingiber officinale, Zingiberis rhizoma

Medicinal use of ginger dates back to ancient China and India. Once its culinary properties were discovered in the 13th century, use of this herb became widespread throughout Europe. In the Middle Ages, it held a firm place in apothecaries for travel sickness, nausea, hangovers, and flatulence. Its pungent properties also contribute to its pharmacologic activities. Ginger contains cardiotonic compounds known as gingerols, volatile oils, and other compounds such as (6)-, (8)-, and (10)-shogaols, (6)- and (10)-dehydrogingerdione, (6)- and (10)-gingerdione, zingerone, and zingibain.

The root has antiemetic effects that result from its carminative and absorbent properties and its ability to enhance GI motility. Large doses exert positive inotropic effects on the cardiovascular system. Anti-inflammatory effects may result from ginger's ability to inhibit prostaglandin, thromboxane, and leukotriene biosynthesis; antimigraine effects, from ginger's ability to inhibit prostaglandins and thromboxane. Antithrombotic effects may result from ginger's ability to inhibit platelet aggregation. The volatile oil may have antimicrobial effects.

Ginger is available as candied ginger root, fresh root, oil, powdered spice, syrup, tablet, tea, and tincture. Common trade names include Alcohol-Free Ginger Root, Caffeine Free Ginger Root, Ginger Aid Tea, Ginger Kid, GingerMax, Ginger Powder, Ginger Root, Quanterra Stomach Comfort, Travellers, Travel Sickness, and Zintona Rhizome.

Reported uses
Ginger is used most commonly as an antiemetic to treat motion sickness, morning sickness, and generalized postsurgical nausea. It's also used to treat colic, flatulence, dyspepsia, and indigestion. Ginger is used as an anti-inflammatory for those with arthritis and as an antispasmodic, and for its antitumorigenic activity in patients with cancer. It's used to treat upper respiratory tract infections, cough, and bronchitis. Topically, fresh juice of ginger is used for treating thermal burns.

Administration
■ As an antiemetic: 2 g of fresh powder by mouth taken with some liquid; total daily recommended dose is 2 to 4 g of dried rhizome powder
■ For arthritis: 1 to 2 g every day
■ For chemotherapy-associated nausea (in the absence of narcotic anesthesia or analgesia): 1 g before chemotherapy
■ For migraine headache or arthritis: Up to 2 g every day
■ For motion sickness: 1 g by mouth 30 minutes before travel, then 0.5 to 1 g every 4 hours; dosage may begin 1 to 2 days before trip

■ Infusion: To prepare, steep 0.5 to 1 g of herb in 150 ml of boiling water, and then strain after 5 to 10 minutes (1 teaspoon = 3 g of drug).

Hazards
Adverse reactions associated with ginger include central nervous system (CNS) depression and increased bleeding time with large doses. It may cause heartburn. Ginger may interfere with hypoglycemic drugs due to its hypoglycemic effects. Use with anticoagulants and other drugs or herbs that can increase bleeding time may further increase bleeding time.

Patients with gallstones or with an allergy to ginger should avoid use. Pregnant women and those with bleeding disorders should avoid using large amounts of ginger. Patients taking a CNS depressant or an antiarrhythmic should use with caution. Patients with diabetes or blood pressure problems should also use with caution.

 SAFETY RISK *The use of ginger in large doses has been associated with cardiac arrhythmias.*

Clinical considerations
■ Adverse reactions are uncommon.
■ Monitor patient for signs and symptoms of bleeding. If patient is taking an anticoagulant, monitor PTT, PT, and INR carefully.
■ Use in pregnant patients is questionable, although small amounts used in cooking are safe. It's unknown if ginger is excreted in breast milk. If patient is pregnant, advise her to consult a knowledgeable practitioner before using ginger medicinally.
■ Ginger may interfere with the intended therapeutic effect of conventional drugs.
■ If overdose occurs, monitor patient for arrhythmias and CNS depression.
■ Educate patient to look for signs and symptoms of bleeding, such as nosebleeds or excessive bruising.
■ Advise patient to keep ginger away from children and pets.

- Tell patient to notify pharmacist of any herbal or dietary supplement that he's taking when obtaining a new prescription.
- Advise patient to consult his health care provider before using an herbal preparation because a conventional treatment with proven efficacy may be available.

Research summary

Clinical trials have examined ginger's antiemetic effects related to kinetosis (motion sickness), perioperative anesthesia, and hyperemesis gravidarum; however, little is known regarding its pharmacology in these settings. Other trials have shown no significant differences among ginger, antiemetics, and placebo with regard to gastric as well as nongastric symptoms. Two separate investigations showed no effect of ginger on CNS impairment caused by kinetosis, as subjects retained the ability to perform certain head and eye movements.

Another placebo-controlled study compared ginger with scopolamine in several subjects. Ginger partially inhibited and stabilized tachygastria but did not effect EGG amplitude. The authors concluded symptoms of motion sickness can be dissociated from gastric electrical activity and that the partial tachygastric effects of ginger offer little to relieve the onset of severity of these symptoms.

In another study, ginger was compared with metoclopromide and droperidol in the prevention of post-operative nausea and vomiting. Findings supported previous studies: ginger and metoclopromide were equally effective and were more effective than placebo in reducing its incidence. The need for post-operative antiemetics was significantly reduced in those receiving ginger over the placebo group.

In studies comparing droperidol and ginger, incidence of post-operative nausea and vomiting was not statistically significant. However, the figures did appear to have potential clinical importance.

Other subjective studies have been done regarding ginger use for hyperemesis gravidarum, with greater symptomatic relief being observed compared to placebo.

Another case report of SSRI administration described the successful use of ginger to alleviate nausea and disequilibrium associated with abrupt discontinuation or intermittent noncompliance of the drugs.

There are currently no reports of severe toxicity in humans from the ingestion of ginger root. However, there is no convincing evidence regarding the safety of ingesting large amounts of ginger by pregnant women. The FDA considers ginger a food supplement, generally recognized as safe.

ginkgo

Ginkgo biloba, kew tree, maiden-hair tree, yinhsing

Medicinal parts of ginkgo include dried or fresh leaves and the seeds separated from the fleshy outer layer. The flavonoids and terpenoids of ginkgo extracts are considered antioxidants that serve as free-radical scavengers. Other suggested mechanisms of action include arterial vasodilation, increased tissue perfusion, increased cerebral blood flow, decreased arterial spasm, decreased blood viscosity, and decreased platelet aggregation. In Germany, standardized ginkgo extracts are required to contain 22% to 27% ginkgo flavonoids and 5% to 7% terpenoids.

Ginkgo may be effective in the management of cerebral insufficiency, dementia, and circulatory disorders. It's available as tablets, capsules, and liquid preparations. Common trade names include Bioginkgo, Gincosan, Ginkgo Go!, Ginkgo Liquid Extract Herb, Ginkgo Nut, Ginkgo Power, Ginkgo Capsules, Ginkyo, and Quanterra Mental Sharpness.

Reported uses

Gingko is primarily used to manage cerebral insufficiency, dementia, and circulatory disorders such as intermittent claudication. It's also used to treat headaches, asthma, colitis, impotence, depression, altitude sickness, tinnitus, cochlear deafness, vertigo, premenstrual syndrome, macular degeneration, diabetic retinopathy, and allergies.

Gingko is used as an adjunctive treatment for pancreatic cancer and schizophrenia. It's also used in addition to physical therapy for Fontaine stage IIb peripheral arterial disease to decrease pain during ambulation.

Administration

■ Tablets and capsules: 40 to 80 mg by mouth three times a day
■ Tincture (1:5 tincture of the crude ginkgo leaf): 0.5 ml by mouth three times a day.

Hazards

Adverse effects of gingko include headache, dizziness, subarachnoid hemorrhage, palpitations, nausea, vomiting, flatulence, diarrhea, and allergic reaction. Administration with anticoagulants, antiplatelets, high-dose vitamin E, and garlic and other herbs that increase bleeding time may increase the risk of bleeding. Ginkgo may potentiate the activity of monoamine oxidase inhibitors. Ginkgo extracts may reverse the sexual dysfunction associated with selective serotonin reuptake inhibitors.

Pregnant or breast-feeding women should avoid use of gingko. Patients with a history of an allergic reaction to ginkgo or any of its components should avoid use, as should patients with risk factors associated with intracranial hemorrhage (hypertension, diabetes). Patients receiving an antiplatelet or an anticoagulant should avoid use because of the increased risk of bleeding. Gingko should be avoided in the perioperative period and before childbirth.

 SAFETY RISK *Gingko has been known to cause GI problems, dizziness, and serious bleeding.*

Clinical considerations

■ Ginkgo extracts are considered standardized if they contain 24% ginkgo flavonoid glycosides and 6% terpene lactones.
■ Treatment should continue for at least 6 to 8 weeks, but therapy beyond 3 months isn't recommended.
■ Monitor patient for possible adverse reactions, such as GI problems, headaches, dizziness, allergic reactions, and serious bleeding.
■ Toxicity may cause atonia and adynamia.
■ Advise patient who plans to take gingko for motion sickness to begin taking it 1 to 2 days before beginning the trip and to continue taking it for the duration of his trip.
■ Inform patient that the therapeutic and toxic components of ginkgo can vary significantly from product to product. Advise him to obtain ginkgo from a reliable source.
■ Advise patient to keep herb out of reach of children.
■ Advise patient to discontinue use at least 2 weeks before surgery.
■ Tell patient to notify pharmacist of any herbal or dietary supplement that he's taking when obtaining a new prescription.
■ Advise patient to consult his a health care provider before using an herbal preparation because a conventional treatment with proven efficacy may be available.

SAFETY RISK *Seizures have been reported in children after ingestion of more than 50 ginkgo seeds.*

Research summary

Both oral and intravenous forms of gingko are available in Europe, where it is one of the most widely prescribed medications. Neither form has been approved for medical use in the United States, although ginkgo is sold as a nutritional supplement.

An extract of the leaves has been shown to have pharmacologic activity in the patients with cerebral insufficiency, dementias, circulatory disorders, and bronchoconstriction. The plant is also known for its antioxidant and neuroprotective effects. Ginkgo extract has not been linked with severe adverse effects, but contact with the fleshy fruit pulp can cause allergic dermatitis, similar to the effect of poison ivy. Limited human data is available on teratogenicity.

ginseng, Asian

American ginseng, Asian Ginseng, Chinese ginseng, dwarf ginseng, five-fingers, Himalayan ginseng, Korean ginseng, Manchurian ginseng, Oriental ginseng, Panax ginseng, P. quinquefolius

Asian ginseng is perhaps the most widely recognized of the plants used in traditional medicine and plays a major role in the herbal health market. It has been used for more than two thousand years. At least six species and varieties of *Panax* have been used in traditional medicine. It is a popular ingredient in herbal teas and cosmetics. It is promoted for its antistress effects.

Ginseng's dried root is medicinal. It contains triterpenoid saponins called ginsenosides that appear to be the active ingredients responsible for the plant's immunomodulatory effects. Ginsenosides seem to increase natural-killer cell activity, stimulate interferon production, accelerate nuclear RNA synthesis, and increase motor activity.

The ginsenosides have been found to protect against stress ulcers, to decrease blood glucose level, to increase high-density lipoprotein level, and to affect central nervous system activity by acting as a de-

pressant, anticonvulsant, analgesic, and antipsychotic.

Ginseng is available as powdered root, tablets, capsules, and tea. Common trade names include Centrum Ginseng, Chikusetsu Ginseng, Gin-Action, Ginsai, Ginsana, Ginseng Manchurian, Ginseng Power Max 004X G-Sana, Ginseng Up, Gin Zip, Herbal Sure Chinese Red Ginseng, Herbal Sure Korean Ginseng, Korean White Ginseng, Lynae Ginse-Cool, Power Herb Korean Ginseng, Premium Blend Korean Ginseng Extract, Sanchi Ginseng, The Ginseng Solution, Time Release Korean Ginseng Power, and Zhuzishen.

Reported uses

Asian ginseng is used to manage fatigue and lack of concentration, and to treat atherosclerosis, bleeding disorders, colitis, diabetes, depression, and cancer. It's also used to help recover health and strength after sickness or weakness.

Administration

■ Powdered root: For a healthy patient, 0.5 to 1.0 g of the root may be taken by mouth, every day, in 2 divided doses for 15 to 20 days. The morning dose is usually taken 1 to 2 hours before breakfast; the evening dose, 2 hours after dinner. If a second course of therapy is desired, patient must wait at least 2 weeks before starting ginseng again. For an elderly or sick patient, 0.4 to 0.8 g of the root by mouth every day taken continuously
■ Solid extracts in tablets and capsules: Dosage is 100 to 300 mg by mouth three times a day
■ Tea: Dosage is 1 cup every day, up to three times a day, for 3 to 4 weeks. The tea is prepared by steeping 3 g (1 teaspoon) of the herb in a cup of boiling water for 5 to 10 minutes.

Hazards

Adverse reactions to Asian ginseng include headache, insomnia, dizziness, restlessness, nervousness, hypertension, hypotension, diarrhea, and vomiting. In women, Asian ginseng may exert estrogenic-like effects, such as vaginal bleeding and mastalgia.

Asian ginseng may decrease the effects of anticoagulants and antiplatelet drugs. Increased hypoglycemic effects may be seen with antidiabetics and insulin. Ginseng may inhibit the CYP 3A4 system, thereby effecting the metabolism of drugs utilizing this system. Headache, irritability, and visual hallucinations may be noted when given with phenelzine or other MAO inhibitors.

Patients with a history of an allergic reaction to the product or any of its components should avoid use, as should patients taking an MAO inhibitor. Although no cases of serious reactions in diabetic patients have been reported, those who must control their blood glucose levels should take ginseng with caution. Patients receiving an anticoagulant or an antiplatelet drug should use with caution.

SAFETY RISK *Reports have circulated of a severe reaction known as ginseng abuse syndrome in patients taking large doses — more than 3 g per day for up to 2 years. Patients experiencing this syndrome report a feeling of increased motor and cognitive activity combined with significant diarrhea, nervousness, insomnia, hypertension, edema, and skin eruptions.*

Clinical considerations

- The German Commission E does not recommend using ginseng for more than 3 months.
- Inform patient that the therapeutic and toxic components of ginseng can vary significantly from product to product. Advise him to obtain ginseng from a reliable source.
- Tell patient to remind pharmacist of any herbal or dietary supplement that he's taking when obtaining a new prescription.
- Advise patient to consult his health care provider before using an herbal preparation because a conventional treatment with proven efficacy may be available.

Research summary

A number of small trials have been reported in eastern Europe and Asia. These studies seem to indicate that ginseng can reduce plasma glucose levels and increase the levels of HDL cholesterol. However, these studies have not been well documented. The establishment of proper dosages and duration of use remains poorly defined. Ginseng is not usually associated with serious adverse reactions, although the potential ginseng abuse syndrome has been reported.

ginseng, Siberian

Acanthopanax senticosus,
Eleutherococcus senticosus

The medicinal portion of Siberian ginseng is derived from the dried root of *Acanthopanax senticosus* and *Eleutherococcus senticosus*. Eleutheroside appears to be the active ingredient responsible for the plant's immunomodulatory effects. It may also affect the pituitary-adrenocortical system and increase T-lymphocyte counts in healthy people. Eleutheroside is believed to strengthen the body and increase resistance to disease.

Siberian ginseng is available as tablets, capsules, liquid (ethanol extract), and tea. Common trade names include Devil's Shrub, Eleuthero Ginseng, Eleuthero Ginseng Root, Pepperbush, Shigoka, Siberian Ginseng Power Herb, Siberian Ginseng Root, Spiny Ginseng, and Wild Pepper.

Reported uses

Siberian ginseng is used to manage fatigue and lack of concentration. It's also used to treat hypotension, diabetes, cancer, and infertility.

Administration
- Capsules: Dosage is 1 g of powdered root in capsule by mouth every day
- Dry root: Dosage is 2 to 3 g by mouth every day for up to 1 month
- Ethanol extract: For a healthy patient, dosage is 2 to 16 ml by mouth every day, up to three times a day, for up to 2 months. For a sick patient, dosage is 0.5 to 6 ml by mouth every day, up to three times a day, for 35 days. A second course of therapy should never be started less than 2 to 3 weeks after the first course ended
- Root decoction: Dosage is 35 ml by mouth twice a day.

Hazards
Adverse effects of Siberian ginseng include drowsiness, anxiety, insomnia, tachycardia, hypertension, pericardial pain, and muscle spasm. When given with anticoagulants or antiplatelet drugs, a decreased effectiveness of these drugs may be noted. Decreased metabolism of barbiturates leads to additive adverse effects. Elevated serum digoxin levels may be seen when given with digoxin.

Patients with a history of allergic reactions to Siberian ginseng or its components should avoid use, as should patients with hypertension. Patients receiving anticoagulant or antiplatelet medications should use with caution.

Clinical considerations
- The German Commission E doesn't recommend using Siberian ginseng for more than 3 months.
- Monitor patient for adverse effects such as tachycardia, hypertension, pericardial pain, drowsiness, anxiety, muscle spasm, and insomnia.
- Siberian ginseng may increase serum alkaline phosphatase, gamma glutamyl transferase, BUN, and serum creatinine levels. It may also decrease serum glucose and serum triglyceride levels. Monitor these laboratory results, as needed.
- Advise patient to consult his a health care provider before using an herbal

preparation because a conventional treatment with proven efficacy may be available.
- Tell patient to notify pharmacist of any herbal or dietary supplement that he's taking when obtaining a new prescription.
- Inform patient that the therapeutic and toxic components of Siberian ginseng can vary significantly from product to product. Advise him to obtain ginseng from a reliable source.

SAFETY RISK *Adulterating ginseng with other herbs, especially substances containing caffeine, is dangerous. Ginseng products, if contaminated with germanium, may cause nephrotoxicity.*

Research summary
The concepts behind the use of Siberian ginseng and the claims made regarding its effects haven't yet been validated scientifically.

glucomannan

Amorphophallus konjac, *koch, konjac, konjac mannan*

Glucomannan is a polysaccharide derived from the underground stems of *Amorphophallus konjac*. Because it absorbs water, glucomannan may increase the viscosity of the intestinal contents, decrease gastric emptying time, act as a barrier to diffusion, delay the absorption of glucose from the intestines, and decrease the need for antidiabetics in diabetic patients. It may also inhibit the active transport of cholesterol in the jejunum and to prevent the absorption of bile acids in the ileum. Glucomannan is available as tablets, capsules, liquid, powder, and hydrophilic gum.

Reported uses
Glucomannan is used to manage constipation, diabetes, obesity, hypercholes-

terolemia, and hyperlipidemia. It's also used to induce weight loss.

Administration
- For diabetes: 3.6 to 7.2 g by mouth every day
- For hyperlipidemia: 3.9 g by mouth every day
- For weight loss: 1 g by mouth three times a day, 2 hours before each meal.

Hazards
Adverse reactions associated with glucomannan include esophageal obstruction, flatulence, diarrhea, and hypoglycemia. Glucomannan may cause significant hypoglycemia when given with oral antidiabetics or insulin. The fiber content of glucomannan may interfere with the absorption of various drugs.

Patients with a history of an allergic reaction to glucomannan or any of its components should avoid use. Patients with GI dysfunction, patients prone to hypoglycemia, and patients with underlying diabetes should use with caution.

Clinical considerations
- Consuming glucomannan may result in a feeling of fullness, thereby decreasing the appetite.
- Monitor patient for adverse effects such as esophageal obstruction, lower GI obstruction, flatulence, diarrhea, and hypoglycemia.
- Monitor patient's weight and serum cholesterol and serum glucose levels.
- Advise patient to avoid using tablet form because it poses an increased risk of esophageal obstruction.
- Inform patient that the therapeutic and toxic components of glucomannan can vary significantly from product to product. Advise him to obtain glucomannan from a reliable source.
- Advise patient to separate administration times by at least 2 hours because glucomannan may interfere with the absorption of medications.
- Tell patient to notify pharmacist of any herbal or dietary supplement that he's

taking when obtaining a new prescription.
- Advise patient to consult his health care provider before using an herbal preparation because a conventional treatment with proven efficacy may be available.

Research summary
Konjac mannan (glucomannan) has been shown to possess many of the pharmacologic characteristics of other polysaccharides. In large doses it has laxative activity and may alter the metabolism of microflora in the intestine. Konjac mannan may be effective in reducing serum cholesterol levels. There is conflicting evidence regarding its use as a weight-reduction aid though it does appear to alter lipid metabolism.

glucosamine sulfate
Chitosamine

Glucosamine, an endogenous amino-monosaccharide, is a simple molecule found in mucopolysaccharides, mucoproteins, and chitin. It stimulates the synthesis of glycosaminoglycans and proteoglycans, both of which are considered building blocks of the cartilage, and has weak anti-inflammatory effects. Glucosamine may inhibit degenerative enzymes responsible for destruction of the cartilage and appears to be effective in reducing pain and improving range of motion in patients with osteoarthritis. It may also slow the process of joint damage. Glucosamine is available as 500-mg tablets.

Reported uses
Glucosamine is used to treat osteoarthritis.

Administration
The average dose is 500 mg by mouth, three times a day. The duration of therapy may be from 2 weeks to 3 months. For

obese patients, dose is 20 mg/kg of body weight.

Hazards

Adverse reactions associated with glucosamine include drowsiness, headache, insomnia, peripheral edema, nausea, vomiting, abdominal pain, diarrhea, tachycardia, bronchopulmonary complications, and skin rash. It may cause increased resistance to hypoglycemics and insulin. Diuretics decrease the effectiveness of glucosamine.

Patients with a history of allergic reaction to glucosamine or any of its components should avoid use. Patients with diabetes mellitus should use with caution.

Clinical considerations

- Glucosamine may increase the adverse effects of diabetes mellitus.
- Monitor patient for possible adverse effects such as peripheral edema, tachycardia, drowsiness, headache, insomnia, nausea, vomiting, abdominal pain, diarrhea, and skin rash.
- Inform patient that the therapeutic and toxic components of glucosamine sulfate can vary significantly from product to product. Advise him to obtain glucosamine sulfate from a reliable source.
- Advise patient that, although limited drug interactions have been reported with use of this product, more potential interactions may exist.
- Inform patient that it may take a minimum of 4 to 6 weeks for benefits to be seen.
- Advise patient to keep the glucosamine sulfate away from children and pets.
- Tell patient to notify pharmacist of any herbal or dietary supplement that he's taking when obtaining a new prescription.
- Advise patient to consult his health care provider before using an herbal preparation because a conventional treatment with proven efficacy may be available.

Research summary

Randomized, placebo-controlled, double-blind studies found that glucosamine is well-tolerated and effective in the treatment of osteoarthritis of the knee. In some studies, pain was reduced, joint flexion abilities were increased, and articular function was restored in patients taking glucosamine, compared with those taking placebo. Investigators concluded that glucosamine rebuilds damaged cartilage, thus restoring articular function in most patients.

At least 15 other studies have shown it to be a safe and effective treatment of various forms of osteoarthritis. Further studies are warranted on various dosage regimens and potential long-term effects.

goat's rue

French honeysuckle, French lilac, Galega officinalis, *Italian fitch*

Goat's rue is derived from the dried, above-ground parts of *Galega officinalis.* It contains lectins, flavonoids, and the alkaloids galegine and paragalegine. May have diuretic and hypoglycemic activity and may also promote weight loss. The effect on blood glucose levels has been attributed to the galegine alkaloid constituent. Goat's rue is available as dried leaves.

Reported uses

Goat's rue is used as a diuretic and lactogenic in breast-feeding patients. It's also used to reduce hyperglycemia and treat plague, fever, and snakebites.

Administration

A tea is prepared by steeping 1 teaspoon of dried leaves in 1 cup of boiling water for 10 to 15 minutes, and then taken by mouth twice a day.

Hazards

Goat's rue has been associated with headache, weakness, and nervousness. It

may interfere with effects of hypoglycemic medications.

Children, pregnant patients, and
breast-feeding patients should avoid use.

 SAFETY RISK *Fatal poisoning has
occurred in animals grazing on
goat's rue. Signs and symptoms of
toxicity include salivation, labored breathing, spasms, and paralysis as well as asphyxiation leading to death.*

Clinical considerations

■ Goat's rue may affect the intended
therapeutic effect of conventional medications.

■ Advise patient that goat's rue isn't recommended for the management of diabetes.

■ If patient is pregnant or breast-
feeding, advise her not to use this herb.

■ Advise patient to keep goat's rue away
from children or pets.

■ Tell patient to notify pharmacist of any
herbal or dietary supplement that he's
taking when obtaining a new prescription.

■ Advise patient to consult his health
care provider before using an herbal
preparation because a treatment with
proven efficacy may be available.

Research summary

Clinical trial data on goat's rue platelet
aggregation inhibiting, lactogogic, or diuretic effects is not yet available.

goldenrod

*Aaron's rod, blue mountain tea,
European goldenrod,*
Solidago canadensis,
S. serotina, S. virgaurea, *sweet
goldenrod, woundwort*

The useful constituents of goldenrod
consist of the above-ground parts of *Solidago virgaurea*, gathered during the
flowering season. The active medicinal
ingredients identified include flavonoids,
saponins, tannins, diterpenes, and
carotenoids. The herb also contains phenol glycosides and caffeic acid derivatives.

Flavonoids and saponins exert a diuretic action on the kidneys. Astringent
properties are derived from tannins. The
herb also has anti-inflammatory activity.
Available as ethanolic and aqueous extracts, dried herbs, and various topical
forms.

Reported uses

Goldenrod is used to treat and prevent
the formation of kidney stones and to
treat inflammatory diseases of the urinary tract. It's also used topically to treat
wound infection or eczema.

German Commission E has approved
goldenrod for use as a diuretic, an anti-
inflammatory, and a mild antispasmodic.

Administration

■ Daily dose: The German Commission
E recommends a daily dose of 6 to 12 g

■ Infusion: Dosage is two to four times a
day, between meals. The infusion is prepared by steeping 1 to 2 tablespoon (3 to
5 g) of dried herb in 5 to 9 oz (150 to
270 ml) of boiling water, and then straining after 15 minutes

■ Liquid extract (1:1 in 25% ethanol):
Dosage is 0.5 to 2 ml by mouth, two to
three times a day

■ Tincture (1:5 in 45% ethanol): Dosage
is 0.5 to 1 ml by mouth two to three
times a day

■ Topical formulations: Apply topical
formulations to affected area as needed.

Hazards

Adverse reactions associated with goldenrod include vomiting after ingestion of
the dried plant, asthma, hay fever,
tachypnea, and contact dermatitis. There
is a risk of disulfiram-like reaction
caused by large amounts of alcohol in
liquid preparations when given with
disulfiram, metronidazole, or cephalosporins. Other central nervous system
(CNS) depressants, including barbitu-

rates and benzodiazepines, could lead to increased CNS depression when given concomitantly.

Pregnant women should avoid use because of risk of miscarriage. Patients with severe coronary heart disease or with severely impaired renal function should avoid using this herb.

 SAFETY RISK *Poisoning resulting from parasites, fungus, and rust in the dried plant may lead to weight loss, leg and abdominal edema, enlarged spleen, and GI hemorrhage.*

Clinical considerations

■ Advise patient with hypertension or kidney stones not to use goldenrod to treat these conditions.

■ Liquid extracts and tinctures may contain up to 45% alcohol and may be unsuitable for children, alcoholics, and patients with liver disease.

■ If patient is taking other drugs that interact with alcohol, tell him to avoid use of the extract and tincture.

■ If patient is pregnant or is planning pregnancy, advise her not to use goldenrod.

■ Caution patient with allergy to any herb in the daisy family not to use this herb.

■ Encourage patient to take in at least 2 qt (2 L) of fluids per day.

■ Tell patient to store the herb away from light and moisture.

■ Tell patient to notify pharmacist of any herbal or dietary supplement that he's taking when obtaining a new prescription.

■ Advise patient to consult his health care provider before using an herbal preparation because a conventional treatment with proven efficacy may be available.

Research summary

Preliminary findings indicate goldenrod may have antifungal and antisperm activities. German health authorities adopted its use as a diuretic agent based on the observations reported by European physicians. However, there are no clinical trials to date confirming its diuretic efficacy. Goldenrod's anti-inflammatory activity has been reported.

golden seal

Eye balm, eye root, ground raspberry, Hydrastis canadensis, *Indian dye, Indian plant, Indian turmeric, jaundice root, orange root, turmeric root, yellow Indian paint, yellow puccoon, yellow root*

Native Americans used golden seal as an eye wash and to relieve stomach problems. Today, it's used to treat menstrual disorders, minor sciatica pain, rheumatic or muscle pain, and as an antispasmodic. It's said to enhance the potency of other herbs as well. The useful portions are derived from the rhizome and roots of *Hydrastis canadensis.* Its principal chemical constituents are the alkaloids hydrastine and berberine; it also contains other alkaloids, volatile oils, chlorogenic acid, phytosterols, and resins.

Golden seal may have anti-inflammatory, antihemorrhagic, immunomodulatory, and muscle relaxant properties. It exhibits inconsistent uterine hemostatic properties. Hydrastine causes peripheral vasoconstriction. Berberine can decrease the anticoagulant effect of heparin. It stimulates bile secretion and exhibits some antineoplastic and antibacterial activity. Berberine can stimulate cardiac function in lower doses or inhibit it at higher doses.

Golden seal is available as capsules, dried ground root and rhizome powder, tablets, tea, tincture, and water ethanol extracts. Common trade names include Golden Seal Power, Nu Veg Golden Seal Herb, and Nu Veg Golden Seal Root.

Reported uses

Golden seal is used to treat postpartum hemorrhage and to improve bile secretion. It's also used as a digestive aid and expectorant. Golden seal is used topically on wounds and herpes labialis lesions.

Administration

- Alcohol and water extract: 250 mg by mouth three times a day
- Dried rhizome: 0.5 to 1 g in 1 cup of water three times a day
- Expectorant: 250 to 500 mg by mouth three times a day
- For symptomatic relief of mouth sores and sore throat: 2 to 4 ml of tincture (1:10 in 60% ethanol), swished or gargled three times a day
- Topical use (cream, ointment, or powder): Applied to wound once a day.

Hazards

Adverse effects associated with golden seal include sedation, reduced mental alertness, hallucinations, delirium, paresthesia, paralysis, hypotension or hypertension, mouth ulderation, nausea, vomiting, diarrhea, GI cramping, contact dermatitis, and megaloblastic anemia from decreased vitamin B absorption.

Golden seal may reduce anticoagulant effect of anticoagulant medications. Increased hypoglycemic effects may be seen with hypoglycemics and insulin. It may reduce or enhance hypotensive effect of antihypertensives. Golden seal may interfere or enhance cardiac effects when given with beta blockers, calcium channel blockers or digoxin. It may enhance sedative effects of central nervous system (CNS) depressants such as benzodiazepines. Disulfiram-like reaction may result when liquid preparations are combined with disulfiram, metronidazole, or cephalosporins.

Patients with hypertension, heart failure, or arrhythmias should avoid use. Pregnant and breast-feeding patients and those with severe renal or hepatic disease should also avoid use. Berberine increases bilirubin levels in infants and shouldn't be given to them.

SAFETY RISK *Life-threatening adverse effects of golden seal include aystole, heart block, leukope-* nia, and respiratory depression. High doses may lead to vomiting, bradycardia, hypertension, respiratory depression, exaggerated reflexes, seizures, and death.

Clinical considerations

- German Commission E has not endorsed the use of golden seal for any condition because of the potential toxicity and lack of well-documented efficacy.
- Monitor patient for signs and symptoms of vitamin B deficiency such as megaloblastic anemia, paresthesia, seizures, cheilosis, glossitis, and seborrheic dermatitis.
- Monitor patient for adverse cardiovascular, respiratory, and neurologic effects. If patient has a toxic reaction, induce vomiting and perform gastric lavage. After lavage, instill activated charcoal and treat symptomatically.
- Advise patient not to use golden seal because of its toxicity and lack of documented efficacy, especially if the patient has cardiovascular disease.
- Warn patient to avoid driving until he knows how golden seal will affect CNS.
- Tell patient to notify pharmacist of any herbal or dietary supplement that he's taking when obtaining a new prescription.
- Advise patient to consult his health care provider before using an herbal preparation because a conventional treatment with proven efficacy may be available.

Research summary

The topical use of golden seal extracts in sterile eye washes persists although there is little clinical evidence for its effectiveness. The plant possesses astringent and weak antiseptic properties that may be effective in treating minor oral problems. While small amounts of the plant can be ingested with no adverse effects as a component of bitter tonics, large doses can be toxic. The effects of the plant and its extracts in pregnant women are inconclusive.

Golden seal is less effective than ergot alkaloids in treating postpartum hemorrhage. Berberine can decrease the duration of diarrhea caused by pathogens such as *Vibrio cholerae*, *Shigella*, *Salmonella*, *Giardia*, and some Enterobacteriaceae.

gossypol

American upland cotton, common cotton, cotton root, upland cotton, wild cotton

First identified as an antifertility agent in China in the 1950s, gossypol is also a component of cottonseed oil, which is used for cooking. It's derived from the stems, roots, and seeds of plants from the Malvaceae family. The cotton plant (*Gossypium* species) is the most common source. Gossypol is the active ingredient found in seeds and other parts of the plant; however, content varies significantly from species to species.

Gossypol exerts antifertility action by inhibiting sperm production and motility. It possesses antitumorigenic activity and may also have anti-human immunodeficiency virus properties. It's available as liquid extracts and tinctures.

Reported uses
Gossypol is used in China as a male contraceptive. It's also used topically as a spermicide.

Administration
Dosage is 20 mg by mouth every day for 2 to 3 months until the sperm count is decreased to less than 4 million/ml. The dosage is reduced to a maintenance ranging from 50 mg weekly to 75 to 100 mg twice a month.

Hazards
Adverse effects associated with gossypol include paralysis, circulatory problems, diarrhea, malnutrition, hypokalemia, muscle fatigue, muscle weakness, and hair discoloration.

Pregnant and breast-feeding patients shouldn't use this herb. Patients with renal insufficiency should use with caution.

SAFETY RISK *Gossypol has been associated with heart failure and nephrotoxicity. There's increased risk of nephrotoxicity when gossypol is given with nephrotoxic drugs. Administration with potassium-wasting diuretics could lead to hypokalemia.*

Clinical considerations
■ The contraceptive effect of gossypol in men is higher than 99%. Fertility usually returns to normal within 3 months of discontinuation; however, inhibition of spermatogenesis may persist in up to 20% of men 2 years after discontinuation.

■ Monitor serum electrolyte levels, especially potassium, creatinine, and BUN levels.

■ Monitor patient for muscle weakness and fatigue.

■ If using formulation containing alcohol, avoid using in patients taking disulfiram, metronidazole, cephalosporins, or any CNS depressants.

■ If patient is pregnant or breast-feeding, advise her not to use gossypol.

■ Inform men of the potential for permanent sterility after using oral gossypol.

■ Advise women who are considering the use of gossypol as a topical spermicide about the lack of adequate information on safety and efficacy. Inform them that there are alternative, safe, and effective contraceptive methods.

■ Advise patient to keep herb out of the reach of children and pets.

■ Tell patient to notify pharmacist of any herbal or dietary supplement that he's taking when obtaining a new prescription.

■ Advise patient to consult his health care provider before using an herbal preparation because a conventional treatment with proven efficacy may be available.

Research summary
Gossypol has been approved to be used as a male contraceptive drug in China due to its ability to inhibit sperm production and motility.

gotu kola

Centella asiatica, *hydrocotyle, Indian pennywort, Indian water navelwort, marsh penny, talepetrako, TECA, thick-leaved pennywort, sheep rot, water pennywort, white rot*

Gotu kola has been widely used to treat a variety of illnesses, especially in traditional Eastern medicine. It's derived from the leaves, stem, and aerial parts of *Centella asiatica*. Gotu kola contains madecassol, madecassic acid, asiatic acid, asiaticentoic acid, centellic acid, centoic acid, isothankuniside, flavonoids including quercetin and kaempferol, and various glycosides such as asiaticoside, brahminoside, brahmoside, centelloside, and madecassoid. It also contains fatty acids, amino acids, phytosterols, and tannin.

Asiaticoside promotes wound healing, brahminoside and brahmoside possess sedative properties, and madecassoid exerts anti-inflammatory action. Gotu kola is available as ampules, capsules, ointment, powder, tablets, tinctures, and extract. Common trade names include Centalase, Centasium, Emdecassol, Gotu Kola Gold Extract, Gotu Kola Herb, and Madecassol.

Reported uses
Gotu kola is used for its anticarcinogenic, antifertility, and antihypertensive effects. It's also used to treat chronic venous insufficiency, chronic hypertension, and chronic hepatic disorders. Gotu kola is used topically to treat psoriasis and burns and to promote wound healing in patients with chronic lesions such as cutaneous ulcers, leprosy sores, fistulas, and surgical and gynecologic wounds.

Administration
- Capsules: 400 to 500 mg by mouth every day
- Creams, ointments: Applied to affected area every day, up to two times a day
- Dried leaves: 0.6 g of dried leaves or infusion by mouth three times a day
- Standardized extract (40% asiaticoside, 29% to 30% asiatic acid and madecassic acid, respectively, and 1% to 2% madecassoside): 20 to 40 mg by mouth three times a day.

Hazards
Adverse effects associated with gotu kola include sedation with higher doses, hypercholesterolemia, hyperglycemia, contact dermatitis, burning, and pruritus. The plant extracts appear to have very little toxicity, although hypersensitivity reactions may still occur. Large doses of gotu kola may interfere with the effect of hypoglycemics. Large doses of gotu kola may interfere with the effect of cholesterol-lowering drugs.

Pregnant patients, breast-feeding patients, young children, and patients with severe renal or hepatic disease should avoid use. Patients with a history of contact dermatitis should use with caution.

SAFETY RISK *Do not confuse gotu kola with kola or kola plant. They are different plants. The latter species has stimulant activities.*

Clinical considerations
- Topical asiaticoside may cause cancer.
- Monitor patient for CNS depression, including drowsiness and increased sleep time.
- Monitor blood glucose and serum cholesterol levels with long-term use.
- Warn patient about potential for sedation. Advise him to avoid driving until he knows how the herb affects him.
- If patient is using the herb for contraception, recommend another method.
- Recommend that patient not use the herb for more than 6 weeks at a time.
- Tell patient to take capsules with meals.

- Advise patient to report planned or suspected pregnancy.
- Tell patient to notify pharmacist of any herbal or dietary supplement that he's taking when obtaining a new prescription.
- Advise patient to consult his health care provider before using an herbal preparation because a conventional treatment with proven efficacy may be available.

Research summary
Studies support claims for gotu kola's efficacy in wound healing, topical uses for psoriasis, antihypertensive effects, effects on varicose veins, and chronic hepatic disorders.

grape seed

Muskat, Vitis vinifera

Obtained by grinding the seeds of red grapes, grape seed extract contains procyanidins, also called proanthocyanidins, or flavonoids, which are free-radical scavengers. Procyanidins inhibit proteolytic enzymes, including collagenase, elastase, beta-glucuronidase, and hyaluronidase, thereby helping to stabilize collagen. Grape seed oil contains essential fatty acids and vitamin E. It has antioxidant properties that are said to be greater than those of vitamin C or vitamin E.

Grape seed extract also has anticarcinogenic effects. It prevents oxidative damage to cholesterol and may lower the serum cholesterol level. It protects collagen lining the walls of the arteries and stabilizes the vasculature. It also protects the eyes against oxidative damage and prevents diabetic retinopathy and macular degeneration. Grape seed may also prevent dental caries by inhibition of *Streptococcus mutans* and glucan formation from sucrose. Grape seed is available as tablets, capsules, grape concentrate liquid, and antistax (capsules, drops, cream).

Common trade names include Mega Juice, NutraPack, and Activin.

Reported uses
Grape seed is used for its antioxidant properties to prevent cardiovascular disease and cancer. It's also used to treat venous insufficiency, bruising, edema, and allergic rhinitis. Grape seed is also used as a chemoprotective agent for cancer treatment.

Administration
- Capsules or tablets: Initial dosage is 75 to 300 mg by mouth every day for 3 weeks, then 40 to 80 mg every day
- Liquid concentrate: Dosage is 1 tablespoon (15 ml) mixed in 1 cup of water by mouth.

Hazards
The use of grape seed could lead to hepatotoxicity. Patients with liver dysfunction should use with caution.

Clinical considerations
- If patient has liver dysfunction, monitor liver enzyme tests.
- Grape seed may interfere with the intended therapeutic effect of conventional drugs.
- Grape seed extract may have antiplatelet effects. If a patient is having elective surgery, it may be prudent to stop the supplement 2 to 3 days before surgery. Monitor PT and INR.
- Warn patients not to treat symptoms of vascular insufficiency or circulatory disorders before seeking appropriate medical evaluation because doing so may delay diagnosis of a potentially serious medical condition.
- Advise patient to keep herb away from children and pets.
- Tell patient to notify pharmacist of any herbal or dietary supplement that he's taking when obtaining a new prescription.
- Advise patient to consult his health care provider before using an herbal

preparation because a conventional treatment with proven efficacy may be available.

Research summary

Grape seed extract has been shown to significantly attenuate acetaminophen-induced liver toxicity. In a clinical trial of 4,729 patients with peripheral vascular disease, the group treated with grape seed extract (150 mg given twice a day for 90 days) demonstrated significant improvement of function and relief of symptoms. Grape seed extract has been observed in humans to protect the retina from pathologic changes due to aging, fatigue, and stress. It's also reported to decrease post-surgery facial edema.

green tea

Camellia sinensis, *Chinese tea,*
Matsu-cha

Green tea is prepared from the steamed and dried leaves of *Camellia sinensis.* (By comparison, black tea leaves are withered, rolled, fermented, and then dried.) Green tea contains the polyphenols epigallocatechin and epigallocatechin-3-gallate, some of the most potent anticarcinogenic substances found in nature.

Green tea's antioxidant activity and its ability to inhibit cell proliferation and induce apoptosis are what give it its anticarcinogenic effects. The caffeine can have stimulatory effects on central nervous system (CNS). The tannins have astringent properties, which provide an antidiarrheal effect. Green tea may also decrease serum cholesterol levels and have antibacterial properties. It's less popular in America and Europe than black tea.

Green tea is available as capsules, dried extract, liquid, tablets, and teas. Common trade names include Chinese Green Tea Bags, Green Tea Extract, Green Tea Power, Green Tea Power Caffeine Free, and Standardized Green Tea Extract.

Reported uses

Green tea is used to prevent cancer, hyperlipidemia, atherosclerosis, dental caries, and headaches, and to treat wounds, skin disorders, stomach disorders, and infectious diarrhea. It's also used as a CNS stimulant, a mild diuretic, an antibacterial and, topically, as an astringent.

Administration

A typical daily dose is 300 to 400 mg of polyphenols (3 cups of green tea contain 240 to 320 mg of polyphenols).

Hazards

Adverse effects associated with green tea include nervousness, insomnia, tachycardia, hyperacidity, GI irritation, decreased appetite, constipation, diarrhea, increased blood glucose and cholesterol levels, asthma, and allergic reactions. Increased stimulatory effects may be seen when administered with ephedrine or any drug that acts as a stimulant because of the caffeine component. Administration with warfarin may lead to a decreased INR. Simultaneous use of green tea and iron supplementation reduce the absorption of iron.

Patients allergic to green tea and breast-feeding patients should avoid use. Green tea shouldn't be used in infants or small children. Pregnant women should avoid or minimize use because of the caffeine. Patients with cardiovascular or renal disease, hyperthyroidism, spasms, and psychic disorders should use with caution.

Clinical considerations

■ Dosage varies with the form of the herb.
■ Advise patient to look for products standardized to 80% polyphenol and 55% epigallocatechin gallate.

- Daily consumption should be limited to fewer than 5 cups, or the equivalent of 300 mg of caffeine, per day to avoid the adverse effects of caffeine.
- Advise patient that heavy consumption may be associated with esophageal cancer secondary to the tannin content in the mixture.
- Prolonged high caffeine intake may cause restlessness, irritability, insomnia, palpitations, vertigo, headache, and adverse GI effects. Monitor patient's intake.
- The adverse GI effects of chlorogenic acid and tannin can be avoided if milk is added to the tea mixture.
- The tannin content in tea increases the longer it's left to brew; this increases the antidiarrheal properties of the tea.
- In children, administering green tea with iron supplements or multivitamins with iron prevents the absorption of iron.
- The first signs of a toxic reaction are vomiting and abdominal spasm.
- Black tea is made from the same resources of green tea but fermented to allow oxidation of polyphenols. The antioxidant activity of green tea is six times greater than black tea. For anti-tumor, antioxidant, or dental caries prevention, black tea cannot be used interchangably.
- Advise patient to consult his health care provider before using an herbal preparation because a conventional treatment with proven efficacy may be available.
- Tell patient to notify pharmacist of any herbal or dietary supplement that he's taking when obtaining a new prescription.

Research summary
The literature regarding green tea and its components is extensive. Preliminary studies indicate that green tea exerts a chemoprotective effect that may contribute to a reduced incidence of cancer and other life-threatening diseases. However, these data are derived from epidemiologic studies that require confirmation.

Green tea's antitumor activities are reported frequently in the literature. Case control studies indicate that green tea consumption is negatively associated with incidence and recurrence of colon cancer, pancreatic cancer, rectal cancer, and breast cancer. In a cohort study, the consumption of extract of green tea that contains polyphenols is associated with significant inhibition of plaque deposition and lower serum cholesterol. The antioxidant activity of green tea extract may be used to prevent ischemic stroke. Green tea is recommended to aid weight reduction. For patients on warfarin therapy, green tea consumption will significantly decrease INR due to its high vitamin K content.

ground ivy

Alehoof, catsfoot, creeping Charlie's cat's paw, gill-go-by-the-hedge, gill-go-over-the-ground, Glechoma hederacea, *haymaids, hedgemaids, lizzy-run-up-the-hedge, robin-run-in-the-hedge, tun-hoof, turnhoof*

Ground ivy contains the sesquiterpenes; volatile oil; pulegone, which has abortifacient, hepatotoxic, and irritant properties; and hydroxy fatty acids, caffeic acid derivatives, and flavonoids. It's available as liquid extract, tincture, and a tea of leaves and flowers.

Reported uses
Ground ivy is used to dry secretions, to treat poorly healing wounds, and to treat upper respiratory tract complaints, including problems with the ears, nose, and throat. It's also used as a decongestant, an anti-inflammatory, and an astringent. Ground ivy may also help with problems in the GI tract, including diarrhea, gastritis, and hemorrhoids. In Chinese medicine, it's used to treat irregular menstrual periods, lower abdominal pain, scabies, carbuncles, dysentery, and jaundice.

Administration
- Dried drug: 2 to 4 g by mouth every day
- Fluid extract (1:1, 25% ethanol): 14 to 28 grains by mouth three times a day
- Topical: Crushed leaves are applied to affected area.

Hazards
Pregnant and breast-feeding patients and children shouldn't use this herb. Patients with renal or hepatic impairment should be monitored closely.

Clinical considerations
- Ground ivy may interfere with the intended therapeutic effect of conventional drugs.
- Patients taking disulfiram, metronidazole, a cephalosporin, or a CNS depressant should avoid formulations containing alcohol.
- Advise patient to keep ground ivy away from children and pets.
- Tell patient to notify pharmacist of any herbal or dietary supplement that he's taking when obtaining a new prescription.
- Advise patient to consult his health care provider before using an herbal preparation because a conventional treatment with proven efficacy may be available.

Research summary
The concepts behind the use of ground ivy and the claims made regarding its effects haven't yet been validated scientifically.

guarana

Brazilian cocoa, guarana bread, guarana gum, guarana paste, guarana seed paste, paullinia, Paullinia cupana, *zoom*

Guarana is the dried paste made from the peeled, dried, roasted, and crushed seeds of *Paullinia cupana*. It contains 3% to 7% caffeine (coffee contains 1% to 2% caffeine); tannins, which provide its astringent taste; and theophylline and theobromine, which are alkaloids that are similar to caffeine.

Guarana plays an important role in the society of Amazonian Indians. It is often taken during periods of fasting to improve tolerance for dietary restrictions. The extract is believed to provide protection from malaria and dysentery. It was listed as an official drug in the U. S. Pharmacopeia until 1910.

Guarana is available as alcohol-containing extracts, capsules, elixirs, syrups, tablets, and teas. It's also available in various soft drinks, weight loss products, energy drinks, and vitamin supplements. Common trade names include Guarana Plus, Guarana Rush, and Superguarana.

Reported uses
Guarana is used to promote weight loss, enhance athletic performance, protect against malaria and dysentery, and treat headaches, dysmenorrhea, and digestion problems. It's used as a stimulant similar to coffee or tea, an aphrodisiac, and a tonic to quiet hunger or thirst. It's also used as a flavoring agent. Guarana is used primarily as a source of caffeine in soft drinks. It stimulates the central nervous system, suppresses the appetite, and inhibits platelet aggregation. It also induces diuresis and relaxes bronchial smooth muscle.

Administration
Dosage is 1 to 2 capsules containing 200 to 800 mg of guarana extract, not to exceed 3 g every day.

Hazards
Adverse reactions associated with guarana include insomnia, irritation, nervousness, anxiety, headache, rapid heart rate, inhibited platelet aggregation, tinnitus, abdominal spasms, vomiting,

diuresis, painful urination, and fibrocystic breast disease.

Interaction with adenosine could lead to a decreased antiarrhythmic effect. Anticoagulants and antiplatelet drugs may increase bleeding tendency. Concomitant use with caffeine-containing analgesics or nonprescription drugs such as NoDoz and Vivarin potentiates the effects of caffeine. Use with cimetidine may decrease the clearance of caffeine from the body, increasing its effects. Ciprofloxacin may decrease the elimination of caffeine from the body, increasing its effects. Ephedrine and phenylpropanolamine can increase stimulant effects and may increase blood pressure.

Large amounts of guarana and caffeine can increase the effects of theophylline. Serum potassium must be monitored if guarana is taken regularly by patients also taking guarana. Hypokalemia induced by excessive guarana use may worsen digoxin toxicity. Additive effects may be seen with guarana and green tea, black tea, or maté.

Pregnant and breast-feeding patients and those with cardiac arrhythmias should avoid use. Patients sensitive to caffeine and patients with cardiovascular or renal disease, hyperthyroidism, spasms, and psychic disorders such as panic attacks or anxiety should use with caution.

 SAFETY RISK *Guarana use has been associated with seizures and arrhythmias.*

Clinical considerations

■ High doses may cause caffeine-like adverse effects.
■ Advise patient that the caffeine content in guarana is higher than in coffee.
■ If patient is sensitive to caffeine, monitor blood pressure and heart rate.
■ If patient is taking an anticoagulant or an antiplatelet, monitor PT and INR.
■ The first signs of a toxic reaction are dysuria, vomiting, and abdominal spasms.

■ Advise patient who is or wants to become pregnant not to use guarana.
■ Tell patient that herb may increase blood pressure, cause arrhythmia, and aggravate hiatal hernia, peptic ulcer disease, gastroesophageal reflux disease, and anxiety or depressive disorders.
■ Tell patient to notify pharmacist of any herbal or dietary supplement that he's taking when obtaining a new prescription.
■ Advise patient to consult his health care provider before using an herbal preparation because a conventional treatment with proven efficacy may be available.

Research summary

Guarana has been shown to inhibit platelet aggregation. Urine analysis showed alleged psychoactive elements in essential oil from guarana estagole and anethole remain unchanged. A double-blind, placebo-controlled study on 45 healthy elderly volunteers didn't demonstrate any alteration of cognition after long term guarana use. An in vitro study showed guarana to be genotoxic and mutagenetic. The clinical importance of the above findings is unclear. Guarana in cola soda has been reported to significantly increase risk of erosion on dental enamel.

guggul

Commiphora molmol, *guggal, gugulipid, gum guggulu*

The useful constituents of guggul, gugulipid and guggulsterone, are derived from *Commiphora molmol.* Guggul may lower serum cholesterol levels by as much as 24%, and triglyceride levels by as much as 23%, by increasing the hepatic binding of LDL cholesterol. Its effects on HDL cholesterol levels are variable, either increasing or decreasing. Guggulsterone stimulates the thyroid gland, has anti-inflammatory properties, may help in weight reduction, and protects against myocardial necrosis resulting from drug toxicity. Guggul is available as capsules and tablets. Common trade names include Guggulow, Guggul Raj, Gugulmax, Gugulplus, and Ultra Guggulow.

Reported uses
Guggul is used primarily for its ability to decrease serum cholesterol levels. It's also used to treat atherosclerosis and high cholesterol and high triglyceride levels. In Ayurvedic medicine, it's used to treat arthritis and to aid in weight loss.

Administration
Daily dose of guggulsterone is 25 mg three times a day, is provided in a 500-mg tablet standardized to contain 5% guggulsterone.

Hazards
Guggul has been associated with diarrhea, anorexia, abdominal pain, and rash. There is potential reduction in the bioavailability of single doses of diltiazem and propranolol when these drugs are given with guggul. The effects of thyroid drugs may be altered because guggul stimulates the thyroid gland. Guggul's lipid-lowering effect is increased when it's used with garlic.

Guggul shouldn't be used by patients with liver or kidney disease. Pregnant and breast-feeding patients should also avoid use.

Clinical considerations
■ Monitor patient with thyroid disease or taking a thyroid supplement because guggul stimulates the thyroid gland.
■ Guggul may interfere with the intended therapeutic effect of conventional drugs.
■ Only preparations with standardized amounts of guggulsterone should be used.
■ Use should be limited to 12 to 24 weeks.
■ Monitor serum cholesterol levels.

■ If patient is pregnant or breast-feeding, or is planning to become pregnant, instruct her not to use guggul.
■ Tell patient that herb isn't a substitute for healthy eating and exercise.
■ Advise patient to keep guggul out of reach of children and pets.
■ Tell patient to notify pharmacist of any herbal or dietary supplement that he's taking when obtaining a new prescription.
■ Advise patient to consult his health care provider before using an herbal preparation because a conventional treatment with proven efficacy may be available.

Research summary
Although the mechanism is unclear, studies show that guggul stimulates the thyroid gland, which may account for its ability to lower serum cholesterol.

RESEARCH *A double-blind, placebo-controlled study of guggul's effects on reducing cholesterol included 61 individuals who were followed for 24 weeks. After 12 weeks of following a healthy diet, half the participants received placebo and the other half received guggul at a dose providing 100 mg of guggulsterones daily. The results after 24 weeks of treatment showed that the treated group experienced an 11.7% decrease in total cholesterol, along with a 12.7% decrease in LDL cholesterol; a 12% decrease in triglycerides; and an 11.1% decrease in the total cholesterol/HDL cholesterol ratio. These results were significantly better than those seen in the placebo group.*

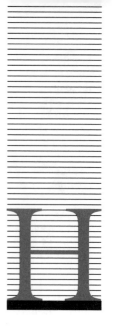

hawthorn

Crataegus laevigata, C. monogyna, *English hawthorn, haw, may, maybush, mayflower*

The use of hawthorn dates back to the ancient Greeks, but the plant became popular in European and American herbal medicine toward the end of the 19th century. The active compounds of hawthorn are obtained from the berries, flowers, and leaves of the *Crataegus* species, most commonly from *C. laevigata* or *C. monogyna*. The primary ingredients responsible for the pharmacologic effects of hawthorn include flavonoids and procyanidins.

Hawthorn flavonoids increase myocardial contraction by dilating coronary blood vessels, reducing peripheral resistance, and reducing oxygen consumption. They also lower blood pressure by inhibiting angiotensin-converting enzyme. The procyanidins slow the heart rate, lengthening the refractory period, and also have mild central nervous system (CNS) depressant effects. Hawthorn's pharmacologic effects usually develop slowly. Hawthorn is available as dried leaves, liquid extract, and tincture, in products such as Hawthorne Formula and Hawthorne Power.

Reported uses
Hawthorn is used to regulate blood pressure and heart rate and to treat atherosclerosis. It's used as a cardiotonic and as

a sedative for sleep. Hawthorn is also used in mild cardiac insufficiency, heart conditions not requiring digoxin, mild stable forms of angina pectoris, and mild forms of bradycardia and palpitations.

Administration

- Dried fruit: 300 mg to 1,000 mg three times a day by mouth
- Liquid extract (1:1 in 25% alcohol): 0.5 to 1 ml three times a day by mouth
- Oral use: 5 g, or 160 to 900 mg of extract
- Tincture (1:5 in 45% alcohol): 1 to 2 ml three times a day by mouth.

Hazards

Side effects of hawthorn may include agitation, dizziness, fatigue, headache, circulatory disturbances, palpitations, GI complaints, nausea, rash on hands, and sweating. The herb's action is similar to that of a class III antiarrhythmic. Use with antiarrhythmics could enhance this action. Increased risk of hypotension when given with antihypertensives or nitrates. Increased risk of cardiac toxicity when used with cardiac glycosides. Additive depressant effects with CNS depressants.

Patients with hypersensitivity to hawthorn or severe renal or hepatic impairment, children, pregnant patients, and breast-feeding patients should all avoid hawthorn use.

Clinical considerations

- High doses may cause hypotension and sedation. Monitor patient for CNS adverse effects, and monitor blood pressure.
- Hawthorn may interfere with digoxin's effects or serum monitoring.
- Hawthorn shouldn't be used for benign arrhythmias.
- If patient has heart failure, he should only use hawthorn under close medical supervision and in combination with other standard treatments, only as prescribed.

- Observe patient closely for adverse reactions, especially adverse CNS reactions.
- Warn patient not to treat cardiac symptoms such as edema or angina before seeking appropriate medical evaluation because doing so may delay diagnosis of a potentially serious medical condition.
- Advise patient to use hawthorn only under medical supervision.
- Advise patient to use caution when performing activities that require mental alertness because of potential CNS adverse effects.
- Warn patient that hawthorn won't stop an angina attack.
- Instruct patient to notify his health care provider if he experiences dizziness, excessive sedation, irregular heartbeats, or any other adverse reactions.
- Instruct patient to seek emergency medical help if he experiences shortness of breath or chest pain.
- Tell patient to remind pharmacist of any herbal or dietary supplement that he's taking when obtaining a new prescription.
- Advise patient to consult his health care provider before using an herbal preparation because a treatment with proven efficacy may be available.

Research summary

Hawthorn has been studied extensively for its benefits in cardiovascular disease. It has also been studied for its vasodilatory action, vasorelaxant effects, and effects in myocardial ischemia. It's been investigated for the prevention and treatment of atherosclerosis, and for hypertension. The ability to effectively treat elective mutism has also been observed. These studies indicate that hawthorn may have beneficial effects in cardiovascular disease such as ischemia, angina, and atherosclerosis. The plant also possesses lipid-lowering and antihypertensive actions.

hellebore, American

*Bear's foot, bugbane, devil's bite,
Earth gall, false hellebore,
green hellebore, Helleborus virdis,
Indian poke, itchweed, swamp hellebore,
tickleweed, white hellebore*

The active ingredients of American hellebore are obtained from the dried rhizome and roots of *Veratrum viride*. The
active components are steroid ester alkaloids that exert their physiologic effects
by lowering arterial blood pressure and
heart and respiratory rates. They also inhibit inactivation of sodium-ion channels in excitable cells, therefore increasing
nerve and muscle excitability, especially
in the cardiac muscles. Hellebore is available as liquid extract, powder, and tincture, in products such as Cryptenamine.

 SAFETY RISK *Medicinal use isn't
recommended because of American hellebore's narrow therapeutic
index and highly toxic adverse effects.*

Reported uses

Hellebore is used to depress the action of
the heart and reduce blood pressure. It's
also used as a diuretic, antispasmodic,
antipyretic, and sedative.

Administration

The tincture (1:10) is administered in 0.3
to 2 ml doses, by mouth, every day.

Hazards

Adverse reactions to hellebore include
syncope, sedation, paralysis, ECG
changes, hypertension, hypotension,
blindness, burning sensations in the
mouth and pharynx, lacrimation, salivation, sneezing, abdominal pain and distention, diarrhea, nausea, vomiting, and
muscular weakness. Use with cardiac
drugs (antiarrhythmics, antihypertensives, cardiac glycosides, and nitrates)
may increase the potential for increased
or decreased effects of these groups of
drugs. Increased sedation and respiratory

depression may be noted with CNS depressants.

SAFETY RISK *American hellebore
has been associated with seizures,
arrhythmias, bradycardia, and
respiratory depression.*

Clinical considerations

■ Advise patient to avoid use because of
toxic adverse effects and narrow therapeutic index.
■ Signs and symptoms of toxic reaction
include burning of mouth and throat, inability to swallow, abdominal pain, cardiac abnormalities, seizures, impaired vision, nausea, shortness of breath, loss of
consciousness, and paralysis. Monitor patient closely for adverse reactions.
■ Advise patient to keep the herb away
from children and pets.
■ Warn patient not to delay seeking appropriate medical evaluation because doing so may delay diagnosis of a potentially serious medical condition.
■ If overdose occurs, perform gastric
lavage and administer activated charcoal,
intravenous diazepam to treat spasms,
and sodium bicarbonate to counteract
acidosis. Patient may need respiratory
support with mechanical ventilation.
■ Tell patient to notify pharmacist of any
herbal or dietary supplement that he's
taking when obtaining a new prescription.
■ Advise patient to consult his health
care provider before using an herbal
preparation because a conventional treatment with proven efficacy may be available.

Research summary

The concepts behind the use of American
hellebore and the claims made regarding
its effects haven't yet been validated scientifically.

hellebore, black

*Black hellebore, Christe herbe,
Christmas rose,* Helleborus niger,
malampode

The active ingredients of black hellebore
are obtained from the rhizome and root
of *Helleborus niger.* The whole black
hellebore plant is considered poisonous.
Black hellebore root contains glycosides
with cardioactive properties similar to
digitalis. It also contains saponins that
can cause irritation to the mucous membranes. Topical application of the plant
may cause serious skin irritation. Black
hellebore is available as liquid extract,
powder, and tincture.

 SAFETY RISK *Medicinal use isn't
recommended because of the poisonous nature of the black hellebore plant and its highly toxic adverse effects. Its use has been associated with
arrhythmias, bradycardia, and respiratory
failure.*

Reported uses
Black hellebore is used to treat nausea,
worm infestations, amenorrhea, and anxiety. It's also used as a laxative and as an
abortifacient. Because of its possible immunostimulatory effects, black hellebore
is used as adjuvant therapy in cancer patients. It's used in homeopathy to treat
eclampsia, epilepsy, meningitis, enceph-
alitis, and mental disorders.

Administration
The average daily dose in one source in
0.05 g, with a maximum single dose of
0.2 g.

Hazards
Adverse reactions to black hellebore include dizziness, irregular pulse, blindness, burning sensations in the mouth
and pharynx, increased salivation, sneezing, abdominal pain, diarrhea, nausea,
vomiting, and shortness of breath. Use
with cardiac drugs such as antiarrhyth-

mics, beta blockers, and cardiac glycosides could increase the potential for increased or decreased effects of these
drugs. Increased sedation and respiratory
depression may be seen with CNS depressants.

Clinical considerations
■ Advise patient that black hellebore is
unsafe for use because it is toxic.
■ Advise patient to keep the herb away
from children and pets.
■ Signs and symptoms of toxic reaction
include burning of mouth and throat, inability to swallow, abdominal pain, cardiac abnormalities, seizures, impaired vision, nausea, shortness of breath, loss of
consciousness, and paralysis. Monitor patient closely for adverse reactions.
■ Tell patient to notify pharmacist of any
herbal or dietary supplement that he's
taking when obtaining a new prescription.
■ Advise patient to consult his health
care provider before using an herbal
preparation because a conventional treatment with proven efficacy may be available.

Research summary
The concepts behind the use of black
hellebore and the claims made regarding
its effects haven't yet been validated scientifically.

Hellerwork

Hellerwork is a type of deep-tissue bodywork developed by Joseph Heller, an
aerospace engineer who studied Rolfing,
Aston-Patterning, and the use of energy
for healing. Heller believed that a person's emotions and way of moving were
just as important as bodywork, and developed his method after deciding that
the other methods he'd investigated
didn't address these issues sufficiently.

Hellerwork encompasses a series of
eleven treatments, each focusing on a different part of the anatomy and all in-

tended to align the body. This alignment is achieved through a series of deep massage techniques focused on fascia and connective tissue. A practitioner of Hellerwork will engage the client in a verbal dialog while performing the bodywork. The dialog focuses on what emotions may have contributed to the client's problem. A session will usually end with some form of movement education in order to help the patient maintain the proper alignment.

Reported uses

Hellerwork is used in the treatment of most common body pains such as backache, knee pain, or neck pain. It's also used to assist in such conditions as asthma, allergies, depression, osteoarthritis, constipation, carpel tunnel syndrome, and other repetitive strain injuries.

How the treatment is performed

Hellerwork is deep-tissue bodywork. The practitioner focuses on a different area of the body during each session (shoulders, legs, chest, etc). The practitioner attempts to align the body by massaging and manipulating fascia and connective tissue. Along with this bodywork, the practitioner will often engage the patient in verbal dialogue as to which emotions might have contributed to his current body state. Following the bodywork session, there is usually time spent on movement education, showing the patient how to sit correctly, stand, or walk.

The series consists of eleven sessions, each having an emotional state attached. For example, session 1 works on ribcage, and the patient might be asked what inspires him. Session 2 focuses on legs, and the patient might be asked about support systems such as friends and family. Session 3 focuses on arms and legs, and the practitioner might ask about anger and self-esteem.

Hazards

The most common adverse effect from Hellerwork is the pain that is occasionally associated with deep-tissue bodywork.

 SAFETY RISK *Hellerwork is contraindicated in patients with fractures, deep-vein thrombosis, and dermatological conditions that may be exacerbated by massage techniques.*

Clinical considerations

Aside from contraindications for patients with fractures, deep-vein thrombosis, or conditions that could be exacerbated by massage techniques, Hellerwork is generally well tolerated.

TRAINING *Training in Hellerwork can be obtained through Hellerwork International training centers located in Japan, New Zealand, Canada, and the United States. To receive certification, the practitioner must complete 1,250 hours of training.*

Research summary

The concepts behind Hellerwork and the claims made regarding its effects haven't yet been validated scientifically.

Homeopathy

The word homeopathy stems from the Greek words *homoios*, meaning similar, and *pathos*, meaning suffering. Homeopathic medicine, a medical system that predates the Western biomedical approach, is based on the principle that "like cures like" — that is, a small amount of the substance that causes a person's symptoms can also relieve them.

Samuel Hahnemann, the German doctor who founded homeopathy in the late 18th century, set out to discover a more humane approach to medical treatment than the primitive methods that were popular in his day, such as bloodletting and purging. He suspected that disease resulted from an imbalance in the body's "vital force" (a concept modern homeopaths believe refers to the immune system) and that with only a small stimulus the balance could be restored, enabling the body to heal itself.

Hahnemann developed his theory while trying to understand how cinchona bark (whose active ingredient is quinine) worked as a cure for malaria. When he tested cinchona on himself, he experienced chills, fever, and weakness — the classic symptoms of malaria. When he stopped taking it, the symptoms disappeared. From this experience, he reasoned that if a substance could cause certain symptoms in a healthy person, a small amount of the same substance given to an ill person with those same symptoms might stimulate the body to fight the disease. Similar theories had been proposed by Hippocrates in the 4th century B.C. and by the Swiss alchemist Paracelsus in the 16th century.

Hahnemann studied hundreds of other substances in the same way, first having volunteers ingest them and then noting the symptoms — physical, mental, and emotional — that each produced. He began treating sick people with small amounts of the particular medicine whose effects most closely resembled their symptoms. Based on the results of these studies, Hahnemann formulated the principles of homeopathy:

- like cures like (the Law of Similars)
- the more diluted a remedy is, the greater its potency (the Law of the Infinitesimal Dose)
- illness is specific to the individual (the model for holistic medicine).

Today, homeopathy is practiced around the world by an estimated 500 million people and is endorsed by the World Health Organization. Homeopathic medicine is especially popular in Europe, its birthplace. In France, pharmacies are required to stock homeopathic remedies, which are used by more than a third of the population; in Britain, homeopathic clinics are a part of the national health system. Homeopathy is also widely practiced in India and Russia.

In the United States, the rise of conventional medicine, with its antagonistic approach to disease, led to the decline of homeopathy, which had been practiced by about 1 in 5 doctors in the United States until the early 1900s. However, homeopathy has seen a resurgence of interest in the past 20 years. Today, about 3,000 health care professionals, including MDs, osteopathic doctors, dentists, veterinarians, acupuncturists, chiropractors, naturopaths, nurse practitioners, and physician assistants are licensed to practice homeopathy. In addition, homeopathic remedies are a multimillion-dollar industry regulated by the Food and Drug Administration.

Reported uses

Homeopathy is used to treat a wide range of chronic conditions, such as headaches, allergies, asthma, eczema, arthritis, and digestive problems; and acute infections, such as bronchitis, influenza, and streptococcal throat infection. Homeopathic remedies are also used to treat colds, rashes, minor skin abrasions, strains, and sprains, and homeopathic first-aid kits are available in many health food stores. (See *Homeopathic first aid*, page 252.) Homeopathy is not an appropriate self-treatment for illnesses involving advanced tissue damage, such as cancer or heart disease; for medical or surgical emergencies; or for severe infections.

How the treatment is performed

Homeopathic practitioners view illness as a disturbance of the vital force that manifests as a whole pattern of physical, mental, and emotional responses unique to each patient. Following Hahnemann's third principle of homeopathy — illness is specific to the individual — homeopaths don't treat all patients with similar symptoms identically. Whereas a conventional doctor typically treats an ordinary headache with analgesics or anti-inflammatory drugs, a homeopathic practitioner tries to get a more complete picture of the patient, analyzing the

HOMEOPATHIC FIRST AID

Homeopathic practitioners recommend that every home contain 10 basic remedies to treat everyday accidents and ailments. The following list groups the remedies by their natural sources and supplies the specific source in parentheses.

From animal sources
Apis (honeybee) — for insect bites and bee stings

From mineral sources
Arsenicum (arsenic) — for upset stomach, food poisoning, vomiting, and diarrhea

From plant sources
■ Aconite (monkshood) — for swelling or fever
■ Arnica (leopard's bane) — for bruises and muscle soreness
■ Belladonna (nightshade) — for sore throats, colds, coughs, headaches, earaches, and fever
■ Gelsemium (yellow jasmine) — for colds and tension headaches
■ Ipecacuanha (ipecac root) — for nausea and bleeding from the nose or other body parts
■ Ledum (marsh tea) — for bites, stings, puncture wounds, eye injuries, and ankle strains
■ Nux vomica (poison nut) — for hangovers
■ Ruta (rue) — for sprains, soreness, and tendinitis (if arnica doesn't work)

about lifestyle, diet, and family dynamics. Emotional and mental symptoms are especially relevant because they're believed to be a good indicator of how the patient generally feels.

When the homeopathic practitioner has sufficient information to identify the patient's overall symptom picture, he matches the pattern revealed to a homeopathic remedy listed in the official compendium, called the *Homeopathic Pharmacopoeia*, using an index that lists all symptoms and their corresponding remedies. This tool helps guide the practitioner to possible remedies, but he must then study the remedies to choose the appropriate one.

Homeopathic medicines are prepared from raw herbs and other natural substances derived from animal and mineral sources. These substances are crushed and dissolved in water or grain alcohol. Each compound is diluted many times, depending on the patient's symptoms. (Homeopaths believe that this process minimizes adverse effects.) After each dilution, the solution is shaken vigorously (a process known as succussion).

A 1:100 dilution means that 1 drop of a plant extract or other substance is placed in 99 drops of water or alcohol. After succussion, 1 drop of the new solution is diluted in another 99 drops of water or alcohol and shaken again. This process may be repeated 20 or 30 times. In the end, the remedy may contain less than one molecule of the original extract; however, homeopathic practitioners believe that each dilution strengthens the solution.

This use of highly diluted remedies is the most controversial aspect of homeopathic medicine. Conventional practitioners question how a solution containing less than a molecule of the medicinal substance can have an effect on the patient's symptoms. The answers haven't been found in conventional pharmacology, but proponents of homeopathy offer a number of theories. (See *Understanding homeopathy.*)

headache's characteristics in that particular person. For example, is the headache affected by cold or heat? Does it improve when the patient changes position?

Seeking not one disease but an overall pattern of symptoms, the homeopathic practitioner elicits as many symptoms as possible from the patient, even those that may not seem to be directly related to his chief complaint. The practitioner asks

Homeopathic remedies are regulated by the Food and Drug Administration, and most are considered safe enough to be sold over the counter in many health food stores. Compounds that are intended for serious conditions must be dispensed by a licensed practitioner.

In homeopathy, the process of healing doesn't end when the initial symptoms are resolved. Instead, the practitioner then attempts to discover and treat older underlying symptoms — residues of fevers, trauma, or other illnesses that were treated incompletely in the past and eventually resulted in the patient's presenting symptoms. This practice of restoring health layer by layer originated with Constantine Hering, the founder of American homeopathy, who believed that healing should proceed in reverse chronological order, from the most recent symptoms to the oldest.

Hazards

Aggravation of presenting symptoms may occur with the use of homeopathic medicine. It is usually brief, lasting from several hours to several weeks. Homeopathic remedies carry precautions similar to conventional medications. Advise patients to store them in a cool, dry place away from the sun, away from strong aromatic substances such as mints, to take nothing by mouth for 15 minutes before and after each dose, and to avoid coffee, home remedies, mints (including mint toothpaste), and over-the-counter drugs during the treatment period.

Clinical considerations

■ Always obtain a thorough history before administering homeopathic remedies. This will help identify not only the patient's current problems but also any potential problems that the therapy could impose. For example, a patient with diabetes mellitus or lactose intolerance shouldn't take homeopathic remedies in tablet form because the tablets contain lactose. Advise such patients to request a liquid form of the medication.

UNDERSTANDING HOMEOPATHY

Of the various theories advanced to explain the therapeutic actions of homeopathic remedies, the most common is the "memory of water" theory, which states that the active ingredient leaves an electromagnetic "imprint" in the water molecules of the homeopathic solution and that shaking the solution prior to administration activates this "memory," thereby stimulating the body's self-healing response.

Conventionally trained scientists say that if water had a memory, it would also "remember" all the other substances (such as minerals) removed during the purification process, some of which might have harmful effects on the patient or might cancel out the beneficial effects of the original extract. However, proponents of homeopathy say magnetic resonance imaging has shown subatomic activity in various homeopathic remedies.

To date, homeopathic practitioners have been unable to provide a research-based explanation of how these remedies work. Several theories exist, but none have been verified by research.

■ Explain the limitations of homeopathic treatment and encourage patients with serious disorders or worsening symptoms to seek further advice from their homeopathic practitioner and their health care provider.
■ Tell recovering alcoholics to make sure the remedies they take are mixed with water, not alcohol.
■ Inform the patient that conventional medications may interfere with the actions of homeopathic remedies and should be avoided unless seriously ill. Consult with a homeopathic practitioner.

Research summary

As with traditional Chinese and Ayurvedic systems of medicine, the whole-person approach used in homeopathic diagnosis and treatment doesn't generally lend itself to placebo-controlled, double-blind studies. In spite of this difficulty, there have been some successful attempts to demonstrate the efficacy and cost effectiveness of specific homeopathic treatments, and to examine patient outcomes.

A 1994 report to the NIH entitled *Alternative Medicine: Expanding Medical Horizons* lists a number of studies published in mainstream medical journals that reported positive effects with homeopathic treatment. Clinical trials in Europe in the 1980s suggested benefits from homeopathic therapy in patients with allergic rhinitis, fibromyalgia, and influenza. A 1986 article in the British medical journal *Lancet* reported that homeopathic remedies were more effective than placebos in treating asthma and hay fever. A double-blind study comparing homeopathic treatment with a placebo for childhood diarrhea, and reported in the May 1994 issue of Pediatrics, found significant improvement in the children who received homeopathic remedies.

German researchers have reported success in treating bronchitis, migraines, influenza, and Parkinson's disease with homeopathic remedies. (Homeopathic practitioners have also claimed success in treating epilepsy, mental and emotional disorders, and premenstrual syndrome, but there is no scientific research to support these claims.) Despite such studies, many in the mainstream medical community still dismiss homeopathy outright, claiming any positive results are a result of the placebo effect.

hops

Common hops, European hops, Humulus lupulus, *lupulin*

Hops extracts have been used for a variety of medicinal purposes throughout the ages, although most of these uses have not persisted to modern times. Hops is used widely in the commercial preparation of beer, where the degradation of its components yields certain flavors. The medicinal parts include the glandular hairs separated from the flowers, the fresh cones, and the fresh or dried female flowers.

The active ingredient in hops, 2-methy-3-butene-2-ol, has sedative-hypnotic properties. The bitter acid constituents lupulone and humulone inhibit the growth of gram-positive organisms by disrupting the primary membrane of the bacteria. The flavonoglucosides have diuretic and antispasmodic activities. Hops is available as liquid extract, tea preparation, and tincture, in products such as Ez, Re-X, and Stress Free.

Reported uses

Hops is used to treat neuralgia, insomnia, nervous tension, restlessness, sleep disturbances, intestinal spasms, anxiety, mood disturbances, and digestive tract disorders involving spasms of the smooth muscle. It's also used as a mild diuretic, appetite stimulant, digestive aid, and aphrodisiac. Topically, hops is used as a mild antibacterial. Hops is also used to preserve beer.

Administration

- As a sedative: Dosage is 500 to 1,000 mg of dried herb by mouth, taken as a single dose. It may also be taken as tea, which is prepared by brewing dried herb in 5 oz of boiling water for 5 to 10 minutes, and then straining
- Liquid extract (1:1 preparation in 45% alcohol): Dosage is 0.5 to 2 ml, taken by mouth as a single dose

■ Tincture (1:5 preparation in 60% alcohol): Dosage is 1 to 2 ml, taken by mouth as a single dose.

Hazards

Side effects of hops include sedation, bronchial irritation and bronchitis after inhalation, contact dermatitis, and allergic reaction. Additive effects occur when used with central nervous system (CNS) depressants. Possible additive effects of hyperthermia may occur when used with phenothiazine-type antipsychotics.

It is generally recommended that pregnant and breast-feeding patients avoid the use of hops preparations, as the effects on infants and children are not well documented. Patients with hypersensitivity to hops and patients with estrogenic-dependent tumors such as breast, uterine, or cervical cancer should avoid use because of possible estrogenic effects. Patients taking a CNS depressant or an antipsychotic should use with extreme caution.

 SAFETY RISK *Hops may cause anaphylaxis.*

Clinical considerations

■ Liquid extract and tincture contain alcohol. Advise patients with liver disease or those taking metronidazole or disulfiram to avoid use.
■ Monitor for adverse effects such as increased sedation and respiratory difficulties.
■ Patient shouldn't inhale smoke from the plant.
■ Warn patient not to treat digestive problems or mood disturbances with hops before seeking appropriate medical evaluation because doing so may delay diagnosis of a potentially serious medical condition.
■ Although hops is botanically related to marijuana, smoking the plant as a substitute may be dangerous because of adverse effects.

■ Warn patient to avoid hazardous activities because of potential CNS adverse effects.
■ Advise patient to notify health care provider immediately if he develops a rash or if he experiences shortness of breath, wheezing, or itching.
■ Advise patient to keep the herb away from children and pets.
■ Tell patient to notify pharmacist of any herbal or dietary supplement that he's taking when obtaining a new prescription.
■ Advise patient to consult his health care provider before using an herbal preparation because a conventional treatment with proven efficacy may be available.

Research summary

Estrogenic or hormone activities in hops haven't been proven in more recent studies. Germany's Commission E authorizes the use of hops for sleep disturbances and discomfort due to restlessness or anxiety.

horehound

Common horehound, hoarhound, houndsbane marrubium, Marrubium vulgare, *marvel, white horehound*

The leaves and flower tops of the horehound have long been used in home remedies for the common cold. They are now used primarily as flavorings in liqueurs, candies, and cough drops. Extracts of the plant have also been used for treating intestinal parasites, as a diaphoretic, and as a diuretic.

The active ingredients are obtained from the leaves and flowers of *M. vulgare.* Horehound's active compound, marrubiin, stimulates secretions in the bronchioles and works as an expectorant. It also contains antiarrhythmic properties, but is of limited use for this purpose because large doses can also cause arrhythmias.

Marrubin acid, derived from marrubiin, stimulates bile secretion. An aqueous extract from horehound may have antagonistic activities toward serotonin. The horehound extract has hypoglycemic effects. Horehound is available as dried herb, liquid extract, lozenges, powder, syrup, and tea.

Reported uses
Horehound is used to treat acute or chronic bronchitis, whooping cough, and sore throat. It's used as an expectorant for treating nonproductive coughs and as a digestive aid. Horehound also may be used for its transient bile secretion-stimulant properties.

Administration
■ Dried herbs: An infusion is prepared by pouring boiling water over 1 to 2 g of the herb and straining after 10 minutes. Dosage is 1 to 2 g by mouth, three times a day
■ Liquid extract (1:1 preparation in 20% alcohol): Dosage is 2 to 4 ml by mouth three times a day
■ Oral use: Average daily dose is 4.5 g of the drug, or 30 to 60 ml of the pressed juice.

Hazards
Horehound may cause diarrhea, hypoglycemia, and contact dermatitis. Antiarrhythmics, some antidepressants, antiemetics, and antimigraine drugs may potentiate the serotonergic effects when used with horehound. Enhanced hypoglycemic effects may be seen with antidiabetics and insulin.

Patients with arrhythmias or diabetes mellitus and patients who are pregnant or breast-feeding should avoid use. Patients with cardiovascular disease should use with caution.

 SAFETY RISK *High doses of horehound may be associated with cardiac arrhythmias.*

Clinical considerations
■ Medicinal use is not recommended.

■ Horehound may interfere with the intended therapeutic effect of conventional drugs.
■ Monitor patient's serum glucose level, and heart rate and rhythm.
■ Monitor patient for changes in bowel habits.
■ Warn patient not to treat chronic cough and dyspepsia before seeking appropriate medical evaluation because doing so may delay diagnosis of a potentially serious medical condition.
■ Advise patients with diabetes or cardiac problems not to use horehound.
■ Advise patient to use less or to stop using horehound if upset stomach or diarrhea occur.
■ Advise patient to seek medical help if cough doesn't improve significantly in 2 weeks, or if a cough brings up brown, black, or bloody phlegm.
■ Advise patient to keep the herb away from children and pets.
■ Tell patient to notify pharmacist of any herbal or dietary supplement that he's taking when obtaining a new prescription.
■ Advise patient to consult his health care provider before using an herbal preparation because a conventional treatment with proven efficacy may be available.

Research summary
The FDA banned the use of horehound in the preparation of OTC cough remedies because of unconvincing evidence to support its effectiveness; however, horehound preparation is still available in sore throat products.

horse chestnut

Aesculus hippocastanum, *buckeye, California buckeye, chestnut, Ohio buckeye, Spanish-chestnut*

The horse chestnut has been used as a traditional remedy for arthritis, rheumatism, and the management of varicose veins and hemorrhoids. The seeds are toxic, and many methods have been used to rid them of toxicity. The herb is more popularly used in Europe.

The useful constituents of horse chestnut are derived from the seeds and bark of the Aesculus tree. Aescin seems to provide some weak diuretic activity and may decrease the permeability of venous capillaries. It also has a tonic effect on the veins and prevents collagen breakdown by inhibiting glycosaminoglycan hydrolases. Sterol content may have some anti-inflammatory activity. The toxic glycoside, aesculin, is a hydroxycoumarin with potential antithrombotic activity; however, the toxin is removed during preparation. Horse chestnut is available as capsules and as creams made from an aescin/cholesterol complex, in products such as Arthro-Therapy, Cell-U-Var Cream, Varicare, Varicosin, VenoCare Ultra-Joint Response, and Venastat.

Reported uses

Horse chestnut is used to treat chronic venous insufficiency, varicose veins, tiredness, and tension, and leg pain, swelling, and edema. The extract is used as a conjunctive treatment for lymphedema, hemorrhoids, and enlarged prostate.

Horse chestnut has been used as an analgesic, anticoagulant, antipyretic, astringent, expectorant, and tonic. It has also been used to treat skin ulcers, phlebitis, leg cramps, cough, and diarrhea.

Administration

■ For symptomatic treatment of chronic venous insufficiency: Dosage is 250 mg by mouth every day, up to three times a day. Some sources recommend taking 450 to 750 mg every day to decrease symptoms, and then decreasing dose to 175 to 350 mg every day
■ Tincture formulation: Dosage is 1 to 4 ml by mouth three times a day.

Hazards

Side effects of horse chestnut include GI irritation (especially with immediate-release products) toxic nephropathy, calf cramps, itching, and skin cancer (topical skin cleansers). Use with anticoagulants may increase anticoagulant effects with increased bleeding and bruising. Increased hypoglycemic effects may occur when horse chestnut is used with antidiabetics and insulin. Aescin binds to plasma proteins and may displace drugs that are protein-bound.

When used with other herbs with anticoagulant or antiplatelet potential, such as feverfew, garlic, ginkgo, and ginseng, horse chestnut may increase anticoagulant effects, bleeding, and bruising. Other herbs with hypoglycemic potential, such as aconite, dong quai, gotu kola, gymnema, sylvestie, and fenugreek, may cause increased hypoglycemic effects when combined with horse chestnut.

The FDA considers whole horse chestnut unsafe. Those with infectious or inflammatory GI conditions shouldn't use horse chestnut because of the potential for GI tract irritation. Patients with severe renal or hepatic impairment, diabetic patients, and patients taking anticoagulants should also avoid the herb, as should pregnant or breast-feeding women.

 SAFETY RISK *Horse chestnut may cause hepatotoxicity and anaphylaxis. High doses and nonstandardized forms can be lethal.*

Clinical considerations

■ The nuts, seeds, twigs, sprouts, and leaves of horse chestnut are poisonous. Standardized formulations remove most of the toxins and standardize the amount of aescin.
■ Signs and symptoms of toxicity include loss of coordination, salivation, hemolysis, headache, dilated pupils, muscle twitching, seizures, vomiting, diarrhea, depression, paralysis, respiratory and cardiac failure, and death.

- Monitor patient for signs of toxicity and discontinue horse chestnut immediately if any occur.
- Monitor blood glucose level in patients taking antidiabetics for hypoglycemia.
- Advise patient to use only a standardized extract containing 16% to 21% aescin, at recommended doses, and to discontinue use if signs of toxic reaction occur.
- Tell patient that this is only symptomatic treatment of chronic venous insufficiency and not a cure.
- Advise patient not to confuse horse chestnut with sweet chestnut, which is used as a food.
- Advise patient to keep the herb away from children. Consumption of amounts of leaves, twigs, and seeds equaling 1% of a child's weight may be lethal.
- Tell patient to notify pharmacist of any herbal or dietary supplement that he's taking when obtaining a new prescription.
- Advise patient to consult his health care provider before using an herbal preparation because a treatment with proven efficacy may be available.

Research summary
FDA considers whole horse chestnut to be an unsafe herb and warns that all parts of the plants in this genus are potentially toxic. However, German Commission E considers it safe. European researchers have evaluated its effectiveness and safety. There are some reports of plants poisonings in Switzerland from 1966 to 1994 in which horse chestnut was responsible for allergic and anaphylactic responses.

Chestnuts of the genus *Aesculus* should be considered toxic and cannot be recommended for internal use. However, recent research suggests that certain components of the horse chestnut may improve venous compliance and reduce edema in patients with chronic venous insufficiency.

horseradish

Armoracia rusticana, *great raifort, mountain radish, pepperrot, red cole*

Horseradish has been cultivated for about 2,000 years. Early settlers brought the plant to America. Early uses included reducing sciatic nerve pain, expelling afterbirth, relieving colic, increasing urination, and killing intestinal worms. Horseradish is one the "five bitter herbs" of Passover.

Topically, the mustard content irritates the skin and stimulates local blood flow, giving relief to minor muscle aches and inflamed joints or tissues. Both the mustard oil and the glucosinolate composition give the root its characteristic pungency, helping to decrease congestion and inflammation of the respiratory tract. Horseradish may also have some antimicrobial activity against both gram-negative and gram-positive bacteria. Horseradish is available as fresh or dried root, ointment with 2% mustard oil from pressed root, and tincture.

Reported uses
Horseradish is used orally to decrease sinus congestion, relieve cough from congestion, and treat edematous conditions. It's also used as an adjunctive treatment for urinary tract infections and kidney stones.

Horseradish is used in foods as a flavoring agent. It's used topically for respiratory congestion and minor muscle aches.

Administration
- Oral use: Typical doses range from 6 to 20 g every day of the root or equivalent preparations
- Topical use: Ointments contain a maximum of 2% mustard oil and are applied as needed.

Hazards

Adverse reactions following use of horse-radish may include mucous membrane inflammation, GI irritation, abdominal pain, diarrhea, decreased thyroid function, skin irritation and blistering, and topical allergic reaction. Bloody vomiting and diarrhea may occur with large doses. Use with anticoagulants or antiplatelet drugs may cause increased bleeding tendencies. When used with levothyroxine or hypothyroid therapy, it may further decrease thyroid function. Concomitant use of horseradish with NSAIDs may increase frequency of GI irritation.

Those with kidney inflammation should avoid using horseradish because of its diuretic effect. Patients with infectious or inflammatory GI conditions or stomach or intestinal ulcers and children younger than age 4 should avoid use. Pregnant patients should avoid taking large oral doses because of the toxic and irritating mustard oil components. Patients with thyroid conditions and those taking an anticoagulant or an NSAID should use horseradish with caution.

Clinical considerations

■ Tincture doses taken regularly and in large amounts may have abortifacient effects.
■ Before applying horseradish topically to a large area, the patient should test it on a small area first to see how he responds.
■ If patient has hypothyroid disease, warn about possible interaction with horseradish and any other plants from the cabbage family.
■ Advise patient to stay within the recommended dose of 20 g per day and to take the herb with meals, to minimize GI irritation and upset.
■ Tell patient to discontinue herb if adverse reactions such as GI irritation and pain occur.
■ Advise patient to keep the herb out of reach of children and pets.
■ Tell patient to remind pharmacist of any herbal or dietary supplement that he's taking when obtaining a new prescription.
■ Advise patient to consult his health care provider before using an herbal preparation because a conventional treatment with proven efficacy may be available.

Research summary

The concepts behind the use of horseradish and the claims made regarding its effects haven't yet been validated scientifically.

horsetail

Bottle-brush, corn horsetail, Dutch rushes, Field horsetail, horsetail grass, horse willow, paddock-pipes, pewterwort, shave grass, toadpipe

Horsetail is used in traditional medicine as a diuretic and an antitubercular drug, and in the treatment of kidney and bladder disturbances. It's been used topically in cosmetics, and as an astringent to stop bleeding and stimulate wound healing.

Horsetail's mild diuretic action is probably the result of the equisetonin and flavonoid glycoside constituents. Horsetail also contains small amounts of pharmacologically active nicotine and inorganic silica components. Horsetail is available as dried extract in powdered form, dried or fresh stem of horsetail plant, infusion, liquid extract (1:1 in 25% alcohol), and tea, in products such as Springtime Horsetail and Wild Countryside.

Reported uses

Horsetail is used orally to treat diuresis, edema, and general disturbances of the kidney and bladder. It's used topically for supportive treatment of burns and wounds. Horsetail has also been used to treat brittle fingernails, rheumatic diseases, gout, frostbite, and profuse menstruation.

Administration

- Diuresis: Dosage is 6 g of the dried stem by mouth every day with plenty of fluids, or 1 cup of tea taken several times between meals, or 1 to 4 ml of liquid extract by mouth three times a day
- Infusion: An infusion is prepared by placing 1.5 g of dried stem in 1 cup of water; dosage is 2 to 4 g by mouth every day
- Tea: A tea is prepared by pouring boiling water over 2 to 3 g of the herb, boiling for 5 minutes, and then straining after 10 to 15 minutes; consumed several times a day between meals
- Topical support for burns or wounds: A compress containing 10 g of stem/L of water may be applied to affected areas.

Hazards

Side effects of horsetail include electrolyte imbalance, skin irritation from topical use, thiamine deficiency from long-term use, and symptoms of nicotine poisoning and toxicity including nausea and vomiting, muscle weakness, abnormal pulse rate, fever, and ataxia. Use of horsetail with benzodiazepines, disulfiram, or metronidazole may cause a disulfiram-like reaction. Horsetail may increase digitalis toxicity as a result of potassium loss with diuretic effect. When it's used with potassium-wasting drugs (including corticosteroids, diuretics, and laxative stimulants), there's an increased risk of hypokalemia. Overuse of licorice with horsetail may increase potassium depletion and risk of cardiac toxicity. Excessive alcohol consumption while horsetail is being used may lead to thiamine deficiency.

Pregnant patients, breast-feeding patients, those with impaired heart or kidney function, those with liver problems, those who are taking a cardiac glycoside, and those who have a history or potential of thiamine deficiency (for example, alcoholic patients) should avoid using horsetail.

 SAFETY RISK *The liquid extract contains 25% alcohol and therefore shouldn't be used with disulfiram, metronidazole, and benzodiazepines.*

Clinical considerations

- Horsetail dosage varies with the formulation. Large amounts may cause a toxic reaction.
- The dried, powdered extract is more concentrated than stem alone.
- Monitor patient's serum potassium level.
- Assess patient for signs and symptoms of hypokalemia, including weakness, muscle flaccidity, and abnormal ECG results.
- Horsetail shouldn't be used for extended periods because of the potential for toxic reaction and thiamine depletion.
- Instruct patients to stop taking horsetail immediately if signs or symptoms of nicotine toxicity (muscle weakness, abnormal pulse rate, fever, ataxia, and cold extremities) or potassium depletion (muscle cramping, irritability, or weakness) occur.
- If patient is pregnant or breast-feeding, advise her not to use horsetail.
- Advise patients taking a potassium-wasting diuretic, a cardiac glycoside (Lanoxin), a corticosteroid, or licorice not to use horsetail.
- Tell patient to notify pharmacist of any herbal or dietary supplement that he's taking when obtaining a new prescription.
- Advise patient to consult his health care provider before using an herbal preparation because a conventional treatment with proven efficacy may be available.

SAFETY RISK *Horsetail should be kept out of reach of children because poisonings have been reported in those that used the stems as blow guns or whistles.*

Research summary

The FDA lists horsetail on its undetermined safety list. Horsetail is still found in some over-the-counter herbal preparations. It has been shown to contain small amounts of nicotine and other active compounds, and is a marginally effective diuretic.

Hoxsey treatment

Derived from an herbal preparation originally used to treat cancer in horses, the Hoxsey treatment is one of the oldest and most controversial alternative therapies for cancer in the United States. The plan consists of powerful herbal remedies (used internally and externally), a dietary program, and vitamin and mineral supplements. The herbal formulas at the center of the plan originated in the 1840s with an American farmer, John Hoxsey, who noticed that one of his horses, which had a leg tumor, recovered after grazing on certain plants and grasses. Hoxsey concocted a salve out of the plants, which he gave to other farmers, and bequeathed the formula to his heirs.

Hoxsey's great-grandson, Harry Hoxsey, opened Hoxsey Cancer Clinics in 17 states between the 1920s and 1940s, and began trying the herbal preparations on humans with cancer. Hoxsey's chief nurse, Mildred Nelson, continued his work at the Biomedical Center in Mexico. The cornerstone of the Hoxsey treatment is an herbal paste that is applied externally (and used primarily for skin cancers) and an herbal tonic taken internally. Other components of the Hoxsey regimen, which is still offered in a Tijuana clinic, include:

- assorted vitamins and calcium supplements
- douches and laxatives
- avoidance of pork, tomatoes, salt, sugar, vinegar, alcohol, refined flour, alcohol, carbonated drinks, artificial sweeteners, bleached flour, and refined sugar.

Reported uses
Despite strong opposition from the American Cancer Society, which placed the Hoxsey treatment on its list of unproven methods in 1968, the regimen has been used as a cancer treatment for nearly 100 years. Hoxsey himself never claimed to understand what caused cancer or how his preparations worked. However, he believed that his therapy normalized and balanced body chemistry.

At least one respected researcher has found a scientific basis for the salve. Frederick Mohs, creator of the Mohs chemosurgical technique for skin cancer excision, reported that Hoxsey's paste contained ingredients that cured most basal cell skin carcinomas. One of the ingredients, bloodroot (*Sanguinaria canadensis*), has been used by Native Americans to treat tumors and warts.

How the treatment is performed
Treatment at the Center is on an outpatient basis only and lasts from one to three days. Patients are given a complete workup including lab tests and X-rays, and have their clinical history taken. They return home with enough Hoxsey medications and supplements to last several months. They are encouraged to make a follow-up visit after three to six months.

The escharotic preparations applied externally reportedly include a yellow preparation containing arsenic sulfide, talc sulfur, a red paste containing antimony trisulfide, zinc chloride and bloodroot, and a clear solution containing trichloracetic acid.

Hazards
The Hoxsey diet may provoke an allergic reaction in susceptible individuals. A topical application of the herbal salve may cause skin irritation, necessitating an end to treatment. No toxicities specifically resulting from the Hoxsey treatment have been reported.

Clinical considerations
Patients on the Hoxsey diet should avoid tomatoes, alcohol, vinegar, and processed

flour because they can negate the effects of the tonic.

Research summary

Medical historian Patricia Spain Ward reported "provocative findings of antitumor properties" in many of the individual Hoxsey herbs when she investigated the Hoxsey regimen in 1988 for the United States Office of Technology Assessment. According to the 1994 report to the National Institutes of Health (NIH), some of the principal herbs in the tonic — pokeweed root, burdock root, buckthorn bark, barberry, stillingia root, and prickly ash — have been shown to have anti-cancer and immunostimulatory effects. The report cites a 1979 study showing that pokeweed root (*Phytolacca americana*) stimulates the production of two cytokines that stimulate the immune system — interleukin-1 and tumor necrosis factor. The report states that although pokeweed is poisonous, "it apparently has been used without serious toxicity problems since the mid-18th century."

The NIH report also cites a 1984 study on burdock root's reported ability to reduce cell mutations and a 1989 World Health Organization report on this plant's reported ability to inhibit human immunodeficiency virus. The report concludes: "Among numerous anecdotal accounts of its effectiveness, some are hard to dismiss out of hand; [the treatment] therefore warrants investigation."

Hydrazine sulfate

Hydrazine sulfate (Sehydrin, HS) is a compound that has been used as first-line treatment for cancer, in combination with other antineoplastic agents, and for treatment of anorexia and cachexia related to cancer. Several large-scale clinical trials have been conducted on hydrazine sulfate over the last 30 years investigating its efficacy in the treatment of lung, brain, and colon cancers. Hydrazine sulfate has been shown to prolong survival,

enhance quality of life, inhibit cachexia, and, when combined with other treatment modalities, to contribute to a complete remission in some cases.

Hydrazine sulfate's mechanism of action hasn't been established, but two theories exist about its potential mechanism. The first theory states that hydrazine sulfate blocks gluconeogenesis in the liver and kidneys through inhibition of phosphoenolpyruvate carboxykinase. It's been proposed that cancer-related cachexia occurs because the body must use its own protein and other sources of energy to meet the demand for glucose by the tumors. Therefore, by blocking gluconeogenesis, hydrazine sulfate interrupts the supply of glucose to tumors, which leads to decreased tumor growth, and inhibition of cachexia.

The second mechanism proposed for hydrazine sulfate involves the inhibition of tumor necrosis factor-alpha (TNF-a). High levels of TNF-a have been observed in cancer patients, which may cause anorexia, increased muscle catabolism, and increased expenditure of energy. TNF-a is a substance produced by white blood cells in response to infection or tissue injury. The breakdown products from the muscle would then be available for gluconeogenesis. Hence, by blocking TNF-a, hydrazine sulfate should inhibit cachexia and tumor growth.

Reported uses

Hydrazine sulfate has been used to treat a variety of cancers, including brain cancer, colon cancer, non-small cell lung cancer (NSCLC), and advanced cancers with disseminated disease (metastases). Other uses include cancer related-cachexia, anorexia, and malnutrition. Because of hydrazine sulfate's inherent ability to starve a tumor of essential nutrients (glucose, etc.) while allowing a patient to regain lost weight, the primary use for it may be in patients with cachexia. Hydrazine sulfate can increase appetite, stabilize albumin, restore energy and quality of life, and prolong survival in end-stage patients. It is also useful to combat the side effects of radiation therapy. Hydrazine sulfate has been used to successfully treat cachexia, brain cancer, lung cancer, colon cancer, and various sarcomas.

How the treatment is performed

Hydrazine sulfate is available in an oral capsule that can be specially prepared by a compounding pharmacist or obtained through certain cancer centers. The most common dosage is 60 mg three times daily; this dosage is maintained as long as the patient is losing weight or has an active case of cancer. Patients continue to receive hydrazine sulfate even when they've had a complete remission (more than 8 years). Because hydrazine sulfate is a monoamine oxidase (MAO) inhibitor, several dietary and lifestyle restrictions must be followed for the therapy to be effective. (See *Dietary restrictions for hydrazine sulfate*, page 264.)

Hazards

A potentially fatal complication of encephalopathy can occur while taking hydrazine sulfate. A patient in New Zealand developed severe encephalopathy while on hydrazine sulfate, but high-dose (5 g, administered intravenously) pyridoxine therapy reversed the encephalopathy.

The side effects associated with hydrazine sulfate have been described as mild to moderate in severity and include nausea/vomiting, dizziness, paresthesias of the upper and lower extremities, impaired fine motor functions (such as, writing), itching, dry skin, insomnia, and hypoglycemia. Most side effects resolve upon discontinuation of hydrazine sulfate.

Precautionary dietary and lifestyle modifications are a must while taking hydrazine sulfate. Hydrazine sulfate is an MAO inhibitor; to avoid risk of hypertensive emergency patients taking it shouldn't use foods and drinks high in tyramine. A special diet is started 3 days prior to taking hydrazine sulfate and

continued for 3 days after discontinuing its use. Substances that must be avoided include sedatives, tranquilizers, alcohol, antidepressants, vitamin B_6 (unless in encephalopathic emergency), and OTC cold and allergy preparations.

 SAFETY RISK *Ensure strict adherence to the dietary restrictions for hydrazine sulfate. Failure to follow the dietary recommendations may precipitate hypertensive crisis.*

Clinical considerations

Strict adherence to the dietary and lifestyle restrictions given for hydrazine sulfate must be ensured to avoid a potentially fatal hypertensive emergency. One report of encephalopathy has occurred with hydrazine sulfate. Proper monitoring of the patient's mental status and other symptoms is crucial. If encephalopathy occurs, high-dose I.V. pyridoxine therapy is recommended.

No special considerations are documented for the use of hydrazine sulfate in pregnant or breast-feeding patients, or for children.

Research summary

Filov et al. performed a study in 1976 on 95 patients with advanced cancer who were treated with hydrazine sulfate after all other therapies were exhausted. No complete responses were found after 1 to 5 months of treatment but there were 3 partial responses (greater than 50% reduction in tumor size for at least 4 weeks or longer). Reductions of less than 50% and stabilized disease (no tumor growth for at least 1½ to 2 months) were seen in 16 of 20 patients (80%).

The same investigators published a continuation of their 1976 study in 1981. This study had 225 patients with advanced cancer that had failed all previous therapies. The 95 patients from the 1976 study were included in the 225 patients in this study. Again, no complete responses were noted, but there were 4 partial responses after 1 to 6 months of treatment. Stabilized disease was noted in

DIETARY RESTRICTIONS FOR HYDRAZINE SULFATE

Food groups	Foods to eat	Foods to avoid
Dairy products	Fresh milk, dry milk, evaporated milk, buttermilk, cottage cheese, cream cheese	Soy milk, sour cream, and yogurt (regular, frozen); cheeses including blue, brick, brie, camembert, mozzarella, Swiss, muenster, American, provolone, parmesan, Romano, and locatelli; snack foods with cheese
Red meat, fish & poultry	Fresh red meat, fish, or poultry	Cured meats, fish, or poultry such as sausage, Italian dry sausage, or liver/blood sausages; deli meats such as salami, ham, bacon, pastrami, and corned beef; smoked meats and fish; pickled herring, pate, fresh liver, and hot dogs; any foods containing MSG or meat tenderizers; and condiments such as ketchup, mustard, or vinegar
Spices	Fresh spices *only*	All Goya™ products (i.e., Sazon-plain, Sofrito-green, etc.); all Adobo™ products; salad dressings; soy sauce and other soy by-products such as soy burgers; teriyaki sauces/marinades; flavor enhancers such as Gravy Master, Worcestershire sauce, Kitchen Bouquet, and so forth
Fruits & vegetables	Fresh, canned, or frozen	Broad bean pods such as English and Chinese pea pods; fava beans, sauerkraut, pickles, bananas, avocados, raisins, figs, dates, any dried fruit
Nuts	None	All
Sugar	Raw, brown, any natural sweetener (i.e., stevia)	NutraSweet, Equal, Sweet'n Low, and so forth
Breads/baked goods	Some breads and baked goods	Any bread or cake containing raisins, figs, dates, or dried fruit
Alcoholic beverages	None	All (including non-alcoholic products)
Other products	Soups (fresh homemade soups with fresh ingredients)	Yeast extracts such as Marmite, Befit, Yeastral, Bovril; brewer's yeast tablets; Miso soup; bouillon cubes (beef, chicken, or vegetable); bean curd

95 of 225 patients (42%). Subjective improvements in appetite, weight gain, and mental outlook were reported in 147 of 225 patients (65%).

A prospective, randomized, double-blind, placebo-controlled study was performed in 1984 on 38 patients with ad-vanced cancer and weight loss to evaluate the effect of hydrazine sulfate (HS) on carbohydrate metabolism in cancer-related cachexia. All patients had 3-day metabolic evaluations including glucose tolerance test, hormonal studies, and total glucose production by infusion. After 30 days of treatment with either 60 mg HS three times a day or placebo, a repeat evaluation was performed. There were frequent reports of abnormal glucose tolerance tests and impaired glucose production on the initial exam. After 30 days of treatment, there were significant improvements in glucose tolerance compared to placebo (169 $^{+/-}$ 24 mg/dl initial HS vs. 128 $^{+/-}$ 12 mg/dl final HS; $P < 0.05$). No improvements in glucose tolerance were seen in patients taking placebo. In addition, the rate of total glucose production was significantly reduced after 30 days compared to placebo (2.46 mg/kg/min HS vs. 3.07 mg/kg/min placebo; $P < 0.05$). Minimal toxic effects were reported.

Chlebowski et al. performed a prospective, placebo-controlled trial in 1990 comparing the influence of hydrazine sulfate on nutritional status and survival in patients with unresectable non-small cell lung cancer (NSCLC). All 65 patients received the same chemotherapy regimen of cisplatin, vinblastine, and bleomycin. Patients were then randomized to receive 60mg HS 3 times daily or placebo. In comparison with patients taking placebo, patients taking hydrazine sulfate showed significantly higher caloric intake and greater albumin maintenance ($P < 0.05$). In addition, survival was significantly longer in the hydrazine sulfate group compared to placebo ($P < 0.05$), while toxicity was comparable in both groups.

Tayek et al. sought to identify the combined metabolic effects of 5-FU and hydrazine sulfate in a 1995 study of 22 patients with advanced colon cancer. The patients had baseline measurements of counter-regulatory hormones, fasting hepatic glucose production (HGP), glucose tolerance test, plasma leucine appearance (LA), and leucine oxidation. Significant findings for the combined therapy include a reduction in fasting glucose levels (98 $^{+/-}$ 2 mg/dl vs. 94 $^{+/-}$ 2 mg/dl; $P < 0.025$), and plasma leucine appearance (63.3 $^{+/-}$ 3 mmol/kg/hr vs. 57.1 $^{+/-}$ 3.9 mmol/kg/hr; $P < 0.025$). Multiple regression analysis later revealed that plasma LA was directly related to length of survival time, while baseline HGP, CEA, and insulin concentration were inversely related to survival time.

Hydrotherapy

Hydrotherapy—the use of water to treat disease and maintain health—has been practiced in one form or another by most cultures throughout history, from the ancient Babylonians, Greeks, and Israelites to the Indians, Chinese, and Native Americans. Today, various water-based treatments are used primarily to treat wounds, burns, and injuries; to aid physical rehabilitation; and to relieve tension. The water can be hot or cold; liquid, frozen, or steam; and applied externally or internally.

There are three types of external hydrotherapy: hot, cold, and contrast. Hot water therapies such as saunas, sweat baths, and application of heat work by dilating the blood vessels and increasing circulation in the area being treated. Increasing the supply of blood to muscles can relieve pain as well as soothing and relaxing the body. These therapies may also stimulate immune system functioning, encouraging white blood cells to leave the blood vessels and migrate into the surrounding tissues, where they scavenge for toxins and help eliminate them from the body. The copious sweat stimulated by these heat treatments is also believed to help release toxins from the body. Cold water therapies such as application of ice and cold packs cause vasoconstriction, which decreases circulation to the body part being treated, thereby reducing swelling and inflammation. Cold water may also tone muscle weakness by stimulating muscle contractions. Alternating between hot and cold application in the same treatment, known as contrast therapy, may stimulate endocrine function, reduce inflammation, decrease congestion, and improve organ function.

Reported uses

Whirlpool baths (heated baths with jets that force water to circulate) are used to assist in the rehabilitation of injured muscles and joints. The water temperature can be either hot or cold, depending on the desired effect; the jets of water act as a massage on soothing muscles. These baths are also used to treat burn patients and to aid healing of skin sores and infected wounds. Patients suffering from paraplegia and polio receive whirlpool baths to increase circulation in atrophied muscles.

A neutral bath is the immersion of the body up to the neck in water that is near body temperature. This soothing bath calms the nervous system and is used to treat emotional disturbances and insomnia. In a sitz bath, the pelvic area is immersed in a tub of warm water; this treatment is used to increase circulation, reduce inflammation, and relieve perianal pain, swelling, or discomfort.

Ice, usually applied locally, is another common therapy used to relieve sprains, strains, and inflammation. Contrast hydrotherapy can be used for trauma relief.

How the treatment is performed

The equipment needed depends on the type of therapy. It may include tub, steam, sauna (a sealed, steam-filled room), pool, hose, hot or cold pack, or Jacuzzi or whirlpool bath. Depending on the type of therapy used, the patient enters the water (hot, cold, or warm) or the sauna and remains in it for the prescribed amount of time. The desired temperature is maintained to prolong the therapy's benefits. If hot or cold packs are used, they're applied to the target body area for the specified length of time and changed as needed to maintain the desired temperature.

Hazards

Any therapy involving heat can produce harmful effects, such as burns, if applied improperly. In addition, very hot treatments can cause elderly people and children to become exhausted or faint. Cold may aggravate painful spasms or acute lung congestion. Some traditional hydrotherapy practitioners consider ice therapies inappropriate and don't use them.

Clinical considerations

■ Hot baths, saunas, and immersion baths are not recommended for pregnant women, children, elderly people, or patients with diabetes, multiple sclerosis, hypertension, or hypotension.

■ Warn patients using hydrotherapy to stop the treatment if they feel lightheaded, dizzy, or faint (possible symptoms of decreased blood pressure).

■ Cold applications are contraindicated for patients with conditions that would be exacerbated by vasoconstriction, such as Raynaud's disease or sickle cell anemia.

■ Use caution when administering a hot bath or steam bath to prevent burns, light-headedness, and falls.

■ Patients shouldn't remain in a sauna for more than 20 minutes and should wipe their faces frequently with a cool cloth to avoid becoming overheated.

■ Many hydrotherapy treatments, such as whirlpool and steam baths, can be performed at home, but more intensive forms are best performed in a clinical setting, where response to the therapy can be monitored by experienced therapists.

Research summary

The concepts behind the use of hydrotherapy and the claims made regarding its effects haven't yet been validated scientifically.

Hyperthermia

Fever therapy, heat therapy,
thermotherapy

Hyperthermia, or fever induction therapy, is used to stimulate the immune system by inducing fever in a patient whose body is too debilitated by a disease to mount a defense on its own. Many alternative practitioners see fever as the body's natural response to a pathogen. Fever has been shown to stimulate immune system production of antibodies and may also enhance the body's excretion of toxins, such as pesticides and drug residues (especially when combined with cold treatments). Hyperthermia can also be effective in relieving muscle aches, combating tiredness, and improving blood circulation.

Exogenous heat sources can be applied to the entire body or a single body part. Whole body application of exogenous heat, commonly referred to as heat therapy, is done with heating sources such as hot baths (see "Hydrotherapy," above), diathermy, or hot air (wet and dry saunas). Local application of exogenous heat, called thermotherapy, uses radiant heating devices that give off infrared rays, and conductive heating devices such as hot water bottles, paraffin baths, moist hot packs, or computerized application of microwaves.

SAFETY RISK *Induced hyperthermia, also called hyperpyrexia or fever therapy, is a state of artificially induced fever. Hyperpyrexia is induced by injecting a pyrogen such as blood products, vaccines, pollens, or benign forms of malaria. This experimental method of inducing general hyperthermia is dangerous and unreliable and is not recommended.*

Reported uses

Hyperthermia is used in a variety of health challenges, ranging from viral and bacterial infections to cancer and ac-
quired immunodeficiency syndrome (AIDS). Therapeutic effects of hyperthermia vary based on the degree of body involved and the modalities used to increase the tissue temperatures. Body involvement may range from the entire body, to the extremities (arms, legs, hands, or feet), to focused tissues (such as, specific tumor tissues). Alternative practitioners have successfully treated acute and chronic infections with simple, whole-body methods of inducing general hyperthermia. The same methods are used to precipitate detoxification — a complementary therapy useful in treatment of chronic illnesses and cancer. High-tech local hyperthermia has gained acceptance as a promising new complementary procedure in cancer therapy.

Bacterial and viral infections

Whole-body hyperthermia is successful in treating both acute and chronic infections such as upper and lower respiratory infections (colds and flu), urinary tract infections, and Lyme disease. Its effects range from potentiation of white cell antimicrobial activity to direct viricidal and bactericidal activity. Hyperthermia alone may not destroy all the invading organisms, but it can significantly reduce their numbers and thus the overall load on the immune system.

HIV infection

Studies have shown the human immunodeficiency virus (HIV) is very sensitive to temperature above the normal body temperature of 98.6° F. Treatment of 107.6° F for 30 minutes showed a 40% decrease the HIV activity. Patients with HIV infections experienced a decrease in night sweats, decreased frequency of secondary infections, and a greater sense of well-being after hyperthermia treatments.

Cancer therapy

The concept of treating cancerous cells with heat began with serendipitous findings of spontaneous tumor regression in patients with smallpox, influenza, tuberculosis, and malaria, who had experienced fevers of 104° F. This lead to a period of experimentation with fever therapy (hyperpyrexia), which is done by injecting blood products, vaccines, pollens, and benign forms of malaria. This method proved to be both unreliable and dangerous, and was rejected by the medical community. Heat therapy was not considered a reliable modality until medical scientist Haim I. Bicher began experimenting with focused microwave diathermy.

How the treatment is performed

Low-tech hyperthermia involves simple techniques of immersion in hot water (baths) followed by wrapping the body in sheets and blankets, exposing the patient to radiant heat by using a heat lamp, or having the patient sit in wet or dry saunas. Treatment can be given on an outpatient basis in the office or clinic, and typically nothing more than a bathtub, heat lamps, sauna, or steam room is needed.

High-tech methods of raising the patient's internal temperature include ultrasound therapy for deep heating of body parts, microwave diathermy for heat directed to specific cells or tissues, and extracorporal heating of the blood, which is invasive and effects the entire body.

Heating and diaphoretics herbs such as *Achillea millefoliu* (yarrow) tea are a helpful in promoting the hyperthermia state and are particularly useful during wholebody hyperthermia therapies.

Immersion hot water baths

This treatment is usually done in a deep, stainless steel tub. The water is typically heated to between 101° and 108° F, although temperatures as high as 115° are sometimes used if the patient can tolerate them. The goal is to keep the body temperature at between 102° and 104° F for about 20 minutes. The typical treatment requires approximately 30 minutes — 10 minutes for the body temperature to rise and 20 minutes of maintained high temperature. The individual is removed from the water and wrapped in a dry sheet and several blankets for 30 more minutes to continue the internal heating.

Treatment frequency and duration depends on the presenting problem. For upper and lower respiratory infections, patients typically undergo only 1 or 2 treatments before improving in a few days. For more serious conditions, however, therapy can take much longer. Cancer patients typically begin with 15 treatments over a 3-week period followed by a 3-week rest. The cycle is then repeated 4 more times, and in cases may continue for as long as a year.

Saunas

General external application of dry or moist heat causes vasodilation (swelling of the arteries) and diaphoresis (sweating), which is the body's attempt to prevent the internal increase in temperature. Superficial vessels in the skin initially contract, increasing the blood pressure. This can make the patient feel as if his head is full and bursting, an uncomfortable effect that dissipates in a short amount of time and can be avoided by applying a cold compress or ice bag to the head. Patients must be monitored carefully; apparent discomfort and the state of pulse, respiration, and skin coloring are observed to be certain the patient doesn't become dehydrated or suffer heat exhaustion.

Ultrasound

In ultrasound, special equipment emits inaudible sound in the frequency range of approximately 20,000 to 10 billion (109) cycles/second. The sound directs its thermal effects deep into the targeted tissues. Ultrasound waves can be transmitted through a coupling agent applied directly onto the skin or through water with the transmitting head held 1 inch from the skin.

Treatment duration varies based on the condition; treatment for acute conditions lasts 4 minutes; for chronic conditions the treatment lasts 10 minutes. Care should be taken when placing the transmitting ultrasound head as these sound waves have the ability to fracture bones, melt myelin sheaths, and burn the periosteum if used incorrectly.

Radiant heat
Radiant heat can be applied with heat lamps and ultraviolet lamps. The body should be kept 30 inches from the ultraviolet lamp source. Treatment durations begin at 15 seconds and increase to 3 minutes as the sessions proceed. Once the 3-minute time frame is reached, the UV lamp can be drawn closer by 2 inches per treatment session until a distance of 18 inches is reached.

Microwave diathermy
Microwave radiation is a high-frequency oscillatory current used to heat specific target cells. All metal must be removed from the general area of treatment to prevent current arcing. The microwave apparatus is placed 1 to 5 inches from the target area. Placement and duration of treatment vary depending on the desired effect. Microwave radiation shouldn't be used over pacemakers or metal implants.

Extracorporeal heating of the blood
Blood is removed from the body, delivered to an external heating device, heated, and returned to the body at the higher temperature. This procedure is used in patients with HIV.

Hazards
Safe and appropriate use of hyperthermia requires an understanding of the safe limits of induced temperature and the contraindications to heat therapy. The lower limit of body temperature for human survival is 74° F; the upper limit is 113° F. Normal cells die at a temperature of 110° F.

Hyperthermia therapists find that adults in good health can tolerate temperatures of 107.6° F for periods of 8 to 10 hours. However, the therapist must take into account the whole presentation of the patient, including age, health status, and past medical history. For example, hyperthermia should be strictly avoided during pregnancy, due to potential danger to the unborn child, and in individuals with temperature regulation problems, especially the very old and very young.

Heat therapy should also be restricted in patients with cardiovascular diseases such as arrhythmias and tachycardia and in those with severe hypertension or hypotension. People with arrhythmias and tachycardia risk increased chance of myocardial infarction from altered blood flow dynamics caused by systemic or local application of heat. Severely hypertensive patients risk hemorrhagic stroke, while severely hypotensive patients risk syncope and tissue ischemic damage.

Heat shouldn't be applied to extremities of patients with peripheral vascular disease such as arteriosclerosis, advanced diabetes, Raynaud's syndrome, or Berger's disease due to their compromised sensation of heat and increased risk of burns. Sensitivity to extreme temperatures is seen in other chronic conditions, such as anemia, heart disease, diabetes, thyroid disease, seizure disorders, and tuberculosis; patients with these conditions may require a reduction in the number of treatments, a reduction in the intensity of heat applied, or another method of treatment.

Patients with acute illness may initially have difficulty tolerating the extreme temperatures, but this usually subsides after hyperthermia is initiated. Use heat therapy with caution in these individuals. Other reported risks in weakened individuals are herpes outbreaks and liver toxicity.

 TRAINING *Licensed naturopathic physicians who graduated from a 4-year training program are*

trained in general and local hyperthermia techniques. However, there are no certification programs for focused microwave hyperthermia. The best option is a licensed conventional physician with at least 1 year of special training in hyperthermia treatments.

Clinical considerations

■ Factors to consider before using heat therapy include age of the patient, his overall health status, and any medications he is currently taking. High temperatures can increase the efficacy of certain drugs to the point of toxicity.

■ Heat therapy can cause or exacerbate internal bleeding. Use extreme caution with patient with anemia, heart disease, and diabetes due to his increased risk of hemorrhage. Periodically take vital signs to catch early signs of increased blood loss and hypovolemic shock.

■ Patient with a history of seizure disorders shouldn't be treated with whole-body hyperthermia methods due to his increased risk of seizure activity and possible nervous system damage.

■ Local hyperthermia can be used with constant monitoring.

■ Patient with tuberculosis has a high risk of reactivation of the latent bacteria due to the increased heat stress on the body.

■ Electrical devices shouldn't be used to heat moist dressings due to the high risk of electrical shock. Microwave diathermy can burn periocular tissues and is contraindicated in people with pacemakers. Radiant heat lamps are safely used to promote local hyperthermia; however, misuse, overexposure, or direct skin contact with the heat lamp can cause blistering, dermal burns, and even heatstroke.

■ Heatstroke is characterized by hyperthermia (42° C), delirium, coma, and anhidrosis, a breakdown of the hypothalamic heat regulatory mechanisms, which has a mortality rate as high as 80% if untreated. Survivors can develop neurological deficits, including cerebellar ataxia and sever dysarthria. Therapists must be alert to changes in the patient and be prepared to rapidly facilitate the dissipation of heat from the individual. Continuous sponging with tepid water and continuous gentle massage promotes cutaneous vasodilation and dissipation of heat.

■ Promoting hyperthermia via fevers induced by injecting blood products, vaccines, pollens, and benign forms of malaria is both unreliable and dangerous. This procedure is not recommended.

 SAFETY RISK *The treatments should be stopped immediately if the patient experiences any side effects. Improvements should be noted after the first few treatments in problems other than cancer or AIDS. If there is not improvement, other forms of therapy should be considered.*

Research summary

Multiple studies have shown that whole-body hyperthermia plays a positive role in several aspects of the healing process — destruction of the invading organism, stimulation of the immune system, and general detoxification of the body — all of which are needed to regain and maintain optimum health. Studies have also shown that focused hyperthermia of specifically targeted tissues can modify cell membranes in a manner that actually protects the healthy cells and makes the cancer cells more susceptible to chemotherapy and radiation treatments. Used as adjunctive therapy, focused microwave diathermy may thus permit lower doses of these potent and toxic forms of therapy.

 RESEARCH *Hyperthermia was given legal status as an approved medical procedure in 1984. Hyperthermic oncology, currently reimbursed by Medicare and most insurance companies, has now joined surgery, radiation, and chemotherapy in the expanding arsenal of proven, effective treatments for both primary cancer and locally recurrent tumors.*

Hypnotherapy

Hypnotherapy applies suggestion and altered levels of consciousness to effect positive changes in behavior and treat a range of health conditions. Under hypnosis, the patient can experience relaxation and changes in respiration, which can lead to a positive shift in behavior and an enhanced sense of well-being. Physiologically, the hypnotic state can give the patient greater control over his autonomic nervous system, functions that would ordinarily be considered beyond his control.

Defined as a state of attentive and focused concentration, hypnosis leaves people relatively unaware of their surroundings. In this state of concentration, a person is very susceptible to suggestion. However, the person must be willing to follow the suggestions offered; he can't be hypnotized to follow suggestions that go against his wishes.

The three major components of hypnosis are absorption, dissociation, and responsiveness. Absorption refers to the rapt attention that the subject pays to the words or images presented by the hypnotherapist. The subject then begins to dissociate from his ordinary consciousness and surroundings and becomes responsive to the therapist's suggestions. To bring the subject to a hypnotic state, the therapist leads him through relaxation, mental imagery, and suggestions. The subject can also be taught to hypnotize himself. The therapist may provide the patient with audiotapes to enable him to practice the therapy at home.

There are actually two states of hypnosis: the superficial state and the deeper somnambulistic state. In the superficial hypnotic state, the patient accepts suggestions but doesn't necessarily carry them out. In the somnambulistic state, the patient is better able to carry out suggestions made during the trance once the session has ended. Although an estimated 90% of the population can be hypnotized, only 20% to 30% are susceptible

---

UNDERSTANDING HYPNOSIS

Under hypnosis, the patient experiences a general decrease in sympathetic nervous system activity, a decrease in oxygen consumption and carbon dioxide elimination, a lowering of blood pressure and heart rate, and an increase in certain types of brain wave activity. These physiologic effects resemble those associated with other forms of deep relaxation.

Exactly how this state of relaxation makes the subject more receptive to suggestion isn't known. One theory, based on the results of a 1978 study, is that the left side of the brain (the center for verbalization) is less active under hypnosis, thereby allowing the right side of the brain to be more receptive to messages that can be used to transform the body.

---

enough to enter the somnambulistic state, making them good candidates for treatment. (See *Understanding hypnosis*.)

Hypnosis has been used for healing since ancient times; its use was central to the practices in early Greek healing temples. Modern applications date back to the 18th century, when Viennese doctor Franz Anton Mesmer used what he called "animal magnetism" to treat psychological and physiologic disorders such as hysterical blindness, paralysis, headaches, and joint pain. Using iron rods along with soothing words and gestures, Mesmer claimed he could realign his patients' "magnetic fluids." Although his magnetism theory was disproved, Mesmer's practices laid the foundation for hypnotherapy by demonstrating that medical conditions could be affected by the power of suggestion. Sigmund Freud also used hypnosis until he became uncomfortable with the powerful emotions it evoked in his patients.

INDICATIONS FOR HYPNOSIS

Hypnotherapy can be used to treat the following conditions:
- Behavioral problems
- Childbirth
- Chronic pain
- Depression
- Facial neuralgia
- Headaches
- Ichthyosis
- Low self-esteem
- Menstrual pain
- Osteoarthritis
- Pain and anxiety associated with dental procedures
- Phobias
- Reflex sympathetic dystrophy
- Rheumatoid arthritis
- Sciatica
- Tennis elbow
- Traumatic memories
- Whiplash

Hypnotherapy can also be used as an adjunct to surgical anesthesia.

The American Medical Association recognized hypnotism as a legitimate practice in 1958. Although it's still not completely understood, hypnosis has become accepted and used by a growing number of doctors, dentists, psychologists, and other mental health professionals in recent years.

TRAINING *The American Society of Clinical Hypnosis is the professional organization for doctors and dentists in the field. Training and certification are provided by the American Institute of Hypnotherapy for hypnotherapists and by the International Medical and Dental Hypnotherapy Association for doctors, dentists, and hypnotherapists. The National Guild of Hypnotists is the oldest certifying guild in the United States.*

Reported uses
Hypnotherapy has therapeutic application for both psychological and physical disorders. A competent hypnotherapist can facilitate profound changes in the patient's respiration and relaxation so that positive shifts in behavior and enhanced physiologic well-being can occur.

Almost any ailment that can be affected by the mind lends itself to treatment with hypnosis. Hypnosis has been shown to be effective in managing pain (including pain associated with dentistry and childbirth), reducing anxiety, and enhancing immune system function. As a method of pain management, hypnosis helps patients gain control over the fear and anxiety typically associated with pain, thereby also reducing the pain. In dentistry, hypnotherapy is used as a replacement for or adjunct to anesthesia, to reduce anxiety and post-procedural discomfort, and to control bleeding.

Pregnant women who receive hypnosis before delivery have reported having shorter, less painful labor and delivery. People with phobias such as fear of flying or stage fright can learn to establish a new response to the trigger activity through hypnosis. Hypnosis has even been used to help people stop smoking and to lessen bleeding in hemophiliacs. (See *Indications for hypnosis*.)

How the treatment is performed
The most essential condition required for successful hypnotherapy is the patient's willingness and desire to be hypnotized. A quiet, private environment that is free from distractions and a comfortable place for the patient to recline are the only types of equipment necessary for hypnotherapy.

Hypnotherapy should be performed only by a qualified practitioner. The hypnotherapist begins by addressing any concerns the patient has and illustrating how suggestion works in everyday life. The therapist also explains what to expect while in the trance — physical relaxation, distraction of the conscious mind, a narrowed focus of attention, increased sensory awareness, reduced awareness of physical surroundings, and increased awareness of internal sensations.

After testing the patient for suggestibility, the therapist asks him to concentrate on an object or the sound of the therapist's voice, guiding the patient into a state of relaxation. The therapist may express suggestions, such as "your eyelids are growing heavy," to help induce the hypnotic state. The sessions usually last from 60 to 90 minutes, depending on the goal and the patient's receptivity.

After the session, the therapist documents any changes in behavior or answers to questions the patient provided while in the hypnotic state. The therapist also documents the patient's response to the session.

Hazards
Because it deals with subconscious areas of the mind, hypnosis may elicit disturbing emotions or memories. If the patient becomes upset or aggressive, or exhibits strong negative emotions, the hypnotherapist should redirect him to a safe memory and terminate the session.

Clinical considerations
■ According to the World Health Organization, patients with psychosis, organic psychiatric conditions, or antisocial personality disorders shouldn't be treated with hypnosis.
■ Although hypnosis sessions usually involve only the therapist and the subject, it may be prudent to have a nurse or assistant sit in on sessions involving opposite sexes as a safeguard against liability.
■ Be aware that some patients experience light-headedness or psychological reactions after hypnosis. Be prepared to deal with these effects if they arise.

Research summary
Controlled studies have shown that hypnosis is effective for the treatment of childhood migraine headaches. A 1989 study of pain in chronically ill patients showed that those who underwent hypnosis increased their pain tolerance by 113%. Studies have also shown positive effects on the immune system, including increased immunoglobulin levels in children and increased white blood cell activity. Other reports have noted success in treating hay fever, asthma, warts, and allergic reactions.

One of the most unusual uses of hypnosis is in the treatment of a genetic skin disorder known as ichthyosis, in which the skin is covered with a hard, wartlike crust. This condition was considered incurable until an anesthesiologist used hypnosis on a teenager he thought had warts. After the hypnosis, the scaly crust fell off, and within 10 days, normal skin replaced it. Since then, hypnosis has often been used to treat this condition, usually resulting in a major improvement, if not a complete cure.

hyssop
Hyssopus officinalis

Hyssop has been used for centuries as an herbal medicine. In ancient times it was used as an insecticide, insect repellant, and pediculicide. Hyssop is obtained from the dried above-ground parts, including leaves and flowering tops, of *H. officinalis*. The oil, which is used in flavorings and extracts, is also made from the above-ground parts of the plant. One of hyssop's glycoside components, marrubiin, stimulates bronchiole secretions. Hyssop has strong antiviral effects, probably because of the caffeic acid, tannin, and high-molecular-weight components present. It may have some activity against human immunodeficiency virus-1 (HIV-1) replication and the herpes simplex virus. Hyssop is available as capsules and extracts.

Reported uses
Hyssop is used orally to treat upset stomach, liver and gallbladder complaints, indigestion, colds, fevers, respiratory and chest ailments, sore throat, asthma, uri-

nary tract inflammation, gas, and colic. It's also used as an expectorant and as an appetite and circulation stimulant.

Hyssop is used topically in a salve or compress to treat skin irritations, burns, bruises, and frostbite. The oil is used as fragrance in soaps and perfumes. It's used to flavor foods and extracts and as a flavoring in alcoholic beverages.

Administration
- Capsules: Two 445 mg capsules by mouth three times a day
- Extract: 10 to 15 gtt in water by mouth two to three times a day
- Tea (1 to 2 tsp dried hyssop tops in 5 oz boiling water): Gargle or consume three times a day.

Hazards
Hyssop may cause uterine stimulation. Using hyssop with anticonvulsants may counteract anti-seizure effects.

Pregnant patients should avoid use of hyssop because of possible uterine stimulation leading to miscarriage and hemorrhaging. Children should avoid use because of reports that 2 to 3 gtt of volatile oil over several days may cause tonic-clonic seizures. Also, patients with seizure disorders shouldn't use hyssop.

 SAFETY RISK *Hyssop has been associated with tonic-clonic seizures and neurotoxicity.*

Clinical considerations
- Only standardized dose forms of hyssop should be used.
- Internal use of hyssop oil is associated with seizures and possible neurotoxicity.
- Hyssop may alter the intended therapeutic effect of conventional drugs.
- If patient is pregnant or breast-feeding or is planning to become pregnant, advise her not to use hyssop.
- Advise patient to use hyssop only at the recommended dosages and to avoid long-term use.
- Inform patient that several other plants have variations of the name hyssop; however, these plants are not related to the genus *Hyssopus*.
- Tell patient to notify pharmacist of any herbal or dietary supplement that he's taking when obtaining a new prescription.
- Advise patient to consult his health care provider before using an herbal preparation because a conventional treatment with proven efficacy may be available.

Research summary
Hyssop appears to be a useful herbal compound. The action of its volatile oil exerts demulcent and expectorant effects. However, it must be used with caution due to its documented convulsive effects. The plant also appears to exhibit strong antiviral activity against HIV-1 in some studies. More studies are needed to verify the therapeutic efficacy of this claim.

Iceland moss

Cetraria islandica,
*eryngo-leaved liverwort, Iceland lichen,
lichen*

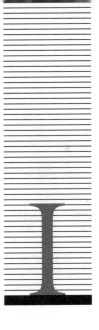

The mucilage components found in Iceland moss, lichenin and isolichenin, may have soothing effects on the oral and pharyngeal membranes. The bitter organic components may stimulate the appetite and promote gastric secretion. Iceland moss is available as dried whole plant of *Cetraria islandica* and as powdered herb extracts.

Reported uses
Iceland moss is used to soothe oral and pharyngeal membranes, relieve dry cough, stimulate appetite, and prevent infection, the common cold, dyspeptic complaints, and fevers. The alcohol-containing extract is used as a flavoring agent in alcoholic beverages.

Administration
- Tea: Simmer 1.5 to 3 g dried plant in 5 oz of boiling water, and then strain
- Extract: 4 to 6 g every day.

Hazards
Iceland moss may cause GI irritation. Using Iceland moss with aspirin or NSAIDS may exacerbate irritation of the gastric mucosa by these medicines. The fiber in Iceland moss can impair the absorption of oral drugs. Instruct patient to separate administration times by at least 2 hours.
   Patients with gastroduodenal ulcers or GI distress or disease should avoid using

Iceland moss because of the potential for mucosal irritation. Pregnant and breast-feeding patients should also avoid use because of potential lead contamination. Iceland moss shouldn't be used in treating children.

 SAFETY RISK *Because of potential lead contamination, the maximum daily dose of Iceland moss is 4 to 6 g.*

Clinical considerations

■ Warn patient not to treat symptoms of respiratory infection before seeking appropriate medical evaluation because doing so may delay diagnosis of a potentially serious medical condition.

■ Tell patient to only take recommended doses of Iceland moss and to discontinue if any GI distress occurs.

■ Advise patient to take Iceland moss at least 1 hour before or 2 hours after any other drugs.

■ Inform patient that taking Iceland moss with food may help prevent GI upset.

■ Advise patient not to delay treatment of an illness that doesn't respond after taking Iceland moss.

■ Advise patient to keep Iceland moss away from children and pets.

■ Tell patient to notify pharmacist of any herbal or dietary supplement that he is taking when obtaining a new prescription.

■ Advise patient to consult his health care provider before using an herbal preparation because a conventional treatment with proven efficacy may be available.

Research summary

The concepts behind the use of Iceland moss and the claims made regarding its effects haven't yet been validated scientifically.

Imagery

Imagery is a mind-body technique in which patients use their imagination to promote relaxation, relieve symptoms (or better cope with them), and heal disease. It isn't limited to visualization (picturing the desired result in one's mind); it can involve mentally hearing, feeling, smelling, or tasting as well. Like alternative therapies such as biofeedback, hypnosis, and meditation, imagery is based on the principle that the mind and body are interconnected and can work together to encourage healing.

Imagery has been used for therapeutic purposes since at least the Middle Ages, when Tibetan monks reportedly tried to visualize the Buddha healing diseases. Today, imagery is successfully used to control pain, to enhance immune function in elderly patients, and as an adjunctive therapy for a number of diseases, including diabetes mellitus. Imagery is widely used in cancer patients to help mobilize the immune system, alleviate the nausea and vomiting associated with chemotherapy, relieve pain and stress, and promote weight gain. It is also used in many cardiac rehabilitation programs and centers specializing in chronic pain.

According to imagery advocates, people with strong imaginations, those who can literally "worry themselves sick," are excellent candidates for using imagery to effect positive changes in their health. Like other relaxation techniques, imagery has documented physiologic effects: It can lower blood pressure, decrease heart rate, and affect brain wave activity; increase oxygen supply to the tissues and promote vascular dilation; and cause changes in skin temperature, cochlear and pupillary reflexes, galvanic skin response, salivation, and GI activity. Advocates believe imagery enhances the effectiveness of conventional medical treatments by allowing them to work in less time and minimizing their adverse effects. (See *Understanding imagery*.)

Palming and guided imagery are two of the more popular imaging techniques. In *palming,* the patient places his palms over his closed eyes and tries to fill his entire field of vision with only the color black. He then tries to picture the black changing to a color he associates with stress, such as red, and then mentally replaces that color with one he finds soothing, such as pale blue. In *guided imagery,* the patient is asked to visualize a goal he wants to achieve and then picture himself taking action to achieve it. An example is the pioneering technique developed by radiation oncologist O. Carl Simonton in the 1970s, in which cancer patients are taught to visualize their white blood cells destroying cancer cells, much like the video game Pac-Man character swallows its victims. This type of therapy is intended to complement traditional cancer treatments, not replace them.

TRAINING *The Academy for Guided Imagery in Mill Valley, California, trains health professionals in the use of interactive guided imagery, publishes a directory of imagery professionals, and provides educational materials and tapes for professionals and lay people. Practitioners who complete a 150-hour program can obtain certification in guided imagery.*

Reported uses

In addition to its documented effectiveness in reducing pain and inducing relaxation, imagery can also be an effective tool for reducing adverse effects of conventional treatments, stimulating the body's healing response, and helping patients tolerate medical procedures. Imagery also facilitates recovery and can strengthen coping skills in patients with acute or chronic illness. It has also been used to help patients clarify attitudes, emotions, behaviors, and lifestyle patterns that may be central to an illness. As an active means of relaxation, imagery is a central part of almost all stress reduction techniques.

Imagery can benefit patients in almost any medical situation in which problem solving, decision making, relaxation, or symptom relief is useful. It has even been used successfully to help people prepare for surgery and to speed post-surgical recovery. Additionally, imagery is a useful self-care tool. With proper instruction,

UNDERSTANDING IMAGERY

Imagery therapy is based on the theory that messages can be sent from the higher centers of the brain, where images are located, to lower centers, which regulate physiologic functions (such as breathing, heart rate, blood flow, blood pressure, digestion, immunity, and temperature). Images that arise from unconscious body processes and memories are believed to be located in the cerebral cortex, whereas images related to smell or feelings may be rooted in more primitive brain centers. The regulation of waking and sleeping rhythms, hunger, thirst, and sexual function may also be affected through imagery.

Picturing brain activity
Using positron emission tomography scanners, scientists have been able to determine which areas of the brain are active as a person performs various tasks. For example, the optic cortex, which is active when a person is looking at something, is also active when he visualizes. The auditory cortex is active not only in the presence of sound, but also when a person imagines a sound, just as the sensory cortex is active both when a person touches or is touched, and he imagines feeling.

Practitioners of guided imagery believe that if the cortex can create these imaginary realities, the lower centers of the nervous system — in the absence of conflicting information — can respond to them. This theory is the basis of sensory recruitment, in which various senses are stimulated simultaneously, increasing the amount of information sent through the lower brain centers and autonomic nervous system and thereby increasing the likelihood of achieving the desired response.

INDICATIONS FOR IMAGERY

The following conditions may be helped by imagery:

- Allergies
- Asthma
- Cancer
- Cardiac arrhythmias (benign)
- Chronic pain
- Cold symptoms
- Dysmenorrhea
- Excessive uterine bleeding
- Fibromyalgia
- Flu symptoms
- Functional urinary complaints
- GI symptoms related to stress
- Headaches
- Hypertension
- Menstrual irregularity
- Multiple sclerosis
- Premenstrual syndrome
- Smoking cessation
- Sprains and strains
- Surgical recovery

---

patients can use imagery to relieve stress, enhance immune function to fight a cold virus, and improve their sense of well-being. (See *Indications for imagery*.)

How the treatment is performed

For imagery to be successful, the patient will need a private, quiet environment that is free from distractions and a comfortable place in which to lie down. If a taped imagery sequence will be used, make sure the tape player is working and that the room has an electrical outlet.

Imagery can be practiced by an individual alone or led by a trained practitioner. Sessions with a therapist usually last 20 to 30 minutes. A variety of imagery techniques and paths can be used. The sample path described below, which focuses on relaxation, is one that most practitioners could conduct in almost any health care setting. For sessions that focus on altering specific disease states, the practitioner should consult with a

professional trained in imagery techniques.

The practitioner gathers any necessary supplies, washes his hands, and helps the patient into a comfortable position. The practitioner then explains the exercise and answers any questions the patient might have. When the patient is comfortable, the practitioner instructs him to close his eyes, and lowers the lights in the room.

Using a steady, soothing, low voice throughout the exercise, the practitioner instructs the patient to take a few deep breaths and imagine that with each breath, he is taking in calmness and peacefulness and releasing tension, discomfort, and worry. The practitioner tells the patient to let his breath find its own natural rate and rhythm, and to continue to breathe in calmness and peacefulness, and breathe out tension and worry.

The practitioner instructs the patient to imagine that he's breathing calmness into his feet and legs and releasing tension with each exhalation. The sequence is continued, moving from feet to head and having the patient breathe calmness into each successive body part. The practitioner reminds the patient not to make any effort during this process, but to let it happen in its own natural way. As each portion of the exercise is completed, the practitioner reminds the patient to let his whole body sink into a peaceful, relaxed state.

Next, the practitioner tells the patient to imagine himself in a place that is peaceful and beautiful. The practitioner suggests that he choose a place he has visited or imagined, or a special place where he would like to be. The practitioner encourages him to notice the details in this place — the colors, shapes, and living things he finds there. The patient should think about the sounds and smells of the place and pay attention to any feelings of peacefulness and relaxation.

The patient is allowed to spend as long as he wants in this place; he's told that when he's ready, he should allow the images to fade and slowly bring himself back to the outer world. The practitioner remains quiet until the patient opens his eyes. If he's willing, the practitioner discusses the experience with him, concentrating on the positive feelings of relaxation and peace. The practitioner documents the length of the session, the imagery path used, and the patient's response.

Hazards

One of the benefits of imagery is the relative absence of complications. Occasionally, an imagery session may lead a person to remember an unpleasant period or event in his life. If that occurs, stop the session and encourage the patient to tell you what he was seeing and feeling. If the patient becomes upset, remain with the patient. Notify a health care provider if necessary.

Clinical considerations

- Imagery is contraindicated in a psychotic patient.
- To enhance the effects of imagery, consider adding a smell to trigger the image that the patient is trying to experience.
- Be aware that a patient with breathing problems may have difficulty controlling his breathing.
- Taking the patient's blood pressure and pulse before and after imagery helps the patient to understand the physiological benefits of it.

Research summary

Numerous studies have referred to imagery's ability to produce the physiologic and biochemical changes listed above. Although most of the research evidence is based on small, unreplicated studies, the 1994 report to the NIH concludes that "there is a relationship between imagery of bodily change and actual bodily change. Without question, imagery calls for further and more precise investigation."

Immunoaugmentative therapy

Immunoaugmentative therapy (IAT) was developed by Lawrence Burton, a cancer researcher at St. Vincent's Hospital in New York City. The goal of his work is to balance four protein components in the blood in order to allow the immune system to fight cancer effectively. Although he originally practiced from a clinic on Long Island, Burton moved his research to the Grand Bahamas in 1977.

Reported uses

Burton's methods are used to cure cancer or prolong life in cancer patients.

How the treatment is performed

IAT treatment consists of giving cancer patients daily injections of a compound of four components — proteins and tumor antibodies — derived from the pooled blood of healthy donors. The four components of the injection are:
- Deblocking protein (DP) – an alpha 2 macroglobulin
- Tumor antibody 1 (TA1) – a combination of alpha 2 macroglobulin with other immune globulins (IgG and IgA)
- Tumor antibody 2 (TA2) – similar to TA1, but differing in potency and possibly in composition
- Tumor complement (TC) – a substance derived from the blood clots of patients with many types of cancer.

The tumor antibodies are used to fight cancer, while the protein component removes a "blocking factor" that prevents the immune system of the patient from recognizing and fighting cancer cells.

Hazards

Adverse reactions of this therapy include abscesses at the injection site and infection.

Clinical considerations

IAT is only available at the IAT clinic in the Bahamas. It is illegal to bring IAT products into the United States.

Research summary
There is no scientific evidence to support the claims of immunoaugmentative therapy. Studies have refuted an important tenet of the theory — that tumors produce "blocks" to hide cancer cells from the immune system.

indigo

Common indigo, Indian indigo, pigmentum indicum

Indigo has been used as an emetic, to purity the liver, reduce inflammation and fever, to alleviate pain, and to treat numerous other ailments from hemorrhoids to scorpion bites. During fermentation of the leaves, indigo is derived from indican, a glucoside constituent of several *Indigofera* species. Little is known about the pharmacologic effects of the herb. Indigo has emetic, anti-inflammatory, and antipyretic properties.

Reported uses
Indigo is used as an emetic; *I. tinctoria*, in particular, is used to treat nematodal infections and malignancies of the ovaries or stomach. Synthetic indigo has commonly been used intravenously or intramuscularly to test kidney function, and used during cystoscopy. In Chinese medicine, indigo is used to detoxify the liver and the blood, reduce inflammation and fever, and relieve pain. Throughout the world, indigo is still used commercially for dyeing wool and cotton.

Administration
The administration of indigo for medicinal purposes isn't well documented.

Hazards
Indigo may cause mild ocular irritation. Pregnant patients should avoid use because some species of *Indigofera* have teratogenic effects; breast-feeding patients should also avoid use. Any patient using indigo should use it with caution because data regarding its effects are lacking.

 SAFETY RISK *Use of indigo can lead to hepatotoxicity and mild ocular irritation.*

Clinical considerations
■ With the exception of *I. tinctoria*, many of the other *Indigofera* species are hepatotoxic. *I. spicata* has caused cleft palate and embryonic death when used by pregnant women.
■ If patient is pregnant or breast-feeding, advise her not to use indigo.
■ Advise patient to use indigo with caution because of risk of liver toxicity.
■ Advise patient to keep indigo away from children and pets.
■ Tell patient to notify pharmacist of any herbal or dietary supplement that he is taking when obtaining a new prescription.
■ Advise patient to consult his health care provider before using an herbal preparation because a conventional treatment with proven efficacy may be available.

 SAFETY RISK *Don't confuse this herbal product with false, wild, or bastard indigo (*Baptisia tinctoria*).*

Research summary
Although indigo has been used for centuries, the concepts behind its use and the claims made regarding its effects haven't yet been validated scientifically.

Irish moss

Carrageenan, carragheen, carrahan, Chondrus crispus, *chondrus extract*

Irish moss is obtained from the dried thallus of *Chondrus crispus*. It's a form of seaweed containing polysaccharides, vitamins, minerals, and iodine. The extract is known as carrageenan, a starch-like substance. This extract can be further differentiated into two types, k-carrageenan and l-carrageenan. The former type is the gelling fraction; the latter form is the non-gelling component.

Irish moss has expectorant, demulcent, anti-inflammatory, anticoagulant, anti-hypertensive, immunosuppressive, and antidiarrheal properties. It also interferes with the absorption of food, and may reduce serum cholesterol and possess antiviral activity. Irish moss is available as dried jellied fruit, jellies, puddings, raw leaves, and teas, in products such as Coreine, Gelcarin, Hydrogel, Seaspen, and Viscarin.

Reported uses

Irish moss is used to soothe irritating coughs that result from various respiratory infections, and to produce bulky stools in patients with chronic diarrhea. Because of its demulcent properties, Irish moss is also used to treat gastritis and peptic ulcer disease. Because it contains ammonium, calcium, magnesium, potassium and sodium esters of galactose and 3-6-anhydrogalactose copolymers it's also used as a nutritional supplement to facilitate recuperation in those with debilitating diseases. Irish moss can also be found as an ingredient in weight-loss products.

Irish moss is used as a skin softener in commercial cosmetic products and lotions. It's used topically to treat anorectal symptoms. In manufacturing, Irish moss can be used as a binder, emulsifier, thickener, and as a stabilizer in drugs, foods, and toothpaste.

Administration

A tea is prepared by boiling 1 oz (28 g) of dried plant in 1 to 2 pints of water for 10 to 15 minutes, and then straining. Dosage is 1 cup two to three times a day. Lemon, honey, ginger, or cinnamon may be added to enhance the flavor.

Hazards

Irish moss may cause bleeding, hypotension, cramping, diarrhea, and infection. There is an increased risk of bleeding when Irish moss is used concomitantly with anticoagulants. Irish moss may potentiate the hypotensive effects of antihypertensives. It may decrease the absorption of drugs. Advise patient to separate administration times by at least 2 hours.

Pregnant or breast-feeding patients should avoid use. Infants shouldn't be given Irish moss because it may suppress the immune system. Patients with underlying bleeding disorders or hypotension should use Irish moss with caution.

Clinical considerations

- Monitor blood pressure regularly during the course of therapy with Irish moss. Patient should also be monitored for signs and symptoms of bleeding.
- In patient receiving warfarin, closely monitor prothrombin time and International Normalized Ratio.
- Tell patient to avoid taking Irish moss within 2 hours of other drugs.
- If patient is taking Irish moss with an antihypertensive, instruct him to notify his health care provider if dizziness, light-headedness, or syncope occurs.
- If patient is using Irish moss to treat diarrhea, advise him to consult his health care provider if the diarrhea persists for longer than 3 to 4 days.
- Caution patient to keep Irish moss out of the reach of children.
- Avoid products that contain the degraded form of Irish moss because it has been known to cause lesions in animals.
- Store in airtight containers in a cool place.
- Tell patient to notify pharmacist of any herbal or dietary supplement that he is taking when obtaining a new prescription.
- Advise patient to consult his health care provider before using an herbal preparation because a conventional treatment with proven efficacy may be available.

Research summary

The concepts behind the use of Irish moss and the claims made regarding its effects haven't yet been validated scientifically.

jaborandi

Arruda brava, arruda do mato, jamguarandi, juarandi, maranhao jaborandi, Pilocarpus microphyllus

Jaborandi is obtained from dried leaves of *Pilocarpus microphyllus*. It contains volatile oils and three alkaloids: pilocarpine, isopilocarpine, and pilocarpidine. Pilocarpine, a parasympathomimetic, is the primary constituent and contributes to the herb's cholinergic properties, including salivation, perspiration, miosis, and increased GI tract motility.

Reported uses
Jaborandi was formerly used to induce sweating and diarrhea, but it's no longer used as a medicinal herb. It is, however, currently used to produce pilocarpine, and approved by the FDA for treating glaucoma.

Administration
Oral use of jaborandi is unsafe. Pilocarpine, a jaborandi constituent, is commercially available by prescription as an ophthalmic solution in various strengths.

Hazards
Adverse reactions to jaborandi may include seizures, hypotension, nausea, vomiting, diarrhea, bronchospasm, dyspnea, increased sweating, and hypersalivation.

Because jaborandi has teratogenic effects and promotes uterine stimulation, pregnant and breast-feeding women shouldn't use it. Oral consumption isn't recommended.

Clinical considerations

■ Patient with cardiac and circulatory diseases is particularly sensitive to adverse CV reactions.

■ Because of potential toxicity, jaborandi isn't recommended for oral or topical use.

■ Symptoms of toxicity can develop after ingestion of 60 mg or more of jaborandi, which is equivalent to 5 to 10 mg of pilocarpine.

■ Don't confuse this herbal product with *P. jaborandi* (*Pernambuco jaborandi*) or *P. pennatifolius* (Paraguay jaborandi).

■ Always advise pregnant and breast-feeding patient to avoid using jaborandi.

■ Warn patient not to take jaborandi before seeking medical attention because doing so may delay diagnosis of a potentially serious medical condition.

■ Tell patient to notify pharmacist of any herbal and dietary supplements that he's taking when obtaining a new prescription.

■ Advise patient to consult his health care provider before using an herbal preparation because a conventional treatment with proven efficacy may be available.

SAFETY RISK *If patient shows signs and symptoms of toxicity, such as bradycardia, bronchospasm, cardiac arrest, seizures, hypotension, dyspnea, nausea, vomiting, diarrhea, increased sweating, and hypersalivation, discontinue use. If toxicity develops, prepare for gastric lavage followed by administration of activated charcoal and atropine. Expect to give diazepam if seizures develop. Give intravenous fluids as directed if hypotension occurs. Patient also may undergo hemodialysis.*

Research summary

The concepts behind the use of jaborandi and the claims made regarding its effects haven't yet been validated scientifically.

Jamaican dogwood

Dogwood, fishfuddle, fish poison bark, fish poison tree, Piscidia piscipula, *West Indian dogwood*

Jamaican dogwood is obtained from the root bark of *P. piscipula* or *P. communis*. It contains isoflavones, organic acids, ichthynone, rotenones, and tannins. Both rotenone and ichthynone have produced toxic effects; rotenone may be carcinogenic. The liquid extract possesses sedative, hypnotic, antitussive, antipyretic, anti-inflammatory, and antispasmodic properties. Jamaican dogwood is available as dried bark and liquid extract.

 SAFETY RISK *Because of its rotenone and ichthynone components, Jamaican dogwood is toxic and should be avoided.*

Reported uses

Jamaican dogwood is used for anxiety, neuralgia, migraines, insomnia, and dysmenorrhea.

Administration

Because of its rotenone and ichthynone components, Jamaican dogwood is toxic and should be avoided. Root bark and liquid extract are no longer used.

Hazards

Adverse reactions of Jamaican dogwood include numbness, tremors, salivation, and sweating. When used with CNS depressants or herbs with sedative properties, such as calamus, calendula, California poppy, capsicum, catnip, celery, couch grass, elecampane, golden seal, gotu kola, hops, kava-kava, lemon balm, sage, sassafras, shepherd's purse, Siberian ginseng, skullcap, St. John's wort, valerian, wild lettuce, and yerba maté, it may enhance sedative effects.

Children shouldn't use Jamaican dogwood because neuromuscular depressant effects are potentiated in this age group. Pregnant and breast-feeding patients should avoid use as well.

Clinical considerations
■ Advise patient not to use Jamaican dogwood because of its potential toxicity and the lack of data regarding its efficacy.
■ Elderly patients are more sensitive to Jamaican dogwood's toxic effects. Suspect toxicity and contact the health care provider if patient complains of numbness, tremors, salivation, and sweating.
■ Don't confuse Jamaican dogwood with American dogwood (*Cornus florida*).
■ Caution patient to keep Jamaican dogwood out of the reach of children.
■ Tell patient to notify pharmacist of any herbal and dietary supplements that he's taking when obtaining a new prescription.
■ Advise patient to consult his health care provider before using an herbal preparation because a conventional treatment with proven efficacy may be available.

Research summary
Studies indicate that Jamaican dogwood is toxic and should be avoided due to its rotenone and ichthynone components.

jambolan

Jambul, jamum, java plum, rose apple, Syzygium cumini

Jambolan is derived from bark and seeds of *S. cumini* or *S. jambolana*. The bark contains gallic and ellagic acid derivatives, flavonoids, and tannins. Tannins in the bark cause astringent effects. Jambolan bark also has antibacterial, hypoglycemic, and sedative activity. The seeds contain fatty oils and tannins and possess hypoglycemic, anti-inflammatory, antipyretic, antispasmodic, sedative, tonic, antidepressant, and aphrodisiac properties. Jambolan is available as dried bark, powdered seeds, and liquid extract.

Reported uses
Jambolan bark is taken orally for nonspecific acute diarrhea. It's also applied to the skin, mouth, or pharynx to decrease mild inflammation. The bark has been used to treat bronchitis, asthma, and dysentery through oral administration, and for ulcers through topical application.

Jambolan seed is used for diabetes, flatulence, constipation, pancreatic and gastric disorders, muscle spasms, fatigue, depression, and anxiety. The seed is also used as an aphrodisiac or diuretic. In India, jambolan seed is used to manage diabetes-induced polydipsia.

Administration
■ Dried bark: 3 to 6 g by mouth every day
■ Liquid extract containing jambolan seed: 4 to 8 ml by mouth every day
■ Powdered seeds: 0.3 to 2 g by mouth every day
■ Tea (simmer 1 to 2 tsp of dried bark in 5 oz of boiling water for 5 to 10 minutes, and then strain)
■ Topical: Warm compress made from jambolan bark tea, applied as needed.

Hazards
The use of jambolan is associated with hypoglycemia. The seed may enhance hypoglycemic effects when used with insulin or oral hypoglycemics.

Pregnant and breast-feeding patients should avoid jambolan because its effects are unknown.

Clinical considerations
■ Monitor blood glucose level closely in diabetic patient who uses jambolan seed, because it may cause hypoglycemia.

■ Advise patient to consult his health care provider if diarrhea persists for longer than 3 or 4 days.

■ Instruct pregnant or breast-feeding patient to avoid using jambolan.

■ Warn patient not to take jambolan for a GI disorder before seeking medical attention because doing so may delay diagnosis of a potentially serious medical condition.

■ Tell patient to remind pharmacist of any herbal and dietary supplements that he's taking when obtaining a new prescription.

■ Advise patient to consult his health care provider before using an herbal preparation because a treatment with proven efficacy may be available.

Research summary
The concepts behind the use of jambolan and the claims made regarding its effects haven't yet been validated scientifically.

jimson weed

Angel tulip, Datura stramonium, *devil's apple, devil's trumpet, Jamestown weed, mad-apple, nightshade, Peru-apple, stinkweed, stinkwort, Stramonium, thorn-apple*

Jimson weed is most commonly used as dried leaves, with or without tips of flowering branches. The ripe seeds and flowers without leaves are also used. Seeds are small, long, flat, and dark yellow to brown. Jimson weed's primary action is anticholinergic, caused by 0.1% to 0.6% atropine, hyoscyamine, and scopolamine. All parts of the plant contain these compounds, but the highest concentration is in the seeds. Anticholinergic levels in other plant parts vary from year to year and from plant to plant. The alkaloids are readily absorbed across GI mucous membranes and across the respiratory tract. Anticholinergic effects usually occur

within 60 minutes and may last 24 to 48 hours because of impaired GI motility.

 SAFETY RISK *Jimson weed is listed as an unsafe herb by FDA. It isn't recommended for routine therapeutic use.*

Reported uses
Jimson weed is used to treat asthma and cough from bronchitis or influenza, usually by smoking cigarettes made from the leaves. It's also used to treat disorders of the autonomic nervous system. Little data exist to support routine therapeutic use of jimson weed.

Illicitly, the seeds have been chewed, the leaves smoked as cigarettes, and a tea brewed and ingested to cause hallucinations and euphoria.

Administration
Dosage and administration aren't well documented.

Hazards
Adverse reactions to jimson weed include headache, confusion, hallucinations, agitation, emotional lability, motor incoordination, restlessness, loss of consciousness, hyperthermia, tachycardia, dilated pupils, blurred vision, photophobia, dry mucous membranes, nausea, vomiting, decreased GI tract motility, dry mouth, urinary retention, tachypnea, dry, flushed skin, and hypertension leading to hypotension.

Additive effects may be seen with anticholinergics such as benzotropine, atropine, scopolamine; with antihistamines such as diphenhydramine; with phenothiazines such as prochlorperazine and promethazine; and with tricyclic antidepressants such as amitriptyline and imipramine. Use of jimson weed with deadly nightshade (belladonna) may cause additive anticholinergic toxicity.

Patients who are pregnant or breast-feeding should avoid use. Those with glaucoma, benign prostatic hyperplasia, urinary retention, tachycardia, or hypersensitivity to jimson weed should also avoid use.

SAFETY RISK *Jimson weed has been associated with seizures, arrhythmias, respiratory depression, and respiratory arrest. Fatal poisonings resulting from respiratory depression and circulatory collapse have been reported from adult doses equal to 10 mg of atropine (15 to 100 g of dried leaves or about 100 [15 to 25 g] of seeds). Fatal doses in children may be much smaller. Fatalities also reported with ingestion of brewed tea.*

Clinical considerations
■ Warn patient that jimson weed isn't recommended for routine therapeutic use.
■ Don't confuse jimson weed with deadly nightshade (*Atropa belladonna*), which has similar effects.
■ Tell patient to report signs and symptoms of anticholinergic toxicity: dilated pupils, impaired vision, dry mouth, heart palpitations, dizziness, confusion, hallucinations, and incoordination.
■ The antidote for anticholinergic toxicity is physostigmine. To avoid profound cholinergic effects, use it only for severe toxicity, including seizures, severe hypertension, severe hallucinations, life-threatening respiratory depression, or arrhythmias. Avoid using sedatives or phenothiazines to treat toxicity because they may have additive anticholinergic effects.
■ Advise patient to keep jimson weed away from children and pets.
■ Tell patient to notify pharmacist of any herbal and dietary supplements that he is taking when obtaining a new prescription.
■ Advise patient to consult his health care provider before using an herbal preparation because a conventional treatment with proven efficacy may be available.

Research summary
Jimson weed is listed as an unsafe herb by the FDA. It isn't recommended for routine therapeutic use.

jojoba

Buxus chinensis, *deernut, goatnut, pignut,* Simmondsia californica, S. chinesis

Jojoba oil has been used for many years as a hair conditioner and restorative, as well as in medicine and cooking. Jojoba is used by the Native Americans of the Southwest, and the Bureau of Indian Affairs has funded many of the research studies into the uses of the herb.

Wax (commonly called oil) from the seeds is odorless and colorless to light yellow. It readily penetrates the skin. Taken orally, it's absorbed, not digested, and stored in intestinal and liver cells. The oil contains 14% erucic acid, which in oral injestion has been reported to cause myocardial fibrosis. Seeds are dark brown, about the size of coffee beans or peanuts. The cosmetic industry uses jojoba in shampoos, conditioners, moisturizers, and sunscreens.

Reported uses
Jojoba is used topically to treat acne, psoriasis, and sunburn. It's also used to unclog hair follicles in the scalp, preventing buildup of sebum, which is believed to contribute to hair loss. Jojoba is a common ingredient in shampoos, conditioners, cosmetics, lotions, sunscreens, and cleaning products. It's used as an industrial lubricant because it doesn't break down at high temperatures.

Administration
Jojoba is used in a variety of topical preparations; administration varies according to product.

Hazards
Jojoba may cause contact dermatitis.

Clinical considerations
■ Minimal toxicity is reported after topical application of jojoba. No routine monitoring after topical application is needed.
■ Symptoms of contact dermatitis include itching, erythema, and occasional vesicle formation. Tell patient to report any skin irritation from jojoba-containing products.
■ Jojoba shouldn't be taken orally because of potential toxicity.
■ Teach proper skin care for the prevention of acne.
■ Teach patient to avoid excessive sun exposure.
■ Tell patient to notify pharmacist of any herbal and dietary supplements that he's taking when obtaining a new prescription.
■ Advise patient to consult his health care provider before using an herbal preparation because a conventional treatment with proven efficacy may be available.

Research summary
Research indicates that jojoba has antioxidant properties. One study in animals produced a 40% reduction of blood cholesterol, although the mechanism was not identified. More long-term studies must be undertaken to investigate this potential. Topical testing in animals resulted in no systemic effects.

Juice therapy

In juice therapy, the fresh, raw juice of vegetables and fruits are used as a means of nourishing and detoxifying the body, stimulating the immune system, and even treating certain health problems. Juice therapy is commonly used as a component of, or complement to, fasting, but it can also serve as a dietary supplement during times of stress or as part of a regular health maintenance program.

Some practitioners prefer juice over solid raw fruits and vegetables because juices require less energy to digest and are more easily absorbed in the body. In addition, the breakdown of fiber that occurs in the juicing process may allow the body to absorb ingredients that would otherwise be excreted. Some critics and nutritionists, however, say that whole fiber is an essential and beneficial component of raw produce that's necessary for proper bowel function and elimination.

Reported uses
Because they contain the same health-enhancing phytochemicals that fresh fruits and vegetables contain, juices provide similar health benefits — such as protection against chronic degenerative diseases — with regular use. However, specific juices may also have medicinal attributes that make them useful in treating certain conditions:
■ Cabbage — iron deficiency
■ Apple — laxative effect (from sorbitol)
■ Papaya — ulcer-healing properties (from papain)
■ Lemon — appetite-stimulating effect
■ Cherry — treatment of gout
■ Pineapple — anti-inflammatory effects (from enzyme bromelain)
■ Cranberry, blueberry — prevention of urinary tract infections.

Juices can be a useful source of nutrition for patients who are weak or have difficulty eating, such as those with cancer or acquired immunodeficiency syndrome.

How the treatment is performed
The two elements required for juice therapy are produce and a juice extractor. Pre-made fresh juices may also be obtained at health food stores and juice bars.

Whenever possible, organically grown produce should be used to ensure the optimal nutritional benefit and prevent in-

JUICING PRECAUTIONS

If your patient is on a juice therapy regimen, make sure he's aware of the following precautions associated with certain fruits and vegetables:

■ Remove the rinds of oranges and grapefruit because they are bitter and contain toxic substances.

■ Don't use the core of the apple because the seeds contain cyanide. (Most other seeds are safe to use.)

■ Remove the greens from carrots and rhubarbs before juicing because that part of the plant contains toxic substances.

■ Always remove the skins of tropical fruits, such as papayas, kiwis, and mangos, because they may contain harmful fungicides and pesticides that are illegal to use in the United States and Canada but permitted in other countries.

■ Very sweet juices (such as those made from grapes, pears, apples, and carrots) can cause bloating and gas and may be hard to digest. Diluting them with equal parts water or a less sweet juice is advisable.

■ When juicing potatoes, avoid those with a green tint, because this indicates the presence of the chemical solanine, which may cause abdominal pain, vomiting, and diarrhea.

■ To prevent GI discomfort, consume green juices gradually and in moderation.

ples could benefit a patient with anemia. Juices made from green vegetables such as dandelion greens, spinach, celery, and alfalfa sprouts are believed to promote detoxification. Fresh apple or carrot juice may be added to dilute or sweeten a green drink.

Most produce can be placed in the juicer with the leaves, stems, and skin intact. However, certain precautions should be followed when juicing some fruits and vegetables. (See *Juicing precautions*.)

After juicing, the fresh juice should be consumed immediately to prevent loss of nutrients. Some juicing advocates recommend drinking fruit and vegetable juices several hours apart to minimize gas and enhance digestion.

Hazards

Excessive juice consumption, or the use of skins or leaves containing toxic substances, can cause abdominal pain, gas, and bloating. Some juices are strong stimulants to the liver and gallbladder and may have a laxative effect.

Juice fasts are not recommended for pregnant or lactating women. Infants, young children, the elderly, and diabetic patients shouldn't use juice therapy unless under the care of a doctor. Juices may be contraindicated for patients with hyperglycemia or hypoglycemia.

Clinical considerations

■ Advise patient to avoid fruits or vegetables to which he's allergic.

■ Inform patient that juices are not considered a substitute for whole fruits and vegetables.

■ Make sure patient understands that frozen, canned, or bottled juices are not recommended for juice therapy because they contain preservatives and other chemicals that decrease nutritional value. Also, the high temperatures used in the pasteurizing process destroy the enzymes in the juice. To ensure optimal benefits, patient should drink juice made with fresh, organic fruits and vegetables.

gestion of pesticides and other chemicals. Bananas, strawberries, green beans, and apples, in particular, tend to have high pesticide residues. If this isn't possible, the produce should be washed using a vegetable brush or one of the various vegetable washes available.

Many different juice recipes are available; some use a variety of fruits or vegetables to provide specific health benefits. For example, an iron-rich juice made with beets, carrots, green pepper, and ap-

Research summary

The concepts behind the use of juice therapy and the claims made regarding its effects haven't yet been validated scientifically.

juniper

Baccae juniperi, *enebro, Genievre, ginepro, juniper berry,* Juniperi fructus, Juniperus communis, *Wacholderbeeren, zimbro*

Juniper berries have long been used as a flavoring in foods and alcoholic beverages such as gin. Gin's original preparation was used for kidney ailments. Immature berries are green, taking 2 to 3 years to ripen to a purplish blue-black. The active component is a volatile oil, which is 0.2% to 3.4% of the berry. The best described effect is diuresis, caused by terpinene-4-ol, which results from a direct irritation to the kidney, leading to increased glomerular filtration rate. Juniper berries are available as ripe berry, also called *berry-like cones* or *mature female cones,* fresh or dried, and as powder, tea, tincture, oil, or liquid extract.

Reported uses

Juniper berries are used to treat urinary tract infections and kidney stones. They're also used as a carminative and for multiple nonspecific GI tract disorders, including dyspepsia, flatulence, colic, heartburn, anorexia, and inflammatory GI disorders.

Juniper berries may be applied topically to treat small wounds and relieve muscle and joint pain caused by rheumatism. The fragrance is inhaled as steam to treat bronchitis. The oil is used as a fragrance in many soaps and cosmetics. Juniper berries are the principle flavoring agent in gin, as well as some bitters and liqueurs.

As a food, maximum flavoring concentrations are 0.01% of the extract or 0.006% of the volatile oil. Other reported effects of juniper include hypoglycemia, hypotension or hypertension, anti-inflammatory and antiseptic effects, and stimulation of uterine activity leading to decreased implantation and increased abortifacient effects.

Administration

- Dried ripe berries: 1 to 2 g by mouth three times a day; maximum 10 g dried berries daily, equaling 20 to 100 mg essential oil
- Liquid extract (1:1 in 25% alcohol): 2 to 4 ml by mouth three times a day
- Oil (1:5 in 45% alcohol): 0.03 to 0.2 ml by mouth three times a day
- Tea (steep 1 teaspoon crushed berries in 5 oz boiling water for 10 minutes, and then strain): three times a day
- Tincture (1:5 in 45% alcohol): 1 to 2 ml by mouth three times a day.

Hazards

Adverse reactions to juniper include local irritation and metrorrhagia. When used with antidiabetics such as chlorpropamide, glipizide, and glyburide, hypoglycemic effects may be potentiated. Concomitant use of juniper and antihypertensives may interfere with blood pressure. Juniper may potentiate the effects of diuretics such as furosemide, leading to additive hypokalemia. A disulfiram-like reaction could occur because of alcohol content of juniper extract.

There may be additive hypoglycemic effects when juniper is combined with other herbs that lower blood glucose level, such as Asian ginseng, dandelion, fenugreek, and Siberian ginseng. Juniper may have additive effects with other herbs causing diuresis, such as cowslip, cucumber, dandelion, and horsetail.

Women who are pregnant or breastfeeding should avoid juniper because of its uterine stimulant and abortifacient properties. Juniper shouldn't be used by those with renal insufficiency, inflammatory disorders of the GI tract (such as Crohn's disease), seizure disorders, or known hypersensitivity. It shouldn't be used topically on large ulcers or wounds because it may cause local irritation.

 SAFETY RISK *Juniper may cause seizures, kidney failure, and spontaneous abortion.*

Clinical considerations

■ Advise patient that he shouldn't take juniper preparations for longer than 4 weeks.

■ Overdose of juniper may cause seizures, tachycardia, hypertension, and renal failure with albuminuria, hematuria, and purplish urine. Monitor blood pressure and potassium, BUN, creatinine, and blood glucose level.

■ Warn patient not to confuse juniper with *cade oil*, which is derived from juniper wood.

■ Advise female patient to report planned or suspected pregnancy before using juniper.

■ Inform patient that urine may turn purplish with higher doses of juniper.

■ Tell patient to avoid applying juniper to large ulcers or wounds because local irritation (burning, blistering, redness, and edema) may occur.

■ Caution against using alcohol while taking juniper.

■ Recommend that patient seek medical diagnosis before taking juniper. Unadvised use of juniper could worsen urinary problems, bronchitis, GI disorders, and other conditions if medical diagnosis and proper treatment are delayed.

■ Tell patient to notify pharmacist of any herbal and dietary supplements that he's taking when obtaining a new prescription.

■ Advise patient to consult his health care provider before using an herbal preparation because a conventional treatment with proven efficacy may be available.

SAFETY RISK *Kidney damage may occur in patients taking juniper for extended periods. This effect may stem from prolonged kidney irritation caused by terpinene-4-ol or by tur-*

pentine oil contamination of juniper products.

Research summary

Juniper may have some benefit in diabetic treatment, but further study is necessary. Juniper has an extensive toxicology profile, and therefore must be used with caution.

karaya gum

Bassora tragacanth, Indian tragacanth, kadaya, kadira, katila, karaya, kullo, mucara, Sterculia gum, Sterculia tragacanth, S. urens, S. villosa

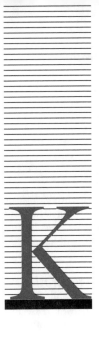

Karaya gum is a soft gum obtained from *Sterculia tragacanth,* a softwood tree cultivated in India and Pakistan. The use of karaya gum became widespread during the early 20th century. Today it's used in a variety of products to provide bulk, including cosmetics, hair sprays, and lotions. Karaya gum absorbs more than 100 times its weight in water; it forms a viscous solution in low concentrations in water and a gel or paste in higher concentrations. When taken orally, it isn't digested or systemically absorbed. In the GI tract, it acts as a bulk-forming laxative to stimulate peristalsis. The dried bark may have astringent properties, and the paste is reputedly antibacterial when applied topically to wounds. Karaya gum is available as a dry powder or paste.

Reported uses
Karaya gum is used industrially as a thickener in pharmaceuticals, cosmetics, hairsprays, lotions, and denture adhesives. It's also used as a binder or stabilizer in foods and beverages. Karaya gum is used orally as bulk-forming laxative akin to psyllium. It's applied topically as powder or paste to treat pressure sores or care for ileostomies or colostomies.

Administration
Karaya gum is generally recognized as safe for ingestion as a food additive.

Hazards
Adverse reactions associated with karaya gum include constipation, abdominal distention, dyspnea, cough, wheezing, and bloating. It may decrease absorption of oral drugs.

Patients with bowel obstruction should avoid using karaya or any other bulk-forming laxative. No information is available on use of karaya gum by pregnant or breast-feeding women.

Clinical considerations
- As with other bulk-forming laxatives, karaya gum may decrease absorption of drugs taken concurrently. This effect should be clinically insignificant with amounts found in food and pharmaceuticals.
- To maximize laxative effect, patient needs adequate fluid intake.
- Karaya gum may cause pain when applied topically to wounds.
- Encourage adequate fluid intake, and teach patient about increasing fiber in diet.
- Instruct patient to separate intake of oral drugs by 2 hours.
- Tell patient to notify pharmacist of any herbal and dietary supplements that he's taking when obtaining a new prescription.
- Advise patient to consult his health care provider before using an herbal preparation because a conventional treatment with proven efficacy may be available.

Research summary
Preliminary studies suggest that karaya gum may normalize blood sugar and plasma lipid levels, but this has not been well substantiated. The demulcent properties make it useful for relieving sore throats. Using karaya gum as a coating applied to dentures has been shown to reduce the adhesion of bacteria by 98%.

Widespread experience with the product throughout the United States and Europe has shown that the gum has not been associated with significant toxicity and is essentially inert when ingested.

kava

Ava, awa, intoxicating pepper, kava-kava, kava pepper, kawa, kawa-kawa, kew, Piper methysticum, *sakau, tonga, yagona*

Kava has been an important part of the Pacific island ceremonial cultures for many centuries, where its main use has been to induce relaxation in kava ceremony participants. Obtained from dried rhizome and root of *Piper methysticum*, a member of the black pepper family (Piperaceae), kava is used to make the beverage of the same name. Kava contains seven major and several minor kava lactones, both aqueous and lipid soluble. Pharmacologic effects result from lipid-soluble lactones. Their mechanism of action differs from that of benzodiazepines and opiate-agonists. Kava affects the limbic system, modulating emotional processes to produce anxiolytic effects. Kava lactones inhibit MAO type B, producing psychotropic effects. They also inhibit voltage-gated calcium and sodium channels, producing anticonvulsant and skeletal muscle relaxant effects. The kava lactone, kawain, inhibits cyclooxygenase and thromboxane synthase, producing antithrombotic effects on human platelets.

Kava is available as liquid extract, capsules, soft gel caps, liquid spray, and tea bags, in products such as Kavacin, Kava Tone, and St. John's Plus Kava Kava.

Reported uses
Kava is used orally to treat nervous anxiety, stress, and restlessness. It's used as a sedative, and to treat headaches, seizure disorders, the common cold, respiratory

tract infection, tuberculosis, and rheumatism. Kava is also used to treat urogenital infections including chronic cystitis, venereal disease, uterine inflammation, menstrual problems, and vaginal prolapse. Some herbal practitioners consider kava an aphrodisiac. Kava is used orally to promote wound healing. Kava juice is used topically to treat skin diseases, including leprosy. It's also used as a poultice for intestinal problems, otitis, and abscesses.

Administration
■ Anxiety: Dosage is 50 to 70 mg purified kava lactones three times a day, equivalent to 100 to 250 mg of dried kava root extract per dose. (By comparison, the traditional bowl of raw kava beverage contains about 250 mg of kava lactones.)
■ Restlessness: Dosage is 180 to 210 mg of kava lactones taken as a tea 1 hour before bedtime, or 1 cup three times a day. Tea is prepared by simmering 2 to 4 g of the root in 5 oz boiling water for 5 to 10 minutes, and then straining.

Hazards
Kava causes mild euphoric changes characterized by feelings of happiness, fluent and lively speech, and increased sensitivity to sounds. Adverse effects of kava include morning fatigue, headache, drowsiness, impairment of motor reflexes, visual accommodation disorders, pupil dilation and disorders of oculomotor equilibrium, mild GI disturbances, mouth numbness, hematuria, increased RBC count, decreased platelets and lymphocytes, pulmonary hypertension, scaly rash with chronic use, and reduced levels of albumin, total protein, bilirubin, and urea with chronic use.

Possible additive effects may occur when kava is used with antiplatelet drugs or MAO type B inhibitors. Kava lactones potentiate the effects of central nervous system (CNS) depressants, leading to toxicity. Kava may cause reduced effectiveness of levodopa therapy in patients with Parkinson's disease, apparently be-

cause of dopamine antagonism. Use of kava with calamus, calendula, California poppy, capsicum, catnip, celery, couch grass, elecampane, German chamomile, golden seal, gotu kola, hops, Jamaica dogwood, lemon balm, sage, sassafras, shepherd's purse, Siberian ginseng, skullcap, stinging nettle, St. John's wort, valerian, wild lettuce, or yerba maté may lead to additive sedative effects. There's an increased risk of CNS depression and liver damage when kava is used with alcohol.

Patients hypersensitive to kava or any of its components should avoid use. Depressed patients should avoid kava because of possible sedative activity; those with endogenous depression should avoid it because of possible increased risk of suicide. Pregnant women should avoid kava because of possible loss of uterine tone; those who are breast-feeding should also avoid it. Children younger than age 12 shouldn't use kava.

Clinical considerations
■ Patients shouldn't use kava with conventional sedative-hypnotics, anxiolytics, MAO inhibitors, other psychopharmacologic drugs, levodopa, or antiplatelet drugs without first consulting health care provider.
■ Adverse effects of kava are minimal at therapeutic dosages, and may occur at start of therapy but are transient.
■ Oral use is probably safe for 3 months or less; use for longer than 3 months may be habit forming.
■ Kava can cause drowsiness and may impair motor reflexes.
■ Patients should avoid taking kava with alcohol because of increased risk of CNS depression and liver damage.
■ Periodic monitoring of liver function tests and CBC may be needed.
■ Heavy kava users are more likely to complain of poor health. Some 20% of these patients are underweight with reduced levels of albumin, total protein, bilirubin, urea, platelets, and lymphocytes. They demonstrate increased HDL cholesterol and RBCs, hematuria, puffy

faces, scaly rashes, and some evidence of pulmonary hypertension. These symptoms resolve several weeks after kava is stopped. Extreme use (more than 300 g per week) may increase gamma-glutamyl transferase levels. Toxic doses can cause progressive ataxia, muscle weakness, and ascending paralysis, all of which resolve when kava is stopped.

■ Encourage patients to seek medical diagnosis before taking kava.

■ Tell patient to notify pharmacist of any herbal and dietary supplements that he's taking when obtaining a new prescription.

■ Advise patient to consult his health care provider before using an herbal preparation because a conventional treatment with proven efficacy may be available.

Research summary
Kava lactones are responsible for its mild sedative effects, which are additive with alcohol or benzodiazepines. Kava root is approved for conditions of nervous anxiety, stress, and restlessness by the German Commission E, and has also been presented in British pharmaceutical journals. However, it shouldn't be used for more than 3 months at a time.

Kelley regimen

An offshoot of the Gerson diet, the Kelley regimen is a metabolic therapy that became one of the most well-known alternative cancer treatments in the 1970s. It was developed in the early 1960s by an orthodontist, William Kelley, after he was told he had terminal pancreatic cancer. After receiving his diagnosis (which wasn't confirmed by a biopsy), Kelley studied the medical literature to try to determine what causes cancer.

He concluded that pollutants and an unhealthy diet impaired the body's ability to metabolize protein, and that this impairment could lead to tumor growth. Kelley believed that this metabolic prob-

lem stemmed from a deficiency of pancreatic enzymes, which were the body's first line of defense against malignant tumors. He began experimenting with doses of vitamins, minerals, and enzymes to develop a corrective diet. Kelley eventually claimed to have cured himself with his diet and began offering his special enzymes to the public.

Reported uses
Nearly all patients with cancer have distinct nutritional deficiencies, which can impair optimal immune function. Cancer patients are also prone to poor appetite and digestion. Many parts of the Kelley program are useful in correcting nutritional status, improving immune function, and optimizing digestion.

How the treatment is performed
Like the Gerson plan, the Kelley regimen includes drinking juices, receiving coffee enemas, and taking nutritional supplements such as pancreatic enzymes. However, because Kelley believed that no single diet was right for all patients, he developed different plans, to be used according to the patient's metabolic profile. Some patients were advised to adhere to a vegetarian diet, others were told to eat lots of red meat, and still others were given a mixed diet.

The basic plan advocates consumption of mostly raw foods (including raw liver), decreased protein intake, elimination of refined foods and additives, regular fasting and colonic irrigation, osteopathic or chiropractic manipulation to provide neurologic stimulation, and a positive spiritual attitude.

Hazards
The intensive nutritional supplements required by the Kelley plan could result in vitamin toxicity and electrolyte imbalances. The raw meats required could expose the patient to bacteria and viruses. Coffee enemas disrupt the GI system's natural balance of flora and can lead to dehydration, fatigue, and malaise.

They've also been associated with dangerous electrolyte imbalances.

Clinical considerations
Advise patients receiving the Kelley treatment to have blood tests periodically to check for nutritional and electrolyte imbalances.

Research summary
Nicholas Gonzalez, a New York immunologist, presented case histories of 50 of Kelley's patients in a 1987 book, *One Man Alone: An Investigation of Nutrition, Cancer, and William Donald Kelley* (out of print). In the early 1990s, the Congressional Office of Technology Assessment asked a panel of six doctors, three of whom were conventional oncologists, to review the 50 case histories presented in Gonzalez' book. The results generally reflected the doctors' medical approaches: The conventional doctors found Gonzalez's findings unconvincing, saying the patients' improvements could be attributed to earlier conventional treatments, while the remaining three doctors found the patient outcomes encouraging and worthy of further study. Investigations into the efficacy of the Kelley regimen continue.

kelp

Laminaria, Laminariae stipites, *seaweed, tangleweed*

Kelp is a dried preparation of various species of seaweed. It's also an ingredient of several dietary supplements and herbal preparations. Kelp is available as a constituent in a variety of products, including Activex 40 Plus, Cellbloc, Fat-Solv, Herbal Diuretic Complex, Kelp Plus 3, Plantiodine Plus, PMT Complex, Vitaforce 21-Plus, and Vitaforce Forti-Plus.

Reported uses
Kelp is used for regulating thyroid function, for goiter, as a bulk laxative, and for obesity. It's also used as an iodine source.

Administration
Oral dosage of kelp varies according to the product in which it's contained; see package inserts for dosage information.

Hazards
Adverse reactions to kelp include restlessness, insomnia, palpitations, hyperthyroidism, and allergic reaction. Kelp may decrease the effectiveness of diuretics because of its high sodium content. Combining kelp with lithium may enhance hypothyroid activity because of kelp's high iodine content. Prolonged ingestion of kelp can reduce iron absorption. Kelp may enhance hypothyroid activity because of its high iodine content. It may interfere with thyroid hormone replacement therapy.

Patients hypersensitive to kelp or any of its components, including iodine, shouldn't use it. Children, and women who are pregnant or breast-feeding, should avoid kelp as well.

Clinical considerations
- Kelp can worsen hyperthyroidism and acne. The high sodium content can worsen conditions that need sodium restriction. Because it inhibits iron absorption, kelp can worsen iron deficiency anemia. Kelp should be used with caution by patients with hyperthyroidism, those who need sodium restriction, and those with iron deficiency anemia.
- Use of kelp has been linked to heavy metal poisoning.
- Kelp may increase serum thyroid-stimulating hormone level, T4 level, and results of thyroid function tests using radioactive iodine uptake.
- Kelp toxicity may cause palpitations, restlessness, insomnia, and other changes.
- Encourage patient to seek medical diagnosis before taking kelp.

- Tell female patient to notify health care provider about suspected, planned, or known pregnancy if she is taking kelp.
- Caution patient to avoid kelp if he takes a diuretic, lithium, thyroid replacement hormones, anticoagulants, or an iron supplement.
- Tell patient to store kelp away from children and pets.
- Tell patient to notify pharmacist of any herbal and dietary supplements that he's taking when obtaining a new prescription.
- Advise patient to consult his health care provider before using an herbal preparation because a conventional treatment with proven efficacy may be available.

Research summary
The concepts behind the use of kelp and the claims made regarding its effects haven't yet been validated scientifically.

kelpware

Black-tang, bladder focus, bladderwrack, blasen-tang, cutweed, fucus, Fucus vesiculosus, knotted wrack, Quercus marina, rockweed, rockwrack, seawrack, tang

Kelpware contains over 600 mcg of iodine per gram of seaweed. A constituent, algin, has bulk laxative and soothing effects. An isolated fraction, fucoidin, has 40% to 50% of the anticoagulation activity of heparin. Live *Fucus* can concentrate heavy metals from seawater. Kelpware is available as dried brown algae plant, liquid extract, tablets, capsules, and soft gel caps, and as a constituent of products including Advantage, Aqua Greens, Atkins Dieters Better Living Multi Vitamins, Daily Essentials, Doctor's Choice, and Osteosupport.

Reported uses
Kelpware is used to treat thyroid disorders, iodine deficiency, lymphadenoid goiter, myxedema, obesity, arthritis, and rheumatism. It's also used for arteriosclerosis, digestive disorders, blood cleansing, constipation, bronchitis, emphysema, GU disorders, anxiety, skin diseases, burns, and insect bites.

Administration
- Dried plant: Usual dose is 5 to 10 g by mouth three times a day.
- Liquid extract (1:1): Typical dose is 4 to 8 ml by mouth three times a day.
- Tea (steep 5 to 10 g in 5 oz of boiling water for 5 to 10 minutes, and then strain): Tea is consumed three times a day.

Hazards
Adverse reactions to kelpware may include restlessness, insomnia, palpitations, anemia, hyperthyroidism or thyrotoxicosis, acne, and allergic reactions. Kelpware may cause a decrease in diuretic effectiveness because of its high sodium content. When kelpware is combined with heparin, low molecular weight heparin, and warfarin, there's an increased risk of bleeding. Prolonged kelpware ingestion can reduce iron absorption. Combining kelpware with lithium may enhance hypothyroid activity because of kelpware's high iodine content. Kelpware's high iodine content may interfere with thyroid hormone replacement therapy.

Patients hypersensitive to kelpware or any of its components, including iodine, shouldn't use it. Kelpware should be used with caution by patients with hyperthyroidism, those who need sodium restriction, and those with iron deficiency anemia. Children and women who are pregnant or breast-feeding should avoid using kelpware.

Clinical considerations
- Kelpware may increase PTT test results, serum thyroid stimulating hormone level, T4 level, and results of thy-

roid function tests that use radioactive iodine uptake.

- A case of heavy metal (arsenic) poisoning has been reported from ingestion of contaminated kelpware.
- Signs and symptoms of kelpware toxicity include palpitations, restlessness, insomnia, and possibly other changes.
- Warn patients not to confuse bladderwrack (kelpware) with bladderwort *(Utricularia)*, a freshwater pond plant.
- Encourage patient to seek medical diagnosis before taking kelpware.
- Tell female patient to notify health care provider about planned, suspected, or known pregnancy.
- Caution patient to avoid using kelpware if taking a diuretic, lithium, thyroid replacement hormones, an anticoagulant, or an iron supplement.
- Tell patient to notify pharmacist of any herbal and dietary supplements that he's taking when obtaining a new prescription.
- Advise patient to consult his health care provider before using an herbal preparation because a conventional treatment with proven efficacy may be available.

Research summary
The concepts behind the use of kelpware and the claims made regarding its effects haven't yet been validated scientifically.

khat

Abyssinian tea, Arabian tea,
Catha edulis, *chaat, gat, kat,*
Kus es Salahin, qut, Somali tea, tchaad,
tohai, tohat, tschut

Khat is a tree *(Catha edulis)* cultivated in southwestern Arabia and eastern Africa. It contains mainly sympathomimetic alkaloids cathinone and cathine (norpseudoephedrine). Cathinone and cathine antagonize the actions of physostigmine, but not those of tubocurarine. Chewing khat causes psychotropic effects from amphetamine-like compounds, which interact with the dopaminergic pathway. Both cathinone and cathine decrease appetite and increase locomotor activity. Khat is available as tender twigs and leaves wrapped in plastic, damp paper, or false banana leaves to avoid wilting and drying.

Reported uses
Khat leaf is used for treating depression, fatigue, obesity, and gastric ulcers. The leaf and stem are chewed by some people in East Africa and the Arabian countries as a euphoriant or appetite suppressant.

Administration
Usually, khat leaves are chewed and the juice is swallowed; the residues are kept in the cheek for up to 2 hours and then expectorated. Sometimes the chewed leaves are also swallowed. Occasionally, khat is brewed as a tea or crushed and mixed with honey to make a paste, which is taken orally.

Hazards
Adverse effects from use of khat may include euphoria, increased alertness, garrulousness, hyperactivity, excitement, aggressiveness, anxiety, manic behavior, insomnia, malaise, lack of concentration, psychotic reactions, migraine, tachycardia, palpitations, increased blood pressure, pulmonary edema, pupil dilation and decreased intraocular pressure, stomatitis, esophagitis, gastritis, constipation, keratosis of the buccal mucosa, temporomandibular joint dysfunction, periodontal disease, increased respiratory rate, hyperthermia, and sweating. Khat may cause increased sexual desire in women and increased libido in men, followed by loss of sexual drive, spermatorrhea, and impotence. Use of khat while taking ampicillin or amoxicillin may decrease the bioavailability of antibiotic drug.

Patients hypersensitive to khat or any of its components should avoid use.

Pregnant women should avoid it because it may reduce birth weight. Breast-feeding mothers should avoid khat because it contains norpseudoephedrine, which passes into breast milk.

 SAFETY RISK *Khat may cause cerebral hemorrhage, myocardial infarction, and cirrhosis.*

Clinical considerations

- Advise patients with diabetes, hypertension, tachyarrhythmias, glaucoma, migraines, GI disorders, or underlying psychotic disorders to use khat with caution.
- Although khat doesn't cause physical dependence, it does cause psychological dependence and can cause serious physical and psychological adverse effects.
- Long-term use of khat may lead to hypertension in young adults, increased susceptibility to infection, insomnia, and disturbed circadian rhythms.
- Khat suppresses the appetite, causing users to skip meals, decrease adherence to dietary advice, and increase consumption of sweetened beverages, potentially leading to hyperglycemia.
- Advise patients to store khat away from children and pets.
- Caution female patient to notify health care provider about planned, suspected, or known pregnancy.
- Tell patient to notify pharmacist of any herbal and dietary supplements that he's taking when obtaining a new prescription.
- Advise patients to consult his health care provider before using an herbal preparation because a conventional treatment with proven efficacy may be available.

Research summary

The concepts behind the use of khat and the claims made regarding its effects haven't yet been validated scientifically.

khella

Ammi daucoides, A. visnaga, *bishop's weed, greater Ammi, khella fruits, visnaga*

Khella is derived from the fruits and seeds of *Ammi visnaga*, a member of the carrot family. One standardized form contains a minimum of 10% gamma-pyrones, calculated as 100 mg khellin. One constituent, visnadin, acts as a mild positive inotrope by dilating coronary vessels and increasing coronary and myocardial circulation. Another component, khellin, is commercially available and used as a vasodilator in treating bronchial asthma and angina pectoris. Khella is available as capsules, tablets, and tea, in products such as Doctor's Choice for Heart Health.

Reported uses

Khella is used orally for angina pectoris, cardiac insufficiency, paroxysmal tachycardia, extrasystoles, hypertonia, asthma, whooping cough, and cramp-like complaints of the abdomen. Khella extracts are used topically for psoriasis.

Administration

- Capsules or tablets: Average daily dose is 20 mg gamma-pyrones by mouth. To increase HDL, take khellin 50 mg four times a day
- Tea: Khella is rarely used as a tea, but it's prepared by pouring boiling water over the powdered fruits, soaking for 10 to 15 minutes, then straining.

Hazards

Adverse reactions associated with khella include dizziness, headache, insomnia, nausea, constipation, lack of appetite, elevated liver transaminases and gamma-glutamyl transferase, cholestatic jaundice, phototoxicity, skin cancer, and itching. Using khella with hepatotoxic drugs may cause additive effects. Using it with digitoxin may decrease therapeutic effect and/or toxicity. Concomitant use of khella and alcohol may lead to hepato-toxicity. Khella may cause photosensitivity reactions.

Patients hypersensitive to khella or any of its components should avoid the herb. It shouldn't be used by women who are pregnant or breast-feeding, by patients with liver disease, or by people who are prone to skin cancer.

Clinical considerations
■ Oral use of khella may raise liver enzyme levels.

■ Although chemical interactions to khella have not been reported in clinical studies, tell patient it may interfere with therapeutic effect of conventional drugs.

■ Warn patient not to take khella for cardiac failure before seeking appropriate medical evaluation because doing so may delay diagnosis of a potentially serious medical condition.

■ Advise patient to store khella away from children and pets.

■ Warn patient against taking khella with alcohol or with hepatotoxic drugs.

■ Tell patient taking khella to protect against sun exposure.

■ Advise female patient to notify health care provider about planned, suspected, or known pregnancy before taking khella.

■ Tell patient to notify pharmacist of any herbal and dietary supplements that he's taking when obtaining a new prescription.

■ Advise patient to consult his health care provider before using an herbal preparation because a conventional treatment with proven efficacy may be available.

Research summary
The concepts behind the use of khella and the claims made regarding its effects haven't yet been validated scientifically.

lady's mantle

Alchemilla vulgaris, *bear's foot,
dew cup, leontopodium, lion's foot,
nine hooks, stellaria*

Lady's mantle is obtained from the root,
stem, leaves, and flowers of the *Alchemilla
vulgaris* plant. The above-ground parts of
Lady's mantle contain tannins, mainly
ellagic acid glycosides (6% to 8%), and
various flavonoids, such as quercetin.
Tannins impart a mild topical astringent
that's useful in treating wounds. It's also
used to treat gastrointestinal ailments.
Lady's mantle is available as tea, tablets,
tincture, ointment, and drops.

Reported uses

Lady's mantle is used as a topical astringent for wounds, ulcers, eczema, and skin
rashes.

The tea is useful in controlling mild diarrhea; it has been used also to reduce
uterine bleeding, ease menstrual cramps,
and regulate the menstrual cycle.

Administration

■ Tablets: For acute diarrhea, 1 tablet is
taken by mouth every 30 to 60 minutes;
for chronic diarrhea, 1 tablet is taken by
mouth one to three times a day
■ Tea (steep 2 to 4 g of dried herb in 5 oz
of boiling water for 10 minutes): Tea is
taken in three divided doses, between
meals
■ Tincture: For acute diarrhea, 5 drops
of tincture are taken by mouth every 30

to 60 minutes; for chronic diarrhea, 5 drops are taken 1 to 3 times a day
- Topical: Apply ointment or fresh or dried roots to the area twice daily.

Hazards
Lady's mantle may cause liver damage in some patients; thus, patients with liver dysfunction should avoid its use. The herb should not be given to pregnant or breast-feeding patients because its safety has not been determined.

Clinical considerations
- Monitor patient's liver function as long-term use may lead to liver dysfunction.
- Advise patient to seek medical attention before taking lady's mantle for diarrhea to avoid delay in diagnosing an illness.
- Warn patient not to take lady's mantle longer than 4 days for control of diarrhea.
- If diarrhea persists for longer than 3 to 4 days, patient should seek medial attention.
- Tell patient to remind prescriber and pharmacist of any herbal or dietary supplement that he's taking when obtaining a new prescription.
- Advise patient to consult his health care provider before using an herbal preparation because a treatment with proven efficacy may be available.

 SAFETY RISK *Don't confuse lady's mantle with Alpine lady's mantle* (A. alpina), *which is unapproved by the German Commission E owing to lack of documented safety and effectiveness.*

Research summary
The concepts behind the use of lady's mantle and the claims made regarding its effects haven't yet been validated scientifically.

lady's slipper

American valerian, bleeding heart, Cypripediium calceolus, *moccasin flower, monkey flower, nerve root, Noah's ark, slipper root, Venus shoe, yellows*

Lady's slipper is obtained from the dried rhizome, with the roots, of the *Cypripedium calceolus*, a member of the orchid family.

Lady's slipper species may contain volatile oils, tannins, and quinones. These constituents may be responsible for the herb's effect on bleeding, diarrhea, menorrhagia, and pruritus. Lady's slipper is usually used in combination with other herbs, especially valerian. It's available as a liquid extract, powdered root, dried root, tea, and tincture.

Reported uses
Lady's slipper is made into a tea for nervousness, headaches, insomnia, and emotional tension. It's also a mild sedative and hypnotic. Its GI antispasmodic effects may be useful in the treatment of diarrhea. Lady's slipper is also used for menorrhagia and topically for pruritus.

Administration
- Dried root made into an infusion: 2 to 4 g by mouth three times a day
- Extract: (1:1 in water or 45% ethanol): 2 to 4 ml by mouth three times a day.

Hazards
Patients using lady's slipper may experience sedation, giddiness, and headache. Hallucinations and restlessness have also been reported, as has contact dermatitis. Lady's slipper prepared with alcohol may cause a disulfiram-like reaction. If used in conjunction with dopamine agonists, there may be risk of increased hallucinations. Because of the sedative effect of lady's slipper, use with other sedatives or hypnotics may cause increased drowsiness.

Lady's slipper shouldn't be used by patients allergic to orchids or those prone to headaches. It shouldn't be used by pregnant or breast-feeding patients.

Clinical considerations

■ Monitor patient for psychotic behavior or headaches related to the use of lady's slipper.

■ Instruct patient to notify his health care provider of any potential allergic reaction.

■ Tell patient to remind prescriber and pharmacist of any herbal or dietary supplement that he's taking when obtaining a new prescription.

■ Advise patient to consult his health care provider before using an herbal preparation because a treatment with proven efficacy may be available.

 SAFETY RISK *Caution patient not to drive or perform hazardous tasks while taking lady's slipper because of the potential for increased sedation.*

Research summary

The concepts behind the use of lady's slipper and the claims made regarding its effects haven't yet been validated scientifically.

lavender

Aspic, Lavandula angustifolia, L. officinalis, L. spica, L. stoechas, L. dentate, L. pubescens, *lavendin, spike lavender*

Lavender is an aromatic evergreen shrub, native to the Mediterranean region, that reaches a height of about 3 feet. The fresh flowering tops produce small blue to purple flowers, which are harvested for their essential oils and extracts. Lavender has been used for many years in folk medicine for a variety of ailments. The volatile oil of lavender (1% to 3%) contains more than 100 monoterpene components, up to 40% linalyl acetate and linalool, and less than 1% camphor. Several coumarins, ursolic acid, flavonoids, and tannins are also found in the plant. Monoterpenes account for the reported antiseptic actions of the oil. Linalool and linalyl acetate account for the central nervous system (CNS) depression associated with its use.

Reported uses

Lavender oil is used as a bath oil and in soaps, other bath products, cosmetics, and candles; the flowers are also added to sachets and potpourri. It's also used as an antiseptic to treat minor scrapes, burns, and cuts. Lavender oil is also used in the topical treatment of functional circulatory disorders. When used orally, topically, or by inhalation, the oil has a calming effect and a mild sedative effect. The flowers have been used as a tea for abdominal complaints, nervous stomach, dyspepsia, Roehmheld syndrome (a rose-colored rash appearing in certain diseases), and intestinal discomfort. Lavender has also been used as a constituent in some commercial herbal antidiabetic preparations.

Administration

■ Dried flowers: 20 to 100 g dried flowers added to a warm bath

■ Oil: 1 to 4 drops by mouth on a sugar cube or diluted in a carrier oil (2% to 5%) as a topical massage

■ Tea (steep 1 to 2 teaspoons dried flowers in 5 oz of hot water): 1 cup of tea three times a day.

Hazards

The use of lavender may be associated with CNS depression, confusion, dizziness, syncope, drowsiness, headache, and neurotoxicity. Respiratory depression and contact dermatitis may also occur. Use of lavender with CNS depressants may potentiate their effect. When lavender is used with alcohol, the patient is at increased risk of CNS depression. Because lavender has antidiabetic properties, and has been shown to lower blood sugar in animals, concomitant administration with antidiabetic medications may lead to hypoglycemia.

Pregnant patients and breast-feeding patients should avoid the use of lavender. Patients with hypersensitivity to lavender should avoid its use.

Clinical considerations

- Advise patient about lavender's drug interactions.
- Monitor patient for an allergic reaction.
- Warn patient to avoid hazardous activities while taking lavender owing to its CNS depressant effects.
- Advise patient to store lavender away from heat and light.
- Warn patient to keep lavender away from pets and children.
- Tell patient to remind prescriber and pharmacist of any herbal or dietary supplement that he's taking when obtaining a new prescription.
- Advise patient to consult with his health care provider before using an herbal preparation because a treatment with proven efficacy may be available.

 SAFETY RISK *Don't confuse true lavender oil with lavendin or spike lavender; the latter two have high levels of camphor and may elicit neurotoxicity.*

Research summary

Studies are ongoing into lavender's efficacy in multiple indications, such as anticancer activity, relief of perineal discomfort related to childbirth, and lowering of blood glucose and cholesterol.

lemon

Citrus limon, limon

Lemon is a common fruit found in many parts of the world. The medicinal parts of the plant include the fruit, fruit juice, peel, and oil expressed from the peel. Expressed oil constitutes 2.5% of the peel,

and consists mainly of monoterpenes (up to 70% limonene); some sesquiterpenes, such as bisabolol; several coumarins and furanocoumarins; and citrus bioflavonoids, such as hesperidan, rutin, and naringoside. The juice contains bioflavonoids plus vitamin C. Pectin is mainly found in the white endocarp of the peel. The bioflavonoids are used to treat vascular insufficiency and problems with capillary fragility by decreasing porosity. Bisabolol possesses some anti-inflammatory activity. The coumarins and furanocoumarins are photodermatoxic. Various monoterpenes produce antispasmodic (1,8 cineole), antimutagenic (limonene), antitumor or chemopreventive (limonene), antioxidant (myrcene), irritant (terpinene-4-ol), and antiviral (a-pinene) actions. Lemon is available as fresh fruit, juice, essential oil, and extract.

Reported uses

Lemon is used extensively as a food and flavoring. The juice is a good source of vitamin C, potassium, and bioflavonoids. Lemon has also been used as a mild diuretic and has a mild anti-inflammatory effect. Lemon scent is often added to soaps, cleaners, and cosmetics.

Administration

Lemon is taken internally as an oil, tincture, and fresh fruit, and may also be applied topically.

Hazards

Patients with known hypersensitivity to citrus should avoid the use of lemon. Ingestion of the expressed oil by pregnant women is contraindicated.

Clinical considerations

- Topical application of lemon to mucous membranes may cause irritation.
- Warn patient that application of lemon oil to skin exposed to sunlight may cause photodermatoxicity.
- Topical products should contain no more than 2% expressed oil to reduce toxicity.

- Alert patient to discontinue use should adverse skin reactions occur.
- Tell patient to remind prescriber and pharmacist of any herbal or dietary supplement that he's taking when obtaining a new prescription.
- Advise patient to consult his health care provider before using an herbal preparation because a treatment with proven efficacy may be available.

Research summary
The concepts behind the use of lemon and the claims made regarding its effects haven't yet been validated scientifically.

lemon balm

Balm, honey plant, cure-all,
dropsy plant, Melissa,
Melissa officinalis,
sweet balm, sweet Mary

Lemon balm is native to southern European countries, where it's planted in gardens to attract bees. It gives off a delicate lemon scent when the leaves are bruised. Lemon balm has been used for the treatment of wounds. It's also effective for the treatment of influenza, insomnia, anxiety, depression, and nervous stomach. The action of lemon balm is a result of volatile oil consisting of 0.1% to 0.2% citral a (gernial) and b (neral), limonene, small amounts of flavonoids, tannins, protocatechuic and caffeic acids, and urosolic and promolic acids. The latter may account for its use as a carminative to settle the stomach. The volatile oil components account for the herb's diaphoretic effects. Limonene, oleaholic acid, and geranial have demonstrated sedative actions. Citral has an estrogenic effect. Rosmarinic acid and the tannins have antiviral actions.

Reported uses
Because lemon balm has antiviral activity, it's used in the treatment of herpes simplex cold sores. It's also used to treat upset stomach and insomnia. Lemon balm is used to treat palpitations related to anxiety or nervousness, vomiting, migraine, and high blood pressure. Lemon balm also exerts an antithyroid effect, and may be useful in treating some psychiatric disorders.

Administration
- Tea: 1.5 to 4.5 g per cup of tea as needed (or the equivalent in other preparations)
- Cream (1% or a 50:1 to 70:1 extract of lemon balm): Apply to herpetic lesion 2 to 4 times a day.

Hazards
Use of lemon balm may cause contact dermatitis. Lemon balm prepared with alcohol may cause a disulfiram-like reaction.

Patients with glaucoma, and those with hypersensitivity to lemon balm or other citrus, should avoid use. Pregnant and breast-feeding women, and patients with benign prostatic hyperplasia or thyroid disorders, should use with caution.

Clinical considerations
- Have patient discontinue use should ocular pain or rash develop.
- Tell patient not to use if allergic to lemon-scented soaps or perfumes.
- Caution patient not to use lemon balm oil orally; brewed tea is more effective and is well tolerated.
- Warn patient about the sedative effects of lemon balm, and caution him to avoid use if driving or doing other potentially hazardous activities.
- Advise patient not to take herb for anxiety or a sleep disorder before seeking medical attention, as doing so may delay diagnosis of a potentially serious medical condition.
- Tell patient to remind prescriber and pharmacist of any herbal or dietary supplement that he's taking when obtaining a new prescription.

■ Advise patient to consult his health care provider before using an herbal preparation because a treatment with proven efficacy may be available.

Research summary
The concepts behind the use of lemon balm and the claims made regarding its effects haven't yet been validated scientifically.

lemongrass

Carmmol, capim-cidrao,
Cymbopogon citratus, C. nardus,
citronella, fevergrass, Indian verbena

Lemongrass is cultivated in Central and South America and Australia. The medicinal parts of the lemongrass plant are the dried leaves, the lemongrass oil of *Cymbopogon citratus*, and the citronella oil of *C. nardus*.

Lemongrass contains alkaloids, a saponin fraction, and cymbopogonol. Fresh leaves contain 0.4% to 0.5% volatile oil that contains citral, myrcene, geranial, and several other fragrant compounds. Myrcene may have some peripheral analgesic activity similar to peripherally acting opiates that directly down-regulate sensitized receptors.

Reported uses
Lemongrass is used topically as an analgesic for neuralgic and rheumatic pain and strains, and as a mild astringent. The crushed leaves are used topically as a mosquito repellent. The essential oil is used as a food additive and also in perfumes. Internally, lemongrass is used as an antispasmodic and for the treatment of nervous and GI disorders.

Administration
■ Oil: Applied topically for pain
■ Tea: Prepared by adding 2 to 4 g of fresh or dried leaves to 5 oz of boiling water.

Hazards
Lemongrass may cause dry mouth, polyuria, allergic reactions, hypotension, and increased liver enzymes. Lemongrass has been found to have a diuretic effect in rats. Concomitant use of lemongrass with a diuretic may cause excess diuresis. Concomitant use of lemongrass with an antihypertensive agent may lead to hypotension. Lemongrass may exert an antimicrobial and antifungal effect. Concomitant use of lemongrass with an antibiotic and/or antifungal may lead to an enhanced effect.

Patients who are pregnant or breast-feeding or with a history of liver dysfunction shouldn't use this herb.

Clinical considerations
■ Tell patient that lemongrass may cause increased frequency of urination.
■ Monitor patient's liver enzymes.
■ Advise patient to keep lemongrass out of reach of children.
■ Tell patient to remind prescriber and pharmacist of any herbal or dietary supplement that he's taking when obtaining a new prescription.
■ Advise patient to consult his health care provider before using an herbal preparation because a treatment with proven efficacy may be available.

Research summary
Studies have shown lemongrass to be useful as an antitumor agent and a fever reducer. There has also been some indication that lemongrass has antiradical and antioxidant activity.

licorice

Glycyrrhiza glabra, *sweet root,*
sweet wood, sweet wort

Licorice is obtained from *Glycyrrhiza glabra*, varieties of which are indigenous to Europe and Asia. The medicinal parts include the unpeeled, dried roots and runners, the peeled dried roots, and the rhizome with the roots.

Licorice contains 7% to 10% glycyrrhizin (glycyrrhizic acid), natural sugars, glucose, mannose, sucrose, flavonoids, isoflavonoids, and sterols (betasitosterol and stigmasterol). Glycyrrhizin is a glycoside 50 times sweeter than sugar. Licorice has been found to stimulate the release of secretin, a potential mediator of antiulcer activity. Carbenoxolene, a semisynthetic ester of glycyrrhetic acid, is an active ingredient for treating stomach ulcers.

Licorice has shown anti-inflammatory and antiarthritic effects by inhibiting prostaglandin activity, which may make it useful in treating pain and inflammation from arthritis. The active ingredient, glycyrrhetinic acid, inhibits 11-beta-hydroxydehydrogenase, an enzyme that prevents cortisol from acting as a mineralocorticoid. Inhibiting this enzyme allows increased mineralocorticoid activity, or aldosterone-like activity, leading to sodium and water retention and potassium excretion. Many reports have been made about severe toxicity caused by these effects. Licorice is available in products such as Herbal Nerve (Canada), Licorice Power, Lightning Cough Remedy, Phyto Power, and Wild Countryside Licorice Root.

Reported uses
Licorice is used to treat stomach ulcers and as an expectorant. It's also used in sweets, soft drinks, medicines, and chewing tobacco as a flavoring agent.

Administration
■ Capsules: 5 to 15 g a day of licorice root (200 to 600 mg glycyrrhizin) by mouth a day; daily intake greater than 50 g of the herb is considered toxic
■ Tea (steep 1 teaspoon of licorice extract in 8 oz boiling water for 5 minutes): 1 cup of tea after each meal
■ Drops: 25 drops taken four times a day.

Hazards
Licorice can cause a variety of adverse reactions, including numbness, tingling, paralysis, hypokalemia, and hypernatremia. There have been reports of hypertension, heart failure, and arrhythmias, most likely due to the effects of hypokalemia and hypernatremia. Licorice may cause edema, myopathy, and muscle cramps. Vision loss has also been reported. Use of licorice with antiarrhythmics such as procainamide and quinidine may cause hypokalemia and torsades de pointes. Use with antihypertensives may render the antihypertensive medication less effective. Use of licorice with corticosteroids may have an additive effect. Patients using licorice with digoxin are at risk for hypokalemia and digoxin toxicity. Use of diuretics with licorice may worsen hypokalemia. Smoking may reduce the metabolism of licorice and lead to potential licorice toxicity.

Patients who are pregnant, breastfeeding, or hypersensitive to licorice, or those with hypokalemia, arrhythmias, diabetes, glaucoma, or history of cerebrovascular accident or renal, hepatic, or cardiac disease should avoid the use of licorice.

Clinical considerations
■ Monitor patient for signs of hypokalemia or hypernatremia.
■ Assess other medications patient is taking for possible interactions.
■ Monitor patient's blood pressure closely.
■ Warn patient to notify his health care provider if he develops swelling, muscle cramps, tiredness, or weakness.
■ Warn patient not to take herb for symptoms prior to speaking with his health care provider, as this may delay medical diagnosis.
■ Tell patient to remind prescriber and pharmacist of any herbal or dietary supplement that he's taking when obtaining a new prescription.
■ Advise patient to consult his health care provider before using an herbal

preparation because a treatment with proven efficacy may be available.

 SAFETY RISK *Warn patient not to take large doses of licorice or use it for longer than 4 weeks at a time, because of the risk of toxicity.*

Research summary

The concepts behind the use of licorice and the claims made regarding its effects haven't yet been validated scientifically.

Light therapy

Light therapy uses the energy of light in a variety of forms to heal. It was used in the temples of ancient Egypt, Greece, China, and India. In ayurvedic medicine, each of the seven chakras, or points of physical and spiritual energy in the body, is associated with a specific color in the spectrum of visible light. The color of the chakra refers to the light's frequency as defined by the wavelength of electromagnetic radiation emitted at that location, as perceived by those who have second sight, or the ability to see *auras*, the luminous radiation that emanates from all living matter (See *Light therapies: A closer look*, page 308.)

Light therapy is based on the understanding that matter consists of energy on a continuum from the ultra high electromagnetic frequencies of gamma rays (pure white light) down to the relatively slow electromagnetic frequencies of apparently solid matter. The lower the frequency, the slower the electron movement in the atoms and the denser the matter. Increasing or decreasing the intensity of the light changes the number of rebounding electrons; changing the color (frequency) of the light changes the velocity of the electrons. As the frequencies (or vibrations) of white light (containing all colors) drop, the colors become visible to the cones in the human eye in the very narrow range of violet to red.

On the theory that disease is the result of imbalance and alteration of the body's energy field, light therapy seeks to restore balance and harmony by administering light in a specific energy frequency or vibration to the whole person or to the specific body part where balance is deemed lacking.

Reported uses

Ultraviolet (UV) light absorbed through the eyes and skin has long been recognized as critical in the production of vitamin D, which the body needs for calcium absorption.

Light therapy consists of a broad range of treatment modalities and indications. For example, full-spectrum light is used in the treatment of seasonal affective disorder (SAD), and color is used to enhance mood and health. Light-triggered photocurrents stimulate the visual cortex and the associative centers of the brain. From the visual cortex, light travels to the limbic system, which controls emotion, learning, memory, sexual behaviors, aggression, and smell perception. Light also stimulates the hypothalamus, which is linked to the pituitary gland, which regulates endocrine glands, such as the thyroid, adrenals, and gonads.

Specific bands of the visible light spectrum have been used to treat certain illnesses. Photobiology researchers in Russia and the United States have used red light to stimulate local regeneration of skin and blood cells, noting an increase in tissue oxygen levels, improved local blood flow, enhanced wound healing, increased nerve stimulation, improved muscle relaxation, and decreased pain, theoretically because of enhanced mitochondrial metabolism.

Red light has been used in photodynamic therapy (PDT) to selectively kill bronchopulmonary tumors through use of light-activated porphyrin dyes that bind to the cancer cells. In China, PDT is administered to basal-cell and squamous-cell skin carcinomas through endoscopes.

LIGHT THERAPIES: A CLOSER LOOK

The following light therapies use various forms of artificial light for therapeutic effects.

Ultraviolet light therapy

Various wavelengths of ultraviolet (UV) light are used to treat specific disorders. For example, UVA-1 is used for systemic lupus erythematosus, and psoralen UVA (commonly called PUVA) is used for pigmentation disorders such as vitiligo (in theory by drawing pigment-producing cells to the skin surface) and psoriasis (by preventing disease cells from dividing). UV light is also used for premenstrual syndrome, high cholesterol, and cancer.

Colored-light therapy

Practitioners of colored-light therapy believe that different colors of light affect specific diseases, perhaps by altering the production of brain chemicals. For example, opaque white or violet light is believed to induce relaxation, thus helping to relieve pain and induce sleep. Monochromatic red light is used to treat headaches, allergies, sore throats, sinus problems, endocrine and GI problems, diabetes, dysmenorrhea, and impotence. Sometimes a flashing pattern of light is used. This form of light therapy is contraindicated in patients with seizure disorders.

Photodynamic therapy

In this therapy for basal and squamous cell skin cancer, a dye that absorbs light is injected directly into the malignant tumor, where it absorbs different wavelengths of external light. The combination of the light and the dye is thought to produce a chemical reaction that causes the cancer cells to die.

Syntonic optometry

The patient sits in a darkened room, where a device called a Lumatron emits rapid flashes of colored lights directed at his eyes. The light signals travel from the eyes to the brain, where they're believed to normalize autonomic nervous system function. This therapy is currently used to treat headaches and traumatic brain injuries. This form of light therapy is contraindicated in patients with seizure disorders.

Cold laser therapy

Cold laser therapy, also called soft or low-level laser therapy, uses a laser beam to induce enzymatic and bioelectric reactions in tissue. This is believed to stimulate a healing process that begins at the cellular level. The treatment has been used in pain management, skin problems, trauma, and dentistry.

Blue light has been used to treat precancerous skin lesions.

Psoralens with ultraviolet A (PUVA) light have been used to treat psoriasis and vitiligo, with reports of inhibited cell division and 90% to 95% improvement following 30 treatments over 10 weeks. UV light has also been used to treat simple infections, to increase cardiac output and cerebral circulation, and to combat black lung disease by helping the body eliminate inhaled dust particles. In the United States, Food and Drug Administration (FDA) approval for some forms of PDT is pending.

In the 1870s, Edwin Babbit used natural and artifical light, colored filters, and solarized water (water exposed to sunlight through colored filters and given to the patient to drink) to treat sprains, bruises, body trauma, sepsis, cardiac lesions, asthma, hay fever, corneal ulcers, eye inflammation, glaucoma, and cataracts, but his work was halted as quackery by the FDA.

In the early 1900s, physicist Dinshah Ghadial noted that every chemical element in an excited state emits a characteristic and distinctive set of colored bands, known as Fraunhofer lines. He devised a set of 12 colored filters to match those of the body and projected light through them onto a patient's affected body area, using purple, scarlet, and magenta for the heart and reproductive systems and indigo for pain, injury, and bleeding. In 1927, Dr. Harry Spitler developed a light-dispensing instrument that delivered colored light of designated frequencies — ruby red and yellow-green — to improve eyesight.

In 1988, California psychologist Helen Irlen used patient-specific tinted spectacles and a range of 140 tints to help nonreading learning disabled children become fluent readers. In 1998, Dr. David Norton of London's Hammersmith Hospital developed a mask containing flickering red lights to treat migraine headache and premenstrual syndrome. Another device, the Photron, uses a gently flickering, colored strobe light focused into the patient's eyes, with green or blue light used to treat posttraumatic stress disorder.

How the treatment is performed

Some methods of light therapy involve full-spectrum lights, colored lights, or, light-emitting apparatus. Some methods of color therapy merely ask the patient to visualize a color and mentally "send" it to the area designated to be healed. Healer Joseph Corvo and clairvoyant Lilian Verner-Bonds developed a system, called Color Zone Therapy, based on 10 body-energy zones of reflexology. It involves localized deep massage of reflexology points combined with visualization of color to an associated body part. The physical manipulation directly stimulates the dysfunctional organ, and the psychically directed color is meant to comple-

ment the massage on an emotional and spiritual level. Some reflexologists have used light from a small handheld light-emitting diode to stimulate reflexology points.

Therapist Pauline Willis uses colored flowers, leaves, and other items to help a patient visualize the color saturating the body. For example, to improve sleep, she might have a patient wear blue pajamas, sleep on blue sheets, and use a blue nightlight, eliminating stimulating colors like red, orange, and yellow. Her theory holds that the colors a person wears influence his mood and health. For example, people with cold hands and feet should wear red socks and underwear because red is a "warm" color.

Dr. Gabriel Cousens feels that the color of the food a person eats resonates with and feeds the subtle color energy of the chakras. He suggests starting the morning with the lower frequency red, orange, and yellow foods and moving up to higher frequency green, blue, and violet foods later in the day.

Hazards
Therapies that use flashing lights may trigger seizures in patients with epilepsy.

Clinical considerations
Fifty years ago, the FDA banned the early forms of colored light therapy as quackery. However, some phototherapy devices, such as the Lumatron for therapeutic use of colors and frequencies of light, and the use of full-spectrum lights for the treatment of SAD have received FDA approval.

Research summary
The relationship between sunlight and mood has been known for longer than 2,000 years, but current study of the healing effects of light began in the 19th century with Nobel Prize winner Niels Finsen, a Danish professor who noticed that tubercular skin lesions were rare in the summer. In the early 20th century, Swiss

doctor Auguste Rollier discovered that the sun's UV light lowered blood pressure for 5 to 6 days. Dr. John Ott's discovery that fluorescent lights in schools increased hyperactivity led to the creation of the first full-spectrum lights. In 1981, Dr. Norman Rosenthal identified SAD and developed the requirements for treatment. Dr. Harry Wohlfarts found that full-spectrum lighting and warm wall colors in a school for handicapped children in Edmonton, Alberta, lowered blood pressure and improved behavior dramatically—in both sighted and blind students. Research into the efficacy of light color therapies continues.

lily-of-the-valley

Convallaria majalis,
Convallariae herba, *convall-lily,
Jacob's ladder, ladder to heaven,
lily constancy, Maiglöckchenkraut,
May bells, May lily, muguet,
Our Lady's tears*

Lily-of-the-valley is a small flowering plant that was introduced into the United States and northern Asia from its native Europe. The medicinal parts are the dried flower tips and the dried inflorescence, the lily-of-the-valley herb, the dried root rhizome with the roots, the flowering aerial parts, and the whole fresh flowering plant.

Lily-of-the-valley has a positive inotropic effect on the heart through natural cardioactive glycosides, including convallatoxin, convalloside, and convallatoxol. The herb has also been found to exhibit negative chromatropic and dromatrophic effects as well as a diuretic effects. Lily-of-the-valley is available as capsules, drops, solutions, tablets, and tinctures.

Reported uses

Lily-of-the-valley is used for mild exertional cardiac failure (New York Heart Association Class I and II), age-related

cardiac complaints, and chronic cor pulmonale.

Administration

No dosage is recommended because of the plant's toxic potential.

 SAFETY RISK *Discourage use of this herb. Warn patient that it's considered poisonous and unsafe by the FDA.*

Hazards

Lily-of-the-valley's inotropic and negative chromatropic effects may cause cardiac arrhythmias, hyperkalemia, nausea, vomiting, abdominal pain, cramping, and diarrhea. Using lily-of-the-valley with beta blockers and/or calcium channel blockers increases the risk of bradycardia or heart block. Use of lily-of-the-valley with calcium salts, digoxin, glucocorticoids, laxatives, and quinidine may cause possible additive effects and increased risk of adverse reactions. Concomitant use of lily-of-the-valley with potassium-depleting diuretics could lead to increased cardiotoxicity. Concomitant use of lily-of-the-valley with either hawthorn or uzara root may potentiate the effects of lily-of-the-valley; either combination should be avioded. Use of lily-of-the-valley and licorice may add to increased cardiotoxicity due to potassium depletion.

Clinical considerations

■ Monitor patient for serious adverse effects, such as increased potassium levels or heart arrhythmias.
■ Inform patient about serious adverse effects, especially when used with digoxin, beta blockers, or calcium channel blockers.
■ Tell patient to notify his health care provider if he develops nausea, vomiting, muscle cramps, or a change in heartbeat. They may indicate serious adverse effects.
■ Tell patient to remind prescriber and pharmacist of any herbal or dietary supplement that he's taking when obtaining a new prescription.

■ Advise patient to consult his health care provider before using an herbal preparation because a treatment with proven efficacy may be available.

Research summary
Research on lily-of-the-valley documents its toxic effects.

linden

Basswood, lime flower, lime tree,
Tilia cordata, T. platyphyllos

The flowers of the linden tree have been used for diaphoretic effect since the Middle Ages. They have also been used as a tranquilizer, and to treat a variety of ailments. The linden is native throughout Europe; it's found both in the wild and under cultivation. The tree has smooth gray bark and heart-shaped leaves. Five-petaled, yellow-white flowers are collected to be dried and preserved for use.

Linden extract contains flavonoid compounds, including kaempferol and quercetin; p-coumaric, caffeic, and chlorogenic acids; and amino acids. The plant contains 0.02% to 0.1% volatile oils, including citral, eugenol, and limonene. The ratio of tannins to mucilage polysaccharides contained in various *Tilia* species accounts for differences in the flavor of teas made from this herb. Quercetin, p-coumaric acid, and kaempferol may cause diaphoretic action. Some species of *Tilia* may posess ligands, which may interact with benzodiazepine receptors. This may explain its anxiolytic effect. The extract of the *Tilia* species has been found to possess antibacterial activity.

Reported uses
Linden is used to induce diaphoresis and to treat various nervous disorders, feverish colds, throat irritation, nasal congestion, infections, and cold-related coughs. Linden is also used as an expectorant and antispasmodic.

Administration
■ Liquid extract: 2 to 4 ml of 1:1 preparation with 25% alcohol
■ Tea (steep 2 to 4 g in boiling water): taken by mouth once a day
■ Tincture: 1 to 2 ml of 1:5 preparation with 45% alcohol.

Hazards
Linden is associated with drowsiness and contact skin allergies. Rarely, frequent use of linden flower teas has been associated with cardiac damage. Linden prepared with alcohol may cause a disulfiram-like reaction. Use of linden with alcohol may cause possible additive effects. Concomitant use of linden with a sedative or hypnotic may increase the risk of dizziness and drowsiness.

Patients hypersensitive to linden and those with a history of heart disease shouldn't use this herb.

Clinical considerations
■ Although no chemical interactions have been reported in clinical studies, consider the herb's pharmacologic properties and the risk that it will interfere with the intended therapeutic effects of conventional drugs.
■ Some patients may be allergic to linden. If signs or symptoms develop, patient should discontinue herb and consult a health care provider.
■ Caution patient with a history of heart disease not to use linden. Frequent use may damage cardiac tissue.
■ Warn patient to contact a health care provider if he develops a rash or swelling, or has trouble breathing.
■ Warn patient to avoid potentially hazardous activities until full effects of herb are known because it may cause drowsiness.
■ Warn patient not to take herb for worrisome symptoms before seeking appropriate medical evaluation because doing so may delay diagnosis of a potentially serious medical condition.

- Tell patient to remind prescriber and pharmacist of any herbal or dietary supplement that he's taking when obtaining a new prescription.
- Advise patient to consult his health care provider before using an herbal preparation because a treatment with proven efficacy may be available.

Research summary

The concepts behind the use of linden and the claims made regarding its effects haven't yet been validated scientifically.

Livingston treatment

Autogenous bacterial vaccine, pleomorphic therapy

The Livingston treatment, a combination of dietary regimen and immunotherapy, is based on laboratory studies performed in the 1940s by Virginia Livingston, a physician and medical researcher. During microscopic examination of diseased tissues, Livingston identified a new bacterium that appeared in various sizes and shapes in the tissue of patients with scleroderma, tuberculosis, leprosy, and all types of cancer. She concluded that this microorganism, which she named *Progenitor cryptocides*, was present in all human beings at birth and normally remained dormant. However, when a person's immune system became weakened (from poor diet, chemical toxins, emotional stress, old age, or genetic predisposition), the microbe could cause cancer.

Livingston developed a vaccine against *P. cryptocides* (derived from a culture of the patient's own bacteria) and began administering it at a clinic she established in California in the 1950s. The vaccine is aimed at increasing the body's resistance to *P. cryptocides* and eliminating the internal conditions that allow it to thrive. Livingston died in 1990, but her regimen is still offered at the Livingston Foundation Medical Center in San Diego.

Reported uses

The vaccine is used to treat a variety of disorders that are caused by a weakened immune system, including cancer and other autoimmune diseases.

How the treatment is performed

Injections of *P. cryptocides* vaccine are given every 3 to 5 days, depending on the patients reaction. Treatment also involves Bacille Calmette-Guérin vaccine to stimulate the immune system and long-term use of antibiotics. In addition, because she believed that diet plays a role in weakening the immune system, Livingston's treatment regimen also contains dietary features, primary elements of which include:

- a modified Gerson diet, including coffee enemas
- megadoses of vitamins, minerals, and digestive enzymes
- a ban on caffeine, alcohol, refined sugar and flour, and all processed foods.

Hazards

Patient may experience soreness or redness at the injection site. Hypersensitivity, fever, and muscle and joint pain have also been reported. Coffee enemas and long-term use of antibiotics can destroy the body's natural flora; enemas can also lead to dehydration, fatigue, malaise, and electrolyte imbalances. Megadoses of vitamins and other supplements can lead to vitamin toxicity.

Clinical considerations

- Inform patient that he may experience reactions to the vaccine, including soreness or redness at the injection site, mild fever, and muscle or joint pain.
- Be alert for superinfections, such as yeast infections, from the long-term use of antibiotics.
- Warn patient about adverse reactions from the prescribed antibiotic.
- Teach your patient the signs and symptoms of dehydration, such as decreased urinary output, dark urine, and increased thirst and skin turgor.

Research summary

According to the University of Pennsylvania's OncoLink web site, "there is no scientific evidence to confirm [Livingston's] theories of cancer or to justify her treatments." This report claims that other researchers have been unable to confirm the existence of *P. cryptocides* and that cultures she submitted to a private organization for study identified her microorganism as *Staphylococcus epidermidis*.

A study conducted by Vincent Speckhardt and Alva L. Johnson at East Virginia School of Medicine found the vaccine useful in reversing the immune-suppressed condition of cancer patients. In a study of 40 patients, several cases of tumor regression were observed, ranging from complete to partial, with no adverse reactions except for an occasional rash. Three patients with advanced cancers showed complete remission, while four others showed dramatic improvement, including shrinkage or disappearance of tumors. Preliminary studies seemed most favorable for localized tumors, such as those of the prostate or breast. However, Livingston vaccines are expensive to produce and are not cost-effective for most practitioners.

lobelia

Asthma weed, bladderpod, emetic herb, emetic weed, eyebright, gagroot, Indian tobacco, Lobelia inflata, *pukeweed, vomitroot, vomitwort, wild tobacco*

Lobelia is an annual or biennial herb with pale green to yellow leaves that's indigenous to northern regions of the United States, Canada, and Kamchatka, although the plant is also cultivated elsewhere. The medicinal part is obtained from the fresh or dried leaves and the seeds. The leaves, which are chewed, have an acrid taste similar to tobacco and have a faintly irritating odor. Lobelia contains 6% alkaloids. Lobeline accounts for most of the herb's effects. Lobelanine, lobelanidine, norlobelanine, and isolobinine are also present. Lobelia acts like nicotine and interacts at the nicotine receptor, stimulating respiratory and emetic centers of the brain. Lobelia is available in homeopathic preparations as tablets and tincture.

Reported uses

Lobelia is used as a constituent of some homeopathic preparations.

Administration

The drug is no longer used aside from its inclusion in some homeopathic preparations; see package information on such preparations for dosage.

 SAFETY RISK *Doses of 600 to 1,000 mg of lobelia leaves are considered toxic; a 4-g dose of lobelia may be fatal.*

Hazards

Lobelia mimics nicotine and interacts with the nicotine receptors, causing adverse effects similar to nicotine, such as anxiety, dizziness, headache, paresthesias, shivering, sweating, and seizures. It causes increased heart rate or bradycardia and may cause either increased or decreased blood pressure. Lobelia causes dry mouth, mouth irritation, abdominal pain, diarrhea, nausea, and vomiting, and may also cause burning of the urinary tract. Respiratory complications such as coughing, a tickling or choking sensation, pain, or burning may occur. Decreased respiration and paralysis of the respiratory center may occur with overdose. Contact allergies of the skin have also been reported. When used in conjunction with GI or respiratory irritants, tobacco products, or nicotine-containing smoking cessation products, there may be an additive toxicity. Advise patient to avoid using lobelia with these products.

Patients with heart disease or hypersensitivity to tobacco or lobelia should avoid using this herb. Women who are pregnant or breast-feeding should also avoid use.

Clinical considerations
- Antacids may decrease the adverse GI effects of lobeline.
- Monitor patient's blood pressure, heart rate, and respiration.
- Tell patient not to take lobelia while smoking or chewing tobacco. Offer other tobacco-cessation options.
- Tell patient to remind prescriber and pharmacist of any herbal or dietary supplement that he's taking when obtaining a new prescription.
- Advise patient to consult his health care provider before using an herbal preparation because a treatment with proven efficacy may be available.

Research summary
Several studies of lobeline for smoking cessation have found little evidence to support its efficacy.

lovage

Aetheroleum levistici,
Angelica levisticum,
Hipposelinum levisticum, *lavose*,
Levisticum officinale, L. radix,
maggi plant, sea parsley, smellage

Lovage is an aromatic perennial that blooms from July to August with yellow-green flowers in thick clusters. It has a strong scent, similar to celery. Lovage is native to the Mediterranean region of Europe and is cultivated in the northeastern United States and Canada. The medicinal components are obtained from roots and seeds of *Levisticum officinale* and *L. radix*. Lovage has been used for longer than 500 years, primarily for its GI effects.

The root contains several compounds that contribute to its aromatic odor and flavor, including butylidenphthalide, butylphthalide, and ligustilide; coumarins; terpenoids; and volatile acids, such as caffeic and benzoic acids. Other compounds include camphene, bergapten, and psoralen. Lovage exerts weak diuretic, spasmolytic, and sedative effects; it also stimulates salivation and gastric secretion.

Reported Uses
Lovage is used for its diuretic properties in treating pedal edema. In Germany, it's approved for irrigation in urinary tract inflammation and for renal calculus prophylaxis. It's also used as a spasmolytic, a sedative, a mucolytic, a carminative (to relieve gastric discomfort and flatulence), and a remedy for menstrual complaints.

Extracts of lovage are also used as an herbal flavoring in liqueur and foods.

Administration
Lovage is usually consumed as tea, which is prepared by pouring 1 cup boiling water over 1.5 to 3 g of finely cut root and straining after 15 minutes. Dosage is 4 to 8 g by mouth every day, taken between meals.

Hazards
Photosensitivity and dermatitis have been reported with the harvesting of lovage, but not with its therapeutic use. Lovage may potentiate the anticoagulant effects of warfarin or other anticoagulants.

Patients with acute renal inflammation or dysfunction should avoid using this herb, as should women who are pregnant or breast-feeding.

Clinical considerations
- Use with caution in patients with a history of photosensitivity reactions and in those with plant allergies.
- Monitor serum electrolyte, blood urea nitrogen, and serum creatinine values periodically while patient is taking lovage.
- Make sure patient maintains adequate fluid intake.
- Lovage may prolong international normalized ratio and prothrombin time if

patient also receives an anticoagulant. Advise against concomitant use.

■ If patient takes lovage for pedal edema, recommend a complete medical evaluation by a health care provider. Explain that pedal edema may indicate a serious underlying cardiovascular or renal disorder mandating medical treatment.

■ Discuss other proven diuretics currently available.

■ Tell patient to notify health care provider about any skin changes or photosensitivity reactions. Emphasize need to avoid prolonged exposure to sunlight while using lovage.

■ Tell patient to remind prescriber and pharmacist of any herbal or dietary supplement that he's taking when obtaining a new prescription.

■ Advise patient to consult his health care provider before using an herbal preparation because a treatment with proven efficacy may be available.

Research Summary

The concepts behind the use of lovage and the claims made regarding its effects haven't yet been validated scientifically.

lungwort

Common lungwort, dage of Jerusalem, Jerusalem cowslip, lungmoss, Pulmonaria officinalis, *spotted comfrey*

Lungwort is a plant common to many parts of Europe. The medicinal parts of the plant are the dried herb and fresh, aerial parts of the flowering plant. Lungwort leaves contain allantoin, which may contribute to its emollient action. Tannins and flavonoids contained in the plant may exert astringent and anti-inflammatory action, and mucilage may act as an antitussive. Other components include ascorbic acid, saponins, potassium and iron salts, and salicylic acid. Lungwort's taste is slightly bitter and has a "slimy" consisten-

cy. Lungwort is available as tablets, syrup, juice, drops, and extracts.

Reported Uses

Lungwort is used as an antitussive, expectorant, and anti-irritant in bronchitis, cough, influenza, and tuberculosis. It's also used for its astringent properties in treating diarrhea, hemorrhoids, GI ulceration, kidney and urinary tract conditions, and excessive menstrual flow. Lungwort is used topically to aid wound healing.

Administration

■ Infusion (1.5 g of dried herb, finely cut, placed in cold water and brought to a rapid boil; or steeped in boiling water for 5 to 10 minutes): three times a day

■ Tincture: 1 to 4 ml by mouth three times a day

■ Liquid extract 1:1 with 25% ethanol.

Hazards

Lungwort is associated with few adverse effects if taken in proper dosage. Common adverse effects that may occur include nausea, contact dermatitis, and prolonged bleeding time. When taking other medications that may prolong bleeding time, such as warfarin or aspirin, there may be a potentiation of effect.

Patients with a history of contact allergies, those taking anticoagulants, and patients who are pregnant or breast-feeding should avoid using lungwort.

Clinical considerations

■ Monitor patient's international normalized ratio and prothrombin time, as needed, because herb may prolong bleeding indexes. Monitor patient for occult blood.

■ If patient has a respiratory disorder, tell him to discuss conventional medical treatments with a health care provider before using lungwort.

■ Warn patient to avoid using herb with an anticoagulant, such as warfarin.

■ Tell patient to notify a health care provider about signs and symptoms of increased bleeding time, such as bruising, bleeding gums, or dark stools.

■ Tell patient to remind prescriber and pharmacist of any herbal or dietary supplement that he's taking when obtaining a new prescription.

■ Advise patient to consult his health care provider before using an herbal preparation because a treatment with proven efficacy may be available.

Research summary
The concepts behind the use of lungwort and the claims made regarding its effects haven't yet been validated scientifically.

Macrobiotic diet

The macrobiotic diet originated in Japan in the middle of the 20th century, not as a cure for any disease, but rather as a lifestyle aimed at enhancing physical and spiritual well-being. It consists primarily of whole-grain cereals, such as wheat, barley, buckwheat, and brown rice, as well as fresh organic vegetables, beans, and nuts. The central concept of this diet is "balance equals health"—a belief that optimal health is the natural result of eating, thinking, and living in balance. The concept of balance extends not only to the selection of food, but also to its preparation.

The original macrobiotic diet was developed by a Japanese teacher, George Ohsawa (1893-1966), who reportedly recovered from a serious illness by changing from the refined diet that had gained popularity in Japan to the traditional Japanese diet that consists primarily of brown rice, sea vegetables, and miso soup (made from soybeans). Ohsawa believed that a simple diet was the key to good health. His plan proceeded in 10 stages, from least stringent (30% vegetables, 15% fruits and salads, 30% animal products, 10% whole grains, 10% soups, 5% desserts, and few beverages) to most stringent (60% cereals, 30% vegetables, 10% soups).

In the 1970s, Michio Kushi, one of Ohsawa's students, took the helm of the macrobiotic movement in the United States. He replaced the 10-stage program with the standard macrobiotic diet practiced today. Kushi uses traditional Chinese medicine's concepts of yin and yang to explain cancer development and to provide a framework for cancer treatment. He maintains that the primary factor responsible for cancer is the consumption of foods that are too yin (expansive) or too yang (contractive). Extremely yin foods include dairy products, tropical fruits, refined sugar, coffee, and alcohol; extremely yang foods include meat, poultry, fish, salty foods, cheese, and eggs. Whole-grain foods are considered ideal — neither too yin nor too yang.

Reported uses

Today, the macrobiotic diet plan is one of the most widely practiced alternative nutritional regimens in the United States, used by healthy people to maintain good health and by patients with serious illnesses, such as cancer, who haven't been helped by conventional therapy or who are combining the diet with conventional medical treatments.

Proponents believe that cancer is the result of prolonged exposure to dietary and environmental toxins, a sedentary lifestyle, and other social and personal factors, most of which are attributable to the patient's own unhealthful practices.

How the treatment is performed

According to Kushi, cancers are classified as predominantly yin or yang (or a combination), depending on where the primary tumor originated. Tumors located in peripheral or upper areas (esophagus, breast, upper stomach, and outer parts of brain) as well as lymphoma and leukemia are considered yin; those in deeper or lower regions (colon, rectum, pancreas, prostate, ovaries, bone, inner parts of brain) are considered yang. Once the cancer is classified, the diet is modified appropriately — emphasizing yang foods for yin cancers, and vice versa — to bring yin and yang back into balance within the body.

Additional measures include engaging in regular exercise; avoiding electromagnetic radiation, chemical fumes, and synthetic fabrics; and maintaining a positive attitude. This essentially vegan regimen emphasizes the intake of complex carbohydrates, high-fiber foods, unsaturated fats, and unrefined foods. Proponents view the plan not simply as a diet but as a sensible approach to daily living. (See *Basic elements of the macrobiotic diet*.)

Hazards

Although the standard macrobiotic diet allows small amounts of fish, people who forego all dairy products and meats may develop frank deficiencies of calcium, vitamin B_{12}, and vitamin D. For children, who need vitamin D for proper growth and development, Kushi advocates fish liver oils, exposure to sunlight, and other foods that contain the vitamin. For teenagers and adults, he advises exposure to sunlight and no supplements unless deficiencies develop.

Clinical considerations

- Suggest periodic blood tests to check for anemia (from protein deficiency) and vitamin and iron deficiencies.
- Be sure patient understands the diet and knows that other treatments may be available.
- Advise patient to notify his health care provider that he is on this diet.

Research summary

By the early 1980s, a number of books (including Kushi's *The Cancer Prevention Diet*) were beginning to claim that the macrobiotic diet could be used not only to enhance well-being but also to prevent cancer and even induce remission. Since then, numerous reports have appeared in the popular media claiming cancer cures after patients switched to the macrobiotic diet. In his book, Kushi says cancers of the breast, colon, cervix, pancreas, liver, bone, and skin have responded best to macrobiotics. Despite substantial anec-

BASIC ELEMENTS OF THE MACROBIOTIC DIET

The standard macrobiotic diet is adjusted from person to person, depending on a number of factors, such as season, geography, and personal factors. Its basic elements include the following:

- 50% to 60% organically grown, cooked whole grains (brown rice, barley, bulghur, millet, oats, corn, rye, wheat, buckwheat, and limited partially processed grains)
- 25% to 30% organically grown, mostly cooked vegetables (classified as those that should be eaten frequently; for example, cabbage, broccoli, cauliflower, bok choy, carrots, pumpkin, collard and dandelion greens, and most types of squash; those that should be eaten occasionally, such as mushrooms, celery, cucumbers, iceberg lettuce, snow peas, and string beans; and those that should be avoided completely, including tomatoes, potatoes, eggplant, zucchini, spinach, asparagus, peppers, avocadoes, and beets
- 5% to 10% (1 to 2 bowls daily) soups made of vegetables, seaweed, grains, or beans, seasoned with miso or tamari soy sauce
- 5% to 10% beans (chickpeas, lentils, and Azuki beans,) bean products (tofu and tempeh), and sea vegetables (wakame, hiziki, kombu, and nori)

- occasional intake (if needed or desired) of fresh white fish, (flounder, haddock, scrod, snapper, sole, cod, trout, and halibut); organically grown, local fruits (dry or cooked); seeds and nuts; and vinegars
- nonstimulating teas or plain water (no ice)
- avoidance of meat and poultry, animal fat, eggs, dairy products, refined sugar, chocolate, tropical fruits, soda, coffee, caffeinated tea, hot spices, alcohol, and all refined, processed, chemically treated, canned, frozen, or irradiated foods

The recommended cooking methods are boiling, steaming, pressure cooking, nisshime (waterless cooking), water sautéing, pressing, and pickling. Foods must be cooked over gas or in a wood-burning stove, and utensils must be made of natural materials. Copper and aluminum pots should be avoided.

When used to treat cancer, the diet is modified according to the principles of yin and yang that are central to Asian medicine. First, the cancer is classified as primarily yin or yang, depending on where in the body the primary tumor occurs. Different foods and cooking styles are recommended based on this classification.

---

dotal evidence, to date there are no clinical data in support of these claims.

Most mainstream doctors and nutritionists are skeptical about claims that the macrobiotic diet (or any other diet) can cure cancer or other diseases. However, Barrie Cassileth, a founding member of the National Center for Complementary and Alternative Medicine's (NCCAM) Advisory Council and currently affiliated with Harvard Medical School, says that certain aspects of the diet "have merit if not carried to extremes." Like other low-fat diets, she says, the macrobiotic diet can lower weight,

blood pressure, and cholesterol levels and may help prevent heart disease and possibly certain cancers. And, like other vegetarian diets, it requires the use of supplements to make up for certain nutritional deficiencies.

A 1993 editorial in the *Journal of the American College of Nutrition* suggests that the macrobiotic diet may be worth examining as a treatment for cancer because of its nutritional inadequacy, noting that "a nutritional regimen clearly deficient in growth-promoting substances might actually be helpful in controlling otherwise untreatable diseases."

madder

Dyer's madder, robbia,
Rubia tinctorum

Madder is a perennial plant indigenous to southern Europe, western Asia, and North Africa and cultivated in other regions. The medicinal part is the dried root, which contains 2% to 4% anthraquinone derivatives and glycosides. Principal components are ruberythric acid, alizarin, pseudopurpurin, rubiadin, lucidin, and lucidin 3-O-primeveroside. Its mechanism of action stems from the Ca^{2+} chelating properties of anthraquinones. Madder may also be mutagenic and carcinogenic because of the lucidin component. It's available as dried root, extract, and capsules.

Reported uses
Madder is used as an antispasmodic, a diuretic, and a prophylactic and treatment for kidney stones. It's also added to foods as a colorant.

Administration
- Capsules: 1 capsule by mouth three times a day for up to 2 months
- Extract: 20 gtt by mouth three times a day for up to 2 months
- Infusion: 1 to 2 g by mouth four times a day for up to 2 months.

Hazards
Madder has been associated with contact dermatitis, cancer, and red discoloration of perspiration, saliva, tears, urine, and bone.
    Women who are pregnant or breastfeeding shouldn't use madder.

 SAFETY RISK *Because of the risk of toxicity, madder is not recommended.*

Clinical considerations
- Warn patient about the possible risks of mutagenic and carcinogenic effects of madder.

- If patient has suspected kidney stones, tell him to discuss conventional treatments with health care provider before using this herb.
- Instruct patient who takes madder to notify health care provider about planned, suspected, or known pregnancy.
- Inform patient that madder may discolor body fluids and objects they touch, such as contact lenses.
- Tell patient to remind prescriber and pharmacist of any herbal or dietary supplement that he's taking when obtaining a new prescription.
- Advise patient to consult his health care provider before using an herbal preparation because a treatment with proven efficacy may be available.

Research summary
Research has confirmed the carcinogenic and mutagenic effects of madder.

Magnetic field therapy

*Biomagnetic therapy,
electromagnetic therapy,
magnet therapy, magnetotherapy*

Magnetic field therapy involves the use of magnetic fields in the prevention and treatment of disease and as first-aid treatment for injuries. Its goal is to restore the body's internal bioelectromagnetic balance. With successful therapy, the patient should learn to maintain this internal balance without the need for continued external intervention.
    Therapeutic magnetism isn't a new idea. Natural mineral magnets, called lodestones, were used for thousands of years in Chinese, Egyptian, and Greek medicine to treat a variety of ailments. Today's magnets consist of iron, iron-containing ceramics, neodymium, or other materials that can be permanently magnetized. (See *Understanding magnetic field therapy*.)

Reported uses

Therapeutic magnets may benefit a wide range of conditions, from acute and chronic pain, strains, and swelling to systemic illness. Magnets and electromagnetic therapy devices are now being used to facilitate the healing of broken bones and counter the effects of stress.

Magnetic field therapy is recognized in sports medicine for its effectiveness in relieving sprains and strains. It's also used in conjunction with other therapies, such as nutrition, herbs, and acupuncture. For example, practitioners believe that having a patient lie on a magnetic mattress enhances the effectiveness of craniosacral therapy.

Although the scientific basis of magnetic field therapy has yet to be established, thousands of patients have reported relief of pain or discomfort from such conditions as arthritis, back pain, pressure ulcers, carpal tunnel syndrome, diabetic neuropathy, gout, rheumatism, shoulder pain, trigeminal neuralgia, toothache, headaches, and ulcers. Magnetic field therapy has been used to treat a variety of orthopedic problems, musculoskeletal disorders, arthritis, and temporomandibular joint pain. It's been applied to diseases such as multiple sclerosis, breast cancer, Parkinson's disease, osteoporosis, joint disease, heart disease, and diabetes to restore electromagnetic field balance. Additionally, practitioners claim that magnetic field therapy may be useful in treating hepatitis, ulcers, epileptic seizures, optic nerve atrophy, migraine headaches, hypertension, and postsurgical swelling.

How the treatment is performed

Handbooks of magnetic field therapy describe the best placement and magnet strength for self-treatment of a variety of illnesses. Treatments are described according to the strength of the magnets used; a magnet's strength is measured in units called *gauss*. High-gauss treatments and those involving prolonged exposure

---

UNDERSTANDING MAGNETIC FIELD THERAPY

One theory of magnetic field therapy suggests that diseased cells have lost their magnetic equilibrium and that topically applied magnets work on a molecular level to restore this equilibrium within the cells. This, in turn, benefits surrounding cells and the entire organism.

Another theory, based on the magnetic nature of red blood cells, suggests a magnetically induced increase in blood and oxygen supply to diseased tissues. This increased blood and oxygen supply accompanies pH adjustment and increased nutrient availability, and relieves congestion and pain through improved circulation.

Reported effects

A survey of magnetic field therapy reports identifies the following specific physiologic effects of treatment with magnets:
- increased blood and oxygen circulation along with the nutrient-carrying potential of blood
- changes in pH balance, often unbalanced in diseased tissues (Bionorth [−] fields promote beneficial alkalinity and biosouth [+] fields promote harmful acidity)
- enhanced migration of calcium ions (to facilitate healing of nerve tissue and bones and help reduce the pathologic buildup of calcium in arthritic joints)
- changes in the production of certain endocrine hormones
- enhanced enzyme activity and other related physiologic processes.

---

to the biosouth (+) pole should be supervised by a qualified practitioner.

The simplest home remedy for pain involves applying a low- to medium-gauss (800-gauss or less) magnet to the

USING MAGNETS FOR BASIC FIRST AID

Magnets may be useful to treat minor complaints. Advise patients to seek medical treatment for serious or nonresponsive burns or injuries. If patient is allergic to insect bites, warn him to keep an anaphylactic kit handy and to seek immediate medical attention for insect bites.

Insect bites
Because bites and stings are acid, practitioners recommend negative magnetic energy to reduce acidity, inflammation, and pain. Magnets are usually applied soon after the bite occurs.

Burns
Practitioners recommend applying negative magnetic energy to burns before tissue deterioration occurs. Either a 2" × 5" (5 cm × 12.5 cm), or a 4" × 6" (10 cm × 15 cm) ceramic magnet is preferred.

Headache
Ceramic magnets or stacked plastiform magnets are applied directly over the painful area. If this brings no relief, the magnets are placed on opposite sides of the head to pull fluid away from the painful area. Alternatively, two ceramic cube magnets or 4" × 6" (10 cm × 15 cm) ceramic magnets may be applied bitemporally. Finally, one plastiform strip and one neodymium round magnet may be applied on the back of the head at the base of the skull, with ceramic or plastiform magnets applied on the forehead at the hairline.

Insomnia
A magnetic bed may help to reduce the stress, muscle tension, and musculoskeletal pain that disrupt sleep.

Muscle spasms
Muscle spasms are treated by placing ceramic magnets, or three or four stacked plastiform magnets, directly over the painful area. Leg cramps may be relieved by placing ceramic magnets under the soles of the feet.

Sprain or strain
Ceramic magnets, or three or four stacked magnetic strips, may be applied directly to the injured area to reduce inflammation and swelling.

---

area of discomfort and leaving it in place until well after the discomfort disappears. The longer the treatment, the quicker the healing and the greater the symptom relief. If the pain decreases with treatment, the magnet is correctly oriented; if the pain increases, even if the magnet's bionorth side is facing the patient, the magnet needs to be turned over. (See *Using magnets for basic first aid*.)

Therapy may be of short duration (1 to 2 hours) if high-gauss magnets are used; magnets may also be used overnight or for 24 hours or longer for maximum effect. Nutrition and diet therapy may be used in addition to magnetic field therapy for optimal healing.

Magnets used for magnetic field therapy should be high-quality medical magnets, which are available in all sizes, shapes, and strengths. Because they aren't regulated as medical devices, quality and consistency may vary from one manufacturer to another. True bionorth (−) and biosouth (+) poles can be determined by using a simple compass; bionorth (−) is south-seeking (attracted to the south, or positive, pole) and biosouth (+) is north-seeking (attracted to the north, or negative, pole). Gauss meters are also available for measuring the external field strength of the magnet. A magnet view device, which is filled with iron particles that respond when placed on a magnet, shows the pattern of plastic strip magnets.

Biomagnetic appliances range from small adhesive pads to belts and mattresses. The typical magnet pad or mattress for a queen-sized bed contains anywhere from 200 to 550 small magnets, spaced from 1½" to 4" (4 to 10 cm) apart, with surface field strength ranging from 75 to 1,075 gauss. The magnets are typically oriented with the bionorth (−) side closest to the person, but may also be oriented with the biosouth (+) side closest to the person. Mattresses are said to be beneficial for promoting restorative sleep, increasing melatonin production, stimulating the body's natural healing ability, and facilitating the rebalancing of the body's electromagnetic flow from the adverse effects of electropollution, such as power lines, cordless telephones, microwave ovens, or photocopiers.

Magnetic insoles are thin, flexible, magnetoform plastic inserts that may be bipolar or unipolar with bionorth (−) on one side and biosouth (+) on the other. They're used to improve circulation and reduce foot discomfort for people who must stand for long periods of time.

Bipolar magnets, in the form of small magnetic pads, come in varying sizes and shapes for easier application over specific areas of discomfort. The bipolar pads often have a metallic foil on the side worn away from the body, which directs the magnetic field more effectively toward the source of discomfort.

Magnetic pads come in various shapes and sizes and can be applied to the back, knees, elbows, wrists, ankles, face, neck, and shoulders. These wraps conveniently hold the magnets in place, directing the magnetic field toward the area of discomfort.

Acuband magnets are tiny (1 to 2 mm in diameter), disk-shaped magnets that are easily attached to the body with round adhesive bandages. Despite their small size, they have impressive internal field strengths ranging from 3,000 to 9,000 gauss. Some discs have marked bionorth (−) poles for easier identification. These magnets are placed on acupressure points and may also be applied at the site of a bone fracture to promote healing.

Hazards

Application of therapeutic magnets is considered relatively safe. However, some experts claim that using the positive pole of a medium- to high-gauss magnet for a protracted time may exacerbate symptoms rather than eliminate them.

Positive (biosouth) magnetic energy should be used only under medical supervision because some investigators believe that overstimulation of the brain may occur, producing seizures, hallucinations, insomnia, hyperactivity, and magnetic addiction. It has also been claimed that positive magnetic energy may stimulate growth of tumors and microorganisms.

A bedridden patient who uses a magnetic bed 24 hours a day risks suppressed adrenal function and slowed energy recovery. A magnetic bed should be used for only 8 to 10 hours at a time.

Because of the vasodilation believed to occur with bipolar magnetic treatment, it's recommended that the treatment be delayed for 24 hours in patients with acute injuries associated with bleeding. Magnetic field therapy isn't recommended for children under age 5 or for pregnant women.

SAFETY RISK *Patients with pacemakers or defibrillators shouldn't use magnetic beds. Magnets should be placed at least 6" (15 cm) away from such devices to avoid interfering with their function.*

Clinical considerations

■ Encourage older patient to continue to seek conventional treatment and to report any alternative therapies he's undergoing.

CARE AND HANDLING OF THERAPEUTIC MAGNETS

The following care measures should be observed when handling magnets (patients should be taught the same principles):

■ Recognize that magnets may alter magnetic instruments, such as pacemakers, battery-powered wristwatches, hearing aids, and other equipment in use around a patient. Keep magnets away from magnetic resonance imaging machines. Also be sure to keep magnets away from patients who have metallic parts in their bodies. Post signs to alert staff and visitors of the presence of magnets.

■ Avoid dropping or rough handling of magnets. Don't heat a magnet above 5,000° F (2,600° C) because this can dissipate its strength.

■ When a U-shaped magnet is not in use, connect the ends with a magnet keeper to prolong its strength.

■ Don't keep different-sized magnets together; it alters the strength of the magnets.

■ Be sure to keep magnets away from computer hard drives and any magnetic media, such as diskettes, audio and video recording tapes, credit or bank cards, and compact discs, to prevent damage or erasure of data. Any item with a magnetic strip on it — for example, a credit card, ATM card, or identification card — can be ruined by exposure to a magnet.

■ Caution patient to use a magnetometer or a compass to check the poles on a magnet he plans to use. With a compass, the tip of the arrow marked N or *north* will point toward the magnet's negative pole.

■ Advise patient to avoid using magnets on the abdomen for 60 to 90 minutes af-

ter meals, in order to allow peristalsis to take place.

■ Monitor patient who's undergoing magnetic field therapy for potential adverse effects and the subsequent need to decrease or discontinue use. The danger exists that people will turn to magnetic field therapy as a cure-all rather than seeking medical attention for significant health problems.

■ Inform patient that using more magnets, or stronger magnets, isn't necessarily better.

■ Warn patient to remove all magnets before undergoing surgery because magnets may cause life-threatening instrument malfunction.

■ Counsel patient about safe magnet use. (See *Care and handling of therapeutic magnets.*)

Research summary

In 1997, investigators at Baylor College of Medicine in Houston, Texas, performed a double-blind, randomized, clinical trial of pain response to static magnetic fields in 50 patients suffering from postpolio syndrome. They found statistically significant evidence of pain relief for the patients who received treatment from an active magnetic device as opposed to those treated with a placebo. The researchers concluded that delivering static magnetic fields of 300 to 500 gauss over a pain trigger point brought significant and prompt relief. This study used bionorth (−) magnets.

Investigations into the efficacy of magnets in treating conditions such as fibromyalgia and phantom limb pain continue. Practitioners report that older people respond especially well to overall energizing effects of magnetic field therapy as well as to specific treatment for chronic pain or illness. No research documents the possible long-term adverse effects of static magnet fields.

male fern

Aspidium oleoresin, bear's paw, bontanifuge, Dryopteris filix-mas, Extractum filicis, E. filicis aethereum, E. filicis maris tenue, *knotty brake, male shield fern, marginal fern, sweet brake, wurmfarn*

Male fern is a plant found in temperate zones of Europe, northern Asia, and North and South America. The medicinal parts are the dried fronds, the dried rhizome collected in autum with the leaf bases, the fresh rhizome, and the fresh aerial parts.

Filicinic and flavaspidic acids are the main active components responsible for herb's anthelmintic properties. Other components include volatile oils, tannin, paraspidin, and desaspidin. Desaspidin and aspidin may have antitumor activity. Male fern is available as extract (1.5% to 22% filicin), draught (4 g of male fern extract), and capsules.

Reported uses

Male fern has long been used as an anthelmintic against pork tapeworm (*Taenia solium*), beef tapeworm (*T. saginata*), and fish tapeworm (*Diphyllobothrium latum*). It's also applied topically for muscle pain, arthritis, sciatica, neuralgia, earache, and toothache.

SAFETY RISK *Male fern is toxic. Ingestion isn't recommended. In poisoning or overdose, optic neuritis, blindness, seizures, psychosis, paralysis, respiratory and cardiac failure, coma, and death may ensue. The patient should seek emergency medical care.*

Administration

- Extract: Initial dosage 6 to 8 g for adults and 4 to 6 g for children over age 4 years. In the case of an unsuccessful cure, the treatment may be repeated, but only after an interim of a few weeks. The single and daily maximum dosage of liquid extract is 3 g
- Oil solution: The maximum daily dosage is 20 g
- Draught: Dosage is 50 ml given by duodenal tube; treatment may be repeated in 7 to 10 days, as needed
- Homeopathic formula: Dosage is 5 drops, 1 tablet, or 10 globules every 30 to 60 minutes (acute) or 1 to 3 times daily (chronic)
- Parenteral: Dosage is 1 to 2 ml subcutaneously, three times a day in acute cases, daily in chronic cases.

Hazards

Therapeutic doses of male fern may cause headache, seizures, queasiness, psychosis, paralysis, and coma. Other possible complications include heart failure, optic neuritis, permanent visual disorders, severe abdominal cramps, diarrhea, nausea, and vomiting. The patient may also experience hepatotoxicity, hyperbilirubinemia, jaundice, dyspnea, respiratory failure, and albuminuria.

Antacids, H_2-blockers (such as famotidine and ranitidine), proton pump inhibitors (including lansoprazole and omeprazole), and other alkalinizing drugs inactive the acid components of male fern. A diet high in fats and oils may cause an increased absorption of male fern and potentiate the risk of toxicity.

Pregnant women should avoid using this herb because it may stimulate uterine muscle. Patients who are breastfeeding, infants, children younger than age 4 years, geriatric patients, and debilitated patients should also avoid use. Patients who are hypersensitive to male fern or its components, and those with anemia, GI ulceration, cardiovascular disease, diabetes, and hepatic or renal failure, should avoid use.

Clinical considerations

- Male fern has a narrow window of intended activity; toxic effects can occur in that window.
- The draught is considered a more effective anthelmintic than capsule form.

- Patients being treated with drugs that affect bilirubin conjugation or alter liver enzyme levels should use herb with caution or avoid it.
- Patient may take a laxative the evening before herb treatment and a second laxative dose with the herb the next morning before eating.
- Monitor patient's liver function tests and renal function.
- Monitor fluid intake and electrolyte loss in patients who develop vomiting and diarrhea.
- Inform patient that toxic effects can occur with normal doses.
- If patient takes an antacid, H_2-blocker, or proton pump inhibitor, tell him to avoid using this herb.
- Tell patient to avoid fats and oils while taking herb.
- Advise patient that conventional anthelmintics for tapeworms are safer than male fern.
- Urge patient to seek medical care for suspected tapeworm before using this herb.
- If patient has persistent abdominal pain or yellowing of the skin and eyes, stress that he should obtain medical care.
- If patient is pregnant or breast-feeding or has anemia, a GI condition, or cardiac, hepatic, or renal impairment, caution against using herb.
- Tell patient to remind prescriber and pharmacist of any herbal or dietary supplement that he's taking whenobtaining a new prescription.
- Advise patient to consult his health care provider before using an herbal preparation because a treatment with proven efficacy may be available.

Research summary
Male fern is considered toxic at therapeutic doses and shouldn't be used.

mallow

Blue mallow, cheeseflower, high mallow, Malva sylvestris, mauls

The mallow is found in subtropical and temperate latitItudes of both hemispheres. The medicinal parts are the dried flowers, the dried leaves, and the whole of the flowering fresh plant.

Mallow contains glycosides, flavonoids, mucilage, anthocyanin, and tannins. The mucilage component, made up largely of glucuronic acid, galacturonic acid, rhamnose, and galactose, is responsible for emollient and demulcent action. It may also act as an astringent and expectorant. Mallow is available as an extract and as dried herb, in products such as Malvedrin and Malveol.

Reported uses
Mallow is used as demulcent to treat oral and pharyngeal mucosal irritation, cough, hoarseness, bronchitis, laryngitis, and tonsillitis. The leaves of the plant are used as a laxative. Mallow is used topically as an emollient for skin irritation and swelling.

Administration
- Dried herb: 5 g every day
- Infusion, mallow flower (*Malvae flos*; 1.5 to 2 g of dried mallow flower added to cold water, boiled, and then strained after 10 minutes)
- Infusion, mallow leaf (*Malvae folium*; 5 oz of boiling water poured over 3 to 5 g and steeped for 2 to 3 hours)

Hazards
No health hazards have been associated with the use of mallow; however, the patient may experience muscle tremors. No interactions have been reported.

Mallow should be avoided by pregnant or breast-feeding patients and by those hypersensitive to it.

Clinical considerations

■ Don't confuse with marshmallow (*Althaea officinalis*).
■ Advise patient to consult a health care provider about a persistent cough and sore throat or mouth pain or irritation.
■ Inform patient that few medicinal data support the use of this herb.
■ Advise patient to report suspected pregnancy.
■ Tell patient to remind prescriber and pharmacist of any herbal or dietary supplement that he's taking whenobtaining a new prescription.
■ Advise patient to consult his health care provider before using an herbal preparation because a treatment with proven efficacy may be available.

Research summary

The concepts behind the use of mallow and the claims made regarding its effects haven't yet been validated scientifically.

marigold

Calendula officinalis, *goldbloom, golds, holligold, Marybud, Marygold, Mary gowles, ruddes*

Marigold is an annual plant grown in central and southern Europe, western Asia, and the United States. The plant has a strong, unpleasant smell. The medicinal components include the flowers, shoots, and leaves. Marigold contains lutein, volatile oils, flavonoids, carotenoid pigments, and sterols. Topical use of its extracts promotes wound healing. The herb has antibacterial, antifungal, antiviral, antimitotic, antimutagenic, antioxidant, cancerostatic, and immunostimulating properties. The extracts also have a systemic anti-inflammatory effect. Marigold is available as ointment, cream, gel, shampoo, tincture, tea, and mouthwash, in products such as Calendula Gel, Calendula Ointment, California Candula Gel, and Kneipp's Calendula Ointment.

Reported uses

Ointments containing marigold are used to treat wounds, burns, insect bites, chapped lips, nipples cracked by breastfeeding, skin inflammation, furunculosis, eczema, acne, and varicose veins. Tinctures and teas are used for peptic ulcers, dysmenorrhea, and sore throat. Extracts are used for cancer therapy and as immunostimulants in viral and bacterial infections. Other reported uses include diuresis and treatment of fever, toothache, and eye inflammation. Volatile oil of marigold is used in perfumes, and plant pigments are used in cosmetics.

Administration

■ Ointment: Apply 2 to 5 g powdered herb in 100 g ointment to affected area
■ Compress: Steep 1 tablespoon herb in 500 ml water for 10 to 15 minutes and apply as a moist compress
■ Homeopathic formula: Dosage is 5 to 10 drops, 1 tablet, or 5 to 10 globules 1 to 3 times per day or 1 ml injection subcutaneously, twice weekly
■ Tea: 1 to 2 g per cup of water daily, ingested or as a gargle.

Hazards

No known reactions have occurred with the use of calendula, although there is a slight possibility that contact dermatitis may occur in some patients.

Women who are pregnant or breastfeeding should avoid using the herb, as should patients who have a history of environmental allergies or hypersensitivity to marigold.

 SAFETY RISK *Don't confuse marigold* (C. officinalis) *with African, Inca, or French marigolds* (Tagetes), *often used in gardens to repel insects.*

Clinical considerations

■ Warn patient about the risk of allergic reaction.
■ Advise women to avoid use while pregnant or breast-feeding. Tell women to notify health care provider about planned, suspected, or known pregnancy.

- Warn patient not to take herb for worrisome symptoms before seeking appropriate medical evaluation because doing so may delay diagnosis of a potentially serious medical condition.
- Be sure patient is using correct dosage and administration route.
- Tell patient to remind prescriber and pharmacist of any herbal or dietary supplement that he's taking whenobtaining a new prescription.
- Advise patient to consult his health care provider before using an herbal preparation because a treatment with proven efficacy may be available.

Research summary

Studies have been conducted on the antiviral and antibacterial components of calendula. It has been found effective in treating human immunodeficiency virus (HIV) and microorganisms such as *Klebsiella pneumoniae* and *Sarcina lutea*. Other studies have found calendula to be a potent anti-inflammatory agent.

marjoram

Origanum majorana

Marjoram (*Origanum majorana*) is a common aromatic herb used in cooking. The medicinal parts are derived from the plant's dried leaves and flowers. Marjoram contains thymol, carvacrol, tannins, flavonoids, hydroquinone, and phenolic glycosides. Its extracts decrease response to acetylcholine, histamine, serotonin, and nicotine. Antiviral, bactericidal, antiseptic, and antifungal effects are attributed to thymol, carvacrol, and marjoram essential oil. Marjoram is available as tea and as an essential oil, extracted by distillation.

Reported uses

Marjoram is used to treat headaches, depression, dizziness, insomnia, motion sickness, conjunctivitis, and GI complaints, such as gastritis, flatulence, and colic. It's also used for symptomatic treatment of rhinitis and colds. The essential oil is used externally for musculoskeletal pain and aromatherapy.

Administration

- Essential oil: Apply externally as needed
- Tea: 1 to 2 teaspoons of dried leaves in 1 cup of boiling water, taken by mouth every day, up to three times a day.

Hazards

Marjoram may cause nausea, vomiting, or diarrhea. Pregnant or breast-feeding women shouldn't use herb in amounts larger than those used in cooking. Children shouldn't use the essential oil. Patients with a history of allergic reaction to oregano or thyme shouldn't use marjoram.

Clinical considerations

- Patient should avoid using essential oil internally.
- Warn patient not to take herb for headaches, insomnia, or depression before seeking medical attention because doing so may delay diagnosis of a potentially serious medical condition.
- Advise patient to stop taking herb if he develops nausea, vomiting, or diarrhea, and tell him to notify his health care provider if these symptoms last longer than 2 or 3 days, as they may indicate toxicity.
- Advise patient to avoid use of volatile oils, or if used, to keep them away from eyes.
- Counsel patient not to use more of the herb than is normally used for cooking.
- Safety in children hasn't been established for amounts greater than those used for cooking.
- Discourage prolonged use due to possible toxic effects of even the low concentrations of thymol, arbutin, and hydroquinone contained in the essential oil.
- Tell patient to remind prescriber and pharmacist of any herbal or dietary supplement that he's taking whenobtaining a new prescription.

■ Advise patient to consult his health care provider before using an herbal preparation because a treatment with proven efficacy may be available.

Research summary

The concepts behind the use of marjoram and the claims made regarding its effects haven't yet been validated scientifically.

marshmallow

Althea, Althaea officinalis, *mallards, Moorish mallow, mortification root, Schloss tea, sweet weed, white maoow, wymote*

Marshmallow is indigenous to Asia, but has spread westward to southeast Europe and eastward to China. In temperate areas, marshmallow is a garden plant. The medicinal components are the dried root, dried leaves, and flowers.

Marshmallow contains mucilage, pectin, and starch. The herb has emollient, demulcent, urinary analgesic, anti-inflammatory, and anticomplement activity. It inhibits mucociliary activity and stimulates phagocytosis and immune activity. Marshmallow also acts as a hypoglycemic agent. It's available as a capsule, extract, syrup, and tea.

Reported uses

Marshmallow is used as a cough suppressant to alleviate irritation of oral and pharyngeal tissue. It's also used to treat inflammation and burns. Marshmallow is used to relieve mild gastric inflammation, irritable bowel syndrome, Crohn's disease, diarrhea, and constipation.

Administration

■ Tea (10 to 15 g steeped for 90 minutes in 150 ml of *cold* water): Dosage is several cups of slightly warmed tea during the day
■ Root: Dosage is 6 g by mouth every day

■ Leaf: Dosage is 5 g by mouth every day
■ Syrup: Taken in a single 10-g dose.

Hazards

No health hazards or adverse effects have been noted with proper dosage and administration of marshmallow. When marshmallow is taken with other medications, absorption may be delayed. When it's taken with insulin or sulfonylureas, there may be an enhanced hypoglycemic effect; patient should monitor blood glucose.

Patients who are hypersensitive to marshmallow should avoid its use, as should patients who are pregnant or breast-feeding.

 SAFETY RISK *Diabetic patients should be warned that marshmallow syrup has a high sugar content.*

Clinical considerations

■ Diabetic patients should use the herb with caution, and should be monitored closely for hypoglycemia.
■ Caution women to avoid using marshmallow during pregnancy or while breast-feeding.
■ Inform diabetic patient about the high sugar content of marshmallow syrup.
■ Advise patient to store marshmallow away from light.
■ Tell patient to separate administration times of marshmallow and other medications.
■ Tell patient to remind prescriber and pharmacist of any herbal or dietary supplement that he's taking whenobtaining a new prescription.
■ Advise patient to consult his health care provider before using an herbal preparation because a treatment with proven efficacy may be available.

Research summary

The concepts behind the use of marshmallow and the claims made regarding its effects haven't yet been validated scientifically.

INDICATIONS FOR THERAPEUTIC MASSAGE

- Chronic pain
- Circulatory problems
- Digestive disorders
- Inflammation
- Intestinal disorders
- Joint mobility disorders
- Muscle tension
- Overstimulated or understimulated nervous system
- Skin conditions
- Swelling.

Massage therapy

Throughout history, human beings have used various forms of touch to help ease pain and promote healing — touching, stroking, and kneading movements are almost automatic when people feel pain or are injured. The importance of touch has given massage its important role in the history of traditional medicine. Today, massage has emerged as a therapeutic discipline in the West, embraced by millions who use it to relieve pain and tension and generally to feel better.

The beginnings of modern massage in the West are often traced to Pehr Henrik Ling, a Swedish physician who developed his own style of massage and exercises in the early 1800s, a style that came to be called Swedish Remedial Massage and Exercise, or Swedish massage. By 1900, modern therapeutic massage techniques were being used throughout the developed world, primarily for rehabilitation. Gertrude Beard, an American nurse who served in the army in World War I, is credited with establishing therapeutic massage as a vital intervention for the stimulation of self-healing in patients.

Most massage therapists in the United States practice some variation of Swedish massage, applying several basic strokes to the body's soft tissue. Beyond this, many individual therapists have developed their own style and techniques.

TRAINING *Massage therapists are licensed in 25 states and the District of Columbia. Licensing requirements vary from state to state; most states require that the therapist undergo at least 500 hours of training from a recognized program and pass an examination. The American Massage Therapy Association in Evanston, Illinois, and the National Certification Board for Therapeutic Massage and Bodywork in McLean, Virginia, provide information and referrals.*

Reported uses

Therapeutic massage is used primarily for stress reduction and relaxation, but it can serve as a complementary therapy for a broad range of conditions. By improving circulation, massage can help relieve the pain and stiffness of arthritic joints. Through its muscle-toning effects, massage stimulates peristalsis, helping relieve constipation and indigestion due to a sedentary lifestyle.

The stress-reducing effects of massage may help people with hypertension or anxiety. Elderly patients may benefit from improved circulation and muscle tone as well as the personal attention and social interaction that a good massage provides. Massage has even been used to reduce irritability in infants. (See *Indications for therapeutic massage.*)

How the treatment is performed

Massage therapy requires a sturdy massage table (or a chair with a head rest for chair massages), lubricating oil, and a quiet room. Some patients may also find that quiet music adds additional relaxing effects.

The patient undresses and covers himself with a sheet or towel. With the patient on the massage table, the therapist may begin playing a tape of quiet, soothing music to induce relaxation. To respect the patient's modesty, the therapist keeps the body fully draped, exposing only the area being worked on.

BASIC MASSAGE TECHNIQUES

Therapeutic massage uses five basic techniques: effleurage, petrissage, friction, tapotement, and vibration.

Effleurage
In effleurage, the therapist performs a long, gliding stroke using the whole hand or the thumb. This motion is a warm-up technique that lets the patient get used to the therapist's hands. The gliding stroke, which should always move toward the heart, improves circulation.

Petrissage
Petrissage is a kneading and compressing motion in which the muscles are grasped and lifted. This motion relieves sore muscles by clearing away lactic acid and increasing circulation to the muscle tissue.

Friction
In friction, the therapist uses the thumbs and fingertips to work around the joints and the thickest part of the muscles. Circular motions break down adhesions

and may also help make soft tissue and joints more flexible. For larger muscles, the therapist may use the palm or heel of the hand.

Tapotement
In tapotement, the therapist uses the sides of the hands, fingertips, cupped palms, or slightly closed fists to make chopping, tapping, and beating motions. These motions invigorate and stimulate the muscles, resulting in a burst of energy. However, when muscles are cramped, strained, or spastic, tapotement performed for a longer period serves to relax the muscles.

Vibration
In vibration, the therapist presses the fingers or flattened hands firmly into the muscle and then "vibrates" (transmits a rapid, trembling motion) the area for a few seconds. This motion is repeated until the entire muscle has been vibrated. This helps to stimulate the nervous system and may increase circulation and improve gland function.

The therapist usually uses a scented oil to prevent friction between his hands and the patient's skin while he kneads various muscle groups in a systematic way from head to toe. (See *Basic massage techniques*.)

Hazards
A trained massage therapist pays close attention to body language as well as the patient's comments to avoid causing pain or discomfort. Other than this, there are no complications from properly performed massage.

Massage is contraindicated for people with diabetes, varicose veins, phlebitis, or other blood vessel problems, because massage to damaged tissue can dislodge a blood clot. It's also contraindicated in pa-

tients with pitting edema or swollen limbs.

Clinical considerations
■ Avoid massaging the abdomen of patient with hypertension or gastric or duodenal ulcers, and massage at least 6" (15 cm) away from bruises, cysts, broken bones, and breaks in skin integrity.
■ Advise patient seeking a massage therapist to get recommendations from satisfied patients, and to be sure the therapist is properly trained, licensed, and a member of a professional organization such as the American Massage Therapy Association.

Research summary
In her classic reference *Beard's Massage*, Gertrude Beard, former Associate Profes-

sor of Physical Therapy at Northwestern University Medical School, summarizes the research findings on massage's therapeutic effects as follows:

- increases blood flow through the muscles, promoting muscle toning and relieving some types of pain
- has a sedative effect on the nervous system
- increases peristalsis
- loosens mucus and induces drainage of sinus fluids from the lungs
- increases lymphatic circulation
- reduces swelling from fractures
- decreases scar tissue, adhesions, and fibrosis due to injury or immobilization.

Mayapple

Devil's apple, duck's foot, ground lemon, hog apple, Indian apple, mandrake, Podophyllum peltatum, raccoon berry, umbrella plant, vegetable Mercury, wild lemon

Mayapple is a perennial plant indigenous to northeastern North America. It has an unpleasant and acrid odor. The medicinal parts are derived from a resin extracted from the dried rhizome.

Mayapple contains podophyllic acid, picropodophyllin, alpha-peltatin and beta-peltatin, and podophyllotoxin. These components demonstrate antimitotic effects, thereby inhibiting tumor growth. Some components decrease mitochondrial cytochrome activity as well. Various anticancer drugs contain a synthetic component of the Mayapple, called podophyllin. The dried root irritates colonic mucosa, acting as purgative cathartic. Mayapple is available as dried roots and rhizomes, powder, and extracted resin, in products such as Condylox, Podocon-25, Podofilm, Podofin, Warix, and Wartex.

Reported uses

Mayapple extracts are included in prescription keratolytics used to treat condylomata acuminata, external and perianal warts, keratoses, laryngeal papilloma, and plantar warts. Some plant components are included in anticancer drugs used to treat testicular, ovarian, and small-cell lung cancer. Mayapple is used as a stimulant laxative, cathartic, purgative, counterirritant, and vermifuge. It's also used to treat tinea capitis, rheumatoid arthritis, and amenorrhea. The topical tincture and extract are FDA-approved for treating warts. Podophyllum is recommended by the Centers for Disease Control and Prevention as an alternative to cryotherapy for external warts.

SAFETY RISK *Mayapple is considered toxic and should be used only under the supervision of a qualified health care provider. Only the ripe fruits are edible.*

Administration

- Dried root: Dosage is 1.5 to 3 g by mouth every day
- Tincture (25% in benzoin): Applied to dry skin with dropper or applicator. A health care provider should apply the solution. To avoid toxicity, the treated area shouldn't exceed 25 cm². Dried resin is removed with soap and water after 1 to 4 hours
- Topical solution (0.5%): Applied two times a day with cotton-tipped applicator to wart surface for 3 days and then discontinued for 4 days. Repeat cycle up to four times.

Hazards

Mayapple is associated with adverse effects, such as changes in mental status, seizures, stupor, dizziness, hallucinations, shortness of breath, tachypnea, hair loss, ulcerative skin lesion and pyrexia, decreased reflexes, peripheral neuropathy, and coma. It may also cause hypotension, tachycardia, conjunctivitis, keratitis, nausea, vomiting, diarrhea, abdominal pain, paralytic ileus, hepatoxicity, nephrotoxicity, urine retention, anemia, hypokalemia, leukopenia, thrombocytopenia, and myelosuppression.

Patients who are pregnant or breastfeeding, and those with a hypersensitivity to it, shouldn't take Mayapple. Those with diabetes mellitus, circulatory problems, inflamed surrounding tissue, or open warts should also avoid its use.

Clinical considerations
- Patient should limit topical use of Mayapple to areas smaller than 25 cm^2 because of the risk of resorptive poisoning.
- Resin extracts of Mayapple are for external use only.
- Topical solutions should be washed off genital and perianal warts after 1 to 4 hours.
- Solution should be washed off meatal warts after 1 to 2 hours.
- Patient should apply occlusive dressing or urea around treated area to avoid contact with healthy skin.
- Advise patient to report any irritation or increase in bleeding or bruising to his health care provider.
- Warn patient not to use Mayapple near the eyes.
- Caution patient about ingesting large amounts of the dried root to avoid excess cathartic effects and poisoning.
- Advise patient to keep the herb out of reach of children and pets.
- Tell patient to remind prescriber and pharmacist of any herbal or dietary supplement that he's taking whenobtaining a new prescription.
- Advise patient to consult his health care provider before using an herbal preparation because a treatment with proven efficacy may be available.

Research summary
Research confirms that Mayapple is toxic. The concepts behind the use of Mayapple and the claims made regarding its effects haven't yet been validated scientifically.

meadowsweet

Bridewort, dolloff, dropwort, Filipendula ulmaria, *lady of the meadow, meadow queen, meadow-wort, meadsweet, meadwort, queen of the meadow,* Spireaea ulmaria

Meadowsweet is a perennial plant found in northern and southern Europe, North America, and northern Asia. The leaves have a very pleasant, almond-like fragrance and smell quite different from the flowers. The medicinal components consist of the dried flowers, the dried aerial parts of the flowering plant, and the fresh underground and aerial parts of the flowering plant.

Meadowsweet contains flavonoids, salicylates, coumarins, tannins, methyl salicylate, mucilage, ascorbic acid, and carbohydrates. It displays analgesic, antipyretic, antiemetic, antiulcer, antirheumatic, antiflatulent, laxative, sedative, diuretic, and anti-inflammatory actions. A heparin complex found in the plant demonstrates in vitro fibrinolytic and anticoagulant properties. Extracts from the flower exhibit in vitro bactericidal activity against *Staphylococcus aureus, S. epidermidis, Escherichia coli, Pseudomonas aeruginosa,* and *Proteus vulgaris.* Astringent properties have been attributed to the tannins in the plant. Extracts demonstrate antitumor, sedative, and urinary antiseptic properties as well. Meadowsweet is available as tablets, infusion, powder, liquid extract, and tincture, in products such as Arkocaps, Artival, Neutracalm, Rheuma-Tee, Rheumex, Santane, and Spireadosa.

Reported uses
Meadowsweet is used as an analgesic and anti-inflammatory for conditions such as toothache, rheumatoid arthritis, headache, tendinitis, and sprains. It's also used for GI complaints such as gastritis, diarrhea, peptic ulcer, heartburn, and irritable bowel syndrome. Meadowsweet is

used as a diuretic or astringent and to relieve cough, colds, and bronchitis.

 SAFETY RISK *Meadowsweet contains methyl salicylate, which is fatal in high doses.*

Administration
- Dried flowers: 2.5 to 3.5 g by mouth every day
- Dried herb: 4 to 5 g by mouth every day
- Infusion (3 to 6 g in 100 ml boiling water, strained after 10 minutes): three times a day by mouth, as needed
- Liquid extract (1:1 in 25% alcohol): 1.5 to 6 ml by mouth three times a day
- Tincture (1:5 in 25% alcohol): 2 to 4 ml by mouth three times a day.

Hazards
Meadowsweet may cause nausea and bronchospasm. Tinctures or extracts prepared with alcohol may cause a disulfiram-like reaction.

Meadowsweet shouldn't be used by patients with a history of salicylate or sulfite sensitivity, patients taking warfarin, or patients with cardiac conditions who take aspirin. It shouldn't be used by children or by pregnant or breast-feeding patients.

Clinical considerations
- Although no chemical interactions have been reported in clinical studies, advise patient that herb may interfere with therapeutic effect of conventional drugs.
- Caution patient to avoid use if he has a history of asthma or sensitivity to aspirin.
- Tell patient to stop using salicylates if using meadowsweet.
- Warn patient not to take herb for chronic or unexplained pain before seeking appropriate medical evaluation because doing so may delay diagnosis of a potentially serious medical condition.
- Advise patient to avoid use during pregnancy and while breast-feeding.
- Tell patient to keep herb out of reach of children because of risk of salicylate poisoning.

- Advise patient to notify health care provider of darkened stools, bleeding gums, or excessive bruising.
- Tell patient to remind prescriber and pharmacist of any herbal or dietary supplement that he's taking when obtaining a new prescription.
- Advise patient to consult his health care provider before using an herbal preparation because a treatment with proven efficacy may be available.

Research summary
Meadowsweet has been studied for its antibacterial effect and for its astringent and anticoagulant properties. It has a low toxic profile.

Meditation

The ancient art of meditation — focusing one's attention on a single sound or image or simply on the rhythm of one's own breathing — has been found to have positive effects on health. By directing attention away from worries about the future or preoccupation with the past, meditation reduces stress, a major contributing factor in many health problems. Stress reduction in turn results in a wide range of physiologic and mental health benefits, from decreased oxygen consumption, heart rate, and respiratory rate to improved mood, spiritual calm, and heightened awareness.

Most meditation approaches fall into one of two techniques, concentrative meditation or mindful meditation. *Concentrative meditation* involves focusing on an image, a sound (called a mantra), or one's own breathing. For example, by concentrating on the continuous rhythm of inhalation and exhalation, the meditating person slows and deepens his breathing — a physiologic benefit — and achieves a state of calm and heightened awareness. Transcendental meditation, a form of concentrative meditation that became popular in the 1960s, arose out of the practice of yoga. In this form of meditation, the individual repeats a mantra over and over while sitting in a comfortable position. The mantra helps concentration; when other thoughts intrude, the individual is taught to notice them and then return to the mantra.

Mindful meditation takes the opposite approach. Instead of focusing on a single sensation or sound, the individual is aware of all sensations, feelings, images, thoughts, sounds, and smells without actually thinking about them. The goal is a calmer, clearer, nonreactive state of mind.

The health benefits of meditation have long been recognized in the East; however, only in the last two decades has meditation become widely accepted in the West, largely as a result of Harvard professor Herbert Benson's pioneering research in the 1970s on the physiologic effects of transcendental meditation. Since that time, instruction in meditation has been added to the curriculum of hundreds of universities and medical schools (including Harvard University, where the Mind-Body Medical Institute is run by Benson). The National Institutes of Health (NIH) now recommends meditation as a first-line treatment for mild hypertension. (See *Relaxation response*, pages 336 and 337.)

Patients interested in learning meditation can get help from many kinds of health care providers, including mental health practitioners, stress-reduction experts, and yoga teachers. Numerous hospitals and clinics offer classes in meditation as part of stress-reduction programs. The Institute of Noetic Sciences in Sausalito, California, is an information resource.

Reported uses

Meditation has a wide variety of indications. It's used to enhance immune function in patients with cancer, acquired immunodeficiency syndrome (AIDS), and autoimmune disorders, and has been successful in treating drug and alcohol addiction as well as posttraumatic stress disorder. Anxiety disorders, pain, and stress are also commonly treated with meditation. Many mainstream medical practitioners recommend meditation in conjunction with dietary and lifestyle changes for patients with hypertension or heart disease.

Because meditation is so well-suited to self-care, an increasing number of healthy people are incorporating it into an overall wellness strategy. According to the 1994 report to the NIH, *Alternative Medicine: Expanding Medical Horizons,* "If practiced regularly, meditation develops habitual, unconscious microbehaviors that produce widespread positive effects on physical and psychological functioning. Meditating for even 15 minutes twice a day seems to bring beneficial results."

How the treatment is performed

Meditation requires a private, quiet environment that's free from distractions, with a comfortable place for the patient to sit or recline.

The procedure is explained to the patient and any questions he has are answered. The patient is assured that he can stop the exercise at any time if he becomes uncomfortable. The patient is helped into a comfortable position; if he's in a sitting position he's advised to keep his back straight and let his shoulders drop.

Using a calm, soothing, low voice, the practitioner instructs the patient to close his eyes if doing so feels comfortable. He's told to focus on his abdomen, feeling it rise and fall with his respirations. He's told to concentrate on his breathing and that if his mind wanders, he should simply bring it back to his breathing. The patient is advised to practice the exercise for 15 minutes every day for a week, after which the benefits are evaluated with the practitioner. The practitioner documents the session, the instructions given the patient, and his response. The practitioner may also record the patient's heart and respiratory rates and blood pressure prior to and after a meditation session. Fi-

RELAXATION RESPONSE

In 1968, a group of Transcendental Meditation (TM) practitioners approached Herbert Benson at his laboratory at Harvard Medical School and asked whether he would study them because they believed that TM could lower their blood pressure. He initially dismissed the idea, but later changed his mind and began a study of volunteers who had been practicing TM for periods from less than 1 month to more than 9 years.

The volunteers were studied for 20 to 30 minute periods, before, during, and after meditation. The results were startling. Benson found that during meditation:

- oxygen consumption decreased markedly
- metabolism decreased
- heart and respiratory rates decreased
- alpha waves (associated with a feeling of well-being) increased in intensity and frequency
- levels of blood lactate (a substance produced by skeletal muscle metabolism and associated with anxiety) decreased.

These physiologic changes were similar to feats observed in highly trained yoga and Zen masters with 15 to 20 years of experience in meditation. The one measurement that was unchanged during meditation was blood pressure. That value was low before, during, and after meditation. Benson reasoned that perhaps the volunteers had low blood pressure because they

Technique	Oxygen consumption	Respiratory rate
Transcendental meditation	Decreases	Decreases
Zen and yoga	Decreases	Decreases
Autogenic training	Not measured	Decreases
Progressive relaxation	Not measured	Not measured
Hypnosis with suggested deep relaxation	Decreases	Decreases

nally, the practitioner may also want to note any change in pain or anxiety level at the end of the session and document any changes.

Hazards

Occasionally, meditation may elicit negative emotions, disorientation, or memories of early childhood abuses and other traumas. Meditation should be used with caution in schizophrenic patients and those with attention deficit disorder.

Clinical considerations

- Reassure patient if he experiences negative emotions, disorientation, or memories of trauma. If possible, find out what the feeling or memory concerns, and direct the patient to a safer, more pleasant thought or memory; otherwise, stop the session and notify the doctor. Stay with the patient until he is calm.
- Remind patient that meditation is not a substitute for medical treatment. Advise patient to continue taking any prescribed medications.
- Be aware that patients with respiratory problems may have difficulty with medi-

practiced meditation. He concluded that if this was true, people with hypertension might be able to lower their blood pressure through meditation.

Protective response to stress
Further experiments over several years led Benson to conclude that the various hypometabolic changes that accompanied TM were part of an integrated response opposite to the fight-or-flight response and that they were in no way unique to TM. Just as humans have an innate way of reacting to stress — the fight-or-flight response — they also have a natural protective mechanism against overstress, which Benson called the relaxation response.

By learning to consciously activate the relaxation response through such techniques as TM and yoga, Benson theorized, humans could offset the negative physiologic effects caused by stress and ultimately prevent stress-related diseases, such as hypertension, strokes, and heart attacks. Benson's work ultimately played a large part in changing the attitudes of conventional medicine toward meditation — from regarding it as a dubious practice to viewing it as a valid technique that could have a positive effect on health. The chart below outlines the practice that produced the physical changes of the relaxation response in Benson's studies.

Heart rate	Alpha waves	Blood pressure	Muscle tension
Decreases	Increases	Decreases in hypertension	Not measured
Decreases	Increases	Decreases in hypertension	Not measured
Decreases	Increases	Inconclusive	Decreases
Not measured	Not measured	Inconclusive	Decreases
Decreases	Not measured	Inconclusive	Not measured

tation techniques that focus on breathing.

Research summary
Since Herbert Benson's studies on transcendental meditation in the 1970s, a number of studies have documented meditation's effectiveness in reducing anxiety, chronic pain, serum cholesterol levels, high blood pressure (in the population at large and in blacks specifically), and substance abuse. It's also been noted in the literature that meditation cuts health care costs and enhances quality of life. Over the past 25 years, Benson and

his colleagues have continued to produce research on the benefits of the relaxation response.

Despite this evidence, most mainstream medical practitioners still regard meditation as an unconventional practice and overlook it as a potential therapy. The NIH report urges them to reconsider, concluding that "given its low cost and demonstrated health benefits, [meditation techniques] may be some of the best candidates among the alternative therapies for widespread inclusion in medical practice and for investment of medical resources."

melatonin

Melatonin is a hormone produced by the pineal gland. Its secretion is stimulated by darkness and inhibited by light. Secretion peaks between 2:00 a.m. and 4:00 a.m., and the degree of excretion diminishes with advancing age. Administering melatonin may regulate circadian rhythms and help regulate body temperature, cardiovascular function, and reproduction. It may also protect cells against oxidation caused by free-radical formation. Melatonin is available as synthetic or animal-derived (pineal tissue) products in tablet or lozenge form. The circadian (controlled-release) form isn't available in the United States. Product names include Mela-T, Melatonex, and Melatonin-Forte (combination).

Reported uses
Melatonin is used to treat insomnia, jet lag, shift-work disorder, blind entrainment, tinnitus, and depression. It's also used to treat benzodiazepine withdrawal in elderly patients with insomnia. Melatonin is also used as a cancer therapy adjuvant, an immune system enhancer, an antiaging product, a contraceptive, and a prophylactic therapy for cluster headaches. Topically, it's used for skin protection against ultraviolet light. It's also been used for cachexia and in treatment of chemotherapy-induced thrombocytopenia.

Administration
- For adjunctive therapy in metastatic lung cancer, dosage is 10 mg by mouth at bedtime
- For benzodiazepine withdrawal in geriatric patients with insomnia, dosage is 2 mg by mouth of controlled-release melatonin at bedtime for 6 weeks. Benzodiazepine dosage is reduced by 50% during week 2 and by 75% during weeks 3 and 4; it's discontinued during weeks 5 and 6. Patient may continue to require melatonin for up to 6 months for insomnia

- As a preventative for jet lag, dosage is 5 to 8 mg by mouth at bedtime for 1 week, beginning 1 to 3 days before the flight
- For other sleep disturbances, dosage is 0.3 to 5 mg by mouth at bedtime
- As supportive treatment for metastatic solid tumors, cachexia, and chemotherapy-induced thrombocytopenia, dosage is 10 to 50 mg by mouth at bedtime
- Transmucosal and sublingual dosage forms more closely mimic endogenous melatonin and bypass first-pass metabolism by the liver; therefore, lower doses may be effective.

Hazards
Melatonin may cause headache, depression, daytime fatigue and drowsiness, dizziness, irritability, reduced alertness, confusion, and dysphoria. Other adverse effects include abdominal cramps, increased hormone levels, mild hypothermia, and pruritus.

Melatonin may interact with other medications. For example, its use with central nervous system (CNS) depressants may cause additive sedation; its use with benzodiazepines may enhance anxiolytic effects; and use with verapamil may increase melatonin secretion. Using melatonin with chlorpromazine may decrease clearance of melatonin, thus increasing its effects. Melatonin may interfere with immunosuppressant therapy by improving immune function. Melatonin interacts with other sedating herbs or supplements, such as 5-HTP, kava-kava, and valerian, causing increased sedation. Patients with hepatic insufficiency may have an increase in melatonin effect due to the extensive hepatic metabolism. Melatonin may increase human growth hormone levels.

Melatonin shouldn't be used by patients taking CNS depressants. It shouldn't be taken by patients using immunosuppressants or by women who are pregnant or breast-feeding. Melatonin shouldn't be used by children because it may inhibit gonadal development. Melatonin is contraindicated in patients with multiple sclerosis and other autoimmune diseases because it may exacerbate symptoms.

Clinical considerations

- Monitor patient for excessive daytime drowsiness.
- Melatonin is designated as an orphan drug for the treatment of circadian rhythm sleep disorders in blind patients with no light perception.
- Warn patient to avoid hazardous activities until full extent of CNS depressant effects is known.
- Advise patient planning to conceive that melatonin may have a contraceptive effect. However, it shouldn't be used as a form of birth control.
- Inform patient that melatonin may interfere with therapeutic effects of conventional drugs.
- Warn patient about possible additive effects if taken with alcohol.
- Advise patient to use only the synthetic form (not the animal-derived product) because of concerns about contamination and viral transmission.
- Advise patient not to use melatonin for prolonged periods because safety data aren't available.
- Caution patient with a history of seizures to consult with a health care provider before using melatonin.
- Tell patient to remind prescriber and pharmacist of any herbal or dietary supplement that he's taking whenobtaining a new prescription.
- Advise patient to consult his health care provider before using an herbal preparation because a treatment with proven efficacy may be available.

Research summary

A variety of randomized, double-blind, placebo-controlled and open-label randomized studies have indicated that melatonin is superior to placebo for indications such as jet lag, sleep disorders, cancer, cachexia, thrombocytopenia, and cluster headaches. Topical use of melatonin isn't well documented.

milk thistle

Cardui mariae fructus, *holy thistle, lady's thistle, Marian thistle, Mary thistle,* Silybum marianum, *silymarin, St. Mary thistle*

Milk thistle was once grown in Europe as a vegetable. The fruit and the seed from the milk thistle are more commonly used than the other aerial parts of the plant. The leaves are used in salads and as a substitute for spinach. The flower portion is eaten similar to an artichoke, and the seeds are roasted as a coffee substitute.

Milk thistle contains silymarin, which consists of hepatoprotective flavonolignans, including silibinin (silybin), silidyanin, and silychristin. Silymarin alters liver cell walls to prevent toxin entry and acts as an antioxidant by scavenging free radicals. It also stimulates protein synthesis in the liver, promoting liver cell generation. Silymarin's anti-inflammatory and immunomodulatory activity may add to its protective actions on the liver. Milk thistle components reduce histamine release from basophils through membrane stabilization, inhibit T-lymphocyte activation, increase neutrophil motility, and alter polymorphonuclear leukocyte function. Silibinin administration decreases biliary cholesterol levels. Milk thistle reduces insulin resistance in patients with cirrhosis resulting from alcoholism.

Milk thistle is available as capsules, soft gels, liquid, extract, and intravenous silbinin (the I.V. form is unavailable in the United States). It's available in products such as Liver Formula with Milk Thistle, Milk Thistle Phytosome, Milk Thistle Power, Milk Thistle Super Complex, Silybin Phytosome, Silymarin Milk Thistle, Simply Milk Thistle, Thisilyn, Liver Maintenance Formula, Liver D-Tox, Liv-R-Actin, Detox Support, and Detoxinal.

Reported uses

Milk thistle has been used for longer than 2,000 years as a medicinal plant for ailments of the liver and GI tract, for varicose veins, and for menstrual problems. It's also used to treat dyspepsia, liver damage from chemicals, and *Amanita* mushroom poisoning, and as supportive therapy for inflammatory liver disease and cirrhosis, loss of appetite, and gallbladder and spleen disorders. Milk thistle is also used as a liver protectant; when taken with hepatotoxic drugs, it may prevent liver damage from butyrophenones, phenothiazines, phenytoin, acetaminophen, and halothane.

Administration

- Oral: Dosage of milk thistle extract varies from 200 to 400 mg of silibinin (70% silymarin extract) by mouth every day, according to the potency. See label for manufacturer's recommendations. For liver dysfunction or ailments, the daily dosage is 140 to 420 mg divided into 2 to 3 doses
- Dried fruit or seed: Dosage is 12 to 15 g by mouth every day
- Tea (3 to 5 g freshly crushed fruit or seed steeped in 5 oz of boiling water for 10 to 15 minutes): Dosage is 1 cup of tea by mouth three to four times a day, 30 minutes before meals
- Injection (not available in the United States): For *Amanita phalloides* mushroom poisoning, dosage is 20 to 50 mg/kg I.V. over 24 hours, divided into four doses infused over 2 hours each.

Hazards

Milk thistle may cause nausea, vomiting, and diarrhea. Milk thistle may improve aspirin metabolism in patients with liver cirrhosis. Products that contain alcohol may cause a disulfiram-like reaction. Silymarin reduces adverse cholinergic effects when given with tacrine; advise patient to use together with caution.

Milk thistle shouldn't be used by patients who are pregnant or breast-feeding, or by patients hypersensitive to it. Its use in decompensated cirrhosis isn't recommended.

SAFETY RISK *Don't confuse milk thistle seeds or fruit with other parts of the plant or with blessed thistle* (Cnictus benedictus).

Clinical considerations

- Tell patient that mild allergic reactions may occur, especially in people allergic to members of the Asteraceae family such as ragweed, chrysanthemums, marigolds, and daisies.
- Silymarin has poor water solubility; therefore, efficacy when prepared as a tea is questionable.
- Advise patient that herb may interfere with therapeutic effect of conventional drugs.
- Warn patient not to take this herb while pregnant or breast-feeding.
- Warn patient not to take herb for liver inflammation or cirrhosis before seeking appropriate medical evaluation because doing so may delay diagnosis of a potentially serious medical condition.
- Advise patient to store the herb out of reach of children and pets.
- Tell patient to remind prescriber and pharmacist of any herbal or dietary supplement that he's taking whenobtaining a new prescription.
- Advise patient to consult his health care provider before using an herbal preparation because a treatment with proven efficacy may be available.

Research summary

Milk thistle has been studied extensively for its efficacy in treatment of liver disease, protection of the liver, treatment of blood disorders, and lipid effects. It has also been evaluated for its effect of preventing diabetic complications. It has been used for many years with few complications.

mistletoe

All-heal, American mistletoe, birdlime, devil's fuge, European mistletoe, mistelkraut, mystyldene, Phoradendron serotinum, *viscid,* Viscum album

Mistletoes are generally grouped into two descriptive classes: the American mistletoe (*Phoradendron* species) and the European mistletoe (*Viscum album* and its related species, *V. abietis* and *V. austriacum*). European mistletoe has been used for centuries in traditional medicine; in the early 1900s, it gained popularity as an anticancer treatment. Mistletoe was used in the past to increase passion during the holidays and is still used today as a holiday decoration. The medicinal parts are the dried leaves, stems, flowers, and fruit.

Phoratoxins and viscotoxins are toxic proteins isolated from American and European mistletoe, respectively. Phoratoxins from American mistletoe can cause hypertension, hypotension, bradycardia, and increased uterine and intestinal motility. Phoratoxins may also cause depolarization of skeletal muscle, smooth muscle contraction, vasoconstriction, and cardiac arrest. Lectins and viscotoxins from European mistletoe may possess anticancer and immunostimulation activity. Other effects include hypotension, bradycardia, and sedation. As an immunomodulator, *V. album* may stimulate DNA repair through lymphokines and cytokines in cancer patients. A lectin from mistletoe extract increases secretion of tumor necrosis factor, interleukin-1, and interleukin-6. Mistletoe is available in products such as Helixor, Iscador, Plenosol, Mistel, Viscysat, Eurixor, Vysorel, ABNOBA viscum, and Isorel. The form used for intravenous injection is unavailable in the United States.

Reported uses
American mistletoe is used as a smooth muscle stimulant for increasing blood pressure and uterine and intestinal contractions. European mistletoe is used to treat hypertension, cancer, internal bleeding, major blood loss, blood purification, arteriosclerosis, epilepsy, gout, and hysteria.

SAFETY RISK *Mistletoe has been proven toxic and is considered unsafe. FDA has forbidden marketing of mistletoe and products containing mistletoe.*

Administration
Administration of mistletoe isn't well-documented.

Hazards
All components of mistletoe, including the berries, are considered toxic and shouldn't be taken by anyone. Severity of adverse reactions correlate with the amount and type of mistletoe plant used. Mistletoe may cause delirium, hallucinations, seizures, bradycardia, hypertension, vasoconstriction, cardiac arrest, double vision, nausea, vomiting, diarrhea, acute gastroenteritis, and hepatitis. European mistletoe may alter efficacy of anticoagulants and antidepressant drug therapy. Blood pressure may be lowered by European mistletoe, which may also interfere with immunosuppressant therapy.

Clinical considerations
■ American mistletoe (*Phoradendron* species) and European mistletoe (*Viscum* species) may have varying pharmacologic effects. Advise patient to avoid American mistletoe.
■ Tell patient to notify health care provider about adverse effects, especially chest pain or tightness, nausea, vomiting, diarrhea, hallucinations, double vision, or slowed heart rate.
■ Store away from light in a dry place.
■ Tell patient to remind prescriber and pharmacist of any herbal or dietary supplement that he's taking when obtaining a new prescription.

- Advise patient to consult his health care provider before using an herbal preparation because a treatment with proven efficacy may be available.

Research summary
The concepts behind the use of mistletoe and the claims made regarding its effects haven't yet been validated scientifically. Mistletoe is considered toxic.

Monascus

Monascus purpureus, *red rice yeast, red yeast, xuezhikang, zhitai*

The use of red yeast dates back to China around 800 AD. It is a mild, non-poisonous yeast, *Monascus purpureus*, grown on cooked, nonglutinous rice. It's used to treat GI problems and circulation. In the late 1970s it was found that Monascus metabolites inhibited 3-hydroxy-3-methyl-glutaryl-coenzyme A (HMG-CoA) reductase, the rate-limiting step in cholesterol biosynthesis. Yeast contains HMG-CoA reductase inhibitors, primarily lovastatin (or monacolin K). Monacolin K is converted in the body to mevinolinic acid, which competitively binds to HMG-CoA reductase in place of the endogenous substance, HMG-CoA, inhibiting cholesterol formation.

Red yeast is available as capsules and extract, in products such as Cholester-Reg, CholesteSure, Cholestin, and Ruby Monascus. Lovastatin is available as a prescription cholesterol-lowering drug.

Reported uses
Red yeast is used to reduce total cholesterol, low-density lipoprotein cholesterol, and triglycerides; to increase high-density lipoprotein in patients with hypercholesterolemia; and to sustain desirable cholesterol levels in healthy people. It's also used for treating indigestion and diarrhea, improving blood circulation, and promoting stomach and spleen health.

Administration
For patients with hypercholesterolemia, the dosage is 1,200 mg (7.2 mg lovastatin, 9.6 mg total HMG Co-A reductase inhibitors) by mouth twice a day with food. Dosage can vary with manufacturer, however; for example, one manufacturer recommends 600 mg once daily and another recommends 1,000 mg daily.

Hazards
Adverse reactions to red yeast include gastritis, abdominal discomfort, nephrotoxicity, elevated liver enzyme levels, rhabdomyolysis, and muscle pain, tenderness, and weakness.

Use of red yeast with cytochrome P450-3A–inhibiting drugs, such as fluconazole, itraconazole, ketoconazole, and theophylline, may increase serum levels and adverse effects. Use with HMG-CoA reductase inhibitors may increase risk of adverse effects without providing added benefit. Grapefruit juice may cause increased bioavailability of lovastatin, thereby increasing the risk of adverse effects. Alcohol may increase risk of liver toxicity.

The manufacturer of the Cholestin brand of Monascus warns patients not to take product if they consume more than two alcoholic drinks per day, have a serious infection, have undergone an organ transplant, have had recent major surgery, or have a serious disease or physical disorder. Patients younger than age 18 should use with caution because safety hasn't been established. Patients at risk for liver disease, with active liver disease, or with a history of liver disease shouldn't take Monascus; pregnant and breastfeeding women should also avoid its use.

Clinical considerations
- Monitor patient closely if he's taking cholesterol-lowering drugs and Monascus concurrently.
- Obtain baseline lipid panel and liver function laboratory studies prior to initi-

ating Monascus and monitor periodically.
- If patient develops muscle pain or weakness, check creatine kinase to test for rhabdomyolysis.
- Review patient's current drug list. Many drugs, including cytochrome P450-3A inhibitors and HMG-CoA reductase inhibitors, may cause drug interactions.
- Tell patient to take herb with food.
- Warn patient with liver disease not to take this drug.
- Recommend that patient abstain from alcohol or limit its use.
- Urge patient to seek medical attention if he experiences brown urine, muscle pain, or weakness.
- Advise patient to take recommended dose of individual commercial products.
- Tell patient to remind prescriber and pharmacist of any herbal or dietary supplement that he's taking when obtaining a new prescription.
- Advise patient to consult his health care provider before using an herbal preparation because a treatment with proven efficacy may be available.

Research summary
The concepts behind the use of Monascus and the claims made regarding its effects haven't yet been validated scientifically.

morinda

Ba ji tian, hog apple, Indian mulberry, mengkudu, mora de la India, Morinda citrifolia, *noni, pain killer, ruibardo caribe, wild pine*

Polynesian healers have used morinda fruits for thousands of years to treat health problems from diabetes to arthritis. The medicinal components are obtained from root, leaves, fruit, and juice of *Morinda citrifolia*. The aerial portions contain essential oils with hexoic and oc-

toic acids, paraffin and esters of methyl, and ethyl alcohols. The root contains anthraquinones, alizarin, morindone, xeronine, and damnacanthal. Xeronine, a digestive enzyme, may be responsible for the herb's action in repairing damaged cells in digestive, respiratory, and skeletal systems, possibly by affecting the shape of protein molecules and by enhancing immune function.

Damnacanthal exerts antitumor activity by inhibiting the reticular activating system oncogene, a protein partially responsible for cell proliferation. Alcoholic extracts have anthelmintic and central analgesic activity. Tannins contained in morinda may have hypoglycemic properties. Morinda is available in many forms, including fruit leather, capsules, oil, fiber, and combination foods such as protein wafers, juices, and nutritional supplements.

Reported uses
Morinda is used to treat diabetes, high blood pressure, aging, and GI and liver conditions. It's also used as a sedative and for chronic fatigue syndrome, premenstrual syndrome, and ankylosing spondylitis. Morinda is used for its immunostimulant, anticancer, and anthelmintic effects. The leaves are used topically to soothe headaches and arthritic joints.

Administration
- Dosage can range from 3 to 6 g daily in two divided doses by mouth, on an empty stomach
- Tea (add 5 to 9 g herb to 3 to 4 cups of water and boil until volume is reduced by half): Dosage is 2 divided doses on an empty stomach
- Tincture (30 to 60 g steeped in 1 L of ethanol for 2 to 3 months): Dosage is 30 ml taken twice a day on an empty stomach, in the afternoon and at bedtime
- Juice: Dosage is 1 oz before meals
- Dried leaves may be used on the chest, stomach, head, or arthritic joints as compresses.

Hazards

Morinda may cause life-threatening hyperkalemia in patients with chronic renal failure. When taken with angiotensin-converting enzyme inhibitors, angiotensin II receptor antagonists, beta blockers, potassium-sparing diuretics, or trimethoprim-sulfamethoxazole, there is an additive effect of hyperkalemia. Morinda may counteract the effects of immunosuppressants.

Pregnant women and those who are breast-feeding shouldn't use morinda. Avoid use in patients with chronic renal failure or end-stage renal disease (the noni juice form contains potassium) or those hypersensitive to it. Morinda shouldn't be used in organ transplant recipients because the risk of rejection may be increased by morinda's immune system–enhancing properties.

Clinical considerations

- Morinda shouldn't replace conventional therapies that are known to be effective in the treatment of cancers and cardiovascular and endocrine disorders.
- Carefully monitor patient for adverse effects. Monitor patient closely for potassium accumulation when herb and drug are used together.
- Advise patient that herb may interfere with therapeutic effect of conventional drugs.
- Caution patient that anthraquinone content in the product may turn urine a pink or rust color.
- Instruct patient to take herb on an empty stomach so intestines may activate the enzyme.
- Because sedation is possible, advise patient not to perform potentially hazardous tasks while taking herb.
- Advise patient with kidney failure that noni juice is a source of potassium and that he shouldn't use it.
- Warn pregnant or breast-feeding patients to avoid using this herb.
- Warn patient not to take herb for worrisome symptoms before seeking appropriate medical evaluation because doing so may delay diagnosis of a potentially serious medical condition.
- Tell patient to remind prescriber and pharmacist of any herbal or dietary supplement that he's taking when obtaining a new prescription.
- Advise patient to consult his health care provider before using an herbal preparation because a treatment with proven efficacy may be available.

Research summary

The concepts behind the use of morinda and the claims made regarding its effects haven't yet been validated scientifically.

motherwort

Leonurus cardiaca, *lion's ear, lion's tail, Roman motherwort, throw-wort*

Motherwort is a perennial indigenous to central Europe and Scandinavia, and is present in temperate areas of Russia and central Asia. The medicinal components are obtained from above-ground parts of *Leonurus cardiaca*. Motherwort contains leocardin, ajugoside (leonuride), ajugol, galiridoside, reptoside, and other constituents, including flavonoids, leonurin, betaine, caffeic acid derivative, tannins, and traces of volatile oil. Alkaloids responsible for major herb activity include stachydrine, betonicine, turicin, leonurine, leonuridin, and leonurinine.

Motherwort has mild negative chronotropic properties, and hypotonic, cardiac-inhibitory, antispasmodic, and sedative actions. Leonurine may stimulate uterine tone and blood flow, and stachydrine may stimulate oxytocin release. Ursolic acid may have antiviral, tumor-inhibiting, and cytotoxic activity. K substance, an extract of motherwort, may decrease blood viscosity through platelet aggregation inhibition and inhibitory effects on cardiac function. Motherwort is available as powdered herb, leaf and flowering tops, fluid extract, solid extract, and alcohol extracts.

Reported uses

Motherwort is used for hyperthyroidism, management of mild to moderate cardiac insufficiency (New York Heart Association classes I and II), arrhythmias such as tachycardia, and other nervous cardiac conditions. It's also used for flatulence, amenorrhea, itching, and shingles, and as a generalized tonic and antiplatelet agent. It's used in combination with other herbs to treat symptoms of benign prostatic hyperplasia. Motherwort is used topically to improve eyesight.

Administration

- Fluid extract 1:1 (g/ml; contains 12% to 15 % organic alcohol): 1 to 2 ml by mouth three times a day as a dietary supplement
- Dried above-ground parts: 2 g by mouth three times a day
- Infusion: 4.5 g herb a day
- Tea (steep 2 g dried above-ground parts in 5 oz boiling water for 5 to 10 minutes, and then strain): 1 cup three times a day
- Tincture 1:5 (g/ml; tincture contains 56% to 62 % grain alcohol): 22.5 ml daily
- Long-term use: 5 gtt, 1 tablet, 10 pellets, by mouth once daily to three times a day
- Acute conditions: 5 gtt, 1 tablet, 10 pellets by mouth every 30 to 60 minutes.

Hazards

Motherwort may cause diarrhea, stomach irritation, uterine bleeding, contact dermatitis, photosensitivity reaction, and allergic reactions. There is risk of increased sedation when motherwort is taken in conjunction with antihistamines or central nervous system depressants. When taken with cardiac glycosides, motherwort may cause additive effects and possible cardiac glycoside toxicity. Caution should be used when taking motherwort with herbs containing cardiac glycosides, such as black hellebore, Canadian hemp root, digitalis leaf, figwort, hedge mustard, lily-of-the-valley roots, oleander leaf, pheasant's-eye plant, pleurisy root, squill bulb leaf scales, strophanthus seeds, and uzara owing to possible cardiac glycoside toxicity. Alcohol and motherwort may potentiate sedative effects. When taken with anticoagulants, there may be an increased risk of bleeding. Photosensitivity reaction may occur; caution should be used with exposure to sunlight.

Motherwort shouldn't be used by pregnant women because of possible uterine-stimulating properties. It should also be avoided by breast-feeding women. Patients currently receiving treatment for cardiac dysfunction or arrhythmias shouldn't use motherwort because of the risk of increased toxicity.

 SAFETY RISK *Avoid preparations containing alcohol in patients concomitantly taking disulfiram or metronidiazole.*

Clinical considerations

- Tinctures, fluidextracts, and flowering tops contain a large amount of alcohol and shouldn't be used by children, alcoholic patients, or patients taking disulfiram or metronidazole.
- Advise patient that motherwort has an unpleasant odor.
- Tell patient to notify health care provider about planned, suspected, or known pregnancy. Discourage taking of herb while breast-feeding.
- Tell patient that doses higher than recommended may cause diarrhea, stomach irritation, or uterine bleeding.
- Warn patient that herb may cause sedation and that he should avoid hazardous activities.
- Tell patient to keep fluidextract, tincture, and flowering tops out of the reach of children.
- Teach patient that motherwort may make him more sensitive to the effects of

sunlight; explain the need for adequate sunscreen when going outdoors.
- Advise cardiac patients to consult with their health care provider prior to using motherwort.
- Tell patient to remind prescriber and pharmacist of any herbal or dietary supplement that he's taking when obtaining a new prescription.
- Advise patient to consult his health care provider before using an herbal preparation because a treatment with proven efficacy may be available.

Research summary
The concepts behind the use of motherwort and the claims made regarding its effects haven't yet been validated scientifically.

mugwort

Artemisiae vulgaris radix, artemisia,
Artemisia vulgaris, carline thistle,
felon herb, hierba de San Juan,
sailor's tobacco, St. John's plant,
wormwood

Mugwort (*Artemisia vulgaris*) is indigenous to Asia and North America, and is also found in many parts of Europe. The medicinal components are obtained from its leaves and roots. Mugwort contains volatile oils (including 1,8-cineol, camphor, linalool, or thujone), sesquiterpene lactones, lipophilic flavonoids, polyenes, umbelliferone, aesculetin, and hydroxy-coumarins. The aqueous extract and essential oil have antimicrobial activity. Thujone may be responsible for uterine stimulant activity. Mugwort is available as leaves, tablets, fluid extract, and powder, and may be found in food products such as pasta.

Reported uses
Mugwort is used for many GI complaints, such as colic, diarrhea, constipation, cramps, weak digestion, and persistent vomiting. It's also used as a laxative for obesity, to stimulate gastric juice and bile secretion, as a therapeutic hand soak, and as a tonic for asthenia. It is used for worm infestations, epilepsy, poor circulation, sedation, and menstrual problems. Mugwort is used in combination with other herbs to treat psychoneuroses, neurasthenia, depression, hypochondria, autonomic neuroses, general irritability, restlessness, insomnia, and anxiety states.

Administration
- Hand soak: 2 handfuls of dried mugwort steeped in 10 oz raw apple cider vinegar. Add 1 to 2 tablespoons of this infusion to warm water and soak hands for 10 minutes
- Tea (steep 1 teaspoon herb in 150 to 200 ml of boiling water for 10 minutes, and then strain): Dosage is 2 to 3 cups before meals every day
- Tincture: Dosages vary depending on formulation and reason for treatment.

Hazards
Mugwort is associated with few adverse effects, seen rarely as sensitization through skin contact. When taken with central nervous system depressants, there may be increased sedative effects. If taken with disulfiram or metronidazole, an adverse reaction may occur because of alcohol content. Alcohol used with mugwort may potentiate sedative effects.

Women who are pregnant should avoid using mugwort because of its uterine-stimulant effects. Breast-feeding women should also avoid use. Patients hypersensitive to members of the *Asteraceae* family (such as ragweed, chrysanthemums, marigolds, daisies, sage, and wormwood) may have an allergic reaction to mugwort and should use the herb with caution. Allergic reactions may also occur in people allergic to tobacco, honey, or royal jelly.

Clinical considerations

■ Allergic IgE-mediated reactions via histamine release may occur in patients with allergies to plants of the same family.

■ Tincture contains significant amount of alcohol and shouldn't be used by children, alcoholic patients, or those taking disulfiram or metronidazole.

■ Advise patient that mugwort root has a pleasant, tangy taste; above-ground parts are aromatic and bitter.

■ Caution patient that he may become sensitized to the herb with skin contact.

■ If patient is allergic to herbs of the *Asteraceae* family (ragweed, chrysanthemums, marigolds, daisies, sage, and wormwood), or to tobacco, honey, or royal jelly, warn of a possible hypersensitivity reaction to mugwort.

■ Advise patient to keep herb out of reach of children.

■ Instruct patient taking this herb to notify a health care provider about planned, suspected, or known pregnancy. Advise against taking herb while breast-feeding.

■ Because it may cause uterine stimulation, avoid during pregnancy.

■ Avoid preparations containing alcohol in patients taking disulfiram or metronidazole.

■ Tell patient to remind prescriber and pharmacist of any herbal or dietary supplement that he's taking when obtaining a new prescription.

■ Advise patient to consult his health care provider before using an herbal preparation because a treatment with proven efficacy may be available.

Research summary

The concepts behind the use of Mugwort and the claims made regarding its effects haven't yet been validated scientifically.

mullein

Aaron's rod, Adam's flannel, ag-leaf, ag-paper, beggar's blanket, blanket herb, blanket-leaf, bouillon blanc, candle-flower, candlewick plant, clot-bur, clown's lungwort, cuddy's lungs, duffle, feltwort, flannelflower, fluffweed, hag's taper, hare's beard, hedge-taper, Jacob's staff, Jupiter's staff, longwort, mullein lobelia, Our Lady's flannel, rag paper, shepherd's club, shepherd's staff, torches, torch weed, velvet plant, Verbascum densiflorum, *wild ice leaf, woollen*

Mullein is a biennial plant found throughout the United States. It has been used for many years as an herbal remedy, particularly in the treatment of respiratory disorders. The medicinal components are obtained from dried flowers and leaves. Mullein contains mucilage, triterpene saponins (including songarosaponin D, E, and F), iridoid monoterpenes, tannins, caffeic acid derivatives, flavonoids, and invert sugar. Tannins, saponins, and mucilage are responsible for herb's effects. Saponins have expectorant actions, mucin has antibiotic actions, and the combination alleviates irritation from colds.

Demulcent properties may be useful for the treatment of sore throats. Mullein extract may have antiviral activity against influenza strains A and B and against herpes simplex virus type 1. Mullein is available as extracts, dried herb, capsules, teas, and oil.

Reported uses

Mullein is used for respiratory tract inflammation, cough, sore throat, bronchitis, and respiratory tract inflammation. It's also used internally as a diuretic, sedative, and narcotic; as an antirheumatic; and for croup, asthma, and tuberculosis. Mullein is used topically for hemorrhoids, burns, bruises, frostbite, and erysipelas. The oil is used to soothe earaches, and leaves are used to soften and protect the skin. Mullein is also used as a flavoring agent in alcoholic beverages.

Administration
- Capsules (330 mg): 2 to 3 capsules by mouth twice a day with meals
- Decoction (1.5 to 2 g of herb placed in 5 to 8 oz cold water, boiled for 10 minutes, and then strained): Taken twice a day
- Fluid extract: 1:1 (g/ml; contains 45% to 55% grain alcohol): 1.5 to 2 ml by mouth twice a day
- Mullein extract: 3 to 4 ml by mouth three times a day, or half this dose for children
- Mullein leaves liquid (alcohol-free): 4 to 8 gtt in a little water by mouth twice a day
- Tea (steep 1.5 to 2 g finely cut petals in boiling water for 10 to 15 minutes, and then strain): 1 cup every day
- Tincture: 1.5 g/ml (7.5 to 10 ml taken by mouth twice a day). May dilute in warm water.

Hazards
When taken with central nervous system depressants, mullein may potentiate sedative effects. When taken with disulfiram or metronidazole, an adverse reaction may occur because of alcohol content. Mullein and alcohol may potentiate sedative effects.

Mullein shouldn't be used by patients who are pregnant or breast-feeding or by those who are hypersensitive to it.

 SAFETY RISK *Don't confuse mullein with goldenrod (Solidago species), which is also known as Aaron's rod.*

Clinical considerations
- Extracts may contain large amounts of alcohol and shouldn't be used by children, alcoholic patients, or those taking disulfiram or metronidazole.
- Advise patient that mullein may interfere with therapeutic effect of conventional drugs.

- Tell patient to store mullein in cool, dry place protected from light. If herb comes into contact with light or moisture, it discolors to brown or dark brown.
- Advise patient to refrigerate mullein extract after opening it.
- Instruct patient taking mullein to notify a health care provider about planned, suspected, or known pregnancy. Caution against taking this herb while breast-feeding.
- Tell patient to remind prescriber and pharmacist of any herbal or dietary supplement that he's taking when filling a new prescription.
- Advise patient to consult with his health care provider before using an herbal preparation because a treatment with proven efficacy may be available.

Research summary
Mullein has been found to have antiviral properties against herpes simplex virus type 1 and influenza strains A and B. No adverse effects are reported with the use of mullein.

Music therapy

Music therapy, a form of sound therapy, uses the universal appeal of rhythmic sound to communicate, relax, encourage healing, and create a general feeling of well-being. It can take the form of creating music, singing, moving to music, or just listening.

Using music for healing dates back to Aristotle, who touted the power of the flute, and Pythagoras, who taught his students that singing and playing musical instruments could erase negative emotions such as worry, fear, sorrow, and anger. Writings dating from the Renaissance describe the influence of music on breathing, blood pressure, digestion, and muscular activity. In 1896, doctors discovered that a young boy's brain, partially exposed from an accident, responded differently when different types of music were played. Cerebral and peripheral circulation increased in response to some music; mental lucidity increased with other types. In the 1940s, Veterans Administration hospitals incorporated music into rehabilitation programs for disabled soldiers returning from World War II. (See *Understanding music therapy*.)

Today, music therapy is used to ameliorate physical, psychological, and cognitive problems in patients with illnesses or disabilities. It is offered in various settings, including general and psychiatric hospitals, rehabilitation facilities, mental health centers, senior centers and nursing homes, hospices, halfway houses, and substance abuse clinics. More than 5,000 registered music therapists practice in the United States today.

TRAINING *The National Association for Music Therapy (NAMT) was established in 1950, around the time that degree programs for professional music therapists were developed. The NAMT maintains curricular programs and training internships, a scientific database, standards of practice, and a code of ethics. It offers a board-certification examination for registered music therapists; candidates are required to have a bachelor's degree in music therapy and to have completed a 6-month internship. The NAMT also sponsors two publications:* Journal of Music Therapy *and* Music Therapy Perspectives.

Reported uses

As a complementary therapy, music therapy benefits patients with developmental disabilities such as mental retardation, and mental health disorders such as anxiety. It's also effective in reducing chronic pain and as an adjunctive therapy for patients with burns, cancer, cerebral palsy, stroke and other brain injuries, Parkinson's disease, and substance abuse problems.

Music thanatology, a new branch of sound therapy focused on psychological mechanisms for coping with death and dying, uses music to ease the emotional and physical pain of terminally ill pa-

---

UNDERSTANDING MUSIC THERAPY

Many different theories exist as to why music affects the body. One theory holds that the resonance emitted by sound waves restores the body's natural rhythm and encourages healing. Another theory proposes that the brain reacts to sound waves by sending out signals to control the heart rate, respiratory rate, and other body functions, which can result in lower blood pressure and decreased muscle tension. Endorphins, which alleviate pain and elevate mood, may also be released in response to the sound impulses. This combination of factors can create a state of total relaxation, possibly allowing the body to heal itself.

In some cases, music therapy may work simply by conjuring up happy memories in the listener. These memories produce positive emotions, which may work to reduce stress and enhance feelings of well-being.

In the Ayurvedic system of medicine, sound waves are believed to balance energy centers, known as chakras, within the body. The body has seven chakras, each of which vibrates at a different frequency, similar to the notes on a scale. When stress or diseases disrupt the chakras, the frequencies are thrown off. Music is one way to re-harmonize the chakras, thereby allowing the body to heal itself.

---

tients. Therapists say music can reduce depression, anxiety, and pain, and improve the overall quality of life for these patients. Music thanatology is used in a wide variety of settings, including homes, hospitals, and hospices.

At the other end of the spectrum, music therapy is used in delivery rooms to enhance the mother's feeling of comfort and security, to reduce the need for medication, and to promote a feeling of personal control over the situation. Studies have shown that premature infants who hear music in the intensive care unit are discharged earlier than infants who aren't exposed to music. In addition, relaxing music played to a fetus still in the womb is believed to improve the newborn's developmental capabilities.

How the treatment is performed

A comfortable environment and enjoyable music are the two necessary ingredients for music therapy. The music should be appropriate for the patient and the goal of the session. Faster music stimulates the patient; slower music has a calming effect. Calming music is usually slower than the patient's pulse (ideally less than 60 beats/minute). Music selection can also be based on the patient's ethnic background. Whatever the choice, the music should be meaningful to the patient.

A music therapy session can involve playing musical instruments, singing, or simply listening to music. It can be directed at a single patient or a group and can be conducted by a music therapist or other trained practitioner. The facilitator may perform, listen with the patients, compose songs, or join in improvisation.

For sessions involving the playing of music, instruments are needed. Tambourines, drums, and kazoos are appropriate for even the most nonmusical participant. Everyday objects like cooking pots may assume the role of percussion instruments. For patients with physical limitations, instruments can be adapted to fit their needs. A person can participate simply by keeping time with a spoon on a tabletop.

For sessions involving singing, the therapist will usually choose music that is familiar to the patient (or group). Lyrics may be provided by recitation or handouts, or displayed using chalkboards or overhead projectors.

Group participants should be introduced to each other. The purpose of the session is explained to them, and they're encouraged to join in as they feel able. The therapist positions himself to observe the patients if the therapy involves listening to music. If the group is performing, the therapist circulates among the participants and offers individual support and praise.

After a session, the participants are encouraged to discuss their feelings. The session and discussion are documented.

Hazards

Complications are rarely associated with music therapy. As with other mind-body therapies, there's a chance that a musical selection will bring back an unpleasant memory or experience. However, in most sessions, the experience will be enjoyable for both the participants and the facilitator.

Clinical considerations

■ Music therapy is especially effective as a means of reminiscence therapy for the elderly. Patients of similar ethnic backgrounds may enjoy music specific to their ethnic group. For children, music therapy is an excellent form of play therapy.
■ If the music evokes an unpleasant memory in a patient, comfort the patient and help him change his focus to more pleasant thoughts.
■ Inform relatives of a patient with Alzheimer's disease that they can use music as a tool to improve communication, especially in the middle phases of the disease. Simple acts, such as tapping the patient's hand in rhythm to speech, reading poetry to music, and playing slow music with language-based phrasing, are often effective.

Research summary

Studies show that music can be an effective complementary therapy for various medical conditions. Music has successfully reduced anxiety in children undergoing surgery, has decreased pain associated with dental and medical procedures, and has improved the rehabilitation of patients experiencing the aftereffects of cerebrovascular accident and those with Parkinson's disease. Patients who listened to classical music before surgery and again in the recovery room reported minimal postoperative disorientation.

Music has also been used successfully to communicate with Alzheimer's patients, autistic persons, and head trauma victims when other approaches failed. Patients who can't communicate verbally or initiate purposeful movement need increased sensory and environmental stimulation, especially that which taps into their remote memory. Music provides both psychological comfort and a means of communication for withdrawn or depressed institutionalized patients. A study of Alzheimer's patients showed that those who listened to big-band music during the day were more alert and happier and had better long-term recollection than the control group. In some cases, music is the only stimulus that elicits a response from these patients.

Myotherapy

Deep tissue therapy, manual ischemic compression, trigger point therapy

Myotherapy is a noninvasive, therapeutic approach developed in 1976 for relief of symptoms associated with muscular pain and dysfunction. Trigger points, localized areas of hyperirritable tissue in muscle, fascia, ligaments, and periosteal tissue, are tender when compressed. If sufficiently hypersensitive, trigger points give rise to referred pain and tenderness, and sometimes to referred autonomic phenomena and distortion of proprioceptions. In addition, trigger points may cause muscle spasm, limited range of movement, numbness, weakness, and fatigue. Therapeutic goals of myotherapy include relaxation of muscle spasms, im-

proved circulation, and pain relief. Myotherapy enhances the function of muscles and joints, improving range of motion and general body tone. Pain relief minimizes the need for muscle relaxants and analgesic drugs.

Bonnie Prudden developed myotherapy in 1976 while working with Desmond Tivy, a trigger-point practitioner who treated chronic pain patients with injection therapy. While preparing patients for treatment, Prudden discovered that compression of trigger points decreased their sensitivity. After testing this theory on a number of patients, she found that ischemic compressions for a period of 5 to 20 seconds would allow passive muscle stretching without procaine injections. Prudden found she could usually return the patient to a normal state of painless activity in fewer than ten sessions.

Trigger points (also called trigger zone, trigger spot, or trigger area) occur when tissue is damaged by accidents, sports activity, occupational stress, and disease conditions. They may also result from nutritional deficiencies. Objective and subjective findings identify trigger points in the absence of laboratory and radiological findings. Objective findings include a palpable firm, tense band of muscle, production of a local twitch response of the muscle during palpation, restricted stretch range-of-motion, weakness without atrophy, and the absence of neurological deficits. Subjective reports of stiffness and easy fatigability, spontaneous pain in a referred pain pattern predictable for the trigger point, and an exquisite, deep tenderness specifically at the trigger point may also occur. Some muscles may produce autonomic concomitants in the pain reference zone, such as localized vasoconstriction, sweating, lacrimation, coryza, salivation, and pilomotor activity (gooseflesh).

These spots become activated by acute or chronic overload of the muscle or when there is undue physical or emotional stress. When the trigger point is activated, it causes the muscle to increase tonus until it induces a painful spasm or cramp—a sharp, disabling pain or deep muscle ache. The pain caused by spasms causes more spasms and the spasm-pain-spasm cycle is set in place. Active trigger points can entrap nerves (sciatica), limit circulation, and pull muscles into a shortened state, which can cause weakness and interfere with coordination. Myotherapy interrupts this spasm-pain-spasm cycle.

TRAINING *Certified Bonnie Prudden myotherapists train for 1,300 hours. After completing the program, students must then pass board examinations to be certified. Forty-five hours of continuing training is required every two years for a myotherapist to maintain certification. Many myotherapists are also licensed massage therapists.*

Reported uses

Myotherapy is useful in relieving pain and dysfunction of any chronic myofascial pain such as chronic back pain, headaches, temporomandibular disorders, carpal tunnel, tendinitis, or bursitis. It is also effective in cases of imbalanced muscle training, acute or repetitive sprain/strain injuries, and occupational injuries or overuse syndromes. The treatment relieves swelling and discomfort in diseases such as lupus, multiple sclerosis, rheumatoid arthritis, osteoarthritis, and fibromyalgia.

How the treatment is performed

A myotherapy patient should be cleared by a physician, nurse practitioner, or physical therapist, or, in the case of temporomandibular joint disease, a dentist, to rule out a pathological condition requiring medical treatment.

The treatment protocol to interrupt the pain-spasm-pain cycle and deactivate trigger points is three-part, as follows: First, a pretreatment assessment is done on the patient; secondly, the trigger point is deactivated, the spasm is released, and the involved muscles are stretched; lastly, a posttreatment prescription of exercise,

nutrition, and stress management is issued.

In the pretreatment assessment, a thorough patient history is taken to develop a customized treatment plan based on the individual's specific medical condition and lifestyle. Locations of the trigger points are identified by palpation of the involved muscles. In trigger point deactivation, a variety of methods may be used to release trigger point spasms. Biofeedback has been successfully used to assist relaxation of the muscles in spasm. Passive stretching and myomassage is performed immediately after the trigger point is released to help lengthen the shortened muscles, thereby increasing movement and flexibility. Deep-stroking myomassage can then be used to advance healing by increasing local blood circulation and lymph drainage.

In *ischemic compression*, direct, firm pressure is applied to the trigger point using knuckles, hands, elbows, or *bodos* (small, wooden dowels with handles). Manual pressure usually releases the muscle spasm, diminishing the patient's experience of pain and allowing for myomassage and passive stretching, which lengthen the involved musculature. Imagery exercises designed to increase skin temperature have been used to help promote warmth and muscle relaxation at trigger point sites, decreasing their pressure-pain sensitivity.

Patients are given a home therapeutic plan delineating corrective exercises to re-educate the involved musculature, suggestions for balanced nutrition, and a stress-management plan. Patients may also be taught self-care methods using ischemic pressure maneuvers to increase the effectiveness of long-term maintenance. A well-designed exercise program incorporates full range of motion for injured muscles, preventing the shortening of newly lengthened muscles; recovers normal muscle activity levels; and maintains an effective level of fitness and function. Stress management is taught to diminish the effects of stress on trigger point activation. And finally, nutritional deficiencies are addressed so the body can achieve the biochemical balance necessary for proper muscle function. Special nutritional concerns with myofascial pain syndromes are vitamins B_1, B_6, B_{12}, folic acid, vitamin C, and calcium, iron, and potassium.

Hazards
Adverse effects may include sensation of pain during trigger-point desensitization. Minor bruising may occur at the site of compression. Bruises tend to occur more often in women, during anticoagulant therapy, and in vitamin C deficiency. Patients should be advised to gradually increase their activity level or risk injury.

Clinical considerations
- Advise patient that bruising may occur following myotherapy.
- Assess patient's pain status before, during, and after treatment.
- Advise patient to alert therapist of any health conditions or medications.

REIMBURSEMENT *Many private insurance companies, personal injury protection plans, and workers' compensation insurance carriers cover myotherapy when it's prescribed by a physician.*

Research summary
The concepts behind the use of myotherapy and the claims made regarding its effects haven't yet been validated scientifically.

myrtle

Myrti aetheroleum, M. folium,
Myrtus communis

Myrtle is an evergreen, bushy shrub indigenous to areas from the Mediterranean to the Himalayas. The medicinal components are obtained from the leaves and branches. *Myrti folium* refers to the dried leaves of *Myrtus communis*, where-

as *Myrti aetheroleum* is the essential oil of *Myrtus communis*. The essential oil is extracted from the leaves and branches by steam distillation. The percentage of oil extracted ranges from 0.1% to 0.5% depending on the month of harvest. Concentration is highest during May and June.

The chief components of myrtle are volatile oils, tannins, tonnic acid, and aceylphloroglucinols. Myrtol is the active constituent. It is absorbed in the intestine, stimulates the mucous membranes of the stomach and, deodorizes the breath. Myrtol also possesses fungicidal, disinfectant, and antibacterial effects. Animal experiments have also demonstrated hypoglycemic effects. Myrtle is available as an oil.

Reported uses
Taken internally, myrtle is used in the treatment of acute and chronic infections of the respiratory tract such as bronchitis, whooping cough, and tuberculosis of the lung. Other uses include bladder conditions, diarrhea, worm infestations, muscle spasms, and hemorrhoids. Externally, myrtle has been used to treat acne and varicose veins.

Administration
- Myrtle oil: 200 mg by mouth daily
- Myrtle leaves (powder from leaves): 5 g by mouth three times a day before meals.

Hazards
Myrtle may cause nausea, vomiting, or diarrhea. When applied to the faces of children, glottal and bronchial spasm has been noted. The tannic acid in myrtle may interfere with glycosides, iron-containing compounds, and alkaloids. When taken with antidiabetic medications, hypoglycemic effects may be enhanced.

Myrtle is contraindicated in patients with gastrointestinal, biliary duct, and liver disease. It shouldn't be used by pregnant or breast-feeding women. Myrtle shouldn't be used topically in children because of the potential for glottal and bronchial spasm.

 SAFETY RISK *Overdoses of myrtle oil (more than 10 g) can lead to a rapid fall in blood pressure and circulatory and respiratory collapse. Vomiting shouldn't be induced owing to the danger of aspiration. Following administration of activated charcoal, use symptomatic treatment for spasms and colic. Intubation may be warranted.*

Clinical considerations

- Caution patient about the potential for overdose.
- Advise patient of the effects of myrtle when taken with other medications.
- Warn patient to store product away from light.
- Advise patient not to use topically on children, and to keep out of reach of children.
- Caution patient to avoid large doses of myrtle as it may lead to hepatic damage, dehydration, and cardiovascular collapse.
- Advise patient that the herb's strength may vary depending on the time it was harvested; highest concentrations of the active component and subsequent higher risk for adverse effects are found in product harvested in May and June.
- Tell patient to remind prescriber and pharmacist of any herbal or dietary supplement that he's taking when obtaining a new prescription.
- Advise patient to consult his health care provider before using an herbal preparation because a treatment with proven efficacy may be available.

Research summary

The concepts behind the use of myrtle and the claims made regarding its effects haven't yet been validated scientifically.

Naturopathic medicine

Naturopathy

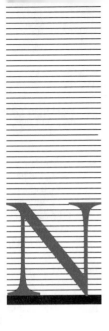

Naturopathy, a distinctly American approach to health care that developed in the late 19th century, emphasizes health maintenance, disease prevention, patient education, and the patient's responsibility for his own health. More a way of life than a system of medicine, naturopathy isn't based on a unique view of human physiology, function, and disease, as the Chinese and Ayurvedic systems are. Naturopathic doctors study the same subjects that conventional doctors do (including anatomy and physiology, pathophysiology, cell biology, and epidemiology). They also use conventional diagnostic methods, such as laboratory tests, to detect pathogens. What differs is their approach to treatment.

Naturopathic medicine evolved from a number of 19th century health movements that emphasized the importance of lifestyle, including good nutrition and avoidance of alcohol and meat, in maintaining health and fighting disease. By the early 1900s, there were more than 20 naturopathic medical schools in the United States, and naturopathic doctors were licensed in most states. The rise of biomedicine, with its emphasis on the pharmaceutical treatment of disease, led to the decline of naturopathic practice. Interest in naturopathy has rekindled in the past few decades, spurred largely by consumer interest in natural remedies. More than 1,000 naturopathic doctors

EIGHT PRINCIPLES OF NATUROPATHY

The following eight basic principles form the foundation of naturopathic medicine:

- The human body has its own inherent healing ability. The doctor must work to restore the patient's own healing system, using medicines that are in harmony with nature.
- Find and treat the cause. The doctor must find and treat the underlying cause of illness, not just the symptoms.
- Use therapies that do no harm. Natural therapies are less likely to cause complications than stronger treatments, such as drugs and surgery.
- The doctor is a teacher. The doctor should educate the patient in how to prevent disease and maintain health.
- Optimal health is the goal. The doctor and patient aim to establish and maintain optimal health and balance, not merely to treat a particular disorder.
- Treat the whole person. An individual is a complex interaction of physical, mental, emotional, spiritual, and environmental systems; the doctor must assess all of these aspects in order to determine a diagnosis and treatment.
- Focus on prevention. Each individual has an inherent state of wellness, even if a disease is present. The doctor must recognize and foster the individual's wellness by encouraging a healthy lifestyle and minimizing risk factors.
- Good nutrition is essential. Good nutrition is an important tool in promoting health and fighting chronic and degenerative disorders.

certain guidelines. The National College of Naturopathic Medicine in Portland, Oregon, and the Bastyr College of Natural Sciences in Seattle are two accredited colleges in the United States for naturopathic doctors. Today, naturopathy includes education and counseling on the benefits of a healthy lifestyle that includes the use of natural food and herbs. It also includes diagnosis and treatment of illness using conventional diagnostic medicines and methods, including minor surgery, if necessary.

The fundamental principle underlying naturopathy is the concept of *vitalism*, the belief that the body has an innate intelligence that strives to maximize health. Naturopathic doctors believe that symptoms aren't directly caused by a pathogen (such as a virus or bacterium) but are a manifestation of the body's effort to defend itself against the pathogen. Like Chinese doctors, they believe that pathogens must land on "fertile soil" in order to produce illness; that is, a person with a strong immune system may be able to fend off illness, while a person with a high stress level or poor nutrition may succumb. Naturopathic doctors strive to understand and support, rather than take over, the body's natural defense efforts.

In naturopathy, the absence of detectable disease doesn't equal health. Health is seen as a dynamic state of being that allows the individual to adapt and thrive in a variety of environments and to cope with the stresses of daily living. Naturopathy places great emphasis on disease prevention through healthful diet and lifestyle. A healthy lifestyle is believed to promote health, while an unhealthy lifestyle leads to degeneration, disability, and early death. (See *Eight principles of naturopathy.*)

TRAINING *There are several schools offering Doctor of Naturopathy (ND) degrees that do not offer the clinical supervision component. Some of the programs are distance learning models. The students receive classroom in-*

are currently licensed to practice in 10 states and the District of Columbia; other states allow naturopathic practice within struction in natural medicine and write a thesis upon completion. There is controversy among some practitioners as to the role of the naturopath. The Coalition for Natural Health resists the conventional model of the naturopathic medical schools. It is important to learn the credentials of the naturopath you choose.

Reported uses

Naturopathic medicine is used to treat a wide range of illnesses, including minor, self-limiting conditions such as the common cold and allergies, and — in combination with conventional medical treatments — life-threatening diseases such as cancer and acquired immunodeficiency syndrome (AIDS). However, naturopathic doctors usually refer patients with emergency cases, or those patients with serious or complicated illnesses, to conventional specialists.

How the treatment is performed

Through questioning and physical examination, the naturopathic doctor learns as much as possible about the patient's overall state of health. He then combines the results of this thorough patient history and physical examination with the results of any necessary radiologic and laboratory tests — conventional tests as well as tests outside of conventional medicine such as a digestive stool analysis — to form a diagnosis and treatment plan. Treatments are aimed at mobilizing the patient's own immune system to combat the disease and to regain and maintain optimal health. The naturopathic doctor may choose from a wide range of available treatments, including the following:

Nutritional therapy

Nutritional therapy uses whole foods, nutritional supplements if needed, and controlled fasting to treat disease and maintain health.

Herbal therapy

Herbal remedies may be taken internally or applied externally to treat the internal conditions that manifest as disease. Naturopathic doctors claim that botanical medicines are safer, more effective, and cheaper than pharmaceutical drugs.

Homeopathic remedies

Homeopathic solutions are very dilute preparations of natural substances that, in large amounts, cause certain symptoms but in small amounts are believed to relieve them. (See Homeopathy, page 250.)

Acupuncture

Commonly used to relieve pain, acupuncture involves the insertion of very fine needles into designated points on the skin to stimulate the body's vital flow of energy, called qi in traditional Chinese medicine. Acupuncture is performed by licensed acupuncturists and is not taught as a basic component of naturopathy. (See Acupuncture, page 30.)

Hydrotherapy

Hydrotherapy involves the use of special baths and other water-based treatments to cure disease and maintain health. In Europe, many patients are sent to spas for rest and rejuvenation. (See Hydrotherapy, page 265.)

Naturopathic manipulative therapy

Physical treatments may include manipulation of the bones and spine (in a manner similar to chiropractic) as well as massage, heat, cold, touch, electricity and sound, ultrasound, diathermy, and therapeutic exercises.

Counseling

Because naturopathic doctors believe that mental and emotional factors play a role in disease, counseling in lifestyle management is an important element of naturopathic treatment. Some naturopathic doctors are specially trained in biofeedback, stress reduction, meditation, yoga, and other techniques aimed at inducing a more balanced and natural lifestyle.

Hazards
Although naturopathy is considered safe, with no known adverse effects, it is important that the patient and provider are able to recognize and acknowledge the necessity for more aggressive treatment, and to act accordingly.

Clinical considerations
- Educate patient about the need to take responsibility for his own health, which may require lifestyle changes. Teach him ways to improve his health through diet and exercise.
- Inform patient that naturopathic doctors don't perform surgery or provide emergency care.
- Obtain patient's medication history to ensure that prescribed botanical remedies don't interact with already prescribed conventional medications.
- Tell recovering alcoholics to make sure that the remedies they take are mixed with water, not alcohol.
- Tell patient to remind prescriber and pharmacist of any herbal or dietary supplement that he's taking whenobtaining a new prescription.
- Advise patient to consult his health care provider before using an herbal preparation because a treatment with proven efficacy may be available.

Research summary
Research has demonstrated positive results in the use of natural (botanical) remedies for cervical dysplasia and as an alternative to estrogen replacement therapy. In a 1993 study on cervical dysplasia, 38 of the 43 women treated naturopathically returned to a normal Papanicolaou (Pap) test and a normal tissue biopsy. In another 1993 study on a substitute for estrogen, 100% of the women treated with the botanical formula showed a significant reduction of symptoms compared with 17% of the placebo group. The effectiveness of acupuncture for pain and dietary changes to reduce the risk of heart disease has been well documented.

nettle
Brennesselkraut, stinging nettle,
Urtica dioica, Urticae herba, U. radix

Nettle is a perennial plant native to Europe and found throughout the United States and in parts of Canada. It's known for its stinging properties. Nettle is used in traditional medicine for a variety of ailments. The medicinal components are obtained from fresh or dried roots and above-ground parts of *Urtica dioica*, *U. urens*, and hybrids of these species. Nettle contains acids, amines, flavonoids, choline acetyltransferase, and lectins. The aqueous extract yields five immunologically active polysaccharides and some lectins, which may also have anti-inflammatory and immunostimulant properties. The lectin agglutinin has antifungal activity. Two of the five polysaccharides have antihemolytic effects. Nettle leaves have diuretic, analgesic, and immunomodulating pharmacologic actions in vivo. It's available as tea, tablets, capsules, tincture, and liquid extract.

Reported uses
Nettle is used in folk medicine for wound healing and for treatment of greasy hair and seborrhea of the scalp. It's believed that nettle may actually stimulate hair growth. Nettle is also used to treat allergic rhinitis, osteoarthritis, rheumatoid arthritis, kidney stones, asthma, and benign prostatic hyperplasia (BPH). It's also used as a diuretic, an expectorant, a general health tonic, a blood builder and purifier, a pain reliever and anti-inflammatory, and a lung tonic for ex-smokers. Nettle is also used to treat eczema, hives, bursitis, tendinitis, laryngitis, sciatica, and premenstrual syndrome.

Administration

- Infusion: 1.5 g powdered nettle in cold water; heated to boiling for 1 minute, then steeped covered for 10 minutes and strained
- Dried leaf: For allergic rhinitis, 150 to 300 mg by mouth a day; for rheumatoid arthritis, 8 to 12 g by mouth a day; for BPH, 4 g root extract taken by mouth four times day, or 600 to 1200 mg encapsulated extract taken by mouth a day.

Hazards

Nettle is considered safe. Although known for its ability to induce topical irritation to exposed skin, this is usually easily treated by washing with mild soap and water. Stinging from nettle may last up to 12 hours or longer unless washed. Occasionally, a more serious reaction, such as urticaria, may require treatment with antihistamines and topical steroids.

Other adverse effects are rare but may include edema, gastric irritation, gingivostomatitis, decreased urine formation, and oliguria. Increased diuresis may occur in patients with arthritic conditions and those with myocardial or chronic venous insufficiency. Interactions may occur in patients who take the liquid extract while using disulfiram, or in those who drink alcohol. Patients taking nonsteroidal anti-inflammatory drugs, particularly diclofene, are at risk for increased effects and potential complications.

Nettle may alter blood glucose; patients on antidiabetic therapy should use this herb with caution. Patients taking diuretics or antihypertensives should use nettle with caution because it may affect urine formation. Patients with fluid retention caused by reduced cardiac or renal activity, those who are hypersensitive to herb, and those who are pregnant or breast-feeding shouldn't use nettle.

 SAFETY RISK *Nettle has been shown to have an abortifacient effect. Warn female patients not to use if pregnant or planning to conceive.*

Clinical considerations

- Nettle is reported to be an abortifacient and may affect the menstrual cycle.
- Adverse effects are rare and allergic in nature.
- Recommend caution if patient takes an antihypertensive or antidiabetic.
- Warn patient that external adverse effects result from skin contact and include burning and stinging that may persist for 12 hours or longer.
- Inform patient that capsules and extracts should be stored at room temperature, away from heat and direct light.
- Instruct women taking herb to notify health care provider about planned, suspected, or known pregnancy. Advise patient not to take this herb while breast-feeding.
- Tell patient to remind prescriber and pharmacist of any herbal or dietary supplement that he's taking whenobtaining a new prescription.
- Advise patient to consult his health care provider before using an herbal preparation because a treatment with proven efficacy may be available.

Research summary

Nettle has been used for years in folk medicine. Studies have shown that nettle possesses antiviral activity against human immunodeficiency virus and cytomegalovirus. It's also been evaluated for its effect on BPH and allergic rhinitis, and its carbohydrate-binding properties. Nettle is also being investigated for treatment of hay fever and irrigation of the urinary tract.

Neural therapy

Neural therapy involves the injection of local anesthetics — most commonly procaine and lidocaine — into various parts of the body to restore the proper flow of electrical energy in the body and thus promote healing. Although not widely used in the United States, neural therapy is popular in Germany and South America, where it's most often used to relieve chronic pain.

An unusual discovery by German doctor Ferdinand Huneke in 1940 laid the foundation for neural therapy. When Huneke injected procaine into a patient's stiff shoulder, the injection had no effect on the shoulder pain, but an old scar on the patient's leg began to itch. Thinking there might be some relation between the itching and the shoulder injection, Huneke then injected the scar with procaine, and the patient's shoulder pain immediately disappeared. From this incident, Huneke began to develop his theory of *interference fields*—disruptions in the flow of electrical energy that he believed were responsible for chronic illnesses. He believed that interference fields in one area could cause problems in other areas of the body, as the shoulder incident had shown, and that injections of anesthetics could destroy the interference fields and allow healing to proceed.

In 1950, Fleckenstein determined that normal body cells and scar tissue have different electric potentials across the cell membrane. In cells that have lost normal potential, ion flux across the membrane stops, allowing toxic substances and abnormal minerals to build up inside the cell. This causes the cell to become unable to heal itself and resume normal functioning. Treatment with a local anesthetic may help restore ion flux for 1 to 2 hours, which is believed to be enough time for the cell to partially repair itself, thereby resuming its normal function.

Another theory holds that scar tissue can act as a battery in the body and send abnormal electric signals that disturb autonomic nerve fibers. The electrical abnormality can disrupt the overall autonomic nervous system, leading to bodily dysfunction. This theory, proposed by Klinghardt and called the *fascial continuity theory*, further states that the fascia or sheaths of connective tissue are all interconnected. If scar tissue is present anywhere in the system, movement is impaired. If a local anesthetic is injected into a scar, movement may be restored.

TRAINING *The American Academy of Neural Therapy in Seattle, Washington, trains doctors in neural therapy techniques and provides referrals to trained practitioners.*

Reported uses
Neural therapy is used to treat allergies, skin disorders, bowel and bladder disorders, and most often, to alleviate chronic pain.

How the treatment is performed
Neural therapy is administered by a physician who has had postgraduate training in the field; it requires a sterile anesthetic for injection (usually procaine), gloves, needle and syringe, alcohol pads, and a receptacle in which to dispose of the contaminated items. After the physician has located the patient's interference fields by taking a detailed medical history, the anesthetic is injected into the appropriate area. The injection site may be an acupuncture point, peripheral nerve, gland, scar, or trigger point (an area that yields sharp pain when pressed). The number of treatments depends on the condition being treated.

Hazards
There are no reports of complications from neural therapy, although complications from local anesthetic may include allergic reaction.

Clinical considerations
- Neural therapy is contraindicated in patients who have cancer, coagulation disorders, renal failure, myasthenia gravis, or diabetes mellitus, and in those allergic to local anesthetics or their derivatives.
- Neural therapy should not be administered to patients receiving morphine, anticoagulants, or antiarrhythmic therapy.

Research summary

The concepts behind the use of neural therapy and the claims made regarding its effects haven't yet been validated scientifically.

Neuro-linguistic programming

Alternative therapy, Bandler method, changework, Ericksonian hypnosis, NLP

Richard Bandler and John Grinder are considered the fathers of neuro-linguistic programming (NLP). They studied under Milton Erickson, a psychologist who pioneered the use of hypnosis and suggestion in psychology. The underlying premise of NLP is that each person has a view of the world based on his or her experiences, and that this view is subjective and may not reflect reality. The experiences that a person has from birth onward have molded him into a set of patterns. For example, someone who is afraid of spiders is molded into a pattern that may be stated as: "I see a spider and I feel terror," whereas other people see a spider without reacting. NLP attempts to change that pattern, giving the patient a new association so that when he sees a spider he is calm instead of frightened.

NLP precipitates change by focusing on behaviors, on the theory that behaviors can be changed if they are broken down into small enough pieces. The patterns individuals use reflect their beliefs about the world—how they stand, walk, talk, and think (the *internal dialog*) are all patterns to an NLP practitioner. NLP works to change these patterns of speech, body movement, and thought in order to recondition and thus change the patterns.

Reported uses

NLP is used for pain management, and to treat psychological conditions such as depression, anxiety, obesity, fears and phobias, and stress. It's also used in business and professional applications for personal change, to improve decision-making ability, to enhance the ability to focus and concentrate, and to condition individuals to achieve success.

TRAINING *NLP training is available through a variety of training centers, seminars, videos, tapes, and books.*

How the treatment is performed

NLP is a unique psychotherapeutic approach in that the patient can be taught to use it on himself, thereby eventually eliminating the need for a practitioner. First, however, the practitioner must lay the groundwork, asking the patient questions that illuminate his world view. The NLP practitioner looks for patterns that help or hurt the patient.

Once the practitioner exposes the harmful patterns, the effort to change those patterns may begin. Patterns are changed through a variety of techniques, called modalities, submodalities, anchoring, transderivational search, chaining states, the *meta model*, meta programs, semantic primes, semantic density, and so forth. Each of these techniques is intended to establish the old patterns as undesirable and replace them with new, helpful patterns of behavior. The patient may be asked to imagine what he's afraid of, and to really feel the fear. Next, the patient is instructed to imagine a time when he's relaxed and calm. The state of calm then, gradually, replaces the state of fear.

Hazards

Disturbing thoughts and memories will surface for the patient as he works to change his patterns of behavior.

Clinical considerations

■ Advise patient seeking NLP to be sure he chooses a properly trained practitioner.

■ If patient is depressed, assess the likelihood of his harming himself prior to starting therapy.

■ Offer reassurance to patient disturbed by unpleasant or traumatic memories during treatment.

■ Determine whether therapy is working for patient, and refer patient to another practitioner if needed for additional psychological treatment.

Research summary

The concepts behind NLP and the claims made regarding its effects haven't yet been validated scientifically.

night-blooming cereus

Cactus grandiflorus,
large-flowered cactus,
Selenicereus grandiflorus,
sweet-scented cactus, vanilla cactus

Night-blooming cereus is a plant indigenous to Central America and cultivated in Mexico. The plant has sweet-smelling flowers that bloom for about 6 hours, and then die. The medicinal components are obtained from fresh or dried flowers and fresh young stems or shoots of *Selenicereus grandiflorus*, a cactus cultivated in greenhouses. The young shoots and flowers are harvested in June and July and preserved in alcohol. Night-blooming cereus contains flavonoids, amines (mainly tyramine, which produces a digitalis effect), and betacyans. It may induce a positive inotropic effect, causing cardiac stimulation and coronary and peripheral vessel dilation. It may also stimulate motor neurons of the spinal cord.

Reported uses

Night-blooming cereus is used for nervous cardiac disorders, angina pectoris, stenocardia, urinary ailments, hemoptysis, menorrhagia, dysmenorrhea, and hemorrhage. Juice of whole plant is used for cystitis, shortness of breath, and edema. Night-blooming cereus is used externally as astringent for rheumatism.

Administration

■ Liquid extract: 0.06 ml to 6 ml by mouth 1 to 10 times a day

■ Tincture: 0.12 ml to 2 ml by mouth two to three times a day

■ Tincture in sweetened water (1:10): 10 gtts by mouth 3 to 5 times a day.

Hazards

Intake of fresh juice of night-blooming cereus may cause some itching and pustules on the skin, along with nausea, vomiting, and diarrhea. Night-blooming cereus may increase the effect of digoxin. There is a potential for cardiac disturbances when it's taken with cardiac medications such as angiotensin-converting enzyme inhibitors, beta blockers, calcium channel blockers, and other anti-arrhythmic agents. When night-blooming cereus is taken with monoamine oxidase (MAO) inhibitors or over-the-counter cold and flu remedies, additive effects may occur.

Women who are pregnant or breast-feeding should avoid using night-blooming cereus, as should patients who are hypersensitive to it.

Clinical considerations

■ Overdose with cereus may cause severe nausea, vomiting, and diarrhea.

■ Night-blooming cereus may decrease heart rate.

■ Advise patient that night-blooming cereus may interfere with therapeutic effect of conventional drugs.

■ Caution patient to immediately notify health care provider about prolonged nausea, vomiting, or diarrhea.

■ Instruct patient taking night-blooming cereus to notify health care provider about planned, suspected, or known pregnancy.

■ Patients who take MAO inhibitors and those with cardiac disorders shouldn't take night-blooming cereus.

■ Tell patient to remind prescriber and pharmacist of any herbal or dietary supplement that he's taking whenobtaining a new prescription.

■ Advise patient to consult his health care provider before using an herbal preparation because a treatment with proven efficacy may be available.

Research summary
The concepts behind the use of night-blooming cereus and the claims made regarding its effects haven't yet been validated scientifically.

nutmeg

Mace, moschata, Myristica fragrans, *myristicea nux*

Nutmeg is an evergreen tree (*Myristica fragrans*) indigenous to the Molucca islands and New Guinea. It has spread to Indonesia, the West Indies, and other tropical areas. The medicinal component is obtained from the nuts and seeds. Nutmeg oil, also known as myristica oil, is distilled from the nuts. The dried aril of the nutmeg seed produces another herbal product, known as mace. The nuts contain 20% to 40% of a fixed oil called nutmeg butter. The oil contains myristic acid and glycerides of laureic, tridecanoic, stearic, and palmitic acids. Also present are starch, protein, saponin, and catechins. The nuts also contain 8% to 15% of an aromatic oil containing d-camphene (60% to 80%), dipentene (8%), and myristicin (4% to 8%), believed to be

partially responsible for nutmeg intoxication. Nutmeg is known for its psychoactive and hallucinogenic properties resulting from central nervous system (CNS) effects. Nutmeg may also play a role in inhibiting prostaglandin synthesis and platelet aggregation. It's available as a spice, and in products such as Vicks Vaporub.

Reported uses
Nutmeg is used internally for diarrhea, indigestion, loss of appetite, colic, flatulence, and insomnia. It's also used as a larvicidal and as a hallucinogen. In Indian medicine, nutmeg is used to treat poor vision, headaches, fever, and malaria. It has also been used for cholera, impotence, and general debility.

Nutmeg is used externally for rheumatoid arthritis. Nutmeg butter is used in soaps and perfumes.

Administration
■ Dried seed powder: 300 mg to 1,000 mg by mouth every day
■ Fluid extract: 10 to 30 gtt by mouth up to four times a day
■ Powder: 5 to 20 grains applied topically to affected area up to three times a day
■ Spirits: 5 to 20 gtt by mouth up to four times a day.

Hazards
Although widely used as a spice and flavoring, nutmeg ingestion may cause flushing, allergic contact dermatitis, nausea, diarrhea, hallucinations, giddiness, disorientation, fear of impending death, loss of feeling in limbs, depolarization, tachycardia, decreased pulse, hypothermia, feeling of pressure in chest, and dry mouth. Nutmeg taken with monoamine oxidase (MAO) inhibitors and other psychoactive drugs may potentiate effects of these drugs via the herb's mild MAO-inhibiting action.

Pregnant or breast-feeding patients, those with cardiac disorders, and those with psychotic disorders should avoid using nutmeg, as should patients who are hypersensitive to it.

SAFETY RISK *Ingestion of several tablespoons of nutmeg can lead to potentially severe, stuporous intoxication. Symptoms of overdose (nausea and violent vomiting) occur 3 to 8 hours after ingestion of the herb. Episodes are characterized by weak pulse, hypothermia, disorientation, giddiness, and a feeling of pressure in the chest or lower abdomen. An extended period of alternating delirium and stupor persists for up to 24 hours, ending in heavy sleep. The patient may have a sensation of loss of limbs and a terrifying fear of death. Gastric lavage and supportive therapy, such as haloperidol, may be warranted. Recovery usually occurs within 24 hours but may take several days.*

Clinical considerations

■ Misuse and abuse of nutmeg is a growing problem. Assess patient's level of use.

■ Caution patient to use nutmeg in moderation because intoxication or death can occur after ingestion of large doses.

■ Warn patient with cardiac problems not to use nutmeg.

■ Advise pregnant or breast-feeding patients not to use nutmeg.

■ Warn patient not to take herb for diarrhea, indigestion, or chronic GI distress before seeking appropriate medical evaluation because doing so may delay diagnosis of a potentially serious medical condition.

■ Tell patient to remind prescriber and pharmacist of any herbal or dietary supplement that he's taking when obtaining a new prescription.

■ Advise patient to consult his health care provider before using an herbal preparation because a treatment with proven efficacy may be available.

Research summary

Nutmeg has been studied for its role in treating diarrhea, and inhibiting both prostaglandin synthesis and platelet aggregation.

oak bark

Quercus alba, Q. robur, *stave oak, stone oak, tanner's oak, white oak*

Quercus robur is a large tree widespread in Europe, Asia Minor, and the Caucasus region. The medicinal components are obtained from the dried bark of young branches and saplings. White oak bark contains the tannin quercitannic acid, which is thought to have astringent, anti-septic, and anti-inflammatory properties. It's also believed to have antiviral and an-thelmintic properties. Oak is available in products such as Alvita White Bark Tea, Conchae Compound, Kernosan Elixir, Menodoron, Peerless Composition Essence, Silvapin, and Traxton.

Reported uses
Oak bark is used as a gargle to treat cough and bronchitis and mild oropha-ryngeal inflammation. It's used topically to treat inflammatory skin diseases and inflammation of genital and anal areas. It's used orally to treat acute diarrhea.

Administration
- Baths (5 g of herb or 1 to 3 teaspoons of bark extract to every 1 L of water): Soak for no longer than 20 minutes
- Rinses, compresses, and gargles (20 g of bark boiled in 1 L of water for 10 to 15 minutes, and then strained): Taken undiluted
- Tea (boil 1 g of powdered bark or 1 to 2 teaspoons of chopped bark in 500 ml of

water for 15 minutes; strain and cool): For diarrhea, 3 g of oak bark powder by mouth every day, or 1 cup of tea three times a day, taken undiluted. Oak bark shouldn't be used for longer than 3 days.

Hazards

Oak bark may cause constipation, nausea or vomiting, stomach upset, abdominal pain, kidney and liver damage, and respiratory failure. It may reduce the absorption of atropine, digoxin, heavy metal salts (such as iron or gold), morphine, nicotine, and quinine.

Patients allergic to oak pollen shouldn't use any products containing oak. Those with skin damage over large areas shouldn't use topical oak products. Patients with weeping eczema, febrile or infectious disease, asthma, chronic obstructive pulmonary disease, renal or hepatic insufficiency, or New York Heart Association class III or IV heart failure shouldn't take full baths containing oak.

Clinical considerations

- Oak and other tannin-containing herbs shouldn't be used for prolonged periods because of an increased risk of cancer and hepatic damage.
- Short-term external use of oak preparations may be effective for skin conditions; however, safety and efficacy of internal use haven't been studied.
- Geriatric patients may be more sensitive to adverse effects.
- Warn patient not to apply topical oak bark preparations on large areas of damaged skin.
- Advise patient to stop taking oak and contact a health care provider if diarrhea lasts longer than 3 days.
- Tell patient to keep oak preparation out of eyes; if contact occurs, advise flushing eyes with water for at least 15 minutes.
- Tell patient to remind prescriber and pharmacist of any herbal or dietary sup-

plement that he's taking when obtaining a new prescription.
- Advise patient to consult his health care provider before using an herbal preparation because a treatment with proven efficacy may be available.

Research summary

The concepts behind the use of oak bark and the claims made regarding its effects haven't yet been validated scientifically.

oats

Avena sativa, *avenae fructus, wild oat herb*

Oats originated in England, France, Poland, Germany, and Russia and are now cultivated worldwide. The medicinal components are derived from the fresh or dried above-ground parts or flowers of *Avena sativa*. Foods are made from the grains (seeds) of the plant, and oat bran is made from the inner husks of the seeds. Oats contain gluten, which forms a sticky mass that holds moisture in skin when mixed with liquid. Oat bran also contains beta-glucan, which may have serum lipid-reducing properties. Oats are available in products such as oat bran, oats and honey, oatstraw, oat straw tea, wild oats, Aveeno soap, lotion, and bath, and Quaker oat bran.

Reported uses

Oats are used topically to treat dry, itchy skin. Dietary oat bran may lower serum cholesterol. Oats are also used to treat opium and cigarette addiction, but the mechanism for this use is unknown.

Administration

- Baths, lotions: Follow package labeling
- For cholesterol reduction: Dosage is 40 to 100 g a day total dietary fiber, taken by mouth.

Hazards

Oats may cause adverse effects such as increased stool bulk, increased defecation, flatulence, and abdominal bloating. There are no reported drug interactions.

Patients allergic to the *Avena sativa* plant should avoid using oat products. Because gluten damages digestive and absorptive cells in the intestines, oats shouldn't be used by patients with celiac disease. Patients with dermatitis herpetiformis should avoid diets high in gluten because they may cause intestinal abnormalities.

Clinical considerations

- Patients with bowel problems should use oat products with caution.
- As with all fiber products, oats should be taken with plenty of fluids to ensure adequate hydration and dispersion of fiber in the GI tract.
- Patient may experience frequent bowel movements, resulting in anogenital irritation.
- Tell patient to drink plenty of water to help regulate bowel movements.
- Caution patient that oat skin-care products shouldn't be used near eyes or on inflamed skin.
- Tell patient to remind prescriber and pharmacist of any herbal or dietary supplement that he's taking when obtaining a new prescription.
- Advise patient to consult his health care provider before using an herbal preparation because a treatment with proven efficacy may be available.

Research summary

The use of oats has been studied extensively for its role in lowering serum cholesterol. Studies evaluating its antifungal properties have also been done; however, this use hasn't yet been validated scientifically.

octacosanol

1-octacosanol, 14c-octacosanol, n-octacosanol, octacosyl alcohol, policosanol

Octacosanol is a type of long-chain alcohol that can be extracted from wheat germ oil, sugar cane wax, and other vegetable oils. It may have ergogenic effects and is thought to increase oxygen use by tissues during workouts; it may also improve glycogen storage in muscles. Octacosanol is available as capsules and concentrate, in products such as Enduraplex, Octa Power, Super Octacosanol, and in combination with other dietary supplements such as Boost, Prometol, and Stamiplex.

Reported uses

Octacosanol is used by athletes to improve cardiac function, stamina, strength, and reaction time. It's also used to treat Parkinson's disease and amyotrophic lateral sclerosis (Lou Gehrig's disease), although little evidence exists to support its use for these disorders.

Administration

- For Parkinson's disease: 5 mg by mouth three times a day with meals
- To enhance athletic performance: 40 to 80 mg by mouth every day.

Hazards

Some patients may experience dizziness, jerky, involuntary movements, and nervousness. Patients taking levodopa-carbidopa along with octacosanol may experience increased dyskinetic activity.

Patients allergic to wheat germ oil or sugar cane shouldn't take octacosanol. Patients with Parkinson's disease should use octacosanol with caution, particularly if they are taking levodopa-carbidopa.

Clinical considerations

- Octacosanol taken with levodopa-carbidopa may worsen dyskinesias.
- Patients allergic to wheat germ oil or sugar cane shouldn't take octacosanol.
- Advise patient of the potential for octacosanol to interfere with the effects of other medications.
- Advise patient with Parkinson's disease or any undiagnosed tremor to consult a health care provider before taking octacosanol.
- Tell patient to remind prescriber and pharmacist of any herbal or dietary supplement that he's taking when obtaining a new prescription.
- Advise patient to consult his health care provider before using an herbal preparation because a treatment with proven efficacy may be available.

Research summary

Octacosanol is being investigated as a herpes antiviral and as a treatment for inflammatory skin diseases. Some studies indicate that its use improves physical endurance.

oleander

Adelfa, laurier rose, Nerium oleander, N. indicum mill, *rosa fancesca, rose laurel, rosebay*

Oleander is an evergreen shrub native to southern Asia and the Mediterranean region and cultivated elsewhere. Although known for its toxic effects, oleander has been used in traditional medicine for centuries for ailments ranging from cardiac disorders to corns. Oleander is a natural cardiac glycoside that has positive inotropic and negative chronotropic effects on cardiac muscle; its actions mimic digoxin. All parts of the plant contain the cardiac glycosides oleandrin and nerlin and the cardenolides gentiobiosyloleandrin and odoroside A. Other pharmacologically active compounds include folinerin, rosagenin, rutin, and oleandomycin. Flavonol glycosides are reported to influence vascular permeability and to possess diuretic properties. Oleander is available as leaf extract and tincture.

Reported uses

Oleander has been used to treat heart and skin diseases.

Administration

Oleander is not recommended for use. Dosages are not well documented.

Hazards

Oleander may cause abdominal pain, appetite loss, nausea, vomiting, bloody diarrhea, respiratory paralysis, enlarged pupils, seizures, irregular pulse, and heart failure. When used with beta blockers, calcium channel blockers, or digoxin, additive effects may occur.

All plant parts are toxic and shouldn't be used. Adults and children have died after ingesting flowers, nectar, and leaves, or from using oleander branches to roast foods. Ingesting water in which the plant has soaked or inhaling smoke from burning oleander wood also may be toxic. The use of oleander in any form should be avoided.

 SAFETY RISK *Don't confuse oleander* (Nerium oleander) *with yellow oleander* (Thevetia peruviana)*, which may also be toxic.*

Clinical considerations

- Patients who ingest oleander may need immediate medical attention. Accidental poisoning may require gastric lavage, activated charcoal, and ipecac syrup. Digoxin immune Fab, used in digoxin overdoses, has been used with some success as an antidote to oleander poisonings. Patients should have continuous electrocardiogram monitoring, and resuscitation equipment should be close at hand.

- Patients who ingest any part of the oleander plant should be advised to contact a poison control center or seek immediate medical attention.
- Warn patient that oleander plants should be kept away from children, pets, and livestock. Plants should be clearly labeled.
- Advise patient not to burn oleander branches and leaves in poorly ventilated areas because smoke is toxic.
- Tell patient to remind prescriber and pharmacist of any herbal or dietary supplement that he's taking when obtaining a new prescription.
- Advise patient to consult his health care provider before using an herbal preparation because a treatment with proven efficacy may be available.

Research summary
The toxicity of oleander is well documented. Its use should be avoided.

olive

Olea europaea, *oleum olivae*

The olive is an evergreen tree native to the Mediterranean region and cultivated in similar climates. The tree produces a fruit from which the oil is extracted. The use of olive oil in traditional medicine dates back to ancient times. The medicinal components, obtained from both the fruit and the leaves, contain the phenolic compound oleuropein, which has anti-inflammatory and antioxidant properties. Oleuropein may exert its anti-inflammatory activity by damping the expression of intercellular adhesion molecule-1, involved in adhesion of leukocytes to endothelial cells. The antioxidant properties of oleuropein may prevent the oxidative modification of low-density lipoprotein cholesterol. Olive oil contains oleic, palmitic, and linoleic acid, which also exert antioxidant, anti-inflammatory, and lipid-lowering prop-

erties. Olive oil also inhibits platelet aggregation. These mechanisms indicate that olive-derived products may help prevent atherosclerosis.

Oleuropein may also have vasodilatory, hypoglycemic, and antimicrobial properties. Although the exact mechanism of vasodilation is unknown, the hypoglycemic activity may result from either a potentiation of insulin release or increased peripheral uptake of glucose. Olive polyphenols have antimicrobial activity against certain gram-positive and gram-negative bacteria. Olives and olive oil are available in a wide variety of forms and products, including Natrol Olive Leaf Extract, Nature's Herb Olive Leaf Powder, Bertolli Olive Oil, and Colavita Olive Oil.

Reported uses
Olive oil is used as an emollient and topical lubricant, to treat skin irritations (such as burns and psoriasis), to soften ear wax, and to relieve constipation. It's also used for dry hair and itchy scalp and to prevent stretch marks caused by pregnancy. Recent evidence suggests that olive oil, when part of a diet high in monounsaturated fats, may lower serum cholesterol. Olive leaf preparations have been used to lower blood pressure, reduce serum glucose level in diabetics, and treat various bacterial, viral, and fungal infections. Olives are eaten either green (unripe) or black (ripe), and olive oil is used in a variety of recipes.

Administration
- For cholesterol reduction: Olive oil is used in moderation as part of a diet low in saturated fats
- Laxative: Dosage is 1 to 2 oz oil by mouth as needed, or 100 to 500 ml olive oil, at body temperature, applied rectally
- For gastrointestinal ulcers: Dosage is 15 to 30 ml by mouth three times a day, at meals

■ For infections: Dosage is 60 to 500 mg olive leaf preparation by mouth every 6 hours

■ For hair and skin problems: Apply undiluted oil to affected area, as needed.

Hazards

The use of olive products may cause hypotension, stomach irritation, and hypoglycemia. When olive products are used with antihypertensives and hypoglycemic agents, potential additive effects may occur. Skin irritation may result when olive oil is applied externally.

Patients allergic to any part of the olive plant shouldn't use these products.

Clinical considerations

■ Patients who are immunocompromised shouldn't use olive leaf products because safety and efficacy data in humans are lacking.

■ Diabetic patients using olive leaf preparations should check blood glucose level more frequently because of the risk of hypoglycemia. Monitor patient's blood pressure and blood glucose levels closely.

■ Olive oil should be part of a diet that's low in saturated fat and cholesterol.

■ Advise patient to consult with his health care provider before using an herbal preparation because a treatment with proven efficacy may be available.

■ Caution patient to consult a health care provider if he has human immunodeficiency virus, other immunosupressed conditions, diabetes, or blood pressure abnormalities.

■ Remind patient to consult a health care provider before self-treating diabetes because it is a serious condition and its management should be overseen by a professional.

■ Review the signs of and treatments for hypoglycemia with the patient.

■ Tell patient to remind prescriber and pharmacist of any herbal or dietary supplement that he's taking when obtaining a new prescription.

■ Advise patient to consult his health care provider before using an herbal preparation because a treatment with proven efficacy may be available.

Research summary

Olive oil has been studied for its serum cholesterol–lowering effects and for cancer prevention. Olive leaf has been found to have mild antihypertensive and hypoglycemic effects, although these are not well documented.

onion

Allii cepae bulbus, Allium cepa

The onion plant is a perennial herb that grows to about four feet in height. The medicinal components are obtained from the underground bulb, which is also used as a food. Onion has been used for centuries to treat a variety of ailments. It contains essential oils, organosulfur compounds, cysteine sulfoxide, quercetin glycosides, thiosulfinates, and diphenylamine. The organosulfur compound may have antimicrobial and anticancer effects. Cysteine sulfoxide is responsible for onion's flavor and lacrimation effects. Quercetin glycosides impart antioxidant properties. Thiosulfinates inhibit mediators of bronchoconstriction such as leukotriene and thromboxane; extracts containing the compound have reduced bronchial constriction in patients with asthma. Onion inhibits platelet aggregation, lowers serum cholesterol levels, decreases blood pressure, enhances fibrinolysis, and has hypoglycemic and antifungal effects.

Reported uses

Onion is used as raw herb to treat appetite loss, stomach gas, furuncles, warts, bruises, bronchitis, asthma, atherosclerosis, diabetes, dyspepsia, fever, colds, hypertension, infection, inflammation, angina, dehydration, and menstruation.

It's also used as a mucolytic agent, an anthelmintic, a diuretic, and a gallbladder stimulant. Onion water is used as tea to relieve sore throat and cough.

Onion is used topically as a poultice for sores, bites, and burns. Fishermen have used onion to treat stingray and fish-spine wounds. Onion is also widely used as a food and food flavoring.

Administration
- Externally: Onion slices or poultices containing onion juice are placed on the affected area and covered with a cloth
- Internally: Typical dosage is 50 g fresh onion or juice from 50 g of fresh onion by mouth daily; 20 g of dried onion per day can also be used. The maximum recommended dose of diphenylamine is 35 mg daily if onion use is intended over several months.

Hazards
The external use of onion is associated with excessive tearing and eczema. Internal use may cause nausea. Patients using onion and antiplatelet drugs may have an increased bleeding risk. When used with diabetic agents, onion may affect blood glucose control. Patients using onions and other herbal supplements that affect platelets and blood glucose may experience additive effects.

Patients hypersensitive to onions should avoid use. Pregnant and breastfeeding women should avoid the use of onion except in foods.

Clinical considerations
- Onion should be used with caution by patients with diabetes, bleeding disorders, and eczema.
- Advise patient at risk of bleeding to use herb with caution. Observe and monitor patient for evidence of bleeding.
- Monitor blood glucose control carefully in patients with diabetes.
- Urge diabetic patient to monitor blood glucose level carefully and to stay alert for

signs of hypoglycemia, such as sweating, a racing heart, hunger, and nausea.
- Tell patient that information on the use of onion during pregnancy and lactation is lacking, and that amounts greater than those used in foods should be avoided.
- Warn patient of potential for flare of eczema.
- Instruct patient to wash hands after handling onion.
- Tell patient to remind prescriber and pharmacist of any herbal or dietary supplement that he's taking when obtaining a new prescription.
- Advise patient to consult his health care provider before using an herbal preparation because a treatment with proven efficacy may be available.

Research summary
Onion has been studied for its antibacterial and antifungal effects. It's also been studied for its use in cardiovascular disease for antiplatelet and hypolipidemic effects. More studies are needed to verify the use of onion in asthma treatment.

oregano

Mountain mint, origan,
Origanum vulgare, *wild marjoram, winter marjoram, wintersweet*

Oregano is a perennial herb commonly found in Europe, North Africa, and throughout Asia. Although oregano is thought of as a common kitchen herb, it has been used for its medicinal properties for many years. The medicinal components are obtained from an oil extracted from oregano leaves. The chief components of oregano oil are carvacrol 40% to 70%, gammaterpinene 8% to 10%, p-cynmene 5% to 10%, alpha-pinen, myrcene, and thymol. Other species of oregano may contain linalool, caryophyllene, or germacren D. Carvacrol has antifungal and antibacterial action against gram-positive and gram-negative bacteria and against yeast. Oregano also has anthelmintic, antispasmodic, irritant, diuretic, bile stimulant, and expectorant properties. Oregano is available as dried leaves, powder, and oil, in products such as Oregamax.

Reported uses
Oregano is used to treat urinary tract disorders, respiratory tract ailments, cough, painful menstruation, arthritis, diuresis, scrofulosis, GI disorders, dyspepsia, and bloating. It's used as an expectorant, a sedative, a diaphoretic, and a stimulant for appetite, digestion, and bile excretion.

Administration
- Tea (steep 1 heaping teaspoon of oregano in 250 ml boiling water for 10 minutes, and then strain): As a beverage, the tea can be sweetened with honey, or may be used unsweetened as a mouthwash or gargle
- Bath (100 g of drug in 1 L water, strained after 10 minutes): Add to a full bath.

Hazards
Adverse effects are rare with proper administration and dosage of oregano. If taken simultaneously, oregano may cause reduced absorption of iron supplements.

Patients who are pregnant or breast-feeding should avoid the use of oregano except in food products. Patients with sensitivity to herbs in the mint family should also avoid use.

 SAFETY RISK *Oregano may cause systemic reactions if the patient has sensitivity to other members of the mint family. If the patient is allergic to mint, thyme, hyssop, basil, marjoram, sage, and lavender, be alert for allergic reactions.*

Clinical considerations
- Patients should take oregano and iron supplements at least 2 hours apart.

- Alert patient of the potential of allergic reaction.
- Tell patient to remind prescriber and pharmacist of any herbal or dietary supplement that he's taking when obtaining a new prescription.
- Advise patient to consult his health care provider before using an herbal preparation because a treatment with proven efficacy may be available.

Research summary
The concepts behind the use of oregano and the claims made regarding its effects haven't yet been validated scientifically.

Oregon grape

Barberry, Berberis aquifolium,
holly-leaved berberis,
Mahonia aquifolium,
Oregon mountain grape

Oregon grape is indigenous to North America and is cultivated in Europe. It was used in North America, well before the arrival of European settlers, to treat a variety of ailments. The medicinal components are obtained from rhizome and root. Physiologic activity stems from alkaloids berberine, berbamine, and oxyacanthine. Berberine and oxyacanthine have antibacterial properties. Berberine is active against amoebas and trypanosomes, and it has anticonvulsant, sedative, and uterine-stimulant properties. Berbamine and berberine may have anticancer activity. Berbamine has a hypotensive effect. Berbamine and oxyacanthine are potent lipoxygenase inhibitors. Oregon grape may also have anti-inflammatory and antifungal activity. It's available in products such as Prime Relief.

Reported uses
Oregon grape is used topically to treat psoriasis, eczema, dry skin, rashes, acne, herpes, and skin eruptions. It's also used

orally to improve appetite and to treat general debility and gall bladder disorders with associated nausea and vomiting. Oregon grape is used in small doses for ulcers, heartburn, diarrhea, and stomach problems, and for parasites and conjunctivitis. Larger doses have a cathartic effect.

Administration
- Powder: Dosage is 0.5 to 1 g by mouth three times a day
- Tincture: Dosage is 2 to 4 ml by mouth three times a day
- Topical: Apply bark extract (10%) ointment to affected areas two or three times a day for psoriasis; massage root extract (10%) cream into affected areas three times a day or as directed by a health care provider.

Hazards
Oregon grape is safe in recommended dosages, although long-term use of standardized extracts shouldn't exceed 2 weeks. Excessive use may lead to toxicity, poisoning, and possibly death.

Minor adverse effects of recommended dosage may include itching, burning, and skin irritation associated with topical use. The patient may experience an allergic reaction. Berberine may cause or worsen kidney irritation. When Oregon grape is used with other herbs containing berberine, including amur cork tree, bloodroot, celandine, Chinese corktree, Chinese goldthread, European barberry, golden seal, and goldthread, there is increased risk of toxicity. Oregon grape may decrease the absorption of tetracyclines.

Pregnant and breast-feeding women shouldn't use Oregon grape. Patients hypersensitive to Oregon grape or to related plants shouldn't use it.

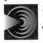 **SAFETY RISK** *Don't confuse Oregon grape with European barberry* (Berberis vulgaris).

Clinical considerations
- Oregon grape may interfere with bilirubin metabolism in infants.

- Oregon grape should be used with caution by patients with kidney problems.
- Tell patient not to use Oregon grape if she's pregnant or breast-feeding.
- Advise patient that poisoning and death have resulted from excessive doses of berberine.
- Advise patient not to use Oregon grape longer than 2 weeks.
- Tell patient to store Oregon grape out of sunlight.
- Tell patient to remind prescriber and pharmacist of any herbal or dietary supplement that he's taking when obtaining a new prescription.
- Advise patient to consult his health care provider before using an herbal preparation because a treatment with proven efficacy may be available.

Research summary
The concepts behind the use of Oregon grape and the claims made regarding its effects haven't yet been validated scientifically.

Orthomolecular therapy

Megavitamin therapy, orthomolecular medicine, orthomolecular nutrition

Orthomolecular therapy is the practice of preventing and treating disease by providing the body with "optimal" amounts of substances that are natural to it. The term was coined in 1968 by Nobel prize recipient Linus Pauling (1901–1994) to denote the use of naturally occurring substances, particularly nutrients, in maintaining health and treating disease. The therapy rests on a vast body of research in the basic foundations of biochemistry, biophysics, physiology, ecology, and clinical nutrition.

Reported uses

Linus Pauling's first use of orthomolecular medicine was megadose niacin therapy in the treatment of schizophrenia (1968). Orthomolecular therapy is now used therapeutically, to treat an entire range of diseases, such as asthma, cardiovascular disease, and hypercholesterolemia. It's also used preventatively to protect against degenerative disease, accelerated aging, cancer, and so forth, and to maintain optimium health.

What began as megavitamin therapy now employs a broad database and a variety of therapies applicable to numerous medical and psychiatric conditions. Diseases such as atherosclerosis, cancer, schizophrenia, and depression are associated with specific biochemical abnormalities, which are either causal or aggravating factors of the illness. Orthomolecular theory states that the provision of vitamins, amino acids, fatty acids, and trace minerals in amounts sufficient to correct biochemical abnormalities will be therapeutic in preventing or treating such diseases. For example, megadose niacin therapy, once considered dangerous and controversial in treating schizophrenia, is now the standard in the treatment of hyperlipidemia.

How the treatment is performed

Doses larger than the RDAs of vitamins, minerals, amino acids, or fatty acids are given, usually by oral administration but sometimes intravenously (such as in high-dose vitamin C administration).

Hazards

Nutritional supplements have a low risk of toxicity, especially when compared with pharmaceuticals. Some supplements may interact with medications, herbal therapies, or diagnostic tests. For example, large doses of vitamin E may, when combined with blood thinners, aspirin, nonsteroidal anti-inflammatory drugs, clopidogrel bisulfate, and ticlopidine, or herbals such as turmeric, ginger, feverfew or gingko biloba, cause increased bleeding times. Large doses of vitamin C can cause false-negative results on hemoccult tests, although the test can be performed accurately if the vitamin is stopped 72 or more hours before the test is performed.

Minerals such as zinc and selenium can lead to immunosuppression if taken in amounts larger than 50 mg and 200 mcg per day, respectively. High doses of vitamin C can lead to diarrhea. Niacin causes flushing of the skin, which can usually be prevented by taking an aspirin 30 minutes before ingesting the niacin.

Persistent or serious adverse effects are rare for water-soluble vitamins, although long-term use of high dose B_6 can lead to neuropathies. Fat-soluble vitamins such as vitamin A have been linked to birth defects in amounts greater than 10,000 IU. High doses of any single mineral, vitamin, or amino acid can lead to a deficiency in nutrients with similar pathways; for example, zinc-deficiency anemia may occur in patients who take large doses of zinc without also increasing their intake of copper.

Clinical considerations

- Every person is biochemically unique and therefore each person's vitamin need is also unique.
- Advise patient to use a balanced approach to supplementation.
- Caution patient about potential drug-supplement interactions.
- Optimal health is a lifetime challenge. Follow-up, repeated testing, and therapeutic trials permit "fine-tuning" of the supplement regimen.
- Taking large doses of any vitamin can lead to problems. This approach to care shouldn't be taken without the guidance of a quailified health care provider.
- Discuss other care options to assure understanding.
- Tell patient to remind prescriber and pharmacist of any herbal or dietary sup-

plement that he's taking when obtaining a new prescription.

 SAFETY RISK *In 1994, Congress passed the Dietary Supplement and Health Education Act (DSHEA), which defined vitamins, minerals, amino acids, and herbals as "dietary supplements." Labels may purport a product's effect on the "structure and function" of the body, but may not make therapeutic claims. The safety of these supplements rests with the manufacturers.*

 TRAINING *Various courses in nutritional therapy exist, ranging from short courses that last a few days and lead to certification in basic nutrition to the four-year, full-time training for naturopaths, which includes anatomy, physiology, biochemistry, pathology, and naturopathic principles (including nutrition). Nutritional consultations may be given by a wide range of practitioners with varying levels of training and experience.*

 REIMBURSEMENT *Most supplements are not covered by insurance unless prescribed by a health care provider and made by a pharmaceutical company. For example, Niaspan is extended-release niacin prescribed for cholesterol lowering.*

Research summary

Scientific research on the optimum intake of specific vitamins traditionally focused on arriving at a standard daily amount necessary to prevent deficiency symptoms; these amounts are known as the Dietary Reference Intakes (DRI; formerly Recommended Dietary Allowances [RDA]). However, scientists are now examining the potential for specific nutrients — including vitamins, minerals, amino acids, and fatty acids — to prevent and treat disease and to enhance physical and mental health and performance. The vast majority of the large-scale studies being done in Europe (particularly Germany and Switzerland).

Osteopathic medicine

Developed in the United States in the late 19th century, osteopathy (derived from the Greek words *osteon*, meaning bone, and *pathos*, meaning suffering) is a health care system that views structural and mechanical problems as the source of disease. Based on the belief that structure directly influences function, osteopathic doctors use various forms of physical manipulation to correct structural anomalies, thereby stimulating the body's own self-healing mechanisms. Osteopathy is closely intertwined with conventional medicine.

Andrew Taylor Still (1828–1917), the founder of osteopathy, was a medical doctor who became disillusioned with orthodox medicine after his father and three of his children died of infectious diseases against which the medicine of the time was ineffective. Still believed that the human body contained the ability to heal itself and that doctors should take steps to elicit that self-healing power. How he came to believe that physical manipulation was the way to unleash that power is unclear; however, he began practicing his new system, which started as a combination of bone setting and the magnetic healing system of Franz Mesmer, in the 1870s.

In 1892, Still founded the American School of Osteopathy in Missouri, which espoused teachings based on the belief that manually restoring structural integrity could improve physiologic function. Eventually, Still and colleagues developed interventions to assist in labor and delivery and to treat disorders such as neck and back pain, migraines, asthma, otitis media, hypertension, coronary artery disease, and diabetes. As currently practiced, osteopathy blends conventional medical and obstetric practices with osteopathic manipulation. Today, there are more than 33,000 licensed doctors of osteopathy in the United States (about

FOUR PRINCIPLES OF OSTEOPATHY

The following four principles form the foundation of osteopathic medicine:

- Each person is an integrated unit consisting of body, mind, and spirit. Because physical, mental, emotional, and spiritual factors are inseparably linked within each person, any stress or alteration in one area will affect all the others. Thus, the doctor must take into account the whole person in both diagnosis and treatment.
- The body is capable of healing itself. Under ideal conditions, the body, mind, and spirit work together to maintain health and to heal. Disease begins when one or more of the body's systems are overwhelmed. The doctor's role is to optimize the patient's own healing process.
- Body structure cannot be separated from function. Abnormal structure leads to abnormal function, and vice versa. When the mechanical structure of the body is corrected, its functioning will also improve.
- Treatment must be based on the preceding three principles. The key to effective care is the recognition that disease isn't the invasion of a host by some external entity, but a breakdown of the body's capacity for self-maintenance.

5% of the country's doctors), providing all aspects of medical care. (See *Four principles of osteopathy*.)

TRAINING *Osteopaths receive the same training as conventional medical practitioners; they must pass the same medical board examinations to become licensed, and have the same ability to prescribe medications. However, their education places considerable emphasis on osteopathic philosophy and principles, including structural diagnosis and manipulative treatment.*

Reported uses

According to osteopathic practitioners, diseases of the internal organs are commonly manifested as musculoskeletal pain. For example, musculoskeletal misalignment over a long period can compromise a coronary artery, leading to angina or myocardial infarction. Detecting and correcting the musculoskeletal dysfunction before major tissue damage has occurred can increase oxygen delivery and decrease venous congestion, thereby preventing a serious cardiac event.

Osteopathic manipulation is commonly used to treat alterations in musculoskeletal structure, such as whiplash injuries, scoliosis, and neck and lower back pain. Other disorders that reportedly respond to osteopathic treatment are arthritis, digestive problems, menstrual problems, chronic pain, cardiac and pulmonary diseases, chronic fatigue, high blood pressure, headaches, sciatica, and various neural disorders.

How the treatment is performed

Osteopaths believe that any restriction in the spine or other bony structures can impair the function of organs and entire body systems. Thus, the musculoskeletal system is the focus of diagnosis and therapy.

Using palpation and inspection, the osteopath evaluates the patient's posture and gait (assessing how he holds himself while sitting, standing, and walking), mobility of moving parts (looking for restricted movements), symmetry of body parts (checking for overuse of one side and for abnormal curvature of the spine), and soft tissues (examining for tenderness, muscle hardening, skin or temperature changes, and signs of fluid retention). The following elements are screened and evaluated as part of the diagnostic procedure:

- posture and gait
- motion (bending, side bending, extension and/or rotation, and so forth)
- symmetry (one-sided use of any body part, possibly with increased or decreased curve to spine)
- soft tissues (noting skin changes, hardening of muscles, tenderness, temperature, excessive fluid retention or reflex activity).

Like practitioners of other complementary therapies, osteopaths take a holistic approach to health care, treating the patient as an integrated whole rather than focusing on a specific symptom or complaint. They believe that given a favorable environment, adequate nutrition, and properly functioning body structures, the body is capable of healing itself. The doctor's task is to assist the body in this process of self-healing.

The osteopath can choose from a number of manipulation techniques. Some require the patient to be passive as the doctor performs the technique; others require the patient to actively perform the technique while the doctor guides and assists him. Some are used alone, while others are combined with conventional treatments. Specific techniques include the following:

- *Gentle mobilization* involves moving a joint slowly through its range of motion while gradually increasing the motion to eliminate restrictions.
- *Articulation* consists of performing a quick thrust (similar to a chiropractic maneuver) to restore joint mobility.
- *Muscle energy technique* involves gently tensing and releasing certain muscles to induce relaxation.
- *Positional release method* involves placing the patient in a specific position to release muscle spasms.
- *Cranial techniques* (also known as craniosacral therapy or cranial manipulation) consist of very gentle manipulation of the cranial and sacral bones. This method is used to treat headaches, spinal injuries, and temporomandibular joint syndrome. (See *Craniosacral therapy*, page 166.)

Osteopaths also teach their patients various self-care practices designed to keep their bodies functioning properly. These may include relaxation techniques, specially designed exercises and stretches, breathing exercises, postural changes, and proper nutrition. Restoring diaphragmatic breathing, stretching, specifically designed exercise, postural correction, and individualized nutritional guidance are all integral parts of an osteopathic program. All of these practices are aimed at reducing stress on joints and muscles, maintaining structural and functional integrity, and teaching the patient how to use his body more efficiently.

Hazards
Soreness and inflammation may occur following treatment.

Clinical considerations
- Caution a patient at risk for injury, such as a pregnant woman or a patient with a prosthetic joint, to inform the doctor of the condition before undergoing osteopathic manipulation.
- Inform the patient that he'll probably need to learn self-care techniques, such as breathing and stretching techniques, to maintain proper body function and alignment.
- Teach the patient how to keep his body functioning in a relaxed state to reduce anxiety and tension.

Research summary
According to the 1994 report to the National Institutes of Health entitled *Alternative Medicine: Expanding Medical Horizons*, extensive research demonstrates that osteopathic techniques can affect physiologic functioning. Of particular interest are the studies dealing with interactions between neuromuscular structures and internal organs, alterations in

reflex thresholds, and effects of manipulation on disease processes and physiologic functioning.

Among the studies showing physiologic effects from manipulation techniques are two that reported changes in postoperative pulmonary flow rates and electromyographic tests. Studies have also documented effects on both visceral and neuromuscular function, including lower back pain, carpal tunnel syndrome, neurologic development in children, collapsed lung, and burning pain in an extremity. Other studies support the usefulness of palpation of musculoskeletal structures to help diagnose visceral disorders; for example, a 1994 report found that diagnoses based on palpation were backed up by X-ray and autopsy results.

Oxygen therapies

Bio-oxidative therapies,
hydrogen peroxide therapy,
ozone therapy

Oxygen is a clear, odorless gas involved with a multitude of body functions. Composing 21% of the earth's atmosphere, oxygen reacts with foods ingested to produce carbon dioxide, water, and energy. The stored energy from this process of combustion is adenosine triphosphate (ATP), which is paramount to survival. According to Sheldon S. Hendler's book, *The Oxygen Breakthrough* (1989), oxygen is the most vital component of ATP within our cells. Hendler states "imbalance or interruption in the production and flow of this substance results in fatigue, disease, disorder, including immune imbalance, cancer, heart disease, and all the degenerative processes we associate with aging."

Oxygen creates energy needed for survival. It's essential for healthy cells and functions to ward off toxins within the body. Many pathogens, including cancer cells, are anaerobic. According to Nobel prize winner Otto Warburg, the key condition for the development of cancer is a lack of oxygen on the cellular level. Bio-oxidative therapy is used to effect the following benefits:

- It stimulates white blood cell production.
- It increases oxygen and hemoglobin disassociation, which in turn increases the delivery of oxygen from the blood to the cells.
- It increases red blood cell distensibility, with consequent improved flexibility and effectiveness.
- It increases the efficiency of the antioxidant enzyme system, which in turn promotes scavenging of excess free radicals.
- Ozone and hydrogen peroxide have viricidal effects.
- Ozone and hydrogen peroxide are both antineoplastic; both substances oxidize and degrade petrochemicals.
- Ozone and hydrogen peroxide therapies increase the production of interferon and tumor necrosis factor.
- Ozone and hydrogen peroxide increase tissue oxygenation.

Bio-oxidative therapeutic effects are based on the relationship of oxygen to human cells. Acceleration of oxygen metabolism and transfer of oxygen atoms from bloodstream to cell are actually facilitated by bio-oxidative therapies. As the level of oxygen increases, potential for disease decreases. As healthy cells not only thrive and multiply, improvement in overall immune function and response is noted.

Bio-oxidative therapies are not a recent discovery. Clinically used by European physicians for more than century, they were initially reported in the United States 1888 in the *Journal of the American Medical Association*. Continued study by various major medical research universities throughout the United States produces abundant annual research.

Reported uses

Bio-oxidative therapies are used to treat cardiovascular disease, gangrene, peripheral vascular disease, Raynaud's disease, temporal arteritis, vascular and cluster headaches, chronic obstructive pulmonary disease, emphysema, *Pneumocystis carinii* infection, acute and chronic viral infections, chronic and unresponsive bacterial infections, Epstein-Barr virus, herpes simplex and zoster, infections related to human immunodeficiency virus (HIV), influenza, parasitic infections, systemic chronic candidiasis, and cancers.

The best-known uses for hyperbaric oxygen therapy are carbon monoxide poisoning, gas gangrene, and tissue decompression. More recently, this therapy has been used for problematic wound healing, anaerobic infections, chronic bone infections, diabetes, vascular diseases, HIV-related disorders, stroke, and chronic fatigue syndrome.

Medical uses for ozone are well known outside the United States. Ozone therapy was first used in 1915 by Berlin physician Albert Wolff, who utilized ozone to treat skin diseases. The German army used ozone in World War I to treat battle wounds and anaerobic infections. Serious consideration and usage of ozone by the scientific community was begun in 1932. Ozone was used by W. Zable to treat cancer in the 1950s. Successful treatment of HIV was noted by H. Kief. He is also thought to be the pioneer of autohomologous immunotherapy using ozone. This treatment procedure is thought to be helpful with those disease entities resistant to conventional medical therapies. Recent Canadian research showed that ozone kills HIV and hepatitis and herpes viruses.

How the treatment is performed

Various treatment modalities are available. Hyperbaric oxygen therapy is performed with 100% pure oxygen and is administered at 2 to 3 times the normal atmospheric pressure in a pressurized chamber. This allows a rise in the body's blood plasma oxygen content and consequent improved tissue oxygenation. Bacterial growth is inhibited and tissue edema is reduced. New blood vessel formation is prompted specifically in areas of decreased circulation. Typical treatment lasts 60 to 90 minutes and is dependent on the exact medical condition. Daily treatments may be necessary dependent on the severity of illness.

One form of ozone therapy is rectal insufflation, pioneered by Payr and Aubourg in the 1930s. This procedure is administered under medical supervision in Germany, Russia, and Cuba. In this therapy, a mixture of ozone and oxygen is introduced into the rectum, from which it's absorbed through the intestine. The procedure takes 90 to 120 seconds and the ozone is retained in the intestine for 10 to 20 minutes. The intestine is thought to be ideal for absorption owing to its enormous surface area. The circulatory system of the intestine is directly connected to the liver through the portal vein, and this is where most of the biochemical, immunologic, and metabolic processes take place. Intramuscular injection is also used to administer ozone therapy; this method is commonly used to treat allergies and inflammatory diseases. Europeans use this method as an adjunct to cancer therapy.

Hydrogen peroxide, like ozone, kills bacteria, fungi, parasites, viruses, and some types of tumor cells. According to Charles H. Farr, one of the leading authorities on the chemical properties and therapeutic applications of hydrogen peroxide, hydrogen peroxide "functions to aid cell membrane transport, acts as a hormonal messenger, regulates thermogenesis, stimulates and regulates immune functions, and regulates energy production in addition to other metabolic functions. It is purposely used by the body to produce hydroxyl radicals to kill bacteria, viruses, fungi, yeast, and a number of

parasites." Farr feels that hydrogen peroxide must be available for our immune
systems to properly function. Granulo-
cytes produce hydrogen peroxide as a
first line of defense against harmful organisms. Hydrogen peroxide is available
in several grades: 3%, 6%, 30%, 35%
food grade, and 90%.

Hazards
Adverse effects from therapy are minimal. Mild discomfort at the injection site
is transient with the intravenous method.
Adverse effects may occur if I.V. infusion
is not administered properly. Hydrogen
peroxide can cause stomach irritation if
taken in doses too high over a long period of time.

TRAINING *The International
Oxidative Medicine Association
(IOMA) conducts training semi-
nars for physicians, funds research in bio-
oxidative therapies, and distributes information about these therapies worldwide.*

Clinical considerations
Specific training should precede patient
treatment.

Research summary
Research done with cancer patients at
Baylor University found that hydrogen
peroxide injected into a vein could
achieve the same effect as hyperbaric
oxygen, at a much lower cost and with
fewer adverse effects. This same group of
researchers also found that hydrogen peroxide had an energizing effect on heart
muscle that could greatly benefit cardiac
patients. Buildup of plaques was also
studied and was found to be significantly
reduced; effects were of long duration.

pansy

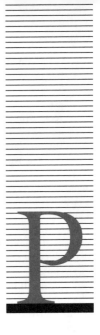

Cuddle me, cull me,
European wild pansy, heartsease,
johnny-jump-up, stiefmütterchenkraut,
three faces under a hood, Viola tricolor

The useful portions of the pansy are obtained from the dried and fresh leaves, stems, and flowers of *Viola tricolor.* It contains flavonoids (0.2%), mucilage (10%), tannins (2% to 5%), and hydroxycoumarins. Pansy has antioxidant and anti-inflammatory properties. Pansy is available as an extract, tea, and poultice.

Reported uses
Pansy is used orally to treat respiratory disorders, as an expectorant and a diuretic, to promote metabolism, and to provide mild laxative effect. It's used topically to treat mild seborrheic skin and scalp disorders, warts, skin inflammation, acne, exanthema, eczema, impetigo, and pruritus vulvae.

Administration
- Poultice: Applied three times a day
- Tea (steep 1.5 g of herb in 5 oz of boiling water for 5 to 10 minutes, and then strain): 1 cup three times a day.

Hazards
There are no reported adverse effects with the use of pansy, and no reported drug interactions. However, pregnant and breast-feeding patients shouldn't use

pansy, as its effects in pregnancy are unknown.

Clinical considerations
- Pansy may be effective for mild seborrheic disorders, but information on its use for other conditions is lacking.
- Tell patient to avoid use while pregnant or breast-feeding.
- Advise patient to store herb in well-sealed container to limit exposure to moisture and light.
- Tell patient to remind prescriber and pharmacist of any herbal and dietary supplement that he's taking when obtaining a new prescription.
- Advise patient to consult his health care provider before using an herbal preparation because a treatment with proven efficacy may be available.

Research summary
The concepts behind the use of pansy and the claims made regarding its effects haven't yet been validated scientifically.

papaya

Baummelonenblätter, Carica papaya, *Caricacacae, mamaerie, melon tree, papaw, pawpaw*

The useful portions of papaya are obtained from leaves and fruits of *Carica papaya.* Its leaf contains 2% papain and carpain. Papain is a mixture of proteolytic enzymes found in the fruit latex and the leaf; it has a fairly broad spectrum of activity. It hydrolyzes proteins, peptides, amides, and some esters. Carpain may have amebicidal properties. Other components of the enzyme blend hydrolyze fats and carbohydrates. Papaya has bacteriostatic and antioxidant activity and may also have antisickling properties. Papaya is available as tablets and tea, and in combination products.

Reported uses
Papaya is used to promote digestion, expel intestinal parasites, and treat inflammation, gastroduodenal ulcers, pancreatic excretion insufficiency, chronic infected ulcers, and keloid scars. Because it can dissolve dead tissue without damaging living cells, it's also used to treat severe wounds and skin ulcers. Papaya is used as a sedative and a diuretic. It's used in preparations to control edema and inflammation from surgical, accidental, or sports trauma. Chymopapain, obtained from papain, is used to treat intervertebral disk hernia in a procedure called chemonucleolysis. Papain is also used as a meat tenderizer.

Administration
To enhance digestion, 10 to 50 mg papain in tablet form may be taken by mouth. Chewable tablets containing 250 mg papaya powder, 150 mg pineapple juice powder, and 10 mg of papain may also be taken, by mouth, three times a day after meals.

Hazards
Adverse effects associated with papaya include gastritis, esophageal perforation (with ingestion of large amounts of papain), asthma attacks, and allergic reactions.

Interactions associated with papaya may include the following:
- Increased International Normalized Ratio may occur with the use of anisindione, dicumarol, and warfarin.
- The effects of papaya may be potentiated with concurrent use of papain because papain is the active ingredient in papaya.

Patients allergic to papaya should avoid using the herb, as should those with a history of Crohn's disease or chronic gastritis.

 SAFETY RISK *Pregnant and breast-feeding patients shouldn't use this herb because papain may be teratogenic and embryotoxic, and it may be an abortifacient.*

Clinical considerations
- Monitor patient for allergic reactions to papaya.
- Warn pregnant patient that papaya may be an abortifacient.
- Urge breast-feeding patient to avoid papaya.
- If patient takes warfarin, tell him to consult his health care provider before taking papaya owing to an increased risk of bleeding.
- Tell patient to remind prescriber and pharmacist of any herbal and dietary supplement that he's taking when obtaining a new prescription.
- Advise patient to consult his health care provider before using an herbal preparation because a treatment with proven efficacy may be available.

Research summary
The concepts behind the use of papaya and the claims made regarding its effects haven't yet been validated scientifically.

pareira

Brava, Chondrodendron tomentosum, Cissampelos pareira, *ice vine, pareira velvet leaf*

The useful constituents of pareira are obtained from fresh or dried bark, roots, and stems of *Chondrodendron tomentosum.* The effects of pareira depend on the toxic derivatives that enter the bloodstream and cause systemic effects. Pareira contains dibenzoyl isoquinoline alkaloids, such as D-tubocurarine, chondrocurarine, curine, chondrofoline, chondrocurine, and isochondrodendrine. These alkaloids have emmenagogic, diuretic, and muscle-relaxing effects. Tubocurarine chloride is used medicinally as a muscle relaxant during anesthesia. It works as a nondepolarizing (competitive) neuromuscular blocker by competing with acetylcholine for cholinergic receptors, thus decreasing the response to acetylcholine and inhibiting skeletal muscle contraction. This effect isn't seen with oral administration unless the amount absorbed is increased because of cuts or ulcers in the mouth or GI tract. Paralysis of the skeletal muscles may occur, except with oral administration. Pareira is available as powder or granules, and in various combination products; however, it isn't commercially available in the United States.

Reported uses
Pareira is used as a laxative, tonic, and diuretic. It's also used to relieve kidney inflammation and induce menstruation. Brazilians use pareira for snakebites; they drink an infusion of the plant and apply bruised leaves to the bite. The herb is also used to make curare, a paralyzing arrow poison used for hunting.

Administration
Dosage information for pareira isn't well documented.

Hazards
Adverse effects associated with the use of pareira include sedation, flushing, hypotension, tachycardia, blurred vision, decreased GI motility, nausea, skeletal muscle relaxation or paralysis, jaw weakness, bronchospasm, and apnea.

Ketamine, quinidine, and procainamide; calcium channel blockers, such as diltiazem and verapamil; anesthetics such as vecuronium; anticonvulsants such as phenytoin; and other drugs containing tubocurarine may potentiate the neuromuscular blocking action of pareira.

 SAFETY RISK *The plant is considered poisonous and shouldn't be consumed.*

Clinical considerations
- Advise patient not to use this poisonous herb.
- Nausea and heavy urine flow have been observed in patients poisoned with tubocurare.

- Tell patient to remind prescriber and pharmacist of any herbal and dietary supplement that he's taking when obtaining a new prescription.
- Advise patient to consult his health care provider before using an herbal preparation because a treatment with proven efficacy may be available.

Research summary

The concepts behind the use of pareira and the claims made regarding its effects haven't yet been validated scientifically.

parsley

Garden parsley, Hamburg parsley, persely, petersylinge, Petroselinum crispum, *rock parsley, umbelliferae*

Parsley is obtained from leaves, roots, and seeds of *Petroselinum crispum*. It contains carotene, iron, calcium, psoralens, flavonoids with anti-inflammatory and antioxidant activity, coumarins with anticoagulant properties, and vitamins B, C, E, and K. It also contains two volatile oils, apiole and myristicin, which are the most active components. The leaves contain 0.3% to 0.5% and the seeds contain 2% to 7% oils.

Myristicin and apiole act as diuretics and strong uterine stimulants. They may act as monoamine oxidase (MAO) inhibitors, causing decreased intracellular metabolism of norepinephrine, serotonin, and other biogenic amines. Sympathetic activity of myristicin and renal irritation of apiole contribute to diuretic effects. Myristicin may be metabolized to compounds with stimulating effects in the body, explaining the central nervous system effects seen with higher doses. Parsley is a rich source of vitamin C. It's available as a dried herb, seeds, liquid extract, capsules, tincture, and tea, and in combination with other herbs, such as garlic.

Reported uses

Parsley is used to treat indigestion, flatulence, dyspepsia, colic, kidney ailments, diuresis, cystitis, liver and spleen disorders, functional amenorrhea, uterine contraction, and dysmenorrhea. It's also used to increase milk production, freshen breath, promote hair growth, and provide antiseptic effects. Parsley is used as an antirheumatic, analgesic, antispasmodic, expectorant, and decongestant.

Administration

- Breath freshener: Dip sprigs into vinegar and chew slowly before swallowing. Effects last up to 3 or 4 hours
- Decoction: Dissolve 1 to 2 teaspoons of dried leaves or root, or 1 teaspoon of bruised seeds dissolved in a cup of water, and infuse for 5 to 10 minutes in a closed container. The decoction is taken by mouth three times a day
- Diuresis: Dosage is 6 g per day of root or leaves by mouth; 1 teaspoon, chopped, equals 2 g of herb
- Dried root: Dosage is 2 to 4 g by mouth or by oral infusion three times a day
- Hair growth promoter: Rub crushed parsley leaves over scalp
- Leaf: Dosage is 2 to 4 g by mouth three times a day
- Leaf capsules: Dosage is 2 capsules (450 mg each) by mouth, two or three times a day, or 3 capsules (455 mg each) by mouth, three times a day
- Liquid extract (1:1 in 25% alcohol): Dosage is 2 to 4 ml by mouth three times a day
- Leaf extract in vegetable glycerin and grain neutral spirit (12% to 14%): Dosage is 10 to 15 gtt with water by mouth, two or three times a day
- Seeds: Dosage is 1 to 2 g by mouth three times a day, or 2 to 3 g in divided daily doses. Protect seeds from light and moisture.

Hazards

Adverse effects associated with the use of parsley include allergic reaction, sedation, headache, loss of balance, seizures, giddiness, hallucinations, hypotension, bradycardia, flushing, tachycardia, hypotension, ventricular arrhythmias, shock, deafness, epistaxis, nausea, vomiting, irritation of stomach and intestines, menstruation, miscarriages, irritation of the kidneys, nephrosis, hemolytic anemia, thrombocytopenic purpura, fatty degeneration of the liver, hepatic dysfunction, paralysis, neuropathy, pruritus, pigmentation, and photosensitivity. Extremely large doses of parsley have been associated with hematologic, hepatic, and renal toxicity.

Herbal products that contain alcohol may cause a disulfiram-like reaction. Parsley may potentiate the effects of MAO inhibitors, such as isocarboxazid, moclobemide, phenelzine, selegiline, and tranylcypromine. Decreased anticoagulant effects may occur if parsley is used with coumadin. Patients should avoid consuming high doses of seed products because of the high volatile oil content.

Pregnant and breast-feeding patients shouldn't use this herb. High doses may also potentiate MAO inhibitor therapy. Patients with kidney and liver disease shouldn't use this herb because some forms may contain alcohol.

Clinical considerations
- Some products may contain alcohol and may not be suitable for use by children, alcoholic patients, patients with liver failure, or patients who take disulfiram or metronidazole.
- Consumption of large amounts of parsley can cause serious adverse effects.
- If patient takes warfarin, monitor him closely for decreased warfarin effects.
- Psoralen raises the risk of photosensitivity.
- Parsley seeds may cause a higher risk of adverse reactions because they contain higher amounts of volatile oils.
- Warn patient that parsley components may cause uterine stimulation and may complicate pregnancy or cause miscarriage.
- Remind patient using parsley to flush out urinary system to drink large amounts of fluid.
- Tell patient to remind prescriber and pharmacist of any herbal and dietary supplement that he's taking when obtaining a new prescription.
- Advise patient to consult his health care provider before using an herbal preparation because a treatment with proven efficacy may be available.

Research summary
The concepts behind the use of parsley and the claims made regarding its effects haven't yet been validated scientifically.

parsley piert
Alchemilla arvensis, Aphanes arvensis, *field lady's mantle, parsley breakstone, parsley piercestone*

Parsley piert is obtained from *Aphanes arvensis*. It contains tannin — an astringent — similar to a related species, *Alchemilla vulgaris* (lady's mantle). Parsley piert may have diuretic and demulcent properties. It's available as dried herb, liquid extract, tincture, and infusion, or in combination with other herbs, such as mullein flowers, sweet flag root, marshmallow root, comfrey root, slippery elm, gravel root, and pellitory.

Reported uses
Parsley piert is used as a diuretic and demulcent, and for dissolving kidney or bladder calculi. Also used for dysuria, edema of renal or hepatic origin, jaundice, bladder inflammation, and recurrent UTI.

Administration
- Dried herb: 2 to 4 g by mouth three times a day
- Infusion: 1 cup three or four times a day; prepared by boiling 1 oz dried herb

in 1 pint of water, simmering for 1 minute, cooling, and straining
- Liquid extract (1:1 in 25% alcohol): 2 to 4 ml by mouth three times a day
- Tincture (1:5 in 45% alcohol): 2 to 10 ml by mouth three times a day.

Hazards
Adverse effects that may be associated with the use of parsley piert in dosages higher than recommended include headache, flushing, tachycardia, hypotension, ventricular arrhythmias, nausea, vomiting, and shock.

Herbal products that contain alcohol may cause a disulfiram-like reaction, such as flushing, headache, nausea, vomiting, tachycardia, hypotension, ventricular arrhythmias, and shock leading to death.

Pregnant and breast-feeding patients shouldn't use this herb because published information is lacking. Liquid extract and tincture contain alcohol and shouldn't be used by patients with liver disease or alcoholism.

 SAFETY RISK *Don't confuse parsley piert with the parsley used in cooking.*

Clinical considerations
- Some products may contain alcohol and may not be suitable for use by children, alcoholic patients, patients with liver failure, or patients who take disulfiram or metronidazole.
- Advise pregnant or breast-feeding patient to avoid using this herb.
- Advise patient not to exceed recommended doses.
- Tell patient to remind prescriber and pharmacist of any herbal and dietary supplement that he's taking when obtaining a new prescription.
- Advise patient to consult his health care provider before using an herbal preparation because a treatment with proven efficacy may be available.

Research summary
The concepts behind the use of parsley piert and the claims made regarding its effects haven't yet been validated scientifically.

passion flower

Granadilla, grenadille, Jamaican honeysuckle, maypop, passiflora, Passiflora incarnata, passion vine, purple passion flower, water lemon

Passion flower is obtained from leaves, fruits, and flowers of *Passiflora incarnata.* It contains indole alkaloids, including harman and harmine, flavonoids, and maltol. Indole alkaloids are the basis of many biologically active substances, such as serotonin and tryptophan. The exact effect of these alkaloids is unknown; however, they can cause central nervous system (CNS) stimulation via monoamine oxidase (MAO) inhibition, thereby decreasing intracellular metabolism of norepinephrine, serotonin, and other biogenic amines. Flavonoids can reduce capillary permeability and fragility. Maltol can cause sedative effects and potentiate hexobarbital and anticonvulsive activity. Passion flower is available as fruits, flowers, extracts, capsules, tincture, and tea, and in a variety of combination products.

Reported uses
Passion flower is used as a sedative, hypnotic, and analgesic. It's also used as an antispasmodic for treating muscle spasms caused by indigestion, asthma, menstrual cramping, pain, or migraines. It's mainly used for insomnia and nervousness, but may also be used to treat neuralgia, generalized seizures, and hysteria. The crushed leaves and flowers are used topically for cuts, bruises, and hemorrhoids.

Administration
- Dried herb: Dosage is 250 mg to 1 g by mouth, 2 to 3 100-mg capsules by mouth twice a day, or one 400-mg capsule by mouth every day, standardized to contain 3.5% isovitoxin per dose
- Extract in vegetable glycerin base (alcohol free): Dosage is 10 to 15 gtt by mouth, two or three times a day
- For cuts and bruises: Crushed leaves and flowers are applied topically, as needed
- For hemorrhoids: A topical poultice is prepared by soaking 20 g dried herb in 200 ml of simmering water, straining, then cooling before application
- Tea infusion: Steep 1 teaspoon of herb in 150 ml of hot water for 10 minutes and then strain; tea is taken two or three times a day, with a final dose about 30 minutes before bedtime
- Liquid extract (1:1 in 25% alcohol): Dosage is 0.5 to 1 ml by mouth three times a day
- Solid extract: Dosage is 150 to 300 mg a day by mouth
- Tincture (1:8 in 45% alcohol): Dosage is 0.5 to 2 ml by mouth three times a day, or ½ to 1 teaspoon by mouth three times a day.

Hazards
Adverse effects that may be associated with improper use of passion flower include drowsiness, headache, flushing, agitation, confusion, psychosis, tachycardia, hypotension, ventricular arrhythmias, nausea, vomiting, asthma, allergic reactions, and shock. Herbal products that contain alcohol may cause a disulfiram-like reaction. If passion flower is used with hexobarbital, increased sleeping time and other barbiturate effects may be potentiated.

The actions of isocarboxazid, moclobemide, phenelzine, selegiline, and tranylcypromine can be potentiated by passion flower. Excessive doses may cause sedation and may potentiate MAO inhibitor therapy.

Pregnant and lactating patients shouldn't take passion flower. Those with liver disease or a history of alcoholism should avoid products that contain alcohol.

Clinical considerations
- Monitor patient for possible adverse CNS effects.
- Some products may contain alcohol and may not be suitable for use by children, alcoholic patients, patients with liver failure, or patients who take disulfiram or metronidazole.
- Because sedation is possible, caution patient to avoid hazardous activities.
- Warn patient not to take herb for chronic pain or insomnia before seeking medical attention because doing so may delay diagnosis of a potentially serious medical condition.
- Caution pregnant patient to avoid using this herb.
- Tell patient to remind prescriber and pharmacist of any herbal and dietary supplement that he's taking when obtaining a new prescription.
- Advise patient to consult his health care provider before using an herbal preparation because a treatment with proven efficacy may be available.

Research summary
The concepts behind the use of passion flower and the claims made regarding its effects haven't yet been validated scientifically.

pau d'arco

Ipe roxo, lapacho,
Tabebuia avellanedae, T. impetiginosa, T. ipe, *taheebo, tahuari, tajy, queshua*

Pau d'arco is obtained from bark and heartwood of *Tabebuia avellanedae.* It contains anthraquinones, naphthoquinones (such as lapachol), flavonoids, alkaloids, and traces of saponins. Lapachol compounds may be effective against psoriasis. Compounds of the lapachol fraction block electron transport in the mitochondria and have shown activity against colon, breast, and lung cancer cells. Lapachol may also interact directly with nucleic acids, thereby blocking DNA replication. Beta-lapachone, a constituent of the extract, stimulates lipid peroxidation, producing toxic derivatives that further weaken cell proliferation.

Pau d'arco is active against *Bacillus subtilis*, *Mycobacterium pyogenes aureus*, *Trypanosoma cruzi*, and certain viruses, such as herpesvirus, avian myeloblastosis, Rous sarcoma, and murine leukemia virus. Lapachol acts as a mild sedative; it has hypotensive action and may be blended with other decongestants. Pau d'arco is available as capsules, extracts, and tea, in products such as Amazon Support, Antifungal Formula, BP-X, Caprylimune, Pau d'arco Power Pack, Red Clover Blend Defense Maintenance, and Trumpet Tree.

Reported uses

Pau d'arco is used to treat ulcers, diarrhea, rheumatism, inflammation, and vaginal infections with *Candida albicans* or *Trichomonas vaginalis*. It's also used to treat influenza, the common cold, and bladder infections. Also used to kill vaginal parasites and to reduce fever and arthritis pain. Its primary use is the treatment of fungal infections.

Administration

■ Capsules: Average daily dose is 250 mg to 1 g by mouth; 5 capsules is usually equal to 2 cups of tea. Duration of treatment may exceed 3 weeks but is usually shorter than 6 months
■ Alcoholic tincture: Dosage is 1.2 to 1.5 ml diluted in a half-cup of warm water by mouth three times a day
■ Bark decoction: Add bark to 1 cup of water, bring to a boil, and simmer for 5 minutes; dosage is ½ to 1 cup one to three times a day
■ Colds and flu: Dosage is 1 or 2 cups of tea every day as a preventive measure. Tea should be freshly prepared each day

■ Vaginal infections: Gauze tampons soaked in the extract are inserted vaginally and changed every 12 hours to heal swollen mucous membranes and kill parasites.

Hazards

Adverse effects associated with the use of pau d'arco may include nausea, diarrhea, vomiting, anemia, and anticoagulation. There is a possible additive effect when pau d'arco is used with anticoagulants. Pau d'arco inhibits the absorption of iodine. Yerba maté may potentiate pau d'arco products.

Pregnant patients and patients with anemia or thyroid disorders shouldn't use this herb.

Clinical considerations

■ Monitor patient's white blood cell count during lapachol treatment; if count changes, advise patient to stop taking the drug.
■ If patient has thyroid problems, tell him to consult his health care provider before taking pau d'arco because lapachol may inhibit iodine utilization. If he takes the herb, tell him to have his thyroid function checked regularly.
■ Adverse reactions occur mainly at doses higher than the recommended amount.
■ Herb may act against vitamin K, causing symptoms of anemia.
■ Advise pregnant or breast-feeding patient to avoid this herb.
■ Tell patient to remind prescriber and pharmacist of any herbal and dietary supplement that he's taking when obtaining a new prescription.
■ Advise patient to consult his health care provider before using an herbal preparation because a treatment with proven efficacy may be available.

Research summary

The concepts behind the use of pau d'arco and the claims made regarding its effects haven't yet been validated scientifically.

peach

Amygdalin, amygdalis persica, laetrile,
Prunus persica, *vitamin B₁₇*

The medicinal constituents of peach are derived from the bark and leaves of the *Prunus persica*. Its mechanism of action is unknown. It contains cyanogenic glycosides (amygdalin), volatile oils that are carminatives and GI irritants, and phloretin. Phloretin may have antibacterial activity against gram-positive and gram-negative organisms. A single peach seed also contains about 2.6 mg of hydrocyanic acid. Peach is available as persic oil, peach kernel oil, seeds, dried bark, leaves, and flowers.

Reported uses

Peach is used to treat constipation, cough, bad breath, blisters, boils, bronchitis, bruises, burns, dysentery, earache, eczema, edema, headache, hemorrhage, hypertension, locked jaw, menstrual pain, minor wounds, nervousness, pain, pinworm, tapeworm, pneumonia, gastritis, bronchitis, whooping cough, scurvy, shingles, skin irritation and inflammation, sore throat, stomach upset, warts, and kidney or liver problems.

 SAFETY RISK *Laetrile, also known as amygdalin or vitamin B₁₇ and touted as an anticancer agent, has been banned by the FDA because of its high cyanide content and potential for overdosing or poisoning.*

Administration

■ Tea: Steep 0.5 oz dried bark or 1 oz dried leaves in 16 oz boiling water for 15 minutes; tea is taken three times a day for indigestion and bladder inflammation
■ Sores and wounds: Peach leaves are applied as a poultice, as needed.

Hazards

Adverse effects associated with peach include peripheral neuropathy, deafness, muscle spasms, and cyanide poisoning

(from pit or bark). There are no reported interactions with peach.

Pregnant patients and those hypersensitive to this herb shouldn't use peach.

SAFETY RISK *Peach should be used with extreme caution because the seeds contain cyanogenic glycosides.*

Clinical considerations

■ Monitor patient for evidence of cyanide poisoning, such as vomiting, severe stomach pain, fainting, drowsiness, seizures, or coma if using oil from the seeds or bark.
■ If cyanide toxicity is suspected, give sodium thiosulfate immediately and monitor patient's cyanide level.
■ Warn patient against high doses or long-term use of seeds because of risk of cyanide poisoning.
■ Tell patient to remind prescriber and pharmacist of any herbal and dietary supplement that he's taking when obtaining a new prescription.
■ Advise patient to consult his health care provider before using an herbal preparation because a treatment with proven efficacy may be available.

Research summary

Peach seed was once thought to be a cancer remedy; however, studies performed by the National Cancer Institute failed to show clinical effectiveness.

pennyroyal

American pennyroyal, European pennyroyal, lurk-in-the-ditch, Mentha pulegium, *mosquito plant, piliolerial, pudding grass, pulegium, run-by-the-ground, squaw balm, squawmint, tickweed*

The leaves and flowering tops of *Mentha pulegium* contain pennyroyal oil. The oil contains D-pulegione (60% to 90%), methone, isomethone, tannins, and flavonoids. Pulegione depletes glutathione in the liver. In high doses, it has abortifacient properties. Pennyroyal is available as a tea, tincture, loose dried herb, and capsules.

Reported uses
In the past, pennyroyal was used to treat digestive disorders, liver and gallbladder disorders, bowel disorders, pneumonia, gout, and colds. It's currently used topically for skin diseases. It's also used as an abortifacient, insect repellent, antiseptic, flavoring agent, and fragrance in detergents, soaps, and perfumes.

Administration
- Dried herb: 1 to 4 g by mouth three times a day
- Insect repellent: Applied sparingly to skin, as needed
- Tea: 1 cup by mouth every day.

Hazards
Adverse effects associated with the use of pennyroyal include lethargy, delirium, unconsciousness, seizures, hallucinations, hypertension, tachycardia, respiratory failure, anesthetic-like paralysis, shock, abdominal pain, nausea, vomiting, miscarriage, irreversible renal damage, hepatotoxicity, severe liver damage, and dermatitis. Herbal products that contain alcohol may cause a disulfiram-like reaction.

 SAFETY RISK *Severe poisoning has been reported after consumption of 5 g of pennyroyal oil as an abortifacient. Overdose may cause vomiting, hypertension, anesthetic-like paralysis, and respiratory failure.*

 SAFETY RISK *Pennyroyal has toxic effects on the liver and isn't recommended for internal use.*

Clinical considerations
- Some products may contain alcohol and may not be suitable for use by children, alcoholic patients, patients with liver failure, or patients who take disulfiram or metronidazole.
- Caution patient about pennyroyal's toxic effects on the liver and warn him to take herb orally only with close supervision by a health care provider.
- If patient uses the oil as a flavoring, warn him to use only small amounts.
- Advise pregnant patient not to use this herb because it has abortifacient properties.
- Warn patient to keep all herbal products away from children and pets.
- Tell patient to remind prescriber and pharmacist of any herbal and dietary supplement that he's taking when obtaining a new prescription.
- Advise patient to consult his health care provider before using an herbal preparation because a treatment with proven efficacy may be available.

Research summary
The concepts behind the use of pennyroyal and the claims made regarding its effects haven't yet been validated scientifically.

pepper, black
Pepper bark, pimenta, piper,
Piper nigrum

Black pepper is obtained from the berries of *Piper nigrum*. The shell is removed and the green fruit is sun-dried or roasted, yielding volatile oils (1.2% to 2.6%), limonene (15% to 20%), sabinene (15% to 25%), caryophyllene (10% to 15%), betaphinene (10% to 12%), alpha-pinene (8% to 12%), acid amides (pungent substances), and fatty oils. Pepper stimulates thermal receptors and increases secretion of saliva and gastric mucus. It may have abortifacient, analgesic, diaphoretic, diuretic, sedative, emetic, hypnotic, mydriatic, narcotic, sudorific, insecticidal, and antimicrobial effects. Black pepper is available as dried berries, powder, and ointment for external use.

Reported uses
Pepper is used to treat constipation, gonorrhea, dyspepsia, colic, headache, cholera, diarrhea, scarlatina, paralytic disorders, asthma, bronchitis, delirium, dysmenorrhea, insomnia, pertussis, tuberculosis, flatulence, nausea, vertigo, and arthritic conditions. It's also used to ease nicotine withdrawal symptoms during smoking cessation. Pepper is used externally for neuralgia and scabies. It's used extensively as a spice and flavoring ingredient for food.

Administration
- To improve digestive function: 1.5 g by mouth every day, divided into doses of 0.3 to 0.6 g
- Scabies: Applied externally, as needed.

Hazards
Adverse effects associated with the use of black pepper include tremors, numbness, eye irritation, mucous membrane irritation, salivation, nausea, gastric pain, skin irritation, and sweating.

Black pepper may cause reduced drug effects of drugs metabolized by the cytochrome P-450 system, such as acetaminophen, erythromycin, ibuprofen, ketoconazole, naproxen, propranolol, and theophylline. It may cause increased absorption of phenobarbital, phenytoin, propranolol, rifampin, and theophylline. Warfarin metabolism may be altered by pepper; monitor patient's International Normalized Ratio closely to maintain therapeutic value.

Pregnant patients and those hypersensitive to black pepper shouldn't use it.

Clinical considerations
- Black pepper is an irritant to the eyes. Flush eyes with water to lessen the irritation.

- Advise patient to be careful of nasal or eye irritation if using powder.
- Exceeding recommended oral dose may cause GI irritation. Tell patient not to exceed recommended amounts without consulting health care provider.
- Monitor patient for altered warfarin metabolism.
- Tell patient to remind pharmacist of any herbal and dietary supplement that he's taking when obtaining a new prescription.
- Advise patient to consult his health care provider before using an herbal preparation because a treatment with proven efficacy may be available.

Research summary
The concepts behind the use of black pepper and the claims made regarding its effects haven't yet been validated scientifically.

peppermint

Brandy mint, lamb mint,
Mentha x piperita

Peppermint is obtained from dried leaves and flowering branch tips of *Mentha x piperita*. The oil contains more than 100 components, including menthol (29% to 48%), methyl acetate (3% to 10%), menthone (20% to 31%), caffeic acid, azulene, and flavonoids. It exerts antibacterial and antiviral actions, as well as spasmolytic effects on smooth muscles. When taken as enteric-coated capsules, peppermint oil may have antispasmodic effects on smooth muscle of the intestines; its antispasmodic activity results from the calcium antagonist effect of menthol. Flavonoids may cause its bile-stimulating effect. Azulene may have anti-inflammatory and antiulcer action. Peppermint is available as an essential oil, ointment, liniment, extract, tincture, leaves, dried herb, and capsules.

Reported uses

Peppermint is used to treat nausea, irritable bowel syndrome (IBS), colitis, colic, ileitis, Crohn's disease, and other spasmodic conditions of the bowel. It's also used in liver and gallbladder complaints, cramps of the upper GI tract and bile ducts, menstrual cramps, colds and flu, inflammation of the oral and pharyngeal mucosa, loss of appetite, dyspepsia, flatulence, and gastritis. Peppermint is used to treat the nausea and vomiting related to pregnancy and motion sickness. It's used externally for myalgia, neuralgia, itching, and skin irritation, and the oil is applied to the forehead to relieve tension and migraine headaches.

Administration

- Enteric-coated capsules: 0.6 ml essential oil in enteric-coated capsules by mouth every day for IBS
- Essential oil: 0.2 ml by mouth every day
- Tincture: (1:10) 5 to 15 g, by mouth two or three times a day
- Infusion: 2 g dried leaf in 150 ml water by mouth two or three times a day
- Dry normalized extract: 0.44 to 0.57 g by mouth two or three times a day
- Fluid extract: 2 ml by mouth two or three times a day
- Liniment: 5% to 20% essential oil in vegetable oil, applied with friction to area of joint or bone pain
- Nasal ointment: 1% to 5% essential oil, applied topically, as needed
- Ointment: 5% to 20% essential oil in petroleum or lanolin used topically, as needed.

Hazards

Adverse effects associated with peppermint include headache, flushing, spasm of tongue, eye irritation, gastroesophageal reflux, respiratory arrest, contact dermatitis, irritation, and allergic reactions.

Calcium channel blockers, such as amlodipine, bepridil, diltiazem, felodipine, isradipine, nicardipine, nifedipine, ni-modipine, nitrendipine, and verapamil, may have decreased effects if used with peppermint. Monitor patient closely.

Patients with gallstones, obstructed bile ducts, gallbladder inflammation, and severe liver damage shouldn't use peppermint. The oil shouldn't be applied to the face or nasal passages of infants or children because of the risk of tongue spasms or respiratory arrest.

Clinical considerations

- Monitor patient with suspected hiatal hernia closely because peppermint weakens the esophageal sphincters.
- The enteric-coated capsule must be used for IBS or other intestinal disorders to ensure that the peppermint oil reaches the intestines in its active form.
- Advise parents not to use peppermint products containing oil on the face, especially around the nares, of infants and children because it may cause glottal or bronchial spasm.
- Stress that patient should consult his health care provider if symptoms don't improve in a reasonable length of time.
- Warn patient that contact dermatitis can occur with topical administration of peppermint oil.
- Peppermint should be stored in a nonplastic container in a dark, cool, dry place.
- Tell patient to remind prescriber and pharmacist of any herbal and dietary supplement that he's taking when obtaining a new prescription.
- Advise patient to consult his health care provider before using an herbal preparation because a treatment with proven efficacy may be available.

Research summary

The concepts behind the use of peppermint and the claims made regarding its effects haven't yet been validated scientifically.

peyote

Anhalonium williamsii,
devil's root, dumpling cactus,
Lophophora levinii Pellote,
L. williamsii, *mescal buttons, mescaline,*
pellote, sacred mushroom

The root and hair tufts of the cactus *Lophophora williamsii* are removed and the mescaline-rich center is sliced and dried to make mescaline buttons. A button contains up to 7% mescaline (trimethoxyphenethylamine), the main active ingredient. It has an emetic and hallucinogenic effect. Mescaline may cause visual, auditory, gustatory, kinesthetic, and synesthetic hallucinations. Peyote is available as buttons, extracts, and tinctures.

Reported uses

Peyote isn't currently used as a medicinal herb. It is used illegally for psychogenic and hallucinogenic effects. It has been used in sacred rituals to promote visions (that is, hallucinations).

Administration

No dosages are available for internal ingestion because herb has no medicinal use.

 SAFETY RISK *Peyote is categorized as controlled substance schedule I and has no proven medicinal use.*

Hazards

Visual, aural, kinesthetic, and synesthetic hallucinations occur when taken in doses of 4 to 12 dried slices. Peyote causes increased sedation if used with sedative drugs. Warn patient not to take peyote.

 SAFETY RISK *Mescaline doses above 20 mg may cause hypotension, bradycardia, vasodilatation, and respiratory depression. Nausea and vomiting may occur 30 to 60 minutes after ingestion.*

Clinical considerations

Advise patient not to take peyote for any reason.

Research summary

The concepts behind the use of peyote and the claims made regarding its effects haven't yet been validated scientifically.

phytoestrogens

Plant estrogens

Phytoestrogens are compounds of plant origin that are usually nonsteroidal but act as partial agonists or antagonists to estrogen receptors. They demonstrate weak estrogen receptor–binding capacity — generally less than one hundredth that of estrogens — and elicit one-thousandth the response in cells compared with endogenous estrogen. These compounds fall into three main classifications: isoflavones, coumestans, and lignans (also known as resorcyclic acid lactones). Isoflavones are found in high abundance in legumes, particularly soy. The main isoflavones are daidzein and genistein. Other isoflavones include biochanin A and formononetin, which undergo fermentation by gut bacteria to genistein and daidzein, respectively. Lignans are compounds found in whole grains, fibers, and flaxseeds; these substances are fermented by gut bacteria to enterolactone and enterodiol, the biologically active phytoestrogens. Equol is another phytoestrogen formed when intestinal bacteria break down formononetin or daidzein. Coumestans are found primarily in clover and legumes.

There are more than 300 foods and herbs that have demonstrated phyto-estrogenic properties. The main dietary sources of phytoestrogens are soybeans, clover and alfalfa sprouts, and oilseeds (such as flaxseed). The seven commonly consumed herbs with the highest estrogen receptor–binding capacity are soy, licorice, red clover, thyme, turmeric, hops, and verbena. Phytoestrogens are available in a variety of over-the-counter products.

Reported uses

Phytoestrogens are used to replace endogenous estrogens, to prevent osteoporosis and breast cancer associated with menopause, and to relieve menopause symptoms such as hot flashes and vaginal dryness.

Administration

See package inserts for dosage instructions.

Hazards

Phytoestrogens found in food are considered safe when consumed in normal amounts. However, soy, in particular, can depress thyroid function in infants and adults. The safety of using soy as an infant formula has been questioned because of its high phytoestrogen content. When using phytoestrogens to treat a specific condition, it is best to consult a qualified health practitioner who specializes in natural treatments.

Clinical considerations

Phytoestrogens have the potential to have additive effects with other estrogens, increasing the potential for adverse effects such as edema and high blood pressure.

Research summary

Studies have shown that post-menopausal women who follow phytoestrogen-rich diets experience fewer hot flashes. Although a negative study of rats showed no change in vaginal epithelium compared with conjugated equine estrogens, studies of women taking phytoestrogens have subjectively shown a decrease in vaginal dryness. Another study demonstrated that phytoestrogens, particularly genistein and daidzein, cause a mild improvement in bone mass.

Results vary in studies of the relationship between phytoestrogens and breast cancer. It is generally believed that phy-

toestrogens block the actions of endogenous estrogens, thereby reducing the deleterious effects of estrogen on breast tissue and estrogen-positive cancers. One study demonstrated a biphasic effect that phytoestrogens have on breast tissue. Estrogen-positive cancer cells were induced to grow when low levels of phytoestrogens were applied, but phytoestrogen inhibited cell reproduction when high levels were applied. A population study of women measured urinary output of phytoestrogens and demonstrated a greater amount of consumption of phytoestrogens in a matched control group without breast cancer. However, in a few studies, soy has been shown to increase breast cancer cell proliferation in vitro. Further research is needed.

pill-bearing spurge

Asthma weed, Euphorbia,
Euphorbia ceritera, E. pilulifera,
garden spurge, milkweed, snakeweed

Pill-bearing spurge contains 0.4% of a glycosidal substance, tannin, fatty acids, phorbic acid, sterols, euphosterol, jambulol, melissic acid, and sugars. It's available as a dried herb, extract, and tincture.

Reported uses

Pill-bearing spurge is used to treat upper respiratory catarrh, bronchial asthma, bronchitis, laryngeal spasm, and intestinal amebiasis.

Administration

- Liquid extract: 1:1 in 45% alcohol, 0.12 to 0.3 ml by mouth
- Tincture: 1:5 in 50% alcohol, 0.6 to 2 ml by mouth
- Dried herb: 120 to 300 mg infusion by mouth.

Hazards

Potential adverse effects associated with the use of pill-bearing spurge include nausea, vomiting, respiratory failure, and contact dermatitis.

Pill-bearing spurge may potentiate the effects of angiotensin-converting enzymne (ACE) inhibitors, such as enalaprilat and quinapril. Decreased drug effects may result when pill-bearing spurge is used with anticholinergics, such as atropine, ipratropium, and scopolamine. Additive effects may occur if pill-bearing spurge is used with anticholinesterases, such as donepezil and edrophonium. Additive effects may occur if used with arecoline, methacholine, muscarine, and muscarinic agonists.

Herbal products that contain alcohol may cause a disulfiram-like reaction. Advise patient to avoid using together. Drugs metabolized by the CYP3A enzyme system, such as cyclosporine and erythromycin, may have decreased absorption if used with pill-bearing spurge. Increased central hypnotic effects may occur if pill-bearing spurge is used with barbiturates, such as phenobarbital. Pill-bearing spurge and warfarin may have potentiated effects. Monitor patient's International Normalized Ratio.

Pregnant and breast-feeding patients shouldn't use this herb. Pill-bearing spurge may decrease platelet aggregation and should be used with caution by alcoholic patients, patients who take anticoagulants, and patients with bleeding disorders or liver disease.

Clinical considerations
■ The FDA does not recognize this herb as a safe and effective treatment of asthma.

■ Monitor patient's blood pressure if taking pill-bearing spurge with ACE inhibitors.

■ Some products may contain alcohol and may not be suitable for use by children, alcoholic patients, patients with liver failure, or patients who take disulfiram or metronidazole.

■ If patient has a bleeding disorder and takes an anticoagulant, tell him not to take herb without consulting his health care provider.

■ Advise pregnant or breast-feeding patient to avoid this herb.

■ Tell patient to remind prescriber and pharmacist of any herbal and dietary supplement that he's taking when obtaining a new prescription.

■ Advise patient to consult his health care provider before using an herbal preparation because a treatment with proven efficacy may be available.

Research summary
The concepts behind the use of pill-bearing spurge and the claims made regarding its effects haven't yet been validated scientifically.

pineapple

Ananas, Ananas comosus, *bromelain, bromelainum, pineapple enzyme*

Pineapple contains bromelain, a proteolytic enzyme used commercially as a meat tenderizer and medically for its soft-tissue anti-inflammatory effect. Bromelain prolongs prothrombin time and bleeding time because it enhances fibrinolytic activity. It also lowers serum bradykinin and kininogen levels. It may influence prostaglandin synthesis, thus explaining its effect in burn debridement and wound healing. It's also active against nematodes and is believed by some to reduce the risk of cancer. Pineapple is available as capsules, syrup, extracts, juices, candy, and whole fruit.

Reported uses
Pineapple is used to treat acute postoperative and posttraumatic swelling, especially in nasal and paranasal sinuses. When combined with trypsin, amylase, and lipase enzymes, it's used to treat dyspepsia and exocrine hepatic insufficiency. Pineapple is also used to treat constipation, jaundice, edema, and inflammation, and for wound debridement. Pineapple also is used in asthma treatment to help reduce the thickness of mucus.

Administration

For acute postoperative or posttraumatic swelling, 80 to 320 mg by mouth two or three times a day for 8 to 10 days.

Hazards

Pineapple may be associated with nausea, vomiting, diarrhea, stomatitis, menorrhagia, uterine contractions, rash, and allergic reactions. Loss of fingerprints may occur after prolonged contact due to bromelain's keratolytic effect.

Bradykinin levels may be altered when pineapple is used with angiotensin-converting enzyme (ACE) inhibitors, such as enalaprilat and quinapril. Increased plasma and urine drug levels may result when used with tetracycline. Pineapple may potentiate the effect of warfarin; monitor patient's International Normalized Ratio levels closely.

Pregnant patients, patients who intend to become pregnant, patients who take anticoagulants, and those hypersensitive to pineapple shouldn't use these products.

Clinical considerations

■ Fruit packers who cut pineapple have reported losing their fingerprints because of bromelain's keratolytic effects.
■ Warn patient not to combine other anticoagulants with pineapple, which also has anticoagulant effects.
■ Caution patient not to take pineapple when taking aspirin.
■ Advise pregnant or breast-feeding patients not to use pineapple.
■ If patient is taking tetracycline, advise him not to use pineapple unless advised by his health care provider.
■ Warn patient not to take pineapple for constipation, inflammation, or edema before seeking medical attention because doing so may delay diagnosis of a potentially serious medical condition.
■ Tell patient to remind prescriber and pharmacist of any herbal and dietary supplement that he's taking when obtaining a new prescription.

■ Advise patient to consult his health care provider before using an herbal preparation because a treatment with proven efficacy may be available.

Research summary

The concepts behind the use of pineapple and the claims made regarding its effects haven't yet been validated scientifically.

pipsissewa

Bitter wintergreen, butter winter, Chimaphila umbellata, *ground holly, King's cure, love in winter, Prince's pine, rheumatism weed, wintergreen*

Pipsissewa is obtained from aboveground parts of *Chimaphila umbellata*. Its active components include ericolin, chimaphilin, ursolic acid, tannin, gallic acid, and arbutin, a hydroquinone glycoside. Arbutin and chimaphilin are reported to function as urinary antiseptics. Pipsissewa is available as a decoction, tincture, extract, and syrup.

Reported uses

Pipsissewa is used to treat tuberculosis of the lymph nodes and cardiac and kidney disease, and as a diuretic and astringent. It's also used to treat chronic gonorrhea, catarrh of the bladder, gallstones, kidney stones, and ascites. It may diminish lithic acid in urine and may be combined with other treatments for edema. Pipsissewa may also have hypoglycemic activity.

Pipsissewa is used topically as a rubefacient. It may be applied to skin ulcers and blisters. It's also used as a flavoring agent in beverages.

Administration

■ Syrup: 1 or 2 tablespoons by mouth
■ Tincture: 1 to 5 grains per dose, by mouth
■ Tubercular sores: Decoction applied topically to external sores, as needed.

Hazards
Adverse effects that may be associated with the use of pipsissewa include hepatotoxicity, redness, vesication, and irritation. There are no reported interactions with pipsissewa.

Patients who are pregnant or breast-feeding shouldn't take this herb. Because it contains the hydroquinone glycoside arbutin, it isn't recommended for long-term use because of risk of hepatotoxicity.

Clinical considerations
- Topical application may cause skin irritation, redness, and vesication.
- Advise patient not to take this herb internally for prolonged periods because of potential liver damage.
- Advise pregnant or breast-feeding patients not to use this herb.
- Warn patient to keep all herbal products away from children and pets.
- Tell patient to remind prescriber and pharmacist of any herbal or dietary supplement that he's taking when obtaining a new prescription.
- Advise patient to consult his health care provider before using an herbal preparation because a treatment with proven efficacy may be available.

Research summary
The concepts behind the use of pipsissewa and the claims made regarding its effects haven't yet been validated scientifically.

plantain

Black psyllium, blond plantago, broad leaf plantain, flea seed, French psyllium, Indian plantago, lance leaf plantain, narrow leaf plantain, Plantago lanceolata, P. ovata, P. psyllium, *ribwort plantain, Spanish psyllium*

Plantain is obtained from the seed of *Plantago ovata, P. psyllium,* and other species. When the seeds are mixed with water, a mucilaginous mass is formed. Seeds provide bulk to aid in treating constipation, while the mucilage — 2% to 6% of glucomannans, arabinogalactane, and rhamnogalacturontane — acts as a mild laxative. Taken in dry form, it decreases intestinal motility and is useful in treating diarrhea and irritable bowel syndrome. Plantain also contains aglycone and aucubigenin, which give psyllium an antimicrobial action. Its cholesterol-lowering action is caused by a polyphenolic compound contained in the herb. Plantain is available as a powder, seeds, extract, infusion, pressed juice, and poultice, and in products such as Effer-Syllium, Ground Psyllium, Hydrocil, Konsyl, Metamucil, and Perdiem.

Reported uses
Plantain is used as a bulk-forming laxative to treat constipation. For irritable bowel syndrome or diarrhea, plantain should be taken without large amounts of water to decrease intestinal motility. Regular internal use helps reduce cholesterol levels. Plantain is also used to treat respiratory catarrh tract and oropharyngeal inflammation, and topically for skin inflammation and insect stings.

Administration
- Compress: Soak a cloth in a solution made by steeping 1.4 g cut herb in 5 oz cold water for 1 to 2 hours. The compress is applied to the affected area, as needed
- Infusion: Prepared by steeping 1.4 g of herb in 5 oz boiled water for 10 to 15 minutes; dosage is 1 cup by mouth three to four times a day
- Powder: Dosage is 3 to 6 g by mouth every day
- Rinse or gargle: To prepare a rinse or gargle, soak 1.4 g cut herb in 5 oz cold water for 1 to 2 hours, stirring often; the liquid is then swished in the mouth three or four times a day. The gargle isn't swallowed
- Tincture (1 g:5 ml): Dosage is 7 ml by mouth three or four times a day.

Hazards

Potential adverse effects associated with the use of plantain include watery eyes, diarrhea, flatulence, GI obstruction, sneezing, chest congestion, and anaphylaxis.

Decreased absorption may occur if plantain is used with carbamazepine or lithium. Advise patient to avoid using together. Decreased iron absorption may occur if plantain is taken with feosol or iron supplements. Advise patient to avoid using together.

Patients hypersensitive to plantain products shouldn't use this herb.

Clinical considerations

- Insufficient water when taking plantain can cause constipation because of the removal of liquid from the GI tract by the herb. Warn patient to drink at least 8 oz of water with each dose.
- Plantain may cause allergic reactions when first used.
- Do not confuse the herb plantain with the edible plantain or banana, *Musa paradisiacal.*
- Advise patient to separate herb ingestion from other oral drugs by at least 2 hours to prevent decreased drug absorption caused by the increased gastric motility.
- Tell patient taking lithium and carbamazepine to speak to his health care provider before taking plantain.
- Inform patient that if allergic symptoms occur, including sneezing, itching, and swollen eyes, he should stop using product and consult his health care provider.
- Tell patient to remind prescriber and pharmacist of any herbal or dietary supplement that he is taking when obtaining a new prescription.
- Advise patient to consult his health care provider before using an herbal preparation because a treatment with proven efficacy may be available.

Research summary

The concepts behind the use of plantain and the claims made regarding its effects haven't yet been validated scientifically.

pokeweed

American nightshade, American spinach, bear's grape, branching phytolacca, cancer-root, cankerroot, coakumchongras, crowberry, garget, inkberry, jalap, Phytolacca americana, *pigeon berry, poke, poke berry, red-ink plant, scoke, Virginia poke*

Pokeweed contains triterpene, saponins, esculinic acid, and pokeweed mitogen. Its mechanisms of action aren't known. Pokeweed mitogen has been linked to blood cell abnormalities. Extracts containing pokeweed mitogens may alter T and B lymphocytes. It may also have anti-inflammatory, antirheumatic, and digestive activity. Pokeweed is available as a powder, liquid, extract, and tincture.

Reported uses

Pokeweed is used as an emetic because of its saponin content. It's also used to treat rheumatism, cough, tonsillitis, itching, laryngitis, and swollen glands.

Pokeweed berries are used as a food coloring. The young spring plant shoots can be used as an edible vegetable, but only after careful boiling.

Administration

- Emetic: Dried root 60 to 300 mg by mouth
- Extract (1:1 in 45% alcohol): 0.1 to 0.5 ml by mouth.

Hazards

Adverse effects associated with the use of pokeweed include dizziness, somnolence, seizures, hypotension, tachycardia, nausea, vomiting, severe stomach cramping, diarrhea, bronchospasm, and apnea. To date, there are no reported interactions with pokeweed.

 SAFETY RISK *Roots, berries, and purple bark of the pokeweed stems are poisonous. Because of its high toxicity, this herb shouldn't be used for any medical conditions. At this time, the FDA has classified pokeweed as an herb of undefined safety with demonstrated narcotic effects. However, herbalists claim that pokeweed, when used carefully, can be very helpful with arthritis, fibrocystic breasts, or as a laxative.*

 SAFETY RISK *Even properly prepared, pokeweed has caused toxicity. Symptoms of poisoning or overdose include nausea, vomiting, diarrhea, stomach cramps, and dizziness. Mild overdose usually subsides within 24 hours, but severe poisoning may last up to 48 hours. Gastric lavage, emesis, and symptomatic and supportive treatment have been suggested.*

Clinical considerations

- Caution patient not to ingest any part of this herb because of its high toxicity.
- Because of blood cell alterations caused by pokeweed mitogens, gloves should be worn when handling this herb.
- Warn patient to keep all herbal products away from children and pets.
- Tell patient to remind prescriber and pharmacist of any herbal and dietary supplement that he's taking when obtaining a new prescription.
- Advise patient to consult his health care provider before using an herbal preparation because a treatment with proven efficacy may be available.

Research summary

Pokeweed is presently under investigation for its antiviral effects in flu, herpes simplex virus-1, and polio.

Polarity therapy

Polarity therapy was created by Randolf Stone, a chiropractor, osteopath, and naturopath who was dissatisfied with the results he achieved by using the methods of conventional medical practice. The relief provided by physical adjustments often proved temporary, with the original symptoms eventually recurring and requiring further correction. Stone traveled to both China and India in the 1930s to study the healing methods of these ancient cultures, and eventually incorporated some of their concepts into his own method. He published his first work in 1947, and by 1954 had completed the seven books containing his findings. Stone reported success when he applied the polarity energy approach in his medical practice.

Polarity therapy is based on the notion that a pattern of energy in the human body forms the blueprint that the body uses when healing itself. Health is viewed as a reflection of the condition of the body's energy field — when injury or disease occurs, the energy pattern becomes distorted. The flow of life energy usually repairs itself when distortions or blockages occur, thereby allowing the body to heal, but if the disruption of the energy pattern — that is, its *polarity* — is too great, or the illness has affected the person's emotional outlook, chronic health problems result. Polarity therapy works to release these energy blocks and balance the flow so that natural healing can take place.

Polarity therapy employs four basic elements to produce balance in the individual: bodywork, improved movement through polarity yoga, diet, and self-awareness. Bodywork is the focal point of the therapy, and a variety of techniques are employed, including massage of deep-tissue pressure points and rhythmical, rocking manipulations. Simple, yoga-like stretches and movements are used to enhance the flow of energy in the body. Daily practice can facilitate higher levels of self-understanding, greater flexibility, and overall body-mind awareness. The nutritional aspect of polarity therapy recommends a diet that includes wholesome vegetarian food and drink. Self-awareness is emphasized as the practitioner encourages the patient to become aware of his physical, mental, and emotional processes. As the patient becomes more able to sense and appreciate his body's energy patterns, he is more capable of self-regulation and less likely to be affected by external factors.

Reported uses

Polarity therapy is used to promote relaxation and balance, and to stimulate energy through the different parts of the body. Specific techniques are used to release energy blockages and reduce pain and discomfort; for example, releasing neck and shoulder tension removes blockages that manifest as pain or tension, sore throat, and laryngitis. Other manipulations are used to reduce pain in the back, sciatic nerve area, and hip. Stimulating energy flow in the colon area relieves constipation and spastic colon.

Polarity therapy uses specific touch and verbal tools for nervous system support and healing. Relieving mental and emotional tension is invaluable in dealing with posttrauma symptoms, in which the sympathetic and parasympathetic systems may be disabled owing to an overwhelming threat that occurred in the past.

How the treatment is performed

Polarity bodywork is performed on a traditional massage table, with the client remaining fully clothed. Each session lasts about an hour, beginning with a general energy balancing session and proceeding along specific principles with a treatment called *manipulations*. Subtle touch moves toward completing energy circuits and overcoming energy blockages in the body. Deep touch is sometimes used to release energy trapped in connective tissue or muscle.

The therapist places both hands on a specific energetic pathway on the client's body to enhance the current flow through that channel. Energy can be pal-

pated by both practitioner and client. The practitioner may feel warming and softening, pulsation, stillness, energetic shaping, and related subtle sensations, as the polarity contact is held. The client may feel relaxation, tingling, wavelike movement, stillness, and similar phenomena during the contact.

The practitioner may also employ verbal skills to support the client's increasing self-awareness of energy movement. A common energetic situation encountered in polarity therapy sessions is what Stone called "fixation at the negative pole." This phenomenon reflects the universal tendency of people to become attached to events, other people, objects, experiences, and thought-forms; in polarity therapy, it's believed that this attachment causes reduced flexibility and adaptability. Polarity therapy contacts are often oriented to relieving this condition by supporting the full cycle of energy — outward from the core of the patient's body to its periphery, and then back to its source. No two sessions follow the same protocol of moves; instead, the sessions are completely dependent on the client's current needs or state.

TRAINING *The American Polarity Therapy Association (APTA) has set standards of practice for the certification of practitioners and schools, which define the minimum level of excellence required to practice as a registered polarity practitioner (RPP) or an associate polarity practitioner (APP). Graduates of approved training programs can become certified by applying to APTA.*

RPP training requires 650 hours for polarity certification. The course of instruction draws on Western, Eastern, Ayurvedic, and Chinese traditions, and on the emerging theories of modern physics. APP training requires 155 hours for polarity certification. This 5-week course offers students a foundation in the core principles and techniques of polarity therapy. Schools and courses are available throughout the United States that teach the certification programs and short courses in the concepts of polarity therapy.

Hazards
The work isn't invasive and no complications have been reported. The usual precautions during any bodywork treatment should be taken, such as not treating areas of inflammation or open wounds, and avoiding tumor sites.

Clinical considerations
If symptoms persist, the patient should check with a conventional practitioner before continuing treatment. Some techniques use points deep in the perineal area, which some patients may find uncomfortable.

Research summary
In one study, a series of gamma detection rate experiments were performed to establish a background and baseline count rate among 10 treatment and 20 control subjects. Marked decreases in gamma counts were found at every anatomical site location for all subjects during polarity therapy, with less change noted during the control sessions. Gamma radiation decreased in 100% of subjects during therapy sessions at every body site tested, regardless of which therapist performed the treatment. This preliminary study suggests a decrease in the number of gamma rays measured in a subject's electromagnetic field during polarity therapy treatments.

polyphenols

Anthrocyanidins, cyanidins, phenolic compounds, phenols, proanthrocyanidins

---

Phenolic compounds are water-soluble, naturally occurring substances, responsible for the brightly colored pigments in many fruits and vegetables. Their prima-

ry function is to protect plants from diseases.

Polyphenols are a class among thousands of phytochemicals with antioxidant properties. High concentrations of polyphenols are found in red wine, green tea, grapes, onions, apples, yams, and a variety of plant sources. Polyphenols are also reported in chocolate and a variety of spices. Bioavailability of polyphenols is dependent on regional growing conditions, ripeness at harvesting, processing, and storing. In humans, polyphenols work to reduce the absorption of certain metal cations such as iron, zinc, and copper. Some of the most promising polyphenols are listed here alphabetically. (See *Polyphenols*, page 402.)

The tea plant (*Camellia sinensis*) has been associated with health benefits since the Chinese started using the leaves of the shrub in ancient times. Green, black, and oolong varieties all come from the same plant; however, the black and oolong varieties are fermented, which oxidizes the tea leaves and destroys much of the polyphenol content. Steaming fresh leaves at high temperatures renders the oxidizing enzymes inactive, thereby leaving the polyphenol content intact. The main catechins or flavonols found in tea are epicatechin, epicatechin-3-gallate, epigallocatechin, and the highly potent epigallocatechin-3-gallate (EGCG). Peppermint and sassafras are two examples of herbal teas.

The polyphenols found in chocolate are the flavan-3-ols (procyanidins), epicatechin and catechin. According to a letter published in *The Lancet*, the catechin content in chocolate is significantly higher than that of tea. Richelle, et al., found that the epicatechin found in chocolate was readily absorbable, possibly even more so than that found in tea.

Reported uses
Polyphenols are reported to protect against heart disease and hypertension by strengthening blood vessels, to prevent certain cancers by acting as free-radical

POLYPHENOLS

Polyphenol	Also known as
Black tea	Theaflavins
Capsaicin (chili pepper)	Trans-8-methyl-N-vanillyl-6-nonenamide
Chocolate	Flavan-3-ol monomeric and dimeric procyanidins
Curcumin (turmeric)	*Curcuma longa L.*, Zingiberaceae
Ginger family	*Zingiber officinale Roscoe*, Zingiberaceae
Green tea	(-)-epigallocatechin gallate (EGCG)
Quercetin (red wine)	quercetin-3-glucoside
Resveratrol (grapes)	3,5,4'-trihydroxytrans-stilbene

scavengers, to protect against infection and viral activity, and to prevent inflammation.

Administration

Polyphenols are available in supplemental form; however, they should be viewed as supplements rather than replacements for whole foods. As with most preventative treatments, the whole-food form supersedes the supplemental form because there are usually other proven benefits from the whole food, such as vitamins, minerals, and trace elements. Also, the whole food may perform interactions in the body that the supplement isn't capable of doing biochemically.

Drinking tea is among the most popular methods of ingesting polyphenols. Consumption of red wine is another way to obtain the benefits of polyphenols. The low incidence of heart disease among the French population, despite the typical high-fat French diet, is often referred to as the "French Paradox." Some health experts believe this is due to a moderate, regular consumption of red wine. Eating a mixed diet rich in fruits, vegetables, nuts, and whole grain cereal should provide adequate antioxidant value.

Hazards

There are no reported complications or significant adverse effects from regular consumption of polyphenols, whether from food sources or supplements. However, a common misconception among consumers is "if some is good, then more is better." For example, consuming high amounts of caffeine-containing green tea, in the hope that doing so will provide enhanced antioxidant benefits, may have a deleterious effect on cardiovascular function in susceptible persons.

Clinical considerations

- Inform the patient that there are no specific recommended dosages.
- Tell patient to remind prescriber and pharmacist of any herbal and dietary supplement that he's taking when obtaining a new prescription.
- Advise patient to consult his health care provider before using an herbal preparation because a treatment with proven efficacy may be available.

Research summary

Multiple studies support the health benefits of polyphenols. The latest evidence supports the intake of red wine, green tea, and other polyphenol-rich foods, such as chocolate, spices, fruits, and vegetables, to help prevent diseases of the heart and certain cancers.

The quantity of polyphenols needed to prevent chronic disease remains a mystery. According to some studies, anywhere from 6 to 10 cups of green tea per day was needed to produce a positive effect. Red wine is usually recommended in the range of 4 to 8 ounces per day for health benefit. Consuming at least 5 fruits and vegetables each day is recommended by nutrition organizations such as the American Dietetic Association, the American Cancer Society, the American Heart Association, and others. Little has been reported for chocolate consumption.

Both chocolate and tea have catechins, though different kinds. Some researchers purport that the catechins in chocolate are more effective in decreasing the oxidation of low-density lipoprotein cholesterol than tea.

Red wine, long studied for its cardioprotective effects, is now being considered for its tumor-arresting ability in breast cancer. One study concluded that ingestion of red wine concentrate could have a beneficial antiproliferative effect on breast cancer cell growth.

Green tea is probably still the most widely studied beverage in polyphenol research. It's acknowledged as a cancer preventative in Japan, and recognition of its benefits is growing in other countries, as well. Although the molecular mechanisms of the cancer chemopreventative effects of the tea polyphenols are not completely understood, caffeine in the tea is considered to play an important role in preventing tumorigenesis. Even black teas have been found to be effective in anticarcinogenic studies, although their activity is often reported as weaker than that of green tea.

pomegranate

Grenadier, Punica granatum

Pomegranate is obtained from the flowers, stems, bark, and rhizomes of *Punica granatum*. It contains tannins (20% to 25%) and piperidine alkaloids (0.4%). Piperidine alkaloids are the basis for its use in treating tapeworm. Tannins may be beneficial in treating hemorrhoids when applied externally. Pomegranate is available as juice, powder, and bark extract.

Reported uses

Pomegranate is used to treat tapeworm and other worm infestations. It's also used as a gargle rinse for sore throat and topically for hemorrhoids. Pomegranate may have abortifacient properties.

Administration

- Juice or extract: Apply topically as needed for hemorrhoids, or 20 g bark juice extract orally, in a single dose, for tapeworm
- Rectal administration: An extract is prepared by combining 60 parts herb and 400 parts water, then macerating for 12 hours to half the initial volume. For tapeworm, instill 65 ml extract by duodenal probe every 30 minutes for 3 doses, followed by a laxative 1 hour after the third dose.

Hazards

Adverse effects associated with pomegranate include dizziness, chills, circulatory collapse, vision disorders, gastric irritation, vomiting, and apnea. There are no reported interactions with pomegranate at this time.

Patients who are pregnant or breastfeeding shouldn't use this herb.

SAFETY RISK *Overdoses of pomegranate rind, stem, or root may lead to emesis, hematemesis, dizziness, chills, visual disturbances (including blindness), circulatory collapse, and death. Treatment includes induced emesis (if pa-*

tient is conscious) or gastric lavage and instillation of activated charcoal. Provide supportive treatment for shock. Patient may need intubation. Monitor renal function closely.

Clinical considerations
■ Patient who uses pomegranate to treat tapeworm needs medical supervision and follow-up by a health care provider.
■ Caution patient to seek medical attention from a health care provider immediately if respiratory, visual, and GI problems develop following ingestion of higher doses.
■ Advise pregnant or breast-feeding patients to avoid using this herb.
■ Warn patient to keep all herbal products away from children and pets.
■ Tell patient to remind prescriber and pharmacist of any herbal and dietary supplement that he's taking when obtaining a new prescription.
■ Advise patient to consult his health care provider before using an herbal preparation because a treatment with proven efficacy may be available.

Research summary
The concepts behind the use of pomegranate and the claims made regarding its effects haven't yet been validated scientifically.

poplar

Black poplar, Canadian poplar, European aspen,
poplar bud (balm of Gilead buds),
Populi cortex et folium, P. gemma, Populus alba, P. gileadensis, P. nigra, P. tremuloides, *quaking aspen, trembling poplar, white poplar*

Poplar is obtained from the bark and leaves of *Populus* species. It contains essential oil, flavonoids, phenol glycosides, and salicylate glycosides. The volatile oil has expectorant properties. Leaves of *P.*

alba may contain up to 6% of glycosides and esters that yield salicylic acid. Populus bark contains about 2% salicylate compounds, such as salicortin and salicin. Salicylate compounds contribute to the herb's analgesic, anti-inflammatory, and antispasmodic properties. Caffeic acid, found in poplar buds, provides antibacterial properties. Zinc lignins contained in poplar may have a beneficial effect on micturition in prostatic hyperplasia. Poplar is available as buds, ointment, extract, powder, and dried bark (in combination products).

Reported uses
Poplar is used to treat pain, rheumatism, and micturition complaints in benign prostatic hyperplasia. It's used topically for superficial skin injuries, external hemorrhoids, frostbite, and sunburn. Poplar is also used as an antiseptic and to stimulate wound healing. It's used for respiratory tract infections and as a gargle for laryngitis.

Administration
■ Dried bark: 1 to 4 g, or as a tea by mouth three times a day
■ Ground drug and galenic preparations of *Populi cortex et folium*: As directed; maximum, 10 g daily
■ Liquid bark extract (1:1 in 25% alcohol): 1 to 4 ml (20 to 80 gtt) by mouth three times a day
■ Topical, semisolid, or ointment preparations containing 5 g of drug or 20% to 30% of drug: Apply as directed.

Hazards
Adverse effects associated with poplar include depression of clotting factors and rash. When poplar is used with antiarthritics and aspirin, there is a possibility of increased bleeding time. Monitor patient for signs of bleeding. Advise patient to avoid using together. Poplar may reduce iron absorption if used with feosol and other iron supplements. There may be an increase in bleeding time if poplar is used with warfarin and other

anticoagulants. Monitor patient's laboratory values.

Patients hypersensitive to poplar products, salicylates, or Peruvian balsam shouldn't take this herb. Herb should be used with caution by patients with heart disease or a history of bleeding disorders.

Clinical considerations

- Closely monitor prothrombin time and International Normalized Ratio if patient takes aspirin, an arthritis medicine, or an anticoagulant.
- Tell patient to stop using topical preparation if it causes a rash or skin irritation.
- Inform patient that poplar contains aspirin-like compounds that can increase the risk of bleeding when taken orally with other drugs.
- Advise patient not to take iron supplements with poplar tea.
- Tell patient to remind prescriber and pharmacist of any herbal and dietary supplement that he is taking when obtaining a new prescription.
- Advise patient to consult his health care provider before using an herbal preparation because a treatment with proven efficacy may be available.

Research summary

The concepts behind the use of poplar and the claims made regarding its effects haven't yet been validated scientifically.

Prayer and mental healing

Prayer and mental healing have been used throughout the ages to seek assistance from a higher being for a wide range of problems, including illness. The earliest faith healers were shamans, priests, and medicine men who used chants and ritual dances to influence evil spirits they believed were responsible for disease. However, seeking divine intervention to heal the sick isn't limited to ancient or primitive cultures. In the United States, the Christian Science Church uses prayer instead of conventional medical treatments. And the hundreds of thousands of pilgrims who flock to Lourdes, France, every year in search of miraculous cures indicate that prayer is still viewed as a powerful tool in healing.

The underlying beliefs of those who use prayer for healing are the same for all religions. They include the belief that a higher power exists, that humans can communicate with this higher power through prayer, and that prayers will be heard and will receive a response. Some modern scientists are trying to confirm whether prayer and mental healing can influence health and illness.

In prayer, the person communicates directly with the divine power, asking for intervention to heal the patient. In mental healing, the divine power's ability to heal is channeled through a healer. Prayer can take the form of silent meditation, or it may be spoken aloud, either by individuals or a group; the person engaging in prayer may seek assistance for himself or for others (intercessory prayer). Most people who use prayer for healing view it as an adjunct to conventional medical treatment.

There are two main categories of mental healing. In type 1 healing, the healer enters into a spiritual level of consciousness where he views himself and the patient as a single being. The healer does not have any physical contact with the patient, and the two do not even need to be in the same location. The healer's role isn't active insofar as administering treatment; he merely tries to achieve a spiritual unity with the patient and the higher power in the hope that love, empathy, and unity will lead to healing. In type 2 mental healing, the healer does touch the patient, attempting to transfer energy from the healer's hands to the diseased parts of the patient's body. Both the healer and the patient commonly report a feeling of heat during this process.

Reported uses

Although the therapeutic uses of prayer and mental healing are limitless, the reliability of these practices still needs to be established. Proponents of prayer argue that even if prayer cannot cure disease, it can at least relieve some of its effects, enhance the effectiveness of conventional medical treatments, and provide comfort to the patient.

How the treatment is performed

No special equipment is needed for prayer or mental healing. If possible, provide the patient with privacy in a quiet, distraction-free environment.

Health care providers can facilitate the use of prayer and mental healing by asking patients a few simple questions, such as, "Is religion important to you?" and, "Is religion important in helping you cope with your illness?"

If the patient answers yes, the practitioner explores his religious practices with him to identify ways in which these practices can be incorporated into the healing regimen. The practitioner may ask whether the patient would like to discuss his faith with a treatment facility chaplain or another member of the clergy. The practitioner remains nonjudgmental and offers to assist with any arrangements for spiritual intervention.

Hazards

One of the benefits of prayer and mental healing is the lack of complications. Patients who have attempted prayer and not seen the results they expected may express a sense of disappointment when the topic of spirituality is discussed. If possible, arrange for a member of the clergy to explore the patient's feelings with him. Ethical questions arise if prayer and mental healing are used without the subject's knowledge or consent.

Clinical considerations

Some health care facilities may not be equipped to allow the full expression of prayer rituals associated with some religions. Rites involving incense, large groups, or loud music and dance may disrupt the care of other patients. Although you should be sensitive to the patient's culture, sometimes a compromise is in order. For example, you could suggest that the patient be taken to an outside area of the facility if incense is involved, or to a conference room away from other patients if noise is an issue or a prayer vigil involves a large number of people.

Advise your patient to consider prayer a complementary therapy rather than a substitute for conventional medical care. However, if the patient's religion advocates the use of prayer as the sole form of treatment, make sure he understands the consequences of foregoing conventional medical treatment so he can make an informed decision.

Research summary

The first scientific study of the connection between prayer and longevity, conducted in the 1870s, showed no demonstrable effect. More recent studies, however, have indicated positive results.

According to a 1994 report to the NIH, numerous studies have demonstrated patients' abilities to influence various biological and cellular systems through mental techniques. The "target systems" included bacteria, blood cells, and cancer cells. Eye and muscle movements, respiration, and brain rhythms have reportedly been affected through mental means.

Recent studies have also shown tangible health benefits in people with strong religious faith. Statistics point to an increased survival rate after open-heart surgery for patients who draw comfort and strength from religion, lower blood pressure in patients who attend religious services, and a lower incidence of depression and anxiety among those who practice some form of religion. Such data are causing doctors and lay people to explore further the relationship between prayer and mental powers and healing.

Although modern science currently has no explanation for type 1 mental healing, the NIH report says the lack of a known mechanism shouldn't lead scientists to dismiss the phenomenon. Pointing out that scientists had no explanation for sunlight until the development of nuclear physics in the 20th century, the report concludes that "mental healing may be valid in the absence of a validating theory."

prickly ash

Northern prickly ash, suterberry, toothache tree, yellow wood, Zanthoxylum americanum, Z. clava-herculis, Z. facara

Prickly ash is obtained from bark and berries of the *Zanthoxylum clava-herculis* tree. It contains volatile oil, resins, pyranocoumarins, such as xanthoxyletin, and isoquinoline alkaloids, including berberine and N-methyl-isocorydin. Prickly ash has anti-inflammatory, antirheumatic, diaphoretic, and circulatory stimulant properties. Prickly ash is available as extract, tablets, or dried bark, and in various combination products.

Reported uses
Prickly ash is used to treat cramps, hypotension, rheumatism, soreness, toothache, poor leg circulation, fever, and inflammation. It's also used topically for treating indolent ulcers and wound healing.

Administration
■ Liquid extract (1:1 in 45% alcohol): 1 to 3 ml (20 to 60 gtt) of extract in a little water by mouth three times a day
■ Dried bark: 1 to 2 g as a tea, by mouth three times a day
■ For toothache: Chewed dried bark or berries, as needed

■ Tincture (1:5 in 45% alcohol): 2 to 5 ml (40 to 100 gtt) by mouth three times a day.

Hazards
There are no reported adverse effects associated with prickly ash. It may potentiate the effects of antihypertensives. Decreased iron absorption may occur if prickly ash is used with iron supplements, such as ferrous sulfate. Prickly ash may potentiate the effects of scopolamine and other muscle relaxants.

Pregnant and breast-feeding patients shouldn't use this herb. Patients with cardiac disease should use it with caution, especially those who take blood pressure drugs. Some prickly ash extracts contain 65% to 70% grain alcohol and should be avoided by alcoholic patients and those with liver disease.

SAFETY RISK *Don't confuse true species of prickly ash trees* (Z. americanum, Z. clava-herculis, Z. facara) *with Devil's walkingstick* (Aralia spinosa), *a shrub also commonly known as prickly ash.*

Clinical considerations
■ If patient has cardiac disease or takes an antihypertensive, monitor vital signs, particularly blood pressure, during and after use of prickly ash.
■ Some products may contain alcohol and may not be suitable for use by children, alcoholic patients, patients with liver failure, or patients who take disulfiram or metronidazole.
■ Caution patient to seek medical attention if his symptoms last longer than 7 days, or if they worsen.
■ Advise pregnant or breast-feeding patient not to use this herb.
■ Tell patient to remind prescriber and pharmacist of any herbal and dietary supplement that he's taking when obtaining a new prescription.
■ Advise patient to consult his health care provider before using an herbal preparation because a treatment with proven efficacy may be available.

Research summary
The concepts behind the use of prickly ash and the claims made regarding its effects haven't yet been validated scientifically.

Pritikin program

The Pritikin program, named after its founder, Nathan Pritikin, is essentially a dietary regimen combined with regular exercise. The diet is very low in fats (less than 10% of daily calories), low in cholesterol, and high in complex carbohydrates. The program also calls for 45 minutes of walking daily.

Pritikin began to study heart disease in the early 1960s after his cardiologist told him he was at high risk for death from myocardial infarction (MI). He developed a low-fat diet similar to that practiced by the people of Uganda, who had practically no incidence of MI-related death. After a few years on the diet, Pritikin's symptoms abated and he decided that the diet had saved his life. In the late 1960s, he founded his clinic in Santa Monica to treat other heart disease patients.

Although the medical establishment rejected Pritikin's basic theory for years, today the American Heart Association and the medical community as a whole have accepted the link between diet, exercise, and heart disease. The Pritikin Longevity Center, run today by Pritikin's son, Robert, offers a 26-day program to initiate patients to the plan and teach them how to prepare meals and exercise.

How the treatment is performed
The Pritikin program consists of a diet that's high in complex carbohydrates and fiber, low in cholesterol, and extremely low in fat. The diet allows 3½ oz (99 g) of animal protein (lean chicken or fish) as well as two glasses of skim milk daily. The program also calls for a 45-minute walk every day.

Hazards
Unlike some more restrictive diets, the Pritikin diet provides adequate protein; however, it might result in a deficiency of iron or other nutrients.

Clinical considerations
■ Because this diet is extremely low in fats, suggest that your patient take a multivitamin while on the plan to ensure that he receives enough vitamins and other nutrients.
■ Some people who've been on the plan for 1 or 2 years have noted the appearance of white vertical ridges on the nails, which may be a sign of an iron or vitamin deficiency. Suggest that your patient have his blood tested periodically to detect such deficiencies.
■ People who are allergic to gluten, the protein portion of grains, would have difficulty maintaining the Pritikin diet because of its emphasis on whole grains.

Research summary
A 1990 analysis of 4,587 participants in the Pritikin residential program showed an average decrease of 23% in total and low-density lipoprotein cholesterol and a 33% drop in triglyceride levels. The Pritikin diet has also shown promise in controlling without drugs newly diagnosed cases of adult-onset diabetes.

Psychotherapy

Psychotherapy is at the root of all mind-body therapies. Derived from the Greek words meaning "healing of the soul," psychotherapy is a method of treating disease by exploring its emotional and behavioral components. The goal of psychotherapy is to enable an individual to correct negative attitudes, emotions, and behaviors that interfere with some aspect of functioning in his life. When used in the treatment of physically ill patients, psychotherapy can improve coping ability and reduce depression and anxiety.

May we have your comments?

Please fill out and mail this postpaid card. Thanks!

Product title _____

Your comments _____

Would you like to be placed on our mailing list? ☐ Yes ☐ No
☐ You have permission to use my name and comments in advertising.
☐ You have my permission to alert me by e-mail of Springhouse savings.

Name _____
                    (please print)

Address _____ Apt. _____

City _____ State _____ Zip _____

E-mail address _____

PROFESSIONAL DATA
Check all applicable boxes.
1. You are an:
☐ RN
☐ LPN/LVN
☐ RN student
☐ LPN student
☐ Librarian
☐ RN inactive
☐ Nurse practitioner
☐ Other

_____
please specify

Visit us at
www.springnet.com

There are a number of different schools of psychotherapy. Any of these therapies can be used either alone or in combination.

■ Psychodynamic (or insight) therapy focuses on the individual and views distress as the result of unresolved unconscious conflicts. The focus of this form of therapy is to bring unconscious conflicts to the surface, allowing modification of the patient's behavior. In psychoanalysis, another form of insight therapy, the unconscious conflicts arise from critical factors in early childhood development. Again, the focus of therapy is to bring these conflicts into the open.

■ Behavioral therapy focuses on very specific behavioral changes, such as learning not to be afraid of flying. Modeling (or operant conditioning) behavioral therapy, rather than looking into the patient's past, focuses on the patient's interactions with his current social environment.

■ Existential therapy focuses on the future, helping the patient see new potential for personal satisfaction and growth.

■ Systems (or family) therapy looks at relationship patterns among family members and tries to activate the family group as a therapeutic force.

■ Body-oriented therapy hypothesizes that emotions are expressed as tension and restriction in any part of the body. Using breathing techniques, movement, and manual pressure and probing, the therapist helps the patient release emotions located in his tissues.

Reported uses
Psychotherapy is generally used to treat people with mental or behavioral problems. It can help patients with psychosis recognize and deal effectively with daily stressors and help patients with neurosis deal with life's unpredictable changes. For patients who are temporarily overwhelmed by daily stressors, psychotherapy can restore emotional equilibrium. Additionally, patients with behavioral problems can be treated with psychother-

apy in an attempt to modify their behavior. However, for the psychotherapy to be successful, the patient must have sufficient motivation to change.

For patients with a physical illness, psychotherapy typically focuses on short-term treatment to deal with the emotions evoked by the disorder. For example, many patients with a serious illness experience depression and anxiety, emotions that can make the illness worse. By helping patients acknowledge their emotions, psychotherapy diminishes the negative effects of the emotions and enhances recovery.

How the treatment is performed
A quiet environment, free from distractions, is essential for psychotherapy. If possible, the room should have a door that can remain closed during the entire session. Adequate seating should be available for the patient, the psychotherapist, and any other participants. Some therapists prefer a desk or table separating them from the patient. Lighting should be even so that the patient does not feel as if he is being interrogated under a spotlight.

Although psychotherapy sessions should be conducted only by a trained psychotherapist, many health care professionals routinely use such interventions, consciously or unconsciously, in dealing with patients. The practitioner who tells a patient "It must be scary here in the ICU" to try to draw him out, who listens supportively to his worries or complaints, and who takes his hand to provide comfort is using psychotherapeutic techniques.

Good listening skills are a key to success in using psychotherapeutic interventions. It's also important to pay close attention to the patient's nonverbal behavior, looking for clues to his underlying emotions. Reflection — repeating to the patient what he has said — is another useful tool. In addition to verifying what the patient said, reflection tells the patient that the practitioner is listening and not passing judgment on what he says.

After the session with a psychotherapist, the patient's response is documented and arrangements for follow-up sessions, if appropriate, are made.

Hazards

Because psychotherapy often deals with suppressed or unexpressed emotions, the patient may be upset or angry after a session. If so, let him discuss his feelings. If you detect signs of agitation or impending violence, keep a safe distance between you and the patient. Consider asking someone else to be present with you until the patient has vented his feelings and is once again calm. Document his responses and any actions taken.

Clinical considerations

■ Be prepared to supply the names and numbers of any support groups that deal with the patient's specific problem. Support groups can provide needed emotional and practical support for patients with chronic or life-threatening illnesses. Positive effects have been seen in patients with cancer, heart disease, asthma, and stroke. Studies have shown that breast cancer patients who participate in a support group survive longer.

■ If your patient is severely depressed, be alert for suicide warning signs.

■ Ensure that your patient continues to take prescribed psychotropic drugs even if he's also receiving psychotherapy.

■ Always maintain patient confidentiality.

Research summary

Studies show that psychotherapy can speed recovery from a medical crisis. In a 1993 study of patients with broken hips, those receiving psychotherapy had a 2-day shorter hospital stay, fewer rehospitalizations, and shorter rehabilitation times. By allowing patients to verbalize their feelings about their health, psychotherapy helps sick people cope with their fears, improve their mood, and

sometimes even improve their outcome. Studies have shown that patients with a medical problem who are also depressed have a much higher mortality rate than those who aren't depressed.

Psychotherapy also benefits people with somatic illnesses — those for which no discernible organic cause for the symptoms can be found. Practitioners believe that these patients are unable to accept an emotional problem and transform it into a physical ailment. In such patients, psychotherapy has been shown to decrease the number of doctor's visits for physical complaints.

pulsatilla

Anemone pulsatilla, Easter flower, meadow anemone, passe flower, pasque flower, Pulsatilla pratensis, P. vulgaris, *Pulsatillae herba*

Pulsatilla is obtained from dried aboveground parts of anemone pulsatilla (*Pulsatilla vulgaris*) and *P. pratensis*. It contains protoanemonin, ranunculin, and degradation products of ranunculin, including anemonin, anemoninic acid, and anemonic acid. Protoanemonin may cause stimulation and paralysis of the central nervous system (CNS); its alkylating action may inhibit cell regeneration, leading to kidney irritation. Protoanemonin also has anti-infective activity. Abortion and birth defects have been reported among grazing animals who consumed large amounts of protoanemonin-containing plants. Pulsatilla is available as a dried herb, pellets, extracts, tincture, and tablets, in products such as Boiron Pulsatilla 9c and Pulsatilla 200ck.

Reported uses

Pulsatilla is used to treat inflammatory and infectious diseases of the skin and mucosa, diseases and functional disorders of the GI tract, and functional urogenital disorders. It's also used to treat neuralgia, migraine, and general restlessness.

Administration

- Dried herb: 100 to 300 mg as a tea by mouth three times a day
- Liquid extract (1:1 in 25% alcohol): 0.1 to 0.3 ml (2 to 6 gtt) by mouth three times a day
- Oral tablets and pellets: by mouth, as directed (see manufacturer package insert)
- Tincture (1:10 in 40% alcohol): 0.5 to 3 ml (10 to 60 gtt) by mouth three times a day.

Hazards

Adverse effects associated with the use of pulsatilla include irritation of mucous membranes, nausea, vomiting, abdominal pain, colic, diarrhea, irritation of kidneys and urinary tract, asphyxiation, and rash. There are currently no reported interactions with pulsatilla.

Pregnant and breast-feeding patients shouldn't use this herb. Alcoholic patients and those with liver disease shouldn't use forms that contain alcohol.

SAFETY RISK *Fresh pulsatilla plant parts can cause severe skin and mucosal irritation in susceptible patients. Irrigate affected area with dilute potassium permanganate solution, and then apply mucilage preparation. Overdose may cause renal and urinary tract irritation and severe stomach irritation with colic and diarrhea. Urge patient to go to the emergency room, where he may undergo gastric lavage with activated charcoal.*

Clinical considerations

- Some products may contain alcohol and may not be suitable for use by children, alcoholic patients, patients with liver failure, or patients who take disulfiram or metronidazole.
- Tell patient that fresh pulsatilla is considered poisonous and shouldn't be ingested or placed on the skin. If patient uses pulsatilla, it should be dried.

- Warn patient that kidney and urinary tract irritation can occur at higher-than-recommended doses.
- If patient is pregnant or planning to get pregnant, caution her not to use this herb.
- Tell patient to consult a licensed health care provider if symptoms last longer than 7 days, or if they worsen.
- Tell patient to remind prescriber and pharmacist of any herbal and dietary supplement that he's taking when obtaining a new prescription.
- Advise patient to consult his health care provider before using an herbal preparation because a treatment with proven efficacy may be available.

Research summary

The concepts behind the use of pulsatilla and the claims made regarding its effects haven't yet been validated scientifically.

pumpkin

Cucurbita pepo, *field pumpkin, pompion, semina cucurbitae, yellow pumpkin*

Pumpkin contains cucurbitacin, tocopherol, and selenium. The seeds contain fatty acids (50%). Cucurbitacin may provide anthelmintic activity. Tocopherol and selenium may inhibit oxidative degradation of lipids, vitamins, hormones, and enzymes. Pumpkin also has anti-inflammatory, diuretic, antioxidative, and antiandrogenic actions. Delta-7 sterols in the fatty oils of the seeds may block dihydrotestosterone from androgen receptors and prevent hyperproliferation of prostate cells in an enlarged prostate. Pumpkin is available as an extract and seeds.

Reported uses

Pumpkin is used to treat irritable bladder and micturition problems associated with benign prostatic hyperplasia (BPH) stages I and II. It's also used as a diuretic and to treat childhood nocturnal enuresis and intestinal worms.

Administration

■ As a dietary supplement: 2 to 4 ml of liquid extract (about 56 to 112 gtt) by mouth three times a day

■ As a diuretic: 200 to 400 g of unpeeled seeds pounded or ground into a pulp and mixed with orange juice, apple juice, or milk and honey to form a porridge, taken orally on an empty stomach in 2 doses in the morning, sometimes followed by castor oil 2 to 3 hours later

■ Whole and coarse-ground seeds: 10 g of ground seeds by mouth, half in the morning and half in the evening, accompanied by 1 to 2 heaping teaspoons of fluid. Outer covering from hard seeds is removed before consumption.

Hazards

There are no known adverse effects associated with pumpkin at this time. There are no known interactions with the use of pumpkin.

Patients hypersensitive to pumpkin or any of its components shouldn't take this herb.

Clinical considerations

■ Inform patient that although pumpkin may relieve irritable bladder and micturition problems caused by BPH stages I and II, it doesn't reduce prostate enlargement and its use requires medical supervision.

■ Advise patient to store pumpkin preparations away from light and moisture.

■ Tell patient to contact a licensed medical practitioner if symptoms last longer than 7 days, or if they worsen.

■ Tell patient to remind prescriber and pharmacist of any herbal and dietary supplement that he's taking when obtaining a new prescription.

■ Advise patient to consult his health care provider before using an herbal preparation because a treatment with proven efficacy may be available.

Research summary

The concepts behind the use of pumpkin and the claims made regarding its effects haven't yet been validated scientifically.

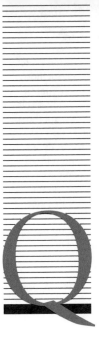

Qigong

Qigong (pronounced "chee gong") is a system of gentle exercise, meditation, and controlled breathing used by millions of Chinese people daily to increase strength and relax the mind. When practiced daily over time, qigong is believed to improve strength and flexibility, reverse damage due to injury or disease, relieve pain, restore energy, and induce relaxation and healing.

Like acupuncture and tai chi chuan, qigong is based on the principles that underlie all of traditional Chinese medicine. The cornerstone is belief in the existence of a vital life force, known as *qi* ("chee"), that flows through the body and is responsible for maintaining health. Qigong, which means "energy work," is believed to enhance or balance the flow of qi through a system of repetitive motions, intense concentration, and breathing exercises.

Qigong is less physically demanding than tai chi chuan and is suitable for people of all ages and physical conditions. Those who are disabled can practice qigong while sitting or lying in bed. In the United States, qigong is taught by qualified instructors in adult education centers, fitness centers, YMCAs, and even some hospitals. It can also be self-taught through videos and books.

There are two forms of qigong: internal and external. Internal qigong focuses on manipulating the qi within one's own body to maintain health and self-healing. This type can consist primarily of meditation and breathing exercises (quiescent qigong), or it can include active, dance-like movements (dynamic qigong). In the quiet form, the body is relaxed while the mind aims to control the qi through breathing and concentration. In the dynamic form, the body is active while the mind is quiet and relaxed.

External qigong is the domain of qigong masters, who have learned through years of practice to transmit the force of their qi to others for healing purposes. Many qigong masters display their skills in exhibitions.

Reported uses

Regular practice of qigong is used to lower heart rate, blood pressure, metabolic rate, and oxygen demand; these effects are known as the relaxation response. Qigong is used to treat a wide range of chronic illnesses and diseases, including nearsightedness, hemorrhoids, coronary artery disease, and arthritis. Chinese practitioners often combine qigong with conventional therapies to treat cancer, bone marrow disease, heart disease, AIDS, and diseases of old age.

How the treatment is performed

No special equipment is required, other than loose, comfortable clothing and an open, flat area in which to practice.

Quiescent qigong is a meditative state that can be achieved sitting, standing, or lying down. The body is relaxed and quiet while the mind controls the qi with breathing, visualization, and mental concentration. The person begins by inhaling as he visualizes a concentration of qi in the abdominal area (believed to be the source of this vital force). As he exhales, he visualizes the qi leaving the abdomen and entering the organs, glands, extremities, and other parts of the body. These thoughts are augmented by deep breathing and relaxation to circulate the healing energy of qi.

In dynamic qigong, the practitioner moves slowly from one posture to another, almost as in a dance. While the body is

in motion and active, the mind is quiet and relaxed. Practitioners believe that both the quiet and active forms of qigong are important, just as in life there must be a balance of activity and relaxation.

Basic qigong exercises can be learned from books or videos; after learning the basics, the patient can design his own daily practice regimen. To receive the full benefits of these exercises, the patient should practice for at least 20 to 30 minutes each morning, with an added afternoon or evening practice if possible. (See *A simple qigong exercise.*)

Hazards

When properly performed, qigong is a gentle and invigorating exercise with no adverse effects.

Clinical considerations

- Be aware that patient with respiratory problems may not be able to perform the breathing exercise aspect of qigong.
- Inform patient with serious illness that qigong may be beneficial as a complementary therapy, but not as a substitute for conventional treatment.
- Tell patient it's best to learn qigong from a qualified teacher rather than from books or videos to ensure that they're doing the movements properly.

Research summary

Chinese researchers have reported success in using qigong to treat numerous conditions, including asthma, insomnia, depression, anxiety, pain, diabetes, and hypertension. Several studies have reported significant improvement in patients with terminal cancer who practiced qigong in addition to receiving chemotherapy.

The Western medical establishment generally hasn't accepted the claims regarding qigong's effectiveness in treating specific diseases. However, an increasing number of conventional practitioners believe that qigong, like meditation and other therapies that induce the relaxation response, may be effective in reducing

A SIMPLE QIGONG EXERCISE

Begin by rubbing your hands together to build up heat, which is thought to increase the flow of qi. Your hands will become warmer if you're relaxed. Stroke your warmed palms across your face, eyes, and forehead as if you were washing your face.

Follow the diagram below, continuing to trace your hands over the tops and sides of your head, down the back of the neck, and forward along the shoulder to the joint; down the rib cage, around the back, and down to the back and sides of the legs; and then out to the sides of the feet. Then, with the same continuous motion, continue the path inside the feet and inner surface of the legs up the front of the torso and back onto the face.

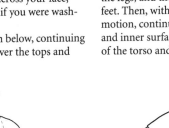
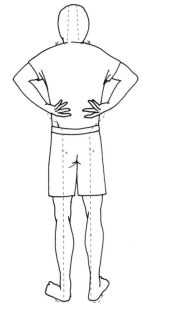

stress and anxiety, relieving pain from arthritis, improving sleep, and enhancing overall well-being.

Queen Anne's lace

Bees' nest, bird's nest, carrot,
Daucus carota, *philtron, wild carrot,*

Queen Anne's lace is obtained from all plant parts of *Daucus carota. D. carota* contains a volatile oil that may have diuretic and hypotensive properties. Queen Anne's lace is available as a tea, seeds, dried herb, infusion, oil, and liquid extract.

Reported uses
Queen Anne's lace is used to treat kidney stones, bladder infections, gout, and swollen joints. The seeds are used to treat flatulence, windy colic, hiccups, dysentery, renal calculi, bowel obstruction, edema, and chronic cough. Poultices made from the root can be used for the pain of cancerous ulcers.

Administration
- Bruised seeds: 1 teaspoon by mouth as needed for flatulence, windy colic, hiccups, dysentery, and chronic cough
- Dried herb: 2 to 4 g as a tea by mouth three times a day
- Infusion: 1 oz of herb in 1 pint of water; 1 glassful twice a day, in morning and evening
- Liquid extract (1:1 in 25% alcohol): 2 to 4 ml (40 to 80 gtt) by mouth three times a day
- Seeds: 1 teaspoon by mouth as needed
- Tea: Brewed from the whole root and taken by mouth twice a day, morning and evening, for gout.

Hazards
Adverse effects associated with Queen Anne's lace include rash and photosensitivity. Possible additive effects may occur when Queen Anne's lace is used with antihypertensives and cardiac drugs.

Pregnant and breast-feeding women shouldn't use this herb.

Clinical considerations
- Inform patient that essential oil may cause a skin rash and increase the risk of sunburn.
- Encourage patient to monitor blood pressure during and after consumption of Queen Anne's lace. Teach patient the symptoms of hypotension, including light-headedness, fatigue, and rapid heart rate.
- Tell patient to remind prescriber and pharmacist of any herbal and dietary supplement that he's taking when obtaining a new prescription.
- Advise patient to consult his health care provider before using an herbal preparation because a treatment with proven efficacy may be available.

Research summary
The concepts behind the use of Queen Anne's lace and the claims made regarding its effects haven't yet been validated scientifically.

quince
Cydonia oblongata

Quince is obtained from fruits and seeds of *Cydonia oblongata*. The fresh fruits and syrup have astringent properties. Seeds contain mucilage and a small amount of amygdalin, a cyanogenic glycoside. When soaked in water, the seeds swell to form a mucilaginous mass or gum that has demulcent properties. Quince is available as a powder, lotion, extract, fruit syrup, and decoction from seeds.

Reported uses
Quince is used as a demulcent to treat digestive disorders and diarrhea. The raw fruits are used to treat diarrhea. A decoction of seeds can be used internally to treat dysentery, diarrhea, gonorrhea, thrush, and mucous membrane irritation.

A decoction can also be used topically as an adjunct to boric acid eyewash and as a compress or poultice for skin wounds and injuries, or inflammation of the joints and nipples.

Administration
- Decoction (boil 2 drams of seed in 1 pint of water in a tightly covered container for 10 minutes, and then strain): Amount of liquid to be ingested varies and should be supervised by a health care provider.
- Poultice: A poultice or compress is prepared from ground, macerated seeds and applied topically.

Hazards
Quince seeds contain cyanogenic glycoside and may therefore be toxic. There are no reported interactions with the herb quince.

Pregnant and breast-feeding women shouldn't use this herb. Geriatric patients and those with a history of immune disorders or peptic ulcers should use it cautiously.

SAFETY RISK *Seeds may be toxic because they contain cyanogenic glycoside.*

Clinical considerations

■ Warn patient not to eat the seeds because they contain cyanogenic glycoside.
■ Warn patient not to take herb for digestive disorders before seeking medical attention because doing so may delay diagnosis of a potentially serious medical condition.
■ Advise pregnant or breast-feeding patient not to use this herb.
■ Advise patient to store herb away from heat and direct sunlight, and to keep all herbal products away from children and pets.
■ Tell patient to remind prescriber and pharmacist of any herbal and dietary supplement that he's taking when obtaining a new prescription.
■ Advise patient to consult his health care provider before using an herbal preparation because a treatment with proven efficacy may be available.

Research summary

The concepts behind the use of quince and the claims made regarding its effects haven't yet been validated scientifically.

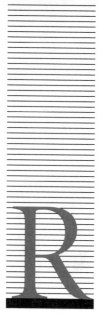

ragwort

Cankerwort, dog standard, ragweed,
Senecio jacoboea, *staggerwort,*
stammerwort, stinking nanny,
St. James wort

Ragwort contains pyrrolizidine alkaloids (0.1% to 0.9%) and a volatile oil. The juice has cooling and astringent properties. Ragwort is available as fresh and dried herb, and lotion.

Reported uses
Ragwort is used as a wash for burns, eye inflammation, sores, bee stings, and cancerous ulcers. It's also used topically to treat rheumatism, painful menstruation, chronic cough, urinary tract inflammation, anemia, anemic headaches, sciatica, and gout. Leaves made into a poultice are applied to painful joints to reduce inflammation and swelling. A solution made with ragwort can be gargled — but not swallowed — for ulcers of the throat and mouth.

Administration
Ragwort lotion is made from 1 part herb and 5 parts 10% alcohol; it's applied topically, as needed, for arthritis.

Hazards
Ragwort may be associated with hepatotoxicity. It may also be carcinogenic, and shouldn't be taken orally. There are currently no reported interactions with ragwort.

Pregnant and breast-feeding women shouldn't use this herb.

 SAFETY RISK *Ragwort may have hepatotoxic and carcinogenic properties from pyrrolizidine alkaloid content.*

Clinical considerations
■ Tell patient the herb is for external use only. Caution patient about the risk of liver failure and cancer if herb is taken orally.
■ Advise pregnant or breast-feeding patient not to use this herb.
■ Warn patient to keep all herbal products away from children and pets.
■ Tell patient to remind prescriber and pharmacist of any herbal and dietary supplement that he's taking when obtaining a new prescription.
■ Advise patient to consult his health care provider before using an herbal preparation because a treatment with proven efficacy may be available.

Research summary
The concepts behind the use of ragwort and the claims made regarding its effects haven't yet been validated scientifically.

raspberry

Bramble of Mount Ida, hindberry, raspbis, Rubus idaeus

Raspberry is obtained from leaves and fruits of *Rubus idaeus.* It contains tannins, flavonoids, vitamin C, crystallizable fruit sugar, fragrant volatile oil, pectin, manganese, citric acid, malic acid, and mineral salts. The tannins have astringent activity. Raspberry is available as a tea, extract, dried leaf, and infusion, in products such as Wild Countryside Red Raspberry Leaves.

Reported uses
Raspberry leaves can be used as a gargle for sore mouths and canker sores and as a wash for wounds and ulcers. An infusion of leaves, taken cold, is used to treat diarrhea. Raspberry is also used to normalize blood glucose level and to treat various disorders of the GI, cardiovascular, and respiratory systems. Leaf tea taken regularly during pregnancy may prevent complications and tone the uterus in preparation for childbirth. Raspberry is reputed to relieve heavy menstrual bleeding and increase lactation.

Administration
■ Dried leaf: 4 to 8 g by mouth three times a day
■ Liquid extract (1:1 in 25% alcohol): 4 to 8 ml (80 to 160 gtt) by mouth three times a day
■ Tea (scald 1.5 g finely cut herb [1 teaspoon = 0.8 g drug], steep for 5 minutes, and then strain): Taken three times a day.

Hazards
No adverse effects are associated with raspberry. Decreased iron absorption may occur if raspberry is used with iron supplements, such as ferrous sulfate.

Patients hypersensitive to raspberry products shouldn't use this herb.

Clinical considerations
■ Advise pregnant or breast-feeding patients, parents of young child, and patient with severe liver or kidney disease that safety of use of raspberry has not been established.
■ Inform patient that little evidence exists to support the use of herbal raspberry during pregnancy, childbirth, or menstruation.
■ If patient has trouble breathing or develops a rash, he may be allergic to raspberry. He should immediately stop taking the herb and seek medical attention.
■ Advise patient taking red raspberry for GI symptoms that other treatments with known safety and efficacy data are available.
■ Warn patient to keep all herbal products away from children and pets, and to store them away from heat and direct sunlight.

- Tell patient to remind prescriber and pharmacist of any herbal and dietary supplement that he's taking when obtaining a new prescription.
- Advise patient to consult his health care provider before using an herbal preparation because a treatment with proven efficacy may be available.

Research summary
The concepts behind the use of raspberry and the claims made regarding its effects haven't yet been validated scientifically.

rauwolfia

Indian snakeroot, Rauwolfia serpentina, *snakeroot*

Rauwolfia contains reserpine, ajmalicine, and numerous other alkaloids. The herb exerts hypotensive and antiarrhythmic effects. The whole extract is more easily tolerated with reserpine than is the isolated substance, indicating the importance of the accompanying substances, or coeffectors. Rauwolfia is available as a dried root, powder, and extracts.

Reported uses
Rauwolfia is used orally to treat nervousness, insomnia, anxiety, tension states, and other psychometric disorders. It's also used to treat flatulence, vomiting, liver disease, hypertension, and eclampsia. Rauwolfia is used topically to treat wounds, snakebite, dysuria, and colic.

Administration
The daily dose is 600 mg (equivalent to 6 mg total alkaloids), by mouth.

Hazards
Adverse effects associated with the use of rauwolfia include depression, fatigue, drowsiness, nightmares, nasal congestion, nausea, vomiting, erectile dysfunction, and decreased libido.

Increased hypotension may occur if rauwolfia is used with antihypertensives.

Monitor patient's blood pressure. Barbiturates and neuroleptic drugs have a synergistic effect when used with rauwolfia. Severe bradycardia may occur if rauwolfia is used with cardiac glycosides. Decreased effect of levodopa may occur if used with rauwolfia. Increased blood pressure may occur if rauwolfia is used with OTC cold medicines, flu remedies, and appetite suppressants. Initial significant increase in blood pressure may occur if rauwolfia is used with sympathomimetics. Increased impairment of motor reactions will occur if rauwolfia is used with alcohol.

Patients hypersensitive to rauwolfia products should avoid this herb, as should pregnant patients, breast-feeding patients, and patients with depression, ulceration, or pheochromocytoma.

Clinical considerations
- Monitor patient's blood pressure closely.
- Warn patient to use caution when taking herb with OTC cough and flu drugs or appetite suppressants.
- Advise patient not to drink alcohol while taking this herb.
- Encourage patient taking rauwolfia not to consume foods or beverages that contain alcohol.
- Warn patient not to take herb for insomnia before seeking medical attention because doing so may delay diagnosis of a potentially serious medical condition.
- Warn patient to keep all herbal products away from children and pets, and to store them away from heat and direct sunlight.
- Tell patient to remind prescriber and pharmacist of any herbal and dietary supplement that he's taking when obtaining a new prescription.
- Advise patient to consult his health care provider before using an herbal preparation because a treatment with proven efficacy may be available.

Research summary
The concepts behind the use of rauwolfia and the claims made regarding its effects haven't yet been validated scientifically.

Reconstructive therapy

Ligament reconstructive therapy, proliferative therapy, prolotherapy, sclerotherapy

Reconstructive therapy is a technique that stimulates the body's own healing capability to regenerate ligaments and tendons, thus restoring function to injured joints. It involves injecting the fibro-osseous junction at an area of ligament or tendon tears with a solution that stimulates fibroblast proliferation. The goal of reconstructive therapy is to complete an incomplete healing process and to restore normal connective tissue length and strength in the affected area. This will restore adequate skeletal support as well as affect the pain cycle.

The solution used is a combination of a natural proliferant (a substance that irritates the tissue) and local anesthetic that provides a biochemical stimulus to the area. By inducing inflammation, it triggers the body's natural healing mechanism. The swelling causes more blood to flow to the area, which produces new collagen to rebuild the tissue within and around the joint. Light exercises allow the new tissue to align correctly with the joint. The result is that the treated joint is stronger than the original joint, providing more support and strength and lowering the potential of future injury.

Reconstructive therapy has been used for centuries to treat chronic joint pain. Hippocrates used cautery of the anterior/inferior shoulder capsule to create scar tissue for chronic dislocations in javelin throwers. In 1937, Earl Gedney began using a technique called sclerotherapy. The term was originally applied to denote the use of a sclerosing agent to aid in the de-velopment of scar tissue that has tightened damaged ligaments. Recent research, however, shows tissue from prereconstructive and postreconstructive therapy to be histologically undifferentiated. The developing tissue is actually new ligament being created over old ligament rather than scar tissue. The term has thus been changed to *prolotherapy*, or *proliferation therapy*.

George Hackett began using prolotherapy in the 1940s. In 1956, he published a book on his procedure, which involved injecting a proliferating agent into torn vertebral ligaments for the treatment of lower back pain. Then, in the 1970s, M. J. Ongley developed the now commonly used solution called P25G — a combination of phenol, glucose, and glycerin.

The rationale behind prolotherapy treatment of low back pain and sciatica is based on the traditional orthopedic principle of stabilization of weakened joints and ligaments. Stretched or torn ligaments and tendons generally don't heal on their own because they lack the influx of good blood supply that is present in uninjured areas of the body. Modern anti-inflammatory drugs further limit the blood flow by blocking the inflammation process that generates the fibroblast cells necessary to the formation of fibrous connective tissue that lays down the collagen. If the ligaments and tendons don't repair fully, an underlying weakness in the tissues occurs. The instability of the underlying ligaments or tendons causes the surrounding muscle to tighten reflexively in order to stabilize the joint, thus creating pain.

Reconstructive therapy is recommended by its proponents as an economical and less risky alternative to surgery that not only gives lasting relief from pain, but also increases endurance and aids in preventing future injury.

Reported uses
Reconstructive therapy is used to treat back pain, herniated disks, sciatica, back fractures, arthritis, fibromyalgia, carpal

tunnel syndrome, and repetitive use syndrome. The treatment is used for shoulder pain and a variety of joint problems: dislocations, a sensation of deep aching or pulling pain in a joint, and grinding, popping, or clicking in a joint. It's used to treat ligament or tendon sprains or incomplete tears. It's also used to treat shooting pains, tingling, or numbness when chiropractic adjustments fail to provide lasting relief, and when muscle relaxants, arthritis medication, cortisone shots, or nerve blocks fail to resolve the problem within 6 weeks.

How the treatment is performed

A structural evaluation is performed and a treatment plan designed. A trained physician uses a needle from 22 to 27 gauge and 2 to 3 inches in length, depending on the area of the body being treated, to inject a proliferative solution into the fibro-osseous junction where damaged ligaments and tendons surround a joint. The most commonly used solution is P25G, which is a combination of glucose, glycerin, phenol, lidocaine or procaine, and sterile water. Several other solution combinations are available. Sodium morrhuate or straight dextrose is also used, but more caution is required with straight dextrose owing to increased infections and concern in treating patients with diabetes.

A fibrosis process begins approximately 15 hours after injection of the solution into the tissues. The fibrous tissue is firm by 7 days and progresses to adult compact bundles in about 18 days. The tissue formation is permanent, and rearrangement into tendinous and ligamentous structures results in the stabilization of previously unstable joints. Treatment also includes joint positioning, proper nutrition, active and passive exercise, and soft-tissue massage.

The American Osteopathic Academy of Sclerotherapy states that maximum benefits are derived when the patient regains full strength and endurance and all other symptoms have been resolved, all examinations are returned with normal results, and the examining physicians note that all ligaments, tendons, and joints have become firm. Reconstructive therapy normally requires between 6 and 12 treatments, sometimes more, depending on the severity of the damaged joint. Treatments are given weekly or every other week.

It is important to emphasize that reconstructive therapy isn't a pain management treatment; rather, it is a strengthening and regeneration treatment. With strengthening, pain is typically reduced.

TRAINING *Reconstructive therapy isn't taught in medical schools, but postgraduate education and certification is offered by both the American Osteopathic Academy of Sclerotherapy, 107 Maple Ave., Wilmington, DE 19809, 302-996-0300; and the American Association of Orthopedic Medicine, 315 Blvd. NE, Suite 336, Atlanta, GA 30312, 800-992-2063; 404-577-5455.*

Hazards

When performed correctly, reconstructive therapy carries a low risk of adverse effects. Some patients experience a sensitivity to the solution in the form of swelling, headache, nausea, and tiredness. The reaction rarely lasts longer than 2 to 4 days after the injection. There is minor risk of infection and hemorrhage.

Clinical considerations

- Reconstructive therapy is generally not used to treat acute injuries.
- Treatment is usually performed at least 4 to 6 weeks after the initial injury.
- Before beginning treatment, check patient's history for allergies to the solution ingredients.
- Make certain that any medications the patient is currently taking won't conflict with the treatments.
- Advise the patient that experiencing soreness and stiffness a couple of days following treatment is normal.

 REIMBURSEMENT *Reconstructive therapy has been practiced for more than 40 years in the United*

States, but is still considered an alternative treatment. There are approximately 250 physicians who are certified and offer it in the United States. Treatments are usually covered by private insurance but are not covered by Medicare.

Research summary

Several studies indicate that reconstructive therapy is effective in treating joint pain. Results of several double-blind studies show that 88% of patients treated with reconstructive therapy improve. Two studies performed by the Department of Orthopedic Surgery at the University of Iowa, in 1983 and 1985, demonstrated similar positive results, with joints treated with reconstructive therapy being stronger than the original joint. Studies show that both ligaments and tendons can increase by up to 40% in strength and size with this therapy.

Other studies demonstrated increased collagen fiber diameter and cellularity on biopsy of injected areas. Disability, range of motion, and pain levels all improved significantly in patients injected after 5 or more years of chronic pain. In human knees with reproducible ligamental laxity, as measured by a computerized knee analysis device, a statistically significant reduction in ligamental laxity was demonstrated.

Randomized, double-blind control studies demonstrated statistically significant improvements in low back pain and disability rating. Typically, when a patient doesn't improve with the therapy, one or more coexisting conditions, such as infection or the use of cortisone, are inhibiting the body's healing process.

red clover

Purple clover, trefoil, Trifolium pratense, *wild clover*

Red clover is obtained from dried and fresh flower heads of *Trifolium pratense.* It contains volatile oil, isoflavones, coumarin derivatives, and cyanogenic glycosides. It has antispasmodic and expectorant effects and promotes skin healing. It also has hormonal effects similar to estrogen and caused by isoflavones. Red clover is available as liquid extract, tinctures, and tea, in products such as EuroQuality Red Clover Blossoms, Nu-Veg Red Clover Concentrate, and Promensil.

Reported uses

Red clover is used orally to treat some cancers, and for coughs and respiratory problems where mucus is lacking (for example, in whooping cough). It's also used to relieve menopausal symptoms. Red clover is used externally to treat chronic skin diseases such as eczema and psoriasis.

Administration

- Dried flower heads: 4 g by mouth, or as a tea, up to three times a day
- Liquid extract (1:1 in 25% alcohol): 1.5 to 3 ml (30 to 60 gtt) by mouth three times a day
- Tincture (1:10 in 45% alcohol): 1 to 2 ml (20 to 40 gtt) by mouth three times a day.

Hazards

Adverse effects associated with red clover include breast tenderness, breast enlargement, weight gain, dyspnea, and allergic reactions, such as hives, swelling, and itching.

Possible increased International Normalized Ratio may occur if red clover is used with heparin or warfarin. Monitor laboratory values and patient closely for bleeding. Possible enhanced estrogen effects may occur if red clover is used with oral contraceptives or hormone replacement therapy.

Pregnant and breast-feeding women should avoid this herb, as should patients hypersensitive to red clover products. Patients shouldn't use this herb for breast or uterine cancer because of possible hormonal effects, which may increase the metabolism of cancer cells. Safety in young children or patients with severe liver or kidney disease hasn't been established.

Clinical considerations
■ Caution patient to watch for signs and symptoms of bleeding, including easy bruising, bleeding gums, black tarry stools, and tea-colored urine, especially when taking large amounts of herb with warfarin or aspirin.
■ Advise pregnant or breast-feeding patient, and patient hypersensitive to red clover products, to avoid use of this herb.
■ Advise patient to watch for estrogen-like effects, such as breast tenderness, breast enlargement, and weight gain.
■ Warn patient to keep all herbal products away from children and pets, and to store them away from heat and direct sunlight.
■ Tell patient to remind prescriber and pharmacist of any herbal and dietary supplement that he's taking when obtaining a new prescription.
■ Advise patient to consult his health care provider before using an herbal preparation because a treatment with proven efficacy may be available.

Research summary
The concepts behind the use of red clover and the claims made regarding its effects haven't yet been validated scientifically.

red poppy

Copperose, corn poppy, corn rose, cup-puppy, headache poppy, headwark, Papaver rhoeas, *rhoeados flos*

Red poppy is obtained from flowers of *Papaver rhoeas*. It contains small amounts of isoquinoline alkaloids (0.1%) and anthocyanin glycosides. Its mechanism of action isn't well defined. Red poppy is available as dried flower petals, powder, and teas.

Reported uses
Red poppy is used to treat respiratory tract diseases and discomforts, for disturbed sleep, for sedation, and for pain relief. It's also used in children's cough syrup and as a tea for insomnia.

Administration
For bronchial irritation, a tea is made by steeping 2 teaspoons of dried petals in 1 cup boiling water for 5 to 10 minutes, and then straining. One cup of tea is taken two or three times a day. It may be sweetened with honey, if desired. (1 teaspoon = about 8 g of red poppy herb.)

Hazards
Adverse effects associated with red poppy include vomiting and stomach pain. There are no reported interactions with the use of red poppy.

Children and pregnant and breast-feeding women shouldn't use this herb.

 SAFETY RISK *Poisoning has occurred in children who consumed fresh leaves and blossoms; symptoms included vomiting and stomach pain. However, the powdered herb has a low alkaloid content and is considered nontoxic.*

Clinical considerations
■ Advise patient to avoid use of red poppy while pregnant or breast-feeding.
■ Warn patient to keep all herbal products away from children and pets.
■ Tell patient to remind prescriber and pharmacist of any herbal and dietary supplement that he's taking when obtaining a new prescription.
■ Advise patient to consult his health care provider before using an herbal preparation because a treatment with proven efficacy may be available.

Research summary
The concepts behind the use of red poppy and the claims made regarding its effects haven't yet been validated scientifically.

RIGHT FOOT REFLEX ZONES

The illustration below, showing the organs and body parts associated with specific regions of the right foot, serves as a map that guides reflexologists in performing therapy.

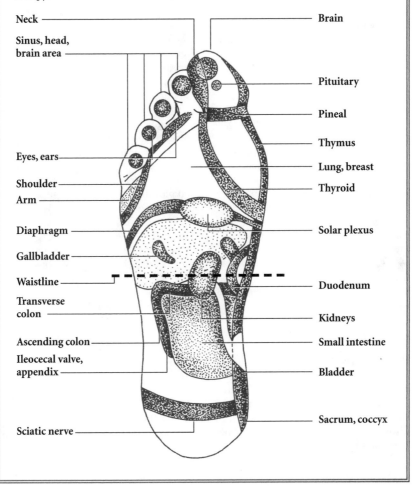

Neck

Sinus, head, brain area

Eyes, ears

Shoulder

Arm

Diaphragm

Gallbladder

Waistline

Transverse colon

Ascending colon

Ileocecal valve, appendix

Sciatic nerve

Brain

Pituitary

Pineal

Thymus

Lung, breast

Thyroid

Solar plexus

Duodenum

Kidneys

Small intestine

Bladder

Sacrum, coccyx

Reflexology

Reflexology is a widely practiced form of manual therapy in which pressure is applied to specific parts of the body, usually the soles of the feet (but sometimes the palms of the hands). It's based on the theory that these areas correspond to, and can therapeutically affect, various or-gans and glands of the body. For example, the top of the big toe is said to connect to the brain, and the arch area to the solar plexus. (See *Right foot reflex zones.*) Some practitioners believe that these points follow the same meridians used in acupuncture.

The roots of reflexology can be traced back 3,000 years to traditional medicine in China, India, and Egypt. The current revival of interest in this technique began in the early 1900s with an American ear, nose, and throat specialist, William Fitzgerald, who discovered that his patients felt less pain when he applied pressure to specific points on their soles or palms before surgery. Fitzgerald's work was expanded on in the 1930s by Eunice Ingham, a physical therapist, who believed that applying varying levels of pressure to certain areas could not only decrease pain but also provide other health benefits. Ingham mapped the specific reflex zones on the feet that reflexologists use today. Reflexologists, who are usually masseurs or physical therapists with special training, say that their technique works by reducing the amount of lactic acid in the feet and breaking up calcium crystals that accumulate in the nerve endings, blocking the flow of energy.

TRAINING *No specific license or certification is needed to practice reflexology. For training or referrals, contact The International Institute of Reflexology, 5650 1st Avenue North, PO Box 12642, St. Petersburg, Florida, 33733-2642; telephone (727) 343-4811.*

Reported uses
Reflexology is used to relieve stress and muscle tension and produce relaxation. Reflexology is used to treat conditions such as skin disorders (eczema, acne), GI disorders (diarrhea, constipation), hypertension, migraines, anxiety, and asthma.

How the treatment is performed
Many health clubs and spas offer reflexology treatments. The therapy requires only a treatment table or chair or a stool to elevate the feet. A quiet environment is preferred.

The patient is either seated comfortably in a reclining chair or placed supine on a treatment table, with feet raised and supported. The therapist is seated facing the soles of the patient's feet. After an initial assessment of the patient's feet for alterations in skin thickness and abnormalities in foot structure, the therapist feels for tender areas and signs of tension or thickening on the sole.

A treatment session typically begins with relaxation techniques designed to release tension and make the patient comfortable with the manipulation of his feet. The therapist uses thumbs and fingers to apply gentle but firm pressure to the reflex zones of the foot, paying more attention to zones that are tender to the touch. Working systematically, the therapist begins with the toes and proceeds in small, creeping movements proximally toward the heel. (For therapy using the hand, the therapist starts with the fingers and moves proximally toward the wrist.) A typical session lasts 20 minutes to 1 hour.

Hazards
Treatments may produce what practitioners call a "healing crisis," consisting of a fever, rash, diaphoresis, or urinary changes or a worsening of symptoms related to the patient's chief complaint — for example, worsening diarrhea or nausea in a patient with a GI disorder. These crises are said to be manifestations of the release of toxins — proof that the treatment is working and the body is healing itself.

Clinical considerations
- Advise patient to postpone reflexology treatments if his feet have cuts, boils, bruises, or other injuries.
- Instruct patient to check with his doctor before trying reflexology if he has diabetes, peripheral vascular disease, or other vascular problems in the legs, such as thrombosis or phlebitis.
- Advise pregnant patient to get her doctor's consent before trying this therapy.
- Many people who claim to perform reflexology are actually providing a simple foot massage. If patient wants treatment for a specific symptom, he should make

sure the practitioner has been trained in reflexology.

Research summary
There is little scientific evidence that reflexology is effective in treating specific illnesses. However, a 1993 randomized, controlled study published in *Obstetrics and Gynecology* found a significant reduction in symptoms after reflexology treatment in 35 women with premenstrual syndrome. Some nurses provide reflexology instead of sleeping pills to older patients; some nurse-midwives say that it can relax women during childbirth and reduce breast engorgement after delivery. Even without scientific evidence of its efficacy, many patients enjoy reflexology and report positive results, including stress reduction and relaxation.

rhatany

Krameria root, Krameria triandra, *mapato, Peruvian rhatany, ratanhiae radix, ratanhiawurzel, red rhatany, rhatania*

Rhatany is obtained from dried root of *Krameria triandra.* It contains high levels of proanthocyanidin tannins, which give the herb astringent properties. Rhatany is available as a powder, tincture, and tea.

Reported uses
Rhatany is used orally as an antidiarrheal for enteritis. It's used topically to treat mild inflammation of the oral and pharyngeal mucosa and gums, as well as fissures of the tongue, stomatitis, pharyngitis, noninfectious canker sores, chilblains, hemorrhoids, and leg ulcers.

Administration
■ Decoction: 1 g of powdered root in 1 cup of water
■ For external sores and ulcers: undiluted tincture painted on affected area, two or three times a day

■ Mouthwash and gargle (simmer 1 to 1.5 g powdered root in 5 oz boiling water for 10 to 15 minutes, and then strain): swished, not swallowed, two or three times a day
■ Tea: scald 1.5 to 2 g (1 teaspoon = about 3 g of powdered rhatany) coarsely powdered rhatany in 1 cup boiling water for 10 to 15 minutes, and then strain
■ Tincture: 5 to 10 gtt in 1 glass of water, swished, not swallowed, two or three times a day.

Hazards
Adverse effects associated with rhatany include digestive complaints and allergic mucous membrane reactions. Herbal products that contain alcohol may cause a disulfiram-like reaction. Decreased absorption of iron may occur if iron supplements, such as ferrous sulfate, are taken with rhatany tea. Possible skin irritation may occur if tretinoin is used with topical rhatany. Milk or cream may inactivate tannins in rhatany tea. Rhatany may potentiate antibiotic activity of echinacea. Rhatany shouldn't be used longer than 2 weeks if taken without medical advice.

Pregnant and breast-feeding women shouldn't use this herb.

Clinical considerations
■ Rhatany is difficult to find, and adulteration with other *Krameria* species is common.
■ Advise patient to avoid use of rhatany while pregnant or breast-feeding.
■ Advise patient not to use rhatany for longer than 2 weeks without a health care provider's advice.
■ Advise patient to avoid alcohol consumption.
■ Tell patient to remind prescriber and pharmacist of any herbal and dietary supplement that he's taking when obtaining a new prescription.
■ Advise patient to consult his health care provider before using an herbal preparation because a treatment with proven efficacy may be available.

Research summary

The concepts behind the use of rhatany and the claims made regarding its effects haven't yet been validated scientifically.

Rolfing

Structural integration

Rolfing, the informal name for structural integration, is a system of bodywork developed in the 1940s by Ida Rolf. Rolf, who was greatly influenced by the principles of yoga and osteopathy, believed that body structure affects all physiologic processes and that maintaining the proper balance of head, torso, and pelvis is the key to improving function and health.

Rolf's work began almost by accident in about 1940, when she met a music teacher who had been injured in a fall and could no longer teach or play the piano. Rolf made a deal with her: If she could help the teacher recover from her injuries, the teacher would give Rolf's children piano lessons. The teacher accepted, and Rolf began to work with her. They started working with yoga exercises, and by the fourth session the woman was able to resume teaching piano. Word spread, and soon Rolf was treating others with the new system she was developing. Rolf's system of bodywork was influenced by three key principles: osteopathy's belief that structure determines function; homeopathy's emphasis on the integration of physical, mental, and emotional aspects of the human being; and yoga's focus on body-lengthening positions to achieve a balanced body.

Rolf built on these three principles, maintaining that repositioning bones wasn't enough to alter body structure; one also needed to focus on the fascia — the fibrous tissue that covers all muscles and organs. She believed that chronic stress, bad posture, and injury cause the fascia to thicken (the feeling of a "knot" in a muscle), restricting movement in the muscles and joints and interfering with proper body alignment. By manipulating the thickened fascial tissues, Rolf believed one could stretch and "unwind" them, restoring the proper alignment of bones and muscles and improving overall body functioning.

TRAINING *The Rolf Institute in Boulder, Colorado, teaches structural integration and certifies instructors. Once certified, instructors become members of the Rolf Institute and are entitled to use the trademarked term Rolfing. Members are required to abide by the Institute's code of ethics and standards of practice. The Institute also provides referrals to certified Rolfers.*

Reported uses

Rolfing practitioners don't claim to cure disease; rather, the method is used to reduce pain and muscle spasms, release tension, and increase range of motion, flexibility, and energy. Rolfing may be most helpful for chronic pain and muscle stiffness related to structural imbalance.

How the treatment is performed

A treatment table may be used for some Rolfing techniques. A mirror may also be used so that the patient can observe how his body moves and see changes as they occur.

Rolfing is usually administered in a series of 10 weekly sessions, each lasting 60 to 90 minutes. The sessions are designed to work systematically on the whole body, beginning at the surface and progressing more deeply into the tissues. Practitioners use their thumbs, fingers, and knuckles — and sometimes their elbows and knees — to apply pressure to the fascia in all areas of the body, gradually releasing tension in overstressed muscles, lengthening muscles, and allowing the skeletal structure to assume its natural position.

As the muscles and fascia move more smoothly together and bones move into a more normal relationship, joints move with greater ease and the body becomes more relaxed and open. According to Rolfing proponents, as the physical body becomes more fluid, blood and lymph circulation improves, and the patient generally experiences a sense of greater well-being.

Hazards
Rolfing may be painful at times, but shouldn't result in any complications when performed by a properly trained practitioner.

Clinical considerations
■ Patient with coagulopathy shouldn't undergo Rolfing because of the risk of bruising.
■ If patient expresses an interest in Rolfing, help him locate a certified practitioner.
■ Inform patient that some aspects of Rolfing may be painful.

Research summary
A study done at UCLA found that patients who experienced Rolfing had smoother, more energetic movements and improved posture. A study done at the University of Maryland found that Rolfing reduced chronic stress, improved neurologic function, and reduced curvature of the spine in patients with lordosis.

rose hip

Brier hip, brier rose, dog rose, heps, hip, hipberry, hip fruit, hip sweet, hopfruit, Rosa canina, R. centifolia, rosehips, sweet brier, wild boar fruit, witches' brier

Rose hip is obtained from fruits (hips) and seeds of various species of *Rosa*. It contains pectins and fruit acids, such as malic and citric acids, which are responsible for diuretic and laxative effects, as well as tannins, vitamin C, carotenoids,

and flavonoids. Fresh rose hip contains 0.5% to 1.7% vitamin C but, because it deteriorates in processing, many natural vitamin supplements have some vitamin C added to them. Rose hip also contains vitamins A, B_1, B_2, B_3, and K. Rose hip is available as capsules, tablets, powder, and tea, and in combination products such as Ascorbate-C, Ester-C 1000, Hi-Potent-C, Honey C Chew Chewable C, and Mega-Stress Complex.

Reported uses
Rose hip is used to treat diarrhea, respiratory disorders such as colds and flu, vitamin C deficiency (scurvy), gastric spasms and inflammation, intestinal diseases, edema, gout, arthritis, sciatica, diabetes, metabolic disorders of uric acid metabolism (including gout), lower urinary tract and gallbladder ailments, gallstones, kidney stones, and inadequate peripheral circulation. It's also used as a diuretic, a laxative, an astringent, and a booster of immune function during exhaustion. Rose hip is also used to treat osteogenesis imperfecta in children.

Administration
■ Osteogenesis imperfecta: 250 to 600 mg/day, by mouth
■ Tea (steep 1 to 2.5 g [1 teaspoon = 3.5 g of herb] of crushed rose hip in 5 oz boiling water for 10 to 15 minutes, and then strain): as a diuretic, as needed.

Hazards
Adverse effects associated with rose hip include insomnia, headache, fatigue, flushing, nausea, vomiting, abdominal cramps, esophagitis, gastroesophageal reflux, diarrhea, kidney stones, severe respiratory allergies (after exposure to herb dust), itching, prickly sensations, and anaphylaxis.

Increased aluminum absorption may occur if rose hip is used with aluminum-containing antacids. Increased excretion of ascorbic acid and decreased excretion of salicylates may occur if rose hip is used with aspirin or salicylates; monitor patient for salicylate toxicity. Barbiturates, estrogens, oral contraceptives, and tetracyclines used with rose hip may increase vitamin C requirements. Rose hip may increase iron absorption; advise patient to avoid using together. Additive effects may occur if rose hip is used with tretinoin. Possible decreased effects may occur if rose hip is used with warfarin; monitor patient's International Normalized Ratio. Milk or cream may inactivate rose hip tea. Rose hip may potentiate the antibiotic activity of echinacea; monitor patient closely.

Pregnant and breast-feeding women shouldn't use more of this herb than is found in foods. Patients with asthma should avoid this herb.

Clinical considerations
■ Rose hip is nontoxic in recommended amounts.
■ Advise pregnant or breast-feeding patient to avoid using this herb.
■ Rose hip interactions depend on the amount of vitamin C present.
■ The German Commission E Monographs lists no known risks of using rose hip, but there have been reports of severe respiratory allergies with mild to moderate anaphylaxis in production workers exposed to rose hip dust during the manufacturing process. Plant fibers may also cause itching and a prickly sensation caused by mechanical irritation rather than allergic reaction.
■ Herb may cause precipitation of urate, oxalate, or cysteine stones, or drugs in the urinary tract, resulting in kidney stones.
■ Rose hip may cause false-negative results for occult blood tests.
■ The following tests may result in false increases: AST that uses color reactions (redox reactions) and Technicon SMA 12/60, bilirubin measured by colorimetric methods or Technicon SMA 12/60, carbamazepine (Tegretol) measured by Ames ARIS method, and urine glucose level measured by Clinitest or serum or urine creatinine.

■ The following tests may result in false decreases: lactic dehydrogenase measured by Technicon SMA 12/60 and Abbott 100 methods, theophylline measured by ARIS system or Ames Seralyzer photometer, and blood glucose level measured by Clinistix or Tes-Tape.
■ Warn patient with asthma to use rose hip with caution and to stop immediately and consult a health care provider if any wheezing or shortness of breath occurs.
■ Inform patient that many rose hip-derived natural vitamin C supplements are fortified with synthetic vitamin C.
■ Tell patient to take rose hip with vitamin C 2 hours before or 4 hours after taking antacids.
■ Tell patient to remind prescriber and pharmacist of any herbal and dietary supplement that he's taking when obtaining a new prescription.
■ Advise patient to consult his health care provider before using an herbal preparation because a treatment with proven efficacy may be available.

Research summary
The concepts behind the use of rose hip and the claims made regarding its effects haven't yet been validated scientifically.

rosemary

Compass plant, compass-weed, old man, polar plant, romero, rosmarinblätter, Rosmarinus officinalis

Rosemary is obtained from leaves of *Rosmarinus officinalis*. It contains 1% to 2.5% of a volatile oil, composed of monoterpene hydrocarbons, camphor, borneol, and cineol. The leaves also contain rosmaricine, various volatile and aromatic components, and the flavonoid pigments diosmin, diosmentin, genkwanin, and related compounds. Diosmin decreases capillary permeability and fragility. Rosemary exerts some antibacterial activity, as well as spasmolytic effects on smooth muscle. It also may have a positive inotropic effect, increasing coronary blood flow. Rosemary may also have antifungal, antioxidant, anticancer, and abortifacient properties as well as stimulant effects on uterine muscle and menstrual flow. When applied topically, rosemary is an irritant and may increase circulation. Rosemary is available as dried leaves, essential oil, lotion, extracts, and tea, in products such as Breast Health Formula, Bright-Eyes, Complete Cleanse, Easy Now, Female Sage, Respi-Oil, RoseOx, and Think-O2.

Reported uses
Rosemary is used to treat flatulence, gout, toothache, cough, and eczema, and as a poultice for poor wound healing. It's also used to aid digestion, ease dyspepsia, promote menstrual flow, induce abortion, increase appetite, and relieve headaches, liver and gallbladder complaints, and blood pressure problems.

Rosemary is used topically as an insect repellent and to treat baldness, circulatory disturbances, joint or musculoskeletal pain, myalgia, sciatica, and neuralgia. It's also popularly used in cooking, cosmetics, and various teas.

Administration
■ Bath: 50 g of leaves added to 1 L hot water and add to bath water
■ Liquid extract (1:1 in 45% alcohol): 2 to 4 ml by mouth three times a day
■ Oral: 4 to 6 g of leaves by mouth every day
■ Tea: Prepared by steeping 1 or 2 g of leaves in 5 oz boiling water for 15 minutes, then straining; 1 cup taken three times a day
■ Topical: 6% to 10% essential oil in semisolid or liquid preparations.

Hazards
Adverse effects associated with rosemary include seizures at high doses, asthma (from repeated occupational exposure), and contact dermatitis. Herbal products that contain alcohol may cause a disulfi-

ram-like reaction. Topical forms of rosemary may cause photosensitivity.

Pregnant and breast-feeding women should avoid this herb, as should children, patients with seizure disorders, and patients hypersensitive to rosemary products.

SAFETY RISK *Undiluted rosemary oil shouldn't be ingested. Overdose may cause spasms, vomiting, gastroenteritis, uterine bleeding, kidney irritation, deep coma, and possibly death.*

Clinical considerations
■ Rosemary is unlikely to have adverse effects when the leaves and oil are used in amounts typically found in foods. The herb is generally recognized as safe by the FDA. Maximum level of leaves is 0.41% in baked goods and 0.003% in oil.
■ Repeated occupational exposure to rosemary may lead to asthma.
■ Warn patient not to ingest undiluted rosemary oil.
■ Advise pregnant patient, patient trying to get pregnant, or breast-feeding patient not to use rosemary in amounts greater than those found in food.
■ Advise patient with seizure disorder not to ingest large amounts of rosemary.
■ Advise parents not to give children amounts greater than those found in food.
■ Advise patient to use sunscreen and limit sun exposure if rosemary is being applied topically.
■ Warn patient to keep all herbal products away from children and pets.
■ Tell patient to inform prescriber and pharmacist of any herbal and dietary supplement that he's taking when obtaining a new prescription.
■ Advise patient to consult his health care provider before using an herbal preparation because a treatment with proven efficacy may be available.

Research summary
The concepts behind the use of rosemary and the claims made regarding its effects haven't yet been validated scientifically.

royal jelly

Royal jelly is obtained from the milky white secretion produced by worker bees of the species *Apis mellifera* for exclusive growth and development of the queen bee. It contains a complex mixture of proteins, sugars, fats, and variable amounts of minerals, vitamins, and pheromones. It's rich in B vitamins, especially pantothenic acid. About 15% of royal jelly is 10-hydroxy-trans-(2)-decenoic acid, which has weak antimicrobial activity. Royal jelly may also have antitumor activity. Royal jelly is available as capsules, creams, lotions, milk baths, and in combination with honey, in products such as Bee Complete, Bee Pollen Complex, Energy Elixir, Pure Energy, Royal Bee Power, Super Energy Up, and Ultra Virile-Actin.

Reported uses

Royal jelly is used orally as a health tonic and to reduce cholesterol, promote rejuvenation, enhance sexual performance, improve the immune system, and treat bronchial asthma, liver disease, kidney disease, pancreatitis, insomnia, stomach ulcers, bone fractures, skin disorders, and hyperlipidemia. It's applied topically as a skin tonic and to stimulate hair growth.

Administration

■ Capsules are available in 62.5-mg, 100-mg, 125-mg, 250-mg, and 500-mg doses. Follow manufacturer's recommendations regarding dosage
■ For hyperlipidemia, 50 to 100 mg is taken by mouth every day.

Hazards

Adverse effects associated with royal jelly include asthma, fatal anaphylaxis, rash, dermatitis, hemorrhagic colitis, and skin irritation. Royal jelly may prolong bleeding times. Avoid use with anticoagulant and antiplatelet therapy.

Pregnant and breast-feeding women should avoid this herb, as should patients hypersensitive to related products and patients with seasonal allergies or dermatitis.

Clinical considerations

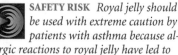 **SAFETY RISK** *Royal jelly should be used with extreme caution by patients with asthma because allergic reactions to royal jelly have led to asthma, anaphylaxis, and death.*

■ One case of severe adverse GI reactions has been reported; it included abdominal pain, hemorrhagic colitis, diarrhea, GI hemorrhage, and mucosal edema of the sigmoid colon.
■ Don't confuse royal jelly with bee pollen and honey bee venom.
■ Tell patient that royal jelly may worsen asthma and lead to anaphylaxis. Warn patient to seek medical attention if shortness of breath develops after taking royal jelly.
■ Advise patient to avoid royal jelly while pregnant or breast-feeding.
■ Advise patient that topical use of royal jelly may worsen existing dermatitis.
■ Tell patient to remind prescriber and pharmacist of any herbal and dietary supplement that he's taking when obtaining a new prescription.
■ Advise patient to consult his health care provider before using an herbal preparation because a treatment with proven efficacy may be available.

Research summary

The concepts behind the use of royal jelly and the claims made regarding its effects haven't yet been validated scientifically.

rue

Herb of grace, herbygrass, rue,
Ruta graveolens

Rue is obtained from above-ground parts of *Ruta graveolens*. It contains essential oils, such as limonene, pinene, anisic acid, and phenol. Flavonoids such as rutin and quercetin may have a strengthening effect on capillaries; the alkaloids arborinine, gamma-fagarine, and graveoline may have antispasmodic and abortifacient activity. Furanocoumarins such as bergapten, psoralen, and xanthotoxin have a photosensitizing effect with topical or oral use. Furanocoumarins are also known mutagens. Chalepensin inhibits fertility, and coumarin derivatives and alkaloids are spasmolytic. Rue also contains hypericin, tannin, pectin, choline, and iron. Rue is available as dried leaves, compresses, capsules, tincture, oil, and tea.

 SAFETY RISK *Rue shouldn't be used for any reason because of its toxic effects. Because of the risk of toxicity, rue is available only from specialty herb suppliers.*

Reported uses
Rue is used orally to treat amenorrhea, Bell's palsy, colic, cough, epilepsy, hypertension, hysteria, multiple sclerosis, skin inflammation, oral and pharyngeal cavities, cramps, hepatitis, dyspepsia, diarrhea, intestinal parasites, and worm infections. It's also used as a uterine stimulant for abortions.

Rue is used externally for backache, ear infection, eye soreness, gout, headache, muscle spasms, varicose veins, sprains, bruising, rheumatism, sore throat, and wounds. It's applied topically as an insect repellent.

Administration
■ Daily oral dosage: 0.5 g to 1 g by mouth every day
■ Tea: 1 heaping teaspoon (about 3 g) to ¼ L of water, by mouth.

Hazards
Adverse effects associated with rue include dizziness, vertigo, tremors, depression, sleep disorders, delirium, melancholic mood, fatigue, bradycardia, phototoxicity, swelling of the tongue, vomiting, epigastric pain, abdominal pain, severe kidney damage, hepatotoxicity, contact dermatitis, clammy skin, and photosensitivity. There are no reported interactions with rue.

Pregnant and breast-feeding women shouldn't use this herb. Large doses of rue used as an abortifacient can be toxic or fatal to the mother.

Clinical considerations
■ Patient should use rue only under strict supervision by a health care provider with extensive herbal experience.
■ Deaths of pregnant women have been reported after using rue for abortion.
■ Advise pregnant or breast-feeding patient to avoid use of this herb.
■ Topical use of rue oil can cause contact dermatitis.
■ Phototoxic reactions causing dermatosis have been reported from the prepared oil and from rubbing fresh leaves on the skin.
■ Large doses may cause photosensitivity.
■ Warn patient to avoid rue because of its potential toxicity and the availability of safer treatments.
■ Warn patient to keep all herbal products away from children and pets.
■ Tell patient to remind prescriber and pharmacist of any herbal and dietary supplement that he's taking when obtaining a new prescription.
■ Advise patient to consult his health care provider before using an herbal preparation because a treatment with proven efficacy may be available.

Research summary
The concepts behind the use of rue and the claims made regarding its effects haven't yet been validated scientifically.

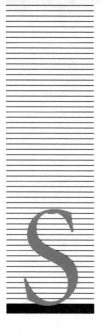

safflower

American saffron, bastard saffron,
Carthamus tinctorius, *dyer's saffron,*
fake saffron, false saffron, hoang-chi,
koosumbha, parrot plant, zaffer

Safflower is obtained from flowers of
Carthamus tinctorius. The oil contains
unsaturated fatty acids, including linoleic
(76% to 79%), oleic (13%), palmitic
(6%), and stearic (3%) acids. The stigmas
also contain lignans, polysaccharides, and
carthamone, a pigment. Linoleic acid is
an omega-6 fatty acid that may help lower cholesterol. Safflower is available as an
oil (from seeds) and as powdered flowers
or stigmas.

Reported uses
Safflower oil is commonly used in cooking as a source of polyunsaturated fats to
help lower dietary cholesterol levels. The
oil is also used as a laxative. Safflower
stigma, or extract, is used to treat
wounds, amenorrhea, stomach tumors,
scabies, arthritis, and chest pain. It's also
used to help stimulate movement of stagnant blood and to help alleviate pain
when used topically and systemically.

Administration
The average daily dose of safflower flower
decoction is 1 g by mouth three times a
day.

Hazards
There are no reported adverse effects associated with safflower oil. Stigma prepa-

rations may prolong blood coagulation time and shouldn't be used with anticoagulant therapy.

Pregnant or breast-feeding women shouldn't use safflower flowers. The purified oil is probably safe to use during pregnancy.

 SAFETY RISK *Safflower flowers shouldn't be used during pregnancy because they may cause abortion by stimulating uterine contractions.*

Clinical considerations

■ Monitor patient's serum cholesterol, as needed.

■ Tell patient to avoid excessive intake of omega-6 oils, such as safflower, without appropriate intake of omega-3 fatty acids.

■ Tell patient to notify health care provider immediately about new or worsened symptoms.

■ Advise patient to notify a health care provider about planned, suspected, or known pregnancy.

■ Warn patient to keep all herbal products away from children and pets.

■ Tell patient to remind prescriber and pharmacist of any herbal and dietary supplement that he's taking when obtaining a new prescription.

■ Advise patient to consult his health care provider before using an herbal preparation because a treatment with proven efficacy may be available.

Research summary

The concepts behind the use of safflower and the claims made regarding its effects haven't yet been validated scientifically.

saffron

Crocus sativus, *nagakeshara, saffron crocus, Spanish saffron, zang hong hua*

Saffron is obtained from flower stigmas and styles of *Crocus sativus,* which is grown mainly in Spain and France. It contains carotenoids and crocetin, the latter of which increases oxygen diffusion in blood plasma and, in turn, may help prevent or treat atherosclerosis. Saffron also contains crocin, a bitter glycoside, vitamins B_1 and B_2, and essential oils such as cineole, safranal, and terpenes. Purified crocetin products in development are more likely than the crude herb to help increase plasma oxygen levels. Saffron is available as dried stigmas, styles, or powder; it's often adulterated with American saffron.

Reported uses

Saffron is used to stimulate digestion and to treat amenorrhea, atherosclerosis, bronchitis, sore throat, headache, vomiting, and fever. It's also used as an abortifacient and a sedative.

Administration

Dosage of saffron isn't well documented.

Hazards

There are no reported adverse effects or interactions with saffron.

 SAFETY RISK *Overdose—that is, doses above 5 g—of saffron may cause central paralysis, dizziness, stupor, vomiting, intestinal colic, bloody diarrhea, and hemorrhaging of skin on the nose, lips, and eyelids. Treatment involves emptying the stomach by gastric lavage and giving activated charcoal, if needed. Symptomatic treatment includes diazepam to control seizures and sodium bicarbonate to correct acidosis. In severe cases, patient may need intubation and artificial respiration. Saffron may be lethal at doses above 12 g.*

Clinical considerations

■ Saffron is generally safe for use as a spice.

■ Caution patient to avoid using saffron medicinally without consulting a qualified health care provider.

■ Instruct patient to promptly notify health care provider about new or worsened symptoms.

■ Warn patient not to take herb before seeking medical attention because doing

so may delay diagnosis of a potentially serious medical condition.
- Warn patient to keep all herbal products away from children and pets.
- Tell patient to remind pharmacist of any herbal and dietary supplements that he's taking when obtaining a new prescription.
- Advise patient to consult his health care provider before using an herbal preparation because a treatment with proven efficacy may be available.

Research summary
The concepts behind the use of saffron and the claims made regarding its effects haven't yet been validated scientifically.

sage

Dalmatian sage, garden sage, meadow sage, Salvia officinalis, *scarlet sage*

Sage contains volatile oils (including thujone, cineole, and camphor), tannins, diterpene bitter principles, triterpenes, steroids, flavones, and flavonoid glycosides. It has antibacterial, fungistatic, virustatic, astringent, antioxidative, carminative, antispasmodic, secretion-promoting, and perspiration-inhibiting properties. Sage is available as dried leaves, extract, tincture, and essential oil.

Reported uses
Sage is used orally to treat loss of appetite, excessive perspiration, laryngitis, tonsillitis, pharyngitis, halitosis, canker sores, gum disease, fatigue, and Alzheimer's disease.

Sage is used topically to treat herpes lesions, shingles, psoriasis, and itching from insect bites. It's used as a vaginal douche to treat vaginal yeast infection, and topically to prevent hair loss and preserve hair color. It's also used in shampoos and conditioners.

Administration
- Dry herb (leaves): 4 g to 6 g by mouth every day
- Essential oil: 0.1 g to 0.3 g by mouth every day
- Fluid extract or tincture (1:2 and 1:5 alcohol): 3 ml to 12 ml by mouth in divided dose, three times a day
- For halitosis: A few leaves chewed occasionally
- For inflammation of bronchial mucous membranes: 50 g of powdered herb mixed with 80 g honey and used as expectorant
- For inflamed mucous membranes: Undiluted alcohol extract, applied as needed
- Gargle or mouth rinse: 2.5 g dry herb or 2 to 3 gtt essential oil in 100 ml of water, or 9 ml of alcoholic extract in 1 glass of water.

Hazards
Adverse effects associated with sage include seizures, vertigo, and tachycardia. Herbal products that contain alcohol may cause a disulfiram-like reaction; advise patient to avoid using together.

Pregnant or breast-feeding women shouldn't use this herb. It should be used with caution by patients with a history of epilepsy or other seizure disorders.

Clinical considerations
- Chemical content of the dry herbal product is likely to vary widely, depending on where the herb is grown, time of harvest, storage time, and drying method used.
- Advise patient to avoid using large amounts of sage, especially tincture or essential oil, because large amounts of thujone may be toxic.
- Advise pregnant or breast-feeding patient to avoid using this herb.
- Advise patient with history of epilepsy to use this herb with caution.
- Warn patient not to take herb before seeking medical attention because doing so may delay diagnosis of a potentially serious medical condition.

- Tell patient to promptly notify health care provider about new symptoms or adverse effects.
- Warn patient to keep all herbal products away from children and pets.
- Tell patient to remind prescriber and pharmacist of any herbal and dietary supplements that he's taking when obtaining a new prescription.
- Advise patient to consult his health care provider before using an herbal preparation because a treatment with proven efficacy may be available.

Research summary

The concepts behind the use of sage and the claims made regarding its effects haven't yet been validated scientifically.

SAM-e

Ademethionine, S-adenosylmethionine, Sammy

SAM-e is a naturally occurring amino acid found in all living cells. It plays an integral role in methylation processes, including DNA methylation, protein methylation (critical for cell growth and repair), and phospholipid methylation, which maintains flexibility of cell membranes. It also helps produce cysteine, an amino acid needed for glutathione, the main antioxidant in the liver.

Reported uses

S-adenosylmethionine is used to treat depression, including postpartum and menopausal types, as well as osteoarthritis, fibromyalgia, fatigue, and liver disorders. It's also used to prevent heart disease.

Administration

- For arthritis, 200 mg to 1,600 mg, taken by mouth every day in divided doses
- For depression, 400 mg once a day or 200 mg twice a day, taken by mouth before breakfast and lunch. Patients sensitive to drugs or supplements may start

with 200 mg every day. Dosage is increased to 800 mg every day or 400 mg twice a day if no improvement occurs after 2 weeks
- For migraine headaches, 200 mg to 400 mg, taken twice a day by mouth.

 SAFETY RISK *Patients taking SAM-e should take additional B_6, B_{12}, and folic acid to help limit homocysteine levels. Increased homocysteine levels may increase the risk of CV disease.*

Hazards

Adverse effects associated with S-adenosylmethionine include headache, diarrhea, nausea, and GI disturbances. There are no reported interactions with SAM-e.

Patients with bipolar disorder should avoid this product because of the risk of inducing mania.

Clinical considerations

- A patient may try to diagnose or treat severe or life-threatening depression on his own. Determine the extent of the patient's depression and make appropriate referrals for psychiatric help, as needed.
- Although no chemical interactions have been reported in clinical studies, consider the pharmacologic properties of the product and the risk that it could interfere with therapeutic effects of conventional drugs.
- SAM-e can be stopped without adverse effects, although depression may recur.
- Advise patient to take additional B_6, B_{12}, and folic acid while taking this herb.
- Tell patient that product should start working within 2 weeks of beginning administration; dosage may need to be increased if no results are seen within that time.
- Instruct patient to have a medical evaluation before taking this product for depression or other symptoms.
- Recommend that patient promptly notify health care provider about new symptoms or adverse effects.
- Warn patient to keep all herbal products away from children and pets.

- Tell patient to remind prescriber and pharmacist of any herbal and dietary supplements that he's taking when obtaining a new prescription.
- Advise patient to consult his health care provider before using this product because a treatment with proven efficacy may be available.

Research summary
The concepts behind the use of SAM-e and the claims made regarding its effects haven't yet been validated scientifically.

santonica

Artemisia cina, *levant, levant wormseed, sea wormwood*

Santonica is obtained from *Artemisia cina*. It contains 1,8 cineole and sesquiterpene lactone beta-santonin, which gives the herb its action against intestinal worms, particularly ascarids. It also may reduce fever. Santonica is available as a powder or lozenges, and in combination products.

Reported uses
Santonica is used to treat intestinal parasites such as *Ascaris* and *Oxyuris* (roundworm, threadworm). It is ineffective against tapeworm.

 SAFETY RISK *Given the toxicity of santonica, other, safer anthelmintic agents should be used instead of this herb.*

Administration
To treat infestation of intestinal worms in adults, 25 mg powder, taken by mouth. In children, the dosage is calculated by the following formula: The child's age in years is multiplied by 2; the result is the dosage amount in milligrams. The herb must be taken with a laxative to ensure expulsion of the worms.

 SAFETY RISK *Fatal poisonings have been reported after ingestion of less than 10 g of this herb.*

Hazards
Adverse effects associated with santonica include headache, muscle twitching, stupor, epileptiform seizures, visual disorders, xanthopsia, gastroenteritis, nausea, vomiting, kidney irritation, and allergic reactions. There are currently no known interactions with santonica.

Patients allergic to members of the Compositae family, which includes ragweed, chrysanthemums, marigolds, and daisies, should avoid this herb. Avoid in pregnancy and while breast-feeding as effects are unknown. Avoid in patients prone to seizures.

Clinical considerations
- To treat intestinal worms, santonica must be taken with a laxative to ensure expulsion.
- Warn patient with seizure disorders not to use santonica.
- Advise patient to avoid using this herb if he's allergic to members of the Compositae family, which includes ragweed, chrysanthemums, marigolds, daisies, and other herbs.
- Advise pregnant or breast-feeding patient not to use this herb.
- Warn patient not to take herb before seeking medical attention because doing so may delay diagnosis of a potentially serious medical condition.
- Instruct patient to promptly notify health care provider about new symptoms or adverse effects.
- Tell patient to remind prescriber and pharmacist of any herbal and dietary supplements that he's taking when obtaining a new prescription.
- Advise patient to consult his health care provider before using an herbal preparation because a treatment with proven efficacy may be available.

Research summary
The concepts behind the use of santonica and the claims made regarding its effects haven't yet been validated scientifically.

sarsaparilla

Anantamul, anantamula, gopakanya,
Indian sarsaparilla, kapuri, khao yen,
naga-jihva, sariva, sarsa, smilax,
Smilax glabra, S. glauca, S. officinalis

Sarsaparilla is obtained from dried root
of Smilax officinalis. It contains saponins, phytosterols, resin, shikimic acid,
terpene alcohols, glycosides, tannins, and
essential oils. The hepatoprotective effect
of sarsaparilla may be based in part on its
ability to bind endotoxins. Antimicrobial
and antipsoriatic activity may be caused
by saponins. It may also act against *Tre-*
ponema pallidum, the organism that
causes syphilis. Sarsaparilla also has diuretic, anti-inflammatory, and hepatoprotective effects. It's available as dried
root, capsules, and tablets, and in products such as EveCare, Renalka, and Sty-
plon.

Reported uses
Sarsaparilla is used to treat psoriasis,
rheumatism, kidney problems (including
kidney stones), other urinary problems,
syphilis, and venereal disease. It's used as
a tonic to improve appetite, digestion, vitality, and virility, and is popular among
body-builders. Sarsaparilla is also used to
improve ailments and excretion of wastes
from the blood, and as a flavoring agent
in medicines.

Administration
- Capsules or tablets: 9 g of dried root by
mouth three times a day, in divided doses
- Decoction: 3 cups by mouth every day,
prepared by placing 1 to 2 teaspoons of
root in 1 cup of water and simmering for
10 to 15 minutes
- Tincture: 1 to 2 ml in 1 cup of warm
water by mouth three times a day.

Hazards
Adverse effects associated with sarsaparilla include GI irritation, nausea, kidney irritation, and occupational asthma from
root dust.

Patients with recurrent kidney stones
should avoid this herb. No one should
take large doses for long periods. Sarsaparilla should be avoided by patients taking hypnotics, digitalis, or bismuth.

Clinical considerations
- If patient takes a drug that contains
digitalis or bismuth, tell him to stop taking sarsaparilla.
- Urge patient to promptly notify a
health care provider about new symptoms or adverse effects.
- Tell patient to remind prescriber and
pharmacist of any herbal and dietary
supplements that he's taking when obtaining a new prescription.
- Advise patient to consult his health
care provider before using an herbal
preparation because a treatment with
proven efficacy may be available.

Research summary
The concepts behind the use of sarsaparilla and the claims made regarding its effects haven't yet been validated scientifically.

sassafras

Ague tree, cinnamon wood,
kuntze saloop, laurus sassafras,
Sassafras albidum, S. officinale,
S. radix, S. variifolia

Sassafras is obtained from root of *Sas-*
safras albidum. The volatile oil contains
safrole (5% to 8%); other constituents
include anethole, asarone, camphor,
eugenol, myristicin, and pinene apiole.
Sassafras elicits a mild antidiuretic response. Safrole and its major metabolite,
1-hydroxysafrole, are carcinogenic and
neurotoxic. Sassafras is available as dried
root bark, and in products such as Saloop, Sassafrax, and Saxifras.

Reported uses

Sassafras is used orally to treat eye or mucous membrane inflammation, catarrh, bronchitis, high blood pressure, kidney disorders, arthritis, cancers, and syphilis; as a sudorific tonic and blood purifier; and as a flavoring agent. It's used topically as an antiseptic and to treat skin eruptions, insect bites and stings, rheumatism, gout, sprains, and swelling.

 SAFETY RISK *Sassafras has been banned by the FDA as a drug or food product; it may be carcinogenic and has caused many adverse reactions, including death.*

Administration

Sassafras has been banned by the FDA and shouldn't be taken.

Hazards

Adverse effects associated with sassafras include ataxia, CNS depression, hallucinations, hot flashes, paralysis, shakes, stupor, exhaustion, spasm, hypertension, tachycardia, CV collapse, dilated pupils, ptosis, vomiting, liver cancer, hypothermia, contact dermatitis, diaphoresis, abortion, carcinogenesis, and hypersensitivity.

Additive effects may occur if sassafras is used with barbiturates and sedatives. Advise patient to avoid using together. Increased metabolism and decreased blood levels of drugs metabolized by cytochrome P-450 and P-488 may occur if phenytoin is used with sassafras. Therapeutic and adverse effects may be enhanced if sassafras is used with herbs with sedative effects, including calamus, calendula, California poppy, capsicum, catnip, celery, couch grass, elecampane, German chamomile, goldenseal, gotu kola, hops, Jamaica dogwood, kava, lemon balm, sage, shepherd's purse, Siberian ginseng, skullcap, stinging nettle, St. John's wort, valerian, wild carrot, and wild lettuce. Potential additive toxicity may occur if sassafras is used with safrole-containing herbs, including basil, camphor, cinnamon, and nutmeg. Alcohol may enhance CNS depressant effects of sassafras.

Because of its carcinogenic potential, sassafras shouldn't be used in any form.

Clinical considerations

- Sassafras will alter phenytoin levels.
- Warn patient not to take herb before seeking medical attention because doing so may delay diagnosis of a potentially serious medical condition.
- Tell patient to remind prescriber and pharmacist of any herbal and dietary supplements that he's taking when obtaining a new prescription.
- Advise patient to consult his health care provider before using an herbal preparation because a treatment with proven efficacy may be available.

Research summary

The concepts behind the use of sassafras and the claims made regarding its effects haven't yet been validated scientifically. Because of its proven toxicity, it shouldn't be used.

saw palmetto

American dwarf palm tree, cabbage palm, fan palm, sabal, scrub palm, Serenoa repens, *shrub palmetto*

Saw palmetto is obtained from berries of *Serenoa repens*. It contains fatty acids, fatty acid esters, sitosterols, and phytosterols. Its mechanism of action is poorly understood, but oleic and linoleic acids may inhibit 5-alpha reductase conversion of testosterone to dihydrotestosterone (DHT), thus reducing prostate enlargement. It may also inhibit androgenic activity by competing with DHT for androgen receptors, thereby affecting testosterone metabolism. Saw palmetto also has anti-inflammatory, immunostimulant, and astringent properties and inhibits prolactin and growth factor-induced cell proliferation. It improves urine flow rate, nocturia, and postvoid residual volume and prostate size in benign prostatic hypertrophy (BPH). Saw palmetto is available as tablets, capsules, fresh and dried berries, and extracts, and in products such as Permixon, PlusStrogen, Propalmex, and Quanterra Prostate.

Reported uses
Saw palmetto is used to treat symptoms of BPH and cough and congestion from colds, bronchitis, or asthma. It's also used as a mild diuretic, urinary antiseptic, and astringent.

Administration
The average daily dose of saw palmetto is 160 mg, taken by mouth twice a day, or 320 mg, taken by mouth once a day (1 to 2 g fresh berries or 320 mg of lipophilic extract).

Hazards
Adverse effects associated with saw palmetto include headache, hypertension, nausea, abdominal pain, diarrhea, urine retention, and back pain. Saw palmetto possibly has estrogenic, androgenic, and alpha-blocking effects. Drug dosages of adrenergics, hormones, and hormone-like drugs may need adjustment if patient takes this herb.

Pregnant or breast-feeding patients and women of childbearing age shouldn't use this herb. Adults and children with hormone-dependent illnesses other than BPH or breast cancer should avoid this herb. Avoid taking with any hormone therapy, including hormone replacement and oral contraceptives.

Clinical considerations
■ Herb should be used with caution for conditions other than BPH because data about its effectiveness in other conditions are lacking.
■ Advise patient that saw palmetto may not alter prostate size.
■ The effects of this herb's lipophilic preparation take 4 to 6 weeks to occur.

■ Warn patient not to take herb for bladder or prostate problems before seeking medical attention because doing so could delay diagnosis of a potentially serious medical condition.
■ Tell patient to take herb with food to minimize GI effects.
■ Caution patient to promptly notify health care provider about new or worsened adverse effects.
■ Warn patient to avoid herb if planning pregnancy, if pregnant, or if breast-feeding.
■ Tell patient to remind prescriber and pharmacist of any herbal and dietary supplements that he's taking when obtaining a new prescription.
■ Advise patient to consult his health care provider before using an herbal preparation because a treatment with proven efficacy may be available.

Research summary
The concepts behind the use of saw palmetto and the claims made regarding its effects haven't yet been validated scientifically.

scented geranium

Pelargonium spp.

Scented geranium is obtained from leaves of certain *Pelargonium* species. It contains l-citronellol, alcohols, esters, aldehydes, and ketones. Its mechanism of antibacterial and antifungal effects is unknown. Scented geranium is available as whole plant and an essential oil.

Reported uses
Scented geranium is used as a mosquito repellent and for antibacterial and antifungal effects. It's also used as an analgesic, antidepressant, expectorant, astringent, diuretic, sedative, flavoring agent, and fragrance.

Administration
Dosage for scented geranium isn't well documented.

Hazards
Adverse effects associated with scented geranium include edema, dermatitis, erythema, vesiculation, and cheilitis. There are no known interactions with scented geranium.

Patients hypersensitive to members of the geranium family should avoid this herb.

Clinical considerations
- Pelargoniums are common annuals and houseplants of many different species and varieties. They shouldn't be confused with plants of the genus Geranium.
- Inform patient that few data are available regarding medicinal use of geraniums. Tell him that scented geranium has questionable efficacy as a topical mosquito repellent and may cause dermatitis.
- Instruct patient to promptly notify health care provider about new or worsened adverse effects.
- Warn patient to keep all herbal products away from children and pets.
- Tell patient to remind prescriber and pharmacist of any herbal and dietary supplements that he's taking when obtaining a new prescription.
- Advise patient to consult his health care provider before using an herbal preparation because a treatment with proven efficacy may be available.

Research summary
The concepts behind the use of scented geranium and the claims made regarding its effects haven't yet been validated scientifically.

schisandra

Gomishi, hoku-gomishi, kita-gomishi, omicha, Schisandra chinensis, schizandra, wu-wei-zu

Schisandra is obtained from *Schisandra chinensis*. It contains 10% organic acids, including carboxylic, malic, citric, tartaric, and nigranoic acids, as well as vitamins E and C. More than 30 lignins have been identified in seeds and fruit (about 2% of fruit by weight), including schizandrin and related compounds and many gomisin compounds. Lignins may have pronounced liver-protecting effects. Herb may have astringent and nervous system stimulant effects. Schisandra is available as dried berries, seeds, and fluid extract, in products such as Clarity, Immunity, NutraPack, ParaCleanse, and Schizandra Plus.

Reported uses
Schisandra is used to treat dry cough, asthma, night sweats, chronic fatigue, nocturnal seminal emissions, chronic diarrhea, and various lung, liver, and kidney disorders. It's also used to improve mental alertness and reflex responses, relieve eye fatigue, increase visual acuity, and ease depression caused by adrenergic exhaustion.

Administration
- Decoction: 1 cup taken every 8 hours, prepared by adding 5 g crushed berries to 100 ml water, boiling, and then simmering
- Liquid extract (1:1 in 12% to 15% grain alcohol or glycerin base): 1.25 to 3 ml by mouth three times a day
- Tea: 2 to 3 cups by mouth every day, prepared by adding 2 to 4 tablespoons dried berries to 2 cups of water, boiling, and then simmering until liquid is reduced to 1 cup.

Hazards

Adverse effects associated with schisandra include restlessness, insomnia, CNS depression, heartburn, altered ALT levels, and dyspnea. Schisandra may potentiate effects of body-strengthening drugs and raise blood pressure.

Pregnant or breast-feeding patients should avoid this herb, as should patients who have epilepsy, peptic ulcers, fever, or high blood pressure.

Clinical considerations

- Patient with peptic ulcer may develop increased acidity.
- Monitor liver function tests.
- Advise patient to avoid taking schisandra before having liver function tests because herb may alter ALT test results.
- Tell patient to take herb with meals to minimize GI upset.
- Advise patient to avoid using this herb when pregnant or breast-feeding.
- Warn patient to keep all herbal products away from children and pets.
- Tell patient to remind prescriber and pharmacist of any herbal and dietary supplements that he's taking when obtaining a new prescription.
- Advise patient to consult his health care provider before using an herbal preparation because a treatment with proven efficacy may be available.

Research summary

The concepts behind the use of schisandra and the claims made regarding its effects haven't yet been validated scientifically.

sea holly

Eryngio herba, Eryngium campestre, *eryngo, sea holme, sea hulver*

Sea holly is obtained from *Eryngium campestre.* Its above-ground parts contain triterpene saponins, caffeic acid esters such as chlorogenic acid and rosmaric acid, and flavonoids. Its roots contain procoumarins, pyranocoumarins, and oligosaccharides. The above-ground plant parts have a mild diuretic effect; the roots have antispasmodic and mild expectorant effects. Sea holly is available as leaves, powdered root, and extract.

Reported uses

Above-ground parts are used to treat UTI, prostatitis, and inflamed bronchial mucous membranes. Roots are used to treat kidney and bladder stones, renal colic, kidney and urinary tract inflammation, urine retention, edema, cough, bronchitis, and skin and respiratory disorders.

Administration

- Decoction: 2 to 3 cups every day, prepared by boiling 4 teaspoons ground root in 1 L water for 10 minutes, steeping 15 minutes, and then straining
- Tea: 3 to 4 cups every day, prepared by steeping 1 teaspoon ground root in 150 ml boiling water until cold, and then straining
- Tincture: 50 to 60 gtt by mouth every day, divided into 3 or 4 doses, prepared by soaking 20 g powdered root in 80 g of 60% alcohol for 10 days.

Hazards

There are no known adverse effects associated with sea holly. Herbal products that contain alcohol may cause a disulfiram-like reaction. Advise patient to avoid using together. Pregnant or breast-feeding women shouldn't use this herb.

Clinical considerations

- Monitor patient's response to herbal therapy.
- Advise pregnant or breast-feeding patient not to use this herb.
- Advise patient to promptly notify health care provider about adverse effects or changes in symptoms.
- Tell patient to remind prescriber and pharmacist of any herbal and dietary supplements that he's taking when obtaining a new prescription.

■ Advise patient to consult his health care provider before using an herbal preparation because a treatment with proven efficacy may be available.

Research summary
The concepts behind the use of sea holly and the claims made regarding its effects haven't yet been validated scientifically.

self-heal

All-heal, blue curls, brownwort, brunella, carpenter's herb, carpenter's weed, heal-all, heart of the earth, Hercules woundwort, hock-heal, hook-heal, Prunella vulgaris, *sicklewort, siclewort, slough-heal, woundwort*

Self-heal is obtained from *Prunella vulgaris*. It contains oleanolic acid, urosolic acid, rutin, hyperoside, caffeic acid, vitamins, carotenoids, tannis, essential oils, and alkaloids. Urosolic acid is cytotoxic against lymphocytic leukemia cells and human lung cancer cells. Also contains rosmarinic acid, an antioxidant, and prunellin, which may have anti-HIV activity. Some marginal cytotoxicity against human colon and mammary tumor cells has also been reported. Self-heal is available as dried herb, capsules, tea, and tincture.

Reported uses
Self-heal is used to treat wounds, stop bleeding, control diarrhea, support the liver, and aid circulation. It's also used as a gargle for mouth and throat infections, as a cooling tea, and as a treatment for tuberculosis, jaundice, infectious hepatitis, bacillary dysentery, pleuritis with effusion, and cancer. It's also used as an antibiotic, antihypertensive, antimutagenic, and antioxidant, especially in patients with HIV and cancer.

Administration
■ Infusion: 6 to 15 g of dried herb steeped for 10 minutes in 8 oz of water, by mouth three times a day
■ Tincture: 1 to 2 ml by mouth three times a day
■ Topical: Juice or poultice applied to affected area.

Hazards
There are no known adverse effects associated with self-heal. Herbal products that contain alcohol may cause a disulfiram-like reaction. Advise patient to avoid using together. Patients hypersensitive to any part of the herb shouldn't take prunella. Pregnant or breast-feeding women shouldn't use this herb. Safety in children isn't known.

Clinical considerations
■ Because entire plant is used, sensitivity reactions are possible.
■ Patient may combine topical and liquid forms of prunella with other herbal products. Read product ingredients carefully.
■ Although no chemical interactions have been reported in clinical studies, consider the pharmacologic properties of the herb and its potential to interfere with therapeutic effects of conventional drugs.
■ Advise patient with allergies to flowers, such as hay fever and ragweed, to use this herb with caution.
■ Advise pregnant or breast-feeding patient to avoid using this herb.
■ Urge patient to consult with health care provider before taking self-heal.
■ Tell patient to promptly notify health care provider about adverse effects or changes in symptoms.
■ Tell patient to remind prescriber and pharmacist of any herbal and dietary supplements that he's taking when obtaining a new prescription.
■ Advise patient to consult his health care provider before using an herbal preparation because a treatment with proven efficacy may be available.

Research summary
The concepts behind the use of self-heal and the claims made regarding its effects haven't yet been validated scientifically.

senega

Milkwort, mountain flax,
Plantula marilandica, *poligala raiz,*
Polygala senega, P. virginiana,
*polygale de virginie, rattlesnake root,
seneca, senegawurzel, snake root,
snakeroot yuan zhi*

Senega is obtained from *Polygala senega.* It contains triterpenoid saponins (senegenin, polygalin, and polygalic acid), which exert expectorant action on the lining of the upper GI tract and stomach. Senega is available as a dried root, liquid extract, infusion, syrup, lozenges, tea, and tincture. It's an ingredient in a variety of preparations, including Antibron, Asthma 6-N, Bronchiplant, Calmarum, Cocillana-Etyfin, Combitorax, Desbly, Dinacode, Hederix, Makatussin, Neo-Codion, Nyl Bronchitis, Patussol, Pectocalamine, Pectoral N, Phol-Tux, Polery, Pulmofasa, Quintopan, and Wampole Bronchial Cough Syrup.

Reported uses
Senega is used with other expectorants for chronic bronchitis and for treating pneumonia or the second stage of acute bronchial catarrh. It is currently used mainly as an expectorant by patients with bronchitis who have poor sputum output. It's also used as an antidote for some poisons, as a poultice for external wounds, and as an abortifacient. It's also used for general ailments.

Administration
■ Fluid extract (1:1 in 60% alcohol): 0.3 to 1 ml (6 to 20 gtt) by mouth three times a day, or 1.5 to 3 g by mouth every day
■ Infusion: 0.5 to 1 g of herb in 1 cup of water by mouth two or three times a day; in severe cases, every 2 hours, as long as patient is being monitored for adverse effects
■ Root: 1.5 to 3 g by mouth every day
■ Tincture (1:4 in 60% alcohol): 2.5 to 5 ml (50 to 100 gtt) by mouth three times a day, or 2.5 to 7.5 g by mouth every day.

Hazards
Adverse effects include nausea, vomiting, GI irritation, diarrhea, increased bronchial secretion, and diaphoresis. Herbal products that contain alcohol may cause a disulfiram-like reaction. Advise patient to avoid using together. Patients hypersensitive to senega shouldn't use this herb. Patients with GI disorders (such as peptic ulcer disease and inflammatory bowel disease) and those who are pregnant or breast-feeding also shouldn't use this herb. Pediatric effects are unknown and such use isn't recommended.

 SAFETY RISK *Be careful not to confuse senega with the herb senna.*

Clinical considerations
■ Prolonged use of seneca has been linked to GI irritation.
■ Monitor patient for nausea, diaphoresis, vomiting, GI complaints, and diarrhea. These problems may indicate an overdose, an adverse reaction, or sensitivity to senega. Emetic properties of the herb at high doses make further toxicity self-limiting.
■ Monitor patient, especially if he has diagnosed respiratory condition, for shortness of breath or other respiratory difficulties from increased bronchial secretions.
■ Tell patient to read product labels carefully because senega is usually taken with other herbs or substances.
■ Caution patient against prolonged use.
■ Recommend that patient stop taking senega if he develops nausea, GI discomfort, vomiting, diarrhea, or increased respiratory problems.

- Tell patient that liquid forms may contain alcohol, which can interact with other drugs.
- Advise pregnant or breast-feeding patient not to use this herb.
- Tell patient to remind prescriber and pharmacist of any herbal and dietary supplements that he's taking when obtaining a new prescription.
- Advise patient to consult his health care provider before using an herbal preparation because a treatment with proven efficacy may be available.

Research summary

The concepts behind the use of senega and the claims made regarding its effects haven't yet been validated scientifically.

senna

Alexandria senna, Cassia acutifolia, C. senna, *India senna, Khartoum senna, sennae folium, tinnevelly senna*

Senna is obtained from dried leaves and pods of *Cassia acutifolia* or *C. angustifolia*. It contains 1.2% to 6% dianthrone glycosides — primarily sennosides A, A1, and B with lesser amounts of C, D, E, F, and G — together with other anthraquinone derivatives that contribute to the laxative effect. Senna increases peristalsis, probably by direct effect on intestinal smooth muscle. It probably either irritates the muscles or stimulates the colonic intramural plexus. Senna is activated in the colon to rheinanthrone. Because activation takes 6 to 12 hours, a bedtime dose typically produces a morning bowel movement. It also promotes fluid accumulation in the colon and small intestine. Senna is available as granules, fluid extract, suppository, syrup, and tablets, and in products such as Black-Draught, Dr. Caldwell Senna Laxative, Fletcher's Castoria, Gentlax,

Senexon Senna-Gen, Senokot, Senolax, and X-Prep Bowel Evacuant.

Reported uses

Senna is used as a laxative to treat constipation or ease bowel evacuation after rectal-anal surgery or if patient has anal fissures or hemorrhoids. It's also used for colon evacuation before rectal and bowel examination or surgery. It's commonly used to treat constipation caused by narcotics. Senna has been investigated as a treatment for fecal soiling, herpes simplex, and infections with *Escherichia coli* or *Candida albicans*.

Administration

The following are general ranges; dosage should be individualized to the smallest dose needed to produce a soft stool. Elderly, debilitated, antepartum, and postpartum patients start with smallest doses. If comfortable elimination doesn't occur by the second day, dosage can be adjusted until evacuation occurs.
- For adults, to evacuate colon for rectal and bowel examinations: Dosage is 75 ml of a standardized senna preparation (1 ml standardized to 26 mg sennoside B)
- For adults with constipation: Dosage is 0.5 to 3.0 g crude herb or 15 to 40 mg sennosides (standardized preparations) taken by mouth, ideally before bed
- For children: Several OTC products are available for children older than age 6 or who weigh more than 60 lb (27 kg). See product labels.

Hazards

Adverse effects associated with senna include arrhythmias, disorders of heart function, rhinoconjunctivitis, GI cramping or gripping, diarrhea, nausea, perianal irritation, aggravated constipation, yellowish-brown or red urine, nephritis, nephropathies, albuminuria, hematuria, damage to renal tubules, hyperaldosteronism, accelerated bone deterioration, muscle weakness, asthma, reversible finger clubbing, IgE-mediated allergy, and loss of fluid and electrolytes, especially potassium.

Overuse or abuse of senna may interfere with the action of antiarrhythmics, cardiac glycosides, including digoxin, and lanoxin via loss of potassium. With extended use, monitor patient's serum potassium levels and heart rate. Senna may increase risk of hypokalemia and potentiation of cardioactive steroids, and may rarely cause heart arrhythmias when used with corticosteroids. With extended concurrent use, monitor patient's serum potassium levels, vital signs, and ECG. When senna is used with estrogen, it may cause decreased serum estrogen levels. NSAIDs may decrease effect of senna. Absorption of some drugs may be decreased by decreased transit time in the colon. Monitor patient for decreased efficacy, especially patients previously well controlled. When used with thiazide diuretics, including furosemide (Lasix), there may be an increased risk of hypokalemia. Senna used with potassium-depleting herbs such as gossypol, horsetail plant, or licorice may increase the risk of hypokalemia. Stimulant laxative herbs such as aloe dried leaf sap, black root, blue flag rhizome, butternut bark, cascara bark, castor oil, colocynth fruit pulp, gamboge bark exudate, jalap root, manna bark exudate, podophyllum, rhubarb root, senna leaves and pods, wild cumber fruit, and yellow dock root may cause an increased risk of hypokalemia.

Senna should be avoided by patients with intestinal obstruction, diarrhea, abdominal pain of unknown origin, fluid and electrolyte imbalance, and acute inflammatory intestinal diseases, such as appendicitis, colitis, Crohn's disease, and irritable bowel syndrome. Those with renal disease should use the herb with caution. There's no consensus in international labeling regarding use of senna by pregnant or breast-feeding women. In Britain and Germany, senna is contraindicated for these conditions. In the United States, no label restrictions appear on standardized OTC products. Studies have not shown that standardized senna products stimulate uterine contractions in pregnant women. The German Commission E doesn't recommend senna for children younger than age 12; however, several OTC products available in the United States provide dose recommendations for children older than age 6 or weighing more than 60 pounds.

Clinical considerations

■ Although senna may be taken as a tea, dosages are difficult to determine or adjust using this unstandardized form. Many OTC products with standardized ingredients and doses are available. Adult dosages for senna can range from 20 to 60 mg of hydroxyanthracene derivatives.

■ Infusions made in cold water may contain less of the compounds suspected to cause abdominal pain.

■ Geriatric patients are usually advised to start with half the typical adult dose.

■ Herb takes effect 6 to 8 hours after administration and isn't suitable for patients with rapid emptying of the bowels.

■ Long-term use is undesirable; however, if patient has chronic constipation, long-term use may be warranted with proper care, including potassium replacement.

■ Long-term use may reduce spontaneous bowel function and lead to "cathartic colon" and laxative-dependency syndrome.

■ Typical symptoms of laxative abuse include abdominal pain, weakness, fatigue, thirst, vomiting, edema, bone pain caused by osteomalacia, fluid and electrolyte imbalance, hypoalbuminemia caused by protein-losing gastroenteropathy, and syndromes that mimic colitis.

■ Evidence of overdose includes vomiting, severe GI spasms, and thin, watery stools. Large overdoses may also cause nephritis.

■ *Melanosis coli* develops in about 5% of people who use anthranoids over the long term (4 to 13 months). It resolves after discontinuation. There's no definite link between anthracene drugs and colon cancer.

- Other anthranoids, such as cassic acid, appear in breast milk in small amounts and may give milk a brownish tint. No data exist to determine whether the anthranoid level is associated with diarrhea in nursing infants.
- Monitor patient's serum potassium during concurrent use of senna and cardiac glycosides, thiazide diuretics, corticosteroids, antiarrhythmics, licorice, potassium-depleting herbs, or other stimulant laxative herbs.
- Encourage patient to first try lifestyle changes — such as increasing dietary fiber, fluid intake, and exercise — to restore normal bowel function. Patient can also use a bulk laxative.
- Tell patient that senna may turn urine yellowish-brown or red.
- Recommend that pregnant or breast-feeding patient consult a health care provider before using senna.
- Inform patient that senna preparations may contain alcohol or sugar; patient should check product label if he has alcohol or sugar restrictions.
- Instruct patient not to take stimulant laxatives for longer than 1 or perhaps 2 weeks without seeking medical advice.
- Advise patient that rectal bleeding or failure to have a bowel movement after using a laxative may indicate a serious condition.
- Instruct patient to stop using senna if he has or develops nausea, vomiting, abdominal pain, loose stools, or diarrhea.
- Tell patient to contact a health care provider if his bowel habits change suddenly for 2 weeks or longer.
- Warn patient to keep all herbal products away from children and pets.
- Tell patient to remind prescriber and pharmacist of any herbal and dietary supplements that he's taking when obtaining a new prescription.
- Advise patient to consult his health care provider before using an herbal preparation because a treatment with proven efficacy may be available.

Research summary

The concepts behind the use of senna and the claims made regarding its effects haven't yet been validated scientifically.

shark cartilage

Shark cartilage is obtained from shredded and dried cartilage of the hammerhead shark (*Sphyrna lewini*) and the spiny dogfish shark (*Squalus acanthias*) captured in the Pacific Ocean. Shark cartilage is purported to have anticancer properties by inhibiting angiogenesis (new blood vessel formation) in tumors. Another hypothesis for the anticancer effect involves a class of proteins normally present in cartilage and bone called tissue inhibitors of metalloproteinases, or TIMPs. TIMPs block enzymes that tumors use to invade surrounding tissue. An inhibitor or a series of inhibitors of neovascularization present in shark cartilage have been identified as guanidine extractable protein. A family of complex carbohydrates and mucopolysaccharides may be the primary anti-inflammatory components. Shark cartilage is available as a powder and capsules, in products such as BeneFin and Cartilade.

Reported uses

Shark cartilage is used to treat or prevent cancer and to treat osteoarthritis, rheumatoid arthritis, psoriasis, lupus, eczema, and enteritis. It's also used to assist in bone and wound healing and to maintain proper bone and joint function. Powder is also used as a retention enema. Data from ongoing studies may help define the role of shark cartilage in the treatment of lung cancer, AIDS-associated Kaposi's sarcoma, and prostate cancer.

Administration

No consensus exists on the dosage for anticancer effects or other uses.
- For benefit of additional cartilage protein and calcium: 6 g powder in 1 glass of water or juice by mouth

■ To maintain proper bone and joint function: 4 g powder in 1 glass of water or juice by mouth.

Hazards

There are no known adverse effects or interactions associated with shark cartilage.

Shark cartilage shouldn't be used by children or by pregnant or breast-feeding women. Patients recovering from MI or CVA shouldn't use this product because inhibition of angiogenesis may interfere with revascularization of an infarcted area.

Clinical considerations

■ No data exist regarding toxicity of shark cartilage.

■ Warn patient not to take shark cartilage before seeking medical attention because doing so may delay diagnosis of a potentially serious medical condition.

■ Tell patient not to use shark cartilage if pregnant or breast-feeding unless advised by a knowledgeable health care provider. Effects of shark cartilage on pregnant or breast-feeding women are unknown.

■ Warn patient not to take shark cartilage after a recent MI or CVA. Explain that shark cartilage may inhibit the body's ability to form new blood vessels, which may obstruct healing in the injured heart or brain area.

■ Tell patient to remind prescriber and pharmacist of any herbal and dietary supplements that he's taking when obtaining a new prescription.

■ Advise patient to consult his health care provider before using an herbal preparation because a treatment with proven efficacy may be available.

Research summary

The concepts behind the use of shark cartilage and the claims made regarding its effects haven't yet been validated scientifically.

shepherd's purse

Blindweed, capsella,
Capsella bursa pastoris, *case-weed, cocowort, lady's purse, mother's heart, pepper-and-salt, pick-pocket, poor man's parmacettie, rattle pouches, sanguinary, shepherd's heart, shepherd's scrip, shepherd's sprout, shovelweed, St. James' weed, toywort, witches' pouches*

Shepherd's purse is obtained from *Capsella bursa pastoris.* It contains the amino acid proline, cardioactive steroids, and a peptide with hemostatic oxytocin-like activity. Also contains saponins, flavonoids, large amounts of potassium salts, oxalates, vitamin C, and sinigrin. Sinigrin can be degraded to allyl isothiocyanate, which is linked to goiter and abnormal thyroid function. Shepherd's purse increases uterine contractions by stimulating smooth muscle. Cardioactive steroids in the seeds cause positive and negative inotropic and chronotropic effects. Muscarine-like, dose-dependent hypertensive and antihypertensive effects are also reported. Shepherd's purse is available as a dried herb and liquid extract.

Reported uses

Shepherd's purse is used internally to treat dysmenorrhea, mild menorrhagia, and metrorrhagia. It's also used for headache, mild cardiac insufficiency, arrhythmia, hypotension, nervous heart complaints, premenstrual complaints, hematemesis, hematuria, diarrhea, and acute catarrhal cystitis. Topically, it's used as a styptic for nosebleeds and other superficial bleeding injuries.

Administration

■ Dried above-ground parts: 10 to 15 g by mouth every day; may be taken as 1 to 4 g of dried herb three times a day

- Fluid extract (1:1 in 25% alcohol): 5 to 8 g or 1 to 4 ml by mouth three times a day
- Tea: 1 to 4 g dried herb steeped in 150 ml of boiling water for 15 minutes and then strained
- Topical form: 3 to 5 g of herb steeped in 180 ml of boiling water for 10 to 15 minutes and then strained; fluid is applied to affected area.

Hazards

Adverse effects associated with shepherd's purse include sedation, palpitations, hypertension, hypotension, increased uterine contractions, abnormal menstruation, and abnormal thyroid function.

Possible reduced effect of antihypertensives and antihypotensives may occur if used with shepherd's purse. Monitor blood pressure closely. Possible reduced effect of CV drugs may occur if used with shepherd's purse. Herbal products that contain alcohol may cause a disulfiram-like reaction. Additive effects may occur if shepherd's purse is used with sedatives. Allyl isothiocyanate may interfere with thyroid therapy. Monitor thyroid function in patients previously well controlled.

Shepherd's purse may have possible additive effects if used with herbs with sedative effects, including calamus, calendula, California poppy, capsicum, catnip, celery, cough grass, elecampane, German chamomile, goldenseal, gotu kola, hops, Jamaica dogwood, kava, lemon balm, sage, sassafras, Siberian ginseng, skullcap, stinging nettle, St. John's wort, valerian, wild carrot, wild lettuce, and yerba maté.

Shepherd's purse is a uterine stimulant and may cause abortion; it shouldn't be used by women planning pregnancy or those who are pregnant or breast-feeding. Patients with a history of kidney stones should use shepherd's purse with caution because of its oxalate content.

 SAFETY RISK *Shepherd's purse commonly harbors endophytic fungi such as* Albugo candida *and* Peronospora parasitica. *Because it may*

contain mycotoxins, patients with compromised immune systems should use the herb with caution.

Clinical considerations

- The use of shepherd's purse instead of ergot for uterine bleeding is inappropriate because of inadequate activity.
- Monitor blood pressure, which may increase or decrease, and thyroid function in patient taking thyroid medication who was previously well controlled.
- Monitor patient for palpitations, especially if susceptible to arrhythmias.
- Warn patient not to use alcohol-containing forms if he takes disulfiram, metronidazole, or any other drug that interacts with alcohol.
- Inform women that shepherd's purse may cause abnormal menstruation.
- Tell patient that this herb may aggravate kidney stones, CV therapy, thyroid therapy, and antihypertensive or antihypotensive therapy. Affected patients should use shepherd's purse with caution and only under direct supervision by a knowledgeable health care provider.
- Advise patient that herb may cause or increase sedation and the adverse effects of other herbs or drugs that cause sedation.
- Caution patient to avoid hazardous tasks until full sedative effects of herb are known.
- Urge patient to promptly notify health care provider about new symptoms or adverse effects.
- Tell patient to store herb away from light and moisture, and to keep it away from children and pets.
- Tell patient to remind prescriber and pharmacist of any herbal and dietary supplements that he's taking when obtaining a new prescription.
- Advise patient to consult his health care provider before using an herbal preparation because a treatment with proven efficacy may be available.

Research summary

The concepts behind the use of shepherd's purse and the claims made regarding its effects haven't yet been validated scientifically.

skullcap

Blue pimpernel, helmet flower, hoodwort, mad-dog weed, madweed, Quaker bonnet, scullcap, Scutellaria lateriflora, *Virginian skull cap*

Skullcap is obtained from the roots and leaves of *Scutellaria lateriflora*. It contains flavonoids such as apigenin, baicalein, baicalin, hispidulin, scutellarein, and scutellarin. Also contains sesquiterpenes such as cadinene, caryophyllene, catapol, limonene, and terpineol. Other compounds include wogonin and its glucuronide, which can inhibit sialidase, an enzyme linked to some cancers. Lignin and various tannins are also present. Extracts from *S. baicalensis* may modulate hematopoiesis, scavenge free radicals, and increase nitric oxide production. Extracts may have some bacteriostatic, bactericidal, anti-inflammatory, and antifungal activity. Skullcap is available as a dried herb, extracts, and capsules.

Reported uses
Skullcap is used as an anticonvulsant, antispasmodic, anti-inflammatory, and sedative. It's also used as an adjunct to chemotherapy to enhance immune response.

Administration
- Dried herb: 1 to 2 g as a tea by mouth three times a day
- Liquid extract (1:1 in 25% alcohol): 2 to 4 ml by mouth three times a day.

Hazards
Adverse effects associated with skullcap include confusion, headache, seizures, arrhythmias, and hepatotoxicity. Herbal products that contain alcohol may cause a disulfiram-like reaction. Advise patient to avoid using together.

Pregnant or breast-feeding women shouldn't use this herb.

Clinical considerations
- Skullcap preparations may be contaminated with other substances.
- Monitor patient for adverse effects and response to herbal treatment.
- Warn patient not to take herb before seeking medical attention because doing so may delay diagnosis of a potentially serious medical condition.
- Advise pregnant or breast-feeding patient not to use this herb.
- Instruct patient to promptly notify health care provider about any new symptoms or adverse effects.
- Advise patient to keep all herbal products away from children and pets.
- Tell patient to remind prescriber and pharmacist of any herbal and dietary supplements that he's taking when obtaining a new prescription.
- Advise patient to consult his health care provider before using an herbal preparation because a treatment with proven efficacy may be available.

Research summary
The concepts behind the use of skullcap and the claims made regarding its effects haven't yet been validated scientifically.

skunk cabbage

Dracontium, meadow cabbage, pole-cat cabbage, polecatweed, skunkweed, Symplocarpus foetidus

Skunk cabbage is obtained from seeds, rhizomes, and roots of *Symplocarpus foetidus*. It contains starch, gum sugar, fixed and volatile oils, iron, various alkaloids, phenolic compounds, glycosides, and tannins. The leaves are also said to contain hydroxytryptamine. The root contains calcium oxalate. Skunk cabbage is available as a powdered root, extract, and tincture.

Reported uses

Skunk cabbage is used for treating chest tightness, as in asthma and bronchitis, and as an antispasmodic, diaphoretic, emetic, expectorant, and sedative.

Administration

- Liquid extract (1:1 in 25% alcohol): 0.5 to 1 ml by mouth three times a day
- Powdered root: 0.5 to 1.0 g in honey, three times a day.

Hazards

Adverse effects associated with skunk cabbage include headache, vertigo, intense burning of oral mucosa, vision impairment, nausea, vomiting, renal damage, inflammation, itching, and irritation.

Herbal products that contain alcohol may cause a disulfiram-like reaction. Advise patient to avoid using together. Oxalates reduce the absorption of iron and calcium.

Pregnant or breast-feeding women shouldn't use this herb. Patients with renal or GI disease should avoid use of this herb.

 SAFETY RISK *Skunk cabbage shouldn't be ingested. It is listed in the AMA's* Handbook of Poisonous and Injurious Plants.

Clinical considerations

- Monitor patient's response to herbal therapy.
- Warn patient not to take herb for asthma or bronchitis before seeking medical attention because doing so may delay diagnosis of a potentially serious medical condition.
- Instruct patient to seek appropriate medical attention if he's short of breath or has a persistent cough.
- Advise pregnant or breast-feeding patient not to use this herb.
- Advise patient with renal or GI disorder not to use this herb.
- Warn patient to keep all herbal products away from children and pets.
- Tell patient to remind prescriber and pharmacist of any herbal and dietary

supplements that he's taking when obtaining a new prescription.
- Advise patient to consult his health care provider before using an herbal preparation because a treatment with proven efficacy may be available.

Research summary

The concepts behind the use of skunk cabbage and the claims made regarding its effects haven't yet been validated scientifically.

slippery elm

American elm, Indian elm, moose elm, red elm, sweet elm, Ulmus rubra

Slippery elm is obtained from the inner bark of *Ulmus rubra*. It contains mucilage composed of hexoses, methylpentosans, pentosans, and polyuronides. Other constituents include phytosterols, sesquiterpenes, calcium oxalate, and tannins that may have astringent activity. Slippery elm is available as a powdered bark, liquid extract, lozenges, and capsules.

Reported uses

Slippery elm is used externally as a demulcent to soothe and soften skin and as an emollient that coats and protects irritated tissues. It's also used to treat wounds, burns, and various skin conditions. It's used internally to treat diverticulitis, gastritis, gastric and duodenal ulcers, herpes, and syphilis. It's also used as an abortifacient, a lubricant to ease labor, and a nutritional source in baby food.

Administration

- Decoction (1:8 with alcohol): 4 to 16 ml by mouth every day
- For GI discomfort: 5 ml liquid extract by mouth three times a day
- Topical use: Poultice is prepared from powdered bark in boiling water. Applied to affected area.

Hazards

Allergic reaction may occur with the slippery elm pollen. Herbal products that contain alcohol may cause a disulfiram-like reaction. Advise patient to avoid using together.

Pregnant or breast-feeding women shouldn't use this herb because safety data are lacking.

Clinical considerations

■ Although no chemical interactions have been reported in clinical studies, consider the pharmacologic properties of the herb and its potential to interfere with therapeutic effects of conventional drugs.
■ Monitor patient's response to herbal therapy.
■ Warn patient not to use herb for burns or wounds before seeking medical attention because doing so may delay diagnosis of a potentially serious medical condition.
■ Instruct patient to promptly notify health care provider about new symptoms and adverse effects.
■ Advise pregnant or breast-feeding patient not to use this herb.
■ Warn patient to keep all herbal products away from children and pets.
■ Tell patient to remind prescriber and pharmacist of any herbal and dietary supplements that he's taking when obtaining a new prescription.
■ Advise patient to consult his health care provider before using an herbal preparation because a treatment with proven efficacy may be available.

Research summary

The concepts behind the use of slippery elm and the claims made regarding its effects haven't yet been validated scientifically.

soapwort

Bouncing bet, bruisewort, crow soap, dog cloves, Fuller's herb, latherwort, old maid's pink, red soapwort root, Saponaria officinalis, *soap root, soapwood, sweet Betty, wild sweet William*

Soapwort is obtained from leaves, roots, and rhizomes of *Saponaria officinalis*. It contains saponin, sapotoxin, saponarine, and other saporins. Other components include flavonoids, resin, and gum. Saponins are cytotoxic compounds that may be active against various cancers, including lymphoma, leukemia, melanoma, and breast cancer. The seeds of *S. officinalis* have ribosome-inactivating activity. Soapwort is available as dried leaves, root, and fluid extract.

Reported uses

Soapwort is used as an expectorant for cough and other respiratory tract disorders, a gargle for tonsillitis, a diaphoretic, and a diuretic. It's also used for GI complaints, liver and kidney disorders, rheumatic gout, and such skin conditions as acne, eczema, psoriasis, and poison ivy. It's also used to alter metabolism. Externally, its lathering action has led to use in shampoo and bath preparations.

Administration

Soapwort herb:
■ Constipation: Decoction of leaves, 2 glasses by mouth every day
■ Daily dose: Aqueous extract, 1 to 2 g every day
Soapwort root:
■ Decoction: 10 to 180 g root added to 1 g sodium carbonate and simple syrup to make 200 g
■ Expectorant: 9 ml (about 2 tsp) of the decoction by mouth every 2 hours
■ Tea: 0.4 g of medium fine cut root; 1 teaspoon contains about 2.6 g of herb.

Hazards

Adverse effects associated with soapwort include neurotoxicity, GI irritation, nausea, vomiting, diarrhea, nephrotoxicity, hepatotoxicity, localized irritation, and mucous membrane irritation. There are no reported interactions with soapwort.

Women who are pregnant or breast-feeding shouldn't use this herb. Patients with GI disorders should avoid using this herb because it irritates the gastric mucosa.

 SAFETY RISK *Internal use of soapwort isn't recommended. Soapwort is listed in the FDA/ CFSAN Poisonous Plant Database.*

Clinical considerations

■ Although no chemical interactions have been reported in clinical studies, consider the pharmacologic properties of the herb and its potential to interfere with therapeutic effects of conventional drugs.
■ Monitor patient's liver and kidney function periodically.
■ If patient takes herb internally, watch for adverse effects, such as vomiting and diarrhea.
■ Observe patient for localized skin reactions.
■ Warn patient not to take herb for extended periods before seeking medical attention because a persistent cough may indicate a potentially serious medical condition.
■ Advise pregnant or breast-feeding patient not to use this herb.
■ Advise patient with GI disorder not to use this herb.
■ Instruct patient to notify a health care provider about adverse effects, such as localized skin reactions or nausea.
■ Tell patient to store herb in a tightly sealed container that protects it from light and moisture.
■ Warn patient to keep all herbal products away from children and pets.
■ Tell patient to remind prescriber and pharmacist of any herbal and dietary supplements that he's taking when obtaining a new prescription.
■ Advise patient to consult his health care provider before using an herbal preparation because a treatment with proven efficacy may be available.

Research summary

The concepts behind the use of soapwort and the claims made regarding its effects haven't yet been validated scientifically.

sorrel

Common sorrel, cuckoo's meate, cuckoo sorrow, dock, garden sorrel, green sauce, green sorrel, Rumex acetosa, R. acetosella, sheep sorrel, sour dock, sourgrass, sour sauce, soursuds

Sorrel is obtained from leaves, winged achenes, and roots of *Rumex acetosa*. It contains oxalates (such as oxalic acid and calcium oxalate) and anthracene derivatives, such as physcion, chryosphanol, emodin, and rhein. Other components include ascorbic acid, tartaric acid, and tannins. Sorrel is available as a tea, liquid extract, and coated tablets.

Reported uses

Sorrel is used for acute and chronic inflammation of nasal passages and the respiratory tract. It's also used as an adjunct to antibacterial therapy and as an antiseptic, an astringent, and a diuretic.

Administration

■ Liquid extract (19% alcohol): 50 gtt by mouth three times a day
■ Tablets: For adults, 2 coated tablets three times a day.

Hazards

Adverse effects associated with sorrel include headache, nausea, flatulence, renal damage, and liver damage. Herbal products that contain alcohol may cause a disulfiram-like reaction. Advise patient to avoid using together. Oxalates reduce the absorption of iron and calcium.

Pregnant or breast-feeding women shouldn't use this herb. Patients with a history of kidney stones should use this herb with caution.

SAFETY RISK *High oxalate salt content may lead to significant toxicity and even death if enough herb is ingested. Such oxalate poisoning can occur with consumption of large quantities of leaves as a salad.*

Clinical considerations
- Advise patient not to consume this herb as its oxalates are toxic.
- Monitor closely patient's response to herbal therapy.
- Warn patient not to take herb for inflammatory or respiratory symptoms before seeking medical attention because doing so may delay diagnosis of a potentially serious medical condition.
- Advise pregnant or breast-feeding patient not to use this herb.
- Instruct patient to promptly notify health care provider about adverse effects or a change in symptoms.
- Warn patient to keep all herbal products away from children and pets.
- Tell patient to remind prescriber and pharmacist of any herbal and dietary supplements that he's taking when obtaining a new prescription.
- Advise patient to consult his health care provider before using an herbal preparation because a treatment with proven efficacy may be available.

Research summary
The concepts behind the use of sorrel and the claims made regarding its effects haven't yet been validated scientifically.

Sound therapy

Sound therapy is based on the theory that certain sounds can have a therapeutic effect on the mind and body. Sound is created by the vibration of objects and travels from one source to another as waves. It enters the body not only through the ears but also as vibrations through other body parts such as the skull.

Pleasant, soothing sounds, such as a babbling brook, birds chirping, or a Mozart sonata, can relax a person and make him feel better. However, sound therapy goes beyond this accepted fact. Practitioners have developed techniques that focus sound waves on targeted areas of the body to achieve specific therapeutic goals. Sound therapists believe that even sounds that aren't loud enough to be heard can still cause a response in the body. Music therapy is probably the most commonly used form of sound therapy. Other forms of sound therapy include the following:

- *Auditory integration training,* a technique developed in the 1950s, uses simulations of the stages of listening development to repattern the hearing range and attention span. The Electronic Ear, developed by French doctor Alfred Tomatis, exercises the muscles of the middle ear, allowing a person to hear a wider range of frequencies. Using this device, patients with dyslexia, autism, learning disabilities, and attention deficit hyperactivity disorder have learned how to listen more effectively. Creativity, musical ability, foreign language learning ability, and organizational abilities are also said to have improved.

Another form of auditory integration training uses a device called the Ears Education and Retraining System (EERS) to desensitize patients who are hypersensitive to high-frequency sounds. This device was developed by another French doctor, Guy Berard, who believed that certain behavioral and cognitive disorders could be traced to distorted perception of sound frequencies. In this technique, sounds — usually music — are filtered to eliminate the frequencies to which the patient is sensitive. The EERS then electronically modulates these frequencies and returns them through headphones to the patient's ears. After listening to the processed sounds, the listener is often able to accept that frequency. This type of training has been successful with autistic children who suffer from hypersensitivity.

■ *Toning* is a technique in which a person tries to release stress by making elongated vowel sounds that are believed to resonate throughout the body. Practitioners claim that toning also improves the speaking and singing voice. Toning is thought to be more beneficial than singing because it moves the vocal chords more slowly, allowing the vibrations to perform their internal massage. Gregorian chant, performed by Benedictine monks as part of their religious ritual, is similar to toning.

■ *Cymatic therapy* involves the use of a computerized instrument to transmit sound waves directly through the skin. This technique is based on the theory that illness is a form of resonant disequilibrium. Practitioners claim that cymatic therapy reestablishes healthy resonance in unhealthy tissues. They explain that cymatic therapy doesn't heal directly, but rather places the body in the proper condition for healing itself. Cymatic therapy is said to help children with learning disorders, such as dyslexia and attention deficit hyperactivity disorder. This technique has been used in the United States since the late 1960s, mainly by nurses, chiropractors, osteopaths, and acupuncturists. Training is necessary if one is to become a cymatic practitioner.

■ The *Infratonic QGM* is a machine that uses sound frequencies to reduce pain and headaches, increase circulatory function, relax muscles, and increase the brain's production of alpha waves. This device, invented by a Chinese scientist, simulates the high-level secondary sound waves emitted from the hands of Chinese qigong masters. It's recognized as a pain management tool in China.

Reported uses

Relief of muscle tension and alleviation of stress are the health problems for which sound therapy is most commonly used. Proponents say that it can also reduce pain, ease anxiety, stimulate the immune system, lower blood pressure, and improve communication in patients with autism, learning disabilities, and Alzheimer's disease. Sound therapy may be most effective for autistic patients. Before sound therapy, treatment options for autism were limited and rarely successful.

How the treatment is performed

Sound therapy can be performed in almost any setting, as long as the environmental needs can be met. The session should take place in a quiet, private room that's free from distractions and has a comfortable place for the patient to sit or recline. The specific equipment needed depend on the form of sound therapy being used.

Most of the more advanced sound therapy techniques are performed by a trained sound therapist. However, you can assist your patient with toning, a simple technique involving only the vocal cords. Begin by explaining the procedure to the patient and answering any questions. Inform him that the vibrations from the elongated vowel sounds, or tones, may help relax him and ease his stress.

When he's ready to start, help him to a comfortable position. Ask him to close his eyes and focus on listening. With his eyes closed, have him take a deep, easy breath and start humming a soft, resonant tone. Explain that the type of sound — high, low, or pretty — doesn't matter. Tell him to continue humming and to concentrate on the vibrations the sound is making in his chest and head. Instruct him to let the sound rise and fall naturally, without effort. After a few minutes, have him place his hands on his cheeks and feel the sound. Tell him to feel the sound in his face and skull as he continues to hum the tone for another 5 minutes. Then have him relax his hands and finish by making another sound, such as "ah," for another 5 minutes.

When the patient is finished, ask him if he notices a relaxation in his body, mind, and breathing. Document the session and the patient's response.

Hazards

Simple sound therapy, such as toning, isn't associated with any complications. The patient may experience an unpleasant sensation — similar to the reaction some people have to fingernails scratching a blackboard — from the more complex forms, such as auditory integration training or cymatic therapy. If the patient has an unpleasant reaction, stop the therapy immediately and notify the doctor. Document the patient's reaction, clinical condition, and response to any interventions you initiate.

Clinical considerations

Cymatic therapy isn't recommended for patients with pacemakers because the resonance of the sound waves may interfere with the pacemaker function. It is also contraindicated for patients with a heart condition because the stimuli can affect the heart rate, and for patients who can't tolerate loud or jarring sounds. Make sure that all equipment is cleaned between patient sessions.

Research summary

The concepts behind most sound therapies (except for music therapy) and the claims made for them haven't yet been validated scientifically.

southernwood

Appleringie, Artemisia abrotanum, *boy's love, garde robe, lad's love, old man, southern wormwood*

Southernwood is obtained from *Artemisia abrotanum*. It contains a volatile essential oil, mostly absinthol, as well as artemisitin, hydroxycoumarins such as umbelliferone and isofraxidin, and tannins. Recently, four flavonols possessing spasmolytic activity have been isolated. Herb has tonic, antiseptic, antimicrobial, anthelmintic, and stimulant effects. Southernwood is available as a dried herb and fluid extract.

Reported uses

Southernwood is used internally to treat fever, infections, and irregular menstruation, as an emmenagogue, and as a bitter to improve digestion. It is applied externally to treat baldness and dandruff, poorly healing or gangrenous wounds, ulcers, and insect bites. It's also used to repel moths, fleas, flies, and mosquitoes.

Administration

- Fluid extract: ½ to 1 dram
- To stimulate menstruation, 1 oz of herb is added to 1 pint boiling water; the resulting tea is taken by mouth three times a day.

Hazards

Adverse effects associated with southernwood include liver damage. Tannic acid may form insoluble complexes if southernwood is used with alkaloids, glycosides, and heavy metal ions such as aluminum and zinc. Altered coagulation may occur if southernwood is used with antiplatelet drugs (such as aspirin), heparin, low-molecular-weight heparin, and warfarin. Monitor PT and International Normalized Ratio closely.

Pregnant or breast-feeding women should avoid this herb, as should patients with a history of liver disease. Using herb to treat burns has caused toxicity.

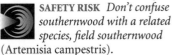 **SAFETY RISK** *Don't confuse southernwood with a related species, field southernwood* (Artemisia campestris).

Clinical considerations

- Southernwood shouldn't be consumed.

- Significant amounts of tannic acid present in the plant may lead to liver damage.
- Advise patient with history of liver disease not to use this herb.
- Monitor patient for signs of bleeding, especially if he takes an anticoagulant.
- Advise pregnant or breast-feeding patient not to use this herb.
- Monitor patient's response to herbal therapy.
- Instruct patient to have a medical evaluation before taking this herb and not to consume large quantities of it.
- Tell patient to consult with his health care provider if he takes the herb for any medical condition that doesn't improve in 2 weeks.
- Tell patient to store herb in a sealed container protected from light.
- Warn patient to keep all herbal products away from children and pets.
- Tell patient to remind prescriber and pharmacist of any herbal and dietary supplements that he's taking when obtaining a new prescription.
- Advise patient to consult his health care provider before using an herbal preparation because a treatment with proven efficacy may be available.

Research summary
The concepts behind the use of southernwood and the claims made regarding its effects haven't yet been validated scientifically.

soy

Glycine max, *Glycine soja, soya, soyabean, soybean*

Soy is obtained from beans (seeds) of *Glycine max*. It contains soy protein, isoflavones, saponins, phenolic acids, lecithin, phytoestrols, amino acids, vitamins A, E, K, and some B; and minerals such as calcium, potassium, iron, and phosphorus. Isoflavones are molecularly similar to natural body estrogens (phytoestrogens). The isoflavones in soy, particularly genistein and daidzen, have antioxidant and phytoestrogenic properties. Saponins enhance immune function and bind to cholesterol to limit its absorption in the intestines. Phenolic acids have antioxidant properties. Phytoestrols and other components, including lecithin, may lower cholesterol levels.

Isoflavones may reduce the risk of hormone-dependent cancers, such as breast and prostate cancer, as well as other forms of cancer. Increased consumption of soy in Asian populations helps account for decreased rates of CV disease. Soy-based diets lead to significant decreases in total cholesterol, HDL levels, and LDL levels. The FDA officially supports the claim that soy protein may decrease blood cholesterol levels.

The mild estrogenic activity of soy isoflavones may help to alleviate menopausal symptoms in some women. However, no clinical data exist concerning the effect of soy on other symptoms of menopause, such as night sweats, insomnia, vaginal dryness, or changes in sexual desire. Soy consumption may also help regulate hormone levels in premenopausal women. Soy may also have a beneficial effect on GI function. Soy is available as soy protein or isoflavone supplements in powder, capsules, or tablets. Also available as beans, flour, and many food items such as sprouts, tofu, tempeh, soy milk, textured and hydrolyzed vegetable protein, meat substitutes, miso, and soy sauce.

Reported uses
Soy is used to treat cancers, CV disease, menopausal symptoms, and osteoporosis. It's also used as a detoxicant, a circulatory stimulant, and a popular dietary protein supplement.

Administration
No consensus exists for the administration of soy. The FDA currently recommends 25 g soy protein by mouth daily. Other sources suggest beneficial CV ef-

fects with doses of 30 to 50 g by mouth daily.

Hazards

Adverse effects that may be related to the use of soy include gastrointestinal effects, such as stomach pain, loose stool, and diarrhea, and asthma and allergic reaction.

Decreased absorption of calcium, iron, and zinc may occur if soy is also being taken. Possible reduced effects of estrogen, raloxifene, and tamoxifen may occur if soy is also being taken.

Patients hypersensitive to soy or soy-containing products shouldn't use this product. High doses of soy protein may have harmful effects in women with breast cancer. Infants shouldn't be fed soy-based formulas because of high isoflavone content. Inhalation of soy dust led to an asthma outbreak in 26 workers exposed to soy powder when unloading the product.

Clinical considerations

■ Soybeans and soybean products are an excellent source of protein, vitamins, and minerals.

■ Monitor patient's response to herbal therapy.

■ If patient takes estrogen, tamoxifen, or raloxifene, tell her to inform a health care provider if she also takes soy. Soy may interfere with therapeutic effects of these drugs.

■ To avoid disturbed absorption, instruct patient to separate consumption of zinc, iron, or calcium supplements by several hours from any soy products.

■ Warn patient to keep all herbal products away from children and pets.

■ Tell patient to remind prescriber and pharmacist of any herbal and dietary supplements that he's taking when obtaining a new prescription.

■ Advise patient to consult his health care provider before using an herbal preparation because a treatment with proven efficacy may be available.

Research summary

The concepts behind the use of soy and the claims made regarding its effects haven't yet been validated scientifically.

spirulina

Blue-green algae, dihe,
Spirulina maxima, S. platensis,
tecuitlatl

Spirulina is obtained from the blue-green algae *Spirulina maxima* and *S. platensis*. It contains about 65% protein and all essential amino acids. Spirulina is a concentrated source of other nutrients, including chlorophyll, beta-carotene, other carotenoids, high levels of B-complex vitamins, including B_{12}, minerals, and essential fatty acids, including gamma linolenic acid and omega-3 fatty acid. Spirulina may enhance disease resistance, inhibit allergic reactions, and exert hepatoprotective and hypocholesterolemic effects. Spirulina contains the blue pigment, phycocyanin, a biliprotein that has been shown to inhibit cancer colony formation. The protein content of spirulina is comparable to other sources, such as meat and milk. Spirulina is available as a powder, flakes, capsules, and tablets.

Reported uses

Spirulina is used as a nutritional supplement and energy booster and to treat obesity, diabetes mellitus, and oral cancers. Also useful in arthritis.

Administration

Average daily dose: 2,000 to 3,000 mg by mouth every day in divided doses.

Hazards

Allergic reaction may occur with the use of spirulina, along with inhibited absorption of vitamin B_{12}. There are no reported interactions with spirulina. Spirulina grown in contaminated water may concentrate such toxic metals as lead, mercury, and cadmium.

Clinical considerations
- Advise patient to store product in a cool, dry place, not to freeze it, and to keep it away from children and pets.
- Tell patient to remind prescriber and pharmacist of any herbal and dietary supplements that he's taking when obtaining a new prescription.
- Advise patient to consult his health care provider before using an herbal preparation because a treatment with proven efficacy may be available.

Research summary
The concepts behind the use of spirulina and the claims made regarding its effects haven't yet been validated scientifically.

squaw vine

Checkerberry, deerberry, deer berry,
Mitchella repens, *one berry,*
partridgeberry, partridge berry,
squawberry, winter clover

Squaw vine is obtained from above-ground parts of *Mitchella repens*. It contains resin, dextrin, mucilage, saponin, wax, alkaloids, glycosides, and tannins. Herb has tonic, antispasmodic, diuretic, and astringent effects. Squaw vine is available as a dried herb, extract, and tincture.

Reported uses
Squaw vine is used to treat dysmenorrhea or amenorrhea and to aid labor and childbirth. It's also used to treat sore nipples and to stimulate lactation. Squaw vine is used to treat insomnia, colitis, dysuria, diarrhea, heart failure, liver failure, and seizures. It's used topically to treat pain, especially with arthritis.

Administration
- For sore nipples: 2 oz of fresh herb is added to 1 pint boiling water, strained, and added to an equal amount of cream. Mixture is boiled to a soft consistency, allowed to cool, then applied to nipples after each breast-feeding session
- Infusion: 1 teaspoon of herb is added to 1 cup boiling water, steeped for 10 to 15 minutes, and taken three times a day
- Strong decoction: 2 to 4 oz of fresh herb is added to 1 pint boiling water, strained, and then cooled; 2 to 4 oz is taken by mouth two or three times a day
- Tincture: 1 to 2 ml is taken by mouth three times a day.

Hazards
Adverse effects associated with squaw vine include liver damage, and, in the case of overdose, severe stomach and kidney irritation. Tannic acid in squaw vine may form insoluble complexes with alkaloid-related substances, such as iron- or zinc-containing products. Squaw vine may increase the effects of cardiac glycosides.

Pregnant or breast-feeding women should use herb with caution.

Clinical considerations
- Human toxicity is rare and is only likely to occur after ingestion of large amounts of tannic acid.
- Advise patient to consult health care provider if taking the herb for any condition that doesn't improve within 2 weeks. Chronic symptoms may indicate a more serious problem.
- Instruct patient to promptly notify a health care provider about new symptoms or adverse effects.
- Tell patient not to exceed recommended dosage.
- Advise patient to store herb in a cool, dry place, not to freeze it, and to keep it away from children and pets.
- Tell patient to remind prescriber and pharmacist of any herbal and dietary supplements that he's taking when obtaining a new prescription.
- Advise patient to consult his health care provider before using an herbal preparation because a treatment with proven efficacy may be available.

Research summary
The concepts behind the use of squaw vine and the claims made regarding its effects haven't yet been validated scientifically.

squill

European squill, Indian squill, Mediterranean squill, red squill, sea onion, sea squill, Urginea indica, U. maritima, *white squill*

Squill is obtained from bulbs of *Urginea maritima* and *U. indica.* It contains several cardioactive steroid glycosides, including scillaren A, glucoscillaren A, scillaridin A, and scilliroside and proscillaridin A, which exert digitalis-like activity. Squill components also have diuretic, natriuretic (increases urinary sodium excretion), stimulant, expectorant, and emetic action. One component, silliglaucosidin, has shown anticancer activity. Squill is available as a powder or syrup.

Reported uses
Squill is used to treat cancer, arthritis, gout, dysmenorrhea, and warts. It's also used to treat mild (New York Heart Association I and II) cardiac insufficiency, arrhythmias, and reduced kidney capacity. However, squill extracts have been superseded by widespread use of digitalis glycosides. Squill is a component of some cough preparations because of its weak expectorant effect.

Red squill has been used externally in hair tonics for dandruff and seborrhea; however, it's mainly used as a rodenticide.

Administration
- Cardiotonic: 0.1 to 0.5 g standardized squill powder by mouth
- Expectorant (Syrup of squill, USP): 30 minims by mouth.

Hazards
Adverse effects associated with squill include fatigue, dizziness, seizures, coma, headache, life-threatening cardiac effects, arrhythmias, bradycardia, hypotension, vomiting, nausea, diarrhea, and loss of appetite.

If squill is used with calcium, digoxin, diuretics, extended glucocorticoid therapy, laxatives, or quinidine, there is an increased risk of digitalis-like toxicity. If squill is used with methylxanthines, such as theophylline; phosphodiesterase inhibitors, including amrinone, cilostazol, and milrinone; quinidine; or sympathomimetics, including epinephrine and phenylephrine, there is an increased risk of cardiac arrhythmias. Monitor ECG closely if these drugs are taken together.

Squill should be avoided by patients with second- or third-degree atrioventricular block, hypercalcemia, hypokalemia, hypertrophic cardiomyopathy, carotid sinus syndrome, ventricular tachycardia, thoracic aortic aneurysm, or Wolff-Parkinson-White syndrome.

 SAFETY RISK *All squill species can cause digitalis-like toxicity, which may lead to nausea, vomiting, diarrhea, fatigue, dizziness, arrhythmias, bradycardia, hypotension, seizures, and coma.*

Clinical considerations
- In patients with GI symptoms and bradyarrhythmias from presumed herbal poisoning, suspect cardiac glycoside poisoning as the cause.
- Because of the narrow therapeutic index of squill glycosides, adverse effects could occur rapidly in some patients even at therapeutic doses.
- Monitor vital signs and ECG, as indicated.
- Instruct patient to consult a health care provider if taking the herb for any condition that doesn't improve within 2 weeks. Chronic symptoms may indicate a more serious medical condition.
- Warn patient to contact a health care provider if he has an irregular heartbeat,

fainting, difficulty breathing, nausea, appetite loss, vomiting, diarrhea, or unusual weakness, tiredness, or drowsiness.

■ Instruct patient to store herb in a cool, dry place, not to freeze it, and to keep it away from children and pets.

■ Tell patient to remind prescriber and pharmacist of any herbal and dietary supplements that he's taking when obtaining a new prescription.

■ Advise patient to consult his health care provider before using an herbal preparation because a treatment with proven efficacy may be available.

Research summary

The concepts behind the use of squill and the claims made regarding its effects haven't yet been validated scientifically.

Static electromagnetic field therapy

Static electromagnetic field (EMF) therapy is another bioelectromagnetic (BEM) treatment that's being applied to cancer. This therapy uses magnets, which create a static EMF, as opposed to electromagnets, which create a pulsed EMF.

Although many substances are known carcinogens, it's been postulated that cancer is a single disease with a single root cause: acid-hypoxia; that is, an acidic, hypoxic environment makes tissues more susceptible to carcinogens. This theory holds that corrective treatment requires the creation of an alkaline-hyperoxic environment.

Therapy with a static bionorth (−) magnetic field is believed to produce such a state. As with cell-specific cancer therapy (CSCT), in static EMF therapy, targeted cancer cells don't revert to a normal state; they die. According to this theory, tumors may still be present after treatment, but they're no longer cancerous.

Reported uses

Practitioners apply static EMF therapy to a variety of cancers. As with conventional cancer treatments, they report that single, nonmetastatic lesions are more successfully treated than obstructive or metastatic lesions.

How the treatment is performed

Static EMF therapy uses high-gauss magnets. The higher the gauss, the better; practitioners prefer high-strength neodymium magnets. Equipment also includes magnetic chair pads, a 5″ × 6″ (12.5 × 15 cm) flexible magnet, and a magnetic mattress.

According to its practitioners, treatment with static EMF therapy consists of continuous, intense therapy with high-gauss magnets for at least 3 months. The bionorth (−) pole of the magnet is placed directly over the lesion, is kept there 24 hours a day for 3 months, and is removed only for bathing. In addition, the patient sits on a magnetic chair pad placed atop still another 5″ × 6″ magnet. When mobile, the patient wears a 5″ × 6″ flexible magnet over the heart. At bedtime, this flexible magnet is placed across the face, and the patient sleeps on a magnetic mattress, adding several other strong magnets as directed.

During the course of intense magnetic exposure, the patient is instructed to avoid toxic substances, such as tobacco, alcohol, pesticides, and other known carcinogens. The patient is also placed on a 4-day rotation diet that reduces exposure to individual foods and eliminates possible allergens, thereby supporting the immune system.

The goal of treatment is to create a more alkaline internal environment and subsequently greater oxygenation of tissues, the opposite of that required by cancer cells, which are anaerobic.

Practitioners believe that placing magnets over the forehead, eyes, and large intestine also helps increase production of melatonin, which is known to have antineoplastic values.

Hazards

Some practitioners believe that prolonged therapy with the biosouth (+) pole of the magnet—especially a high-gauss magnet—can overstimulate tissues and worsen the pain and symptoms of infection.

Clinical considerations

- Patients with pacemakers or defibrillators shouldn't use magnetic beds; furthermore, no magnets should be placed closer than 6″ (15 cm) from such devices to avoid interfering with their function.
- Older patients, children, and pregnant patients may be more sensitive and may require shorter and milder treatment.
- Pregnant patient should never use magnets on the abdominal area.
- Patient should avoid using magnets on the abdomen for 60 to 90 minutes after meals.
- To ensure patient safety, caution patient to seek practitioners who are affiliated with a medically supervised magnetic therapy research project.

Research summary

Similar to CSCT, practitioners justify static EMF therapy as being in line with current knowledge of cancer. It's considered noninvasive and nondestructive of healthy tissue but requires further and independent research.

St. John's wort

Amber, goatweed, hardhay, herb John, hexenkraut, Hypericum perforatum, *Johanniskraut, John's wort, klamath weed, millepertuis, Saint John's word, tipton weed, titson weed*

St. John's wort is obtained from *Hypericum perforatum.* It contains naphthodianthrones, including hypericin and pseudohypericin; hyperoside; quercitrin; rutin; isoquercitrin; bioflavonoids, including amentoflavone; 1,3,6,7-tetrahydroxy-xanthone; hyperforin; adhyperforin; aliphatic hydrocarbons, including 2-methyloctane and undecane; dodecanol; monoterpenes and sesquiterpenes, including alphapinene and caryophyllene; 2-methyl-3-but-3-en-2-ol, oligomeric procyanidines; catechin tannins; and caffeic acid derivatives, including chlorogenic acid. St. John's wort may have a slight inhibitory effect on MAO inhibitors and reuptake of serotonin. Hypericin has antiviral activity and also inhibits catechol O-methyltransferase and receptors for adenosine, benzodiazepines, GABA-A, GABA-B, and inositol triphosphate. Certain constituents have also shown antibacterial activity. St. John's wort is available as tablets, pellets, capsules of standardized extract, powdered or dried herb, liquid extract, tincture, and transdermal forms, in products such as Alterra, Hypercalm, Kira, Quanterra Emotional Balance, St. John's Wort Extracts, Tension Tamer, and various combination products.

Reported uses

St. John's wort is used orally for mild to moderate depression, anxiety, psychovegetative disorders, sciatica, and viral infections, including herpes simplex virus types 1 and 2, hepatitis C, influenza virus, murine cytomegalovirus, and poliovirus. St. John's wort has also been used to treat bronchitis, asthma, gallbladder disease, nocturnal enuresis, gout, and rheumatism, although it hasn't proven effective in these cases. It's used topically for contusions, inflammation, myalgia, burns, hemorrhoids, and vitiligo. In traditional Chinese medicine, St. John's wort has been used externally as a gargle for tonsillitis and as a lotion for dermatoses.

Administration

- Capsules or tablets for mild to moderate depression: Initially, 900 mg by mouth every day; for maintenance, 300 to 600 mg by mouth every day

- For depression: 2 to 4 g dried herb by mouth every day, or 0.2 to 1 mg hypericin
- For wounds, bruising, and swelling: Applied topically to affected area
- Liquid extract: (1:1) 2 to 4 ml by mouth every day
- Tea: 2 to 3 g of dried herb in boiling water
- Tincture:(1:10) 2 to 4 ml by mouth every day.

Hazards

Adverse effects associated with St. John's wort include fatigue, neuropathy, restlessness, headache, digestive complaints, fullness sensation, constipation, diarrhea, nausea, abdominal pain, dry mouth, photosensitivity reaction, pruritus, and delayed hypersensitivity.

Decreased effectiveness of St. John's wort, requiring possible dosage adjustment, may occur if used with amitriptyline, chemotherapy drugs, cyclosporine, digoxin, drugs metabolized by the cytochrome P-450 enzyme system, oral contraceptives, protease inhibitors, theophylline, and warfarin. Decreased sedative effects may occur if barbiturates are used with St. John's wort. St. John's wort may increase effects and cause possible toxicity and hypertensive crisis if used with MAO inhibitors, including phenelzine and tranylcypromine. Increased sedative effects of narcotics may occur if used with St. John's wort. Antagonized effects of reserpine may occur if used with St. John's wort. If St. John's wort is used with selective serotonin reuptake inhibitors, such as citalopram, fluoxetine, paroxetine, and sertraline, there is an increased risk of serotonin syndrome.

St. John's wort, used with tyramine-containing foods such as beer, cheese, dried meats, fava beans, liver, yeast, and wine, may cause hypertensive crisis when used together. Advise patient to separate administration times.

Herbs with sedative effects, such as calamus, calendula, California poppy, capsicum, catnip, celery, couch grass, elecampane, German chamomile, goldenseal, gotu kola, Jamaica dogwood, kava, lemon balm, sage, sassafras, skullcap, shepherd's purse, Siberian ginseng, stinging nettle, valerian, wild carrot, and wild lettuce, if taken with St. John's wort, may result in possible enhanced effects of either herb. Monitor patient closely, and advise to avoid using together. Possible increased sedative effects of alcohol may occur if used with St. John's wort. There is an increased risk of photosensitivity reactions when St. John's wort is used.

Pregnant patients and men and women planning pregnancy shouldn't take St. John's wort because of mutagenic risk to developing cells and fetus. Transplant patients maintained on cyclosporine therapy should avoid this herb because of the risk of organ rejection.

Clinical considerations

- Monitor patient for response to herbal therapy, as evidenced by improved mood and lessened depression.
- By using standardized extracts, patient can better control the dosage. Clinical studies have used formulations of standardized 0.3% hypericin as well as hyperforin-stabilized version of the extract.
- St. John's wort interacts with many other products; they must be considered before patient takes it with other prescription or OTC products.
- Serotonin syndrome may cause dizziness, nausea, vomiting, headache, epigastric pain, anxiety, confusion, restlessness, and irritability.
- Because St. John's wort decreases the effect of certain prescription drugs, watch for signs of drug toxicity if patient stops herb. Drug dosage may need reduction.
- St. John's wort has mutagenic effects on sperm cells and oocytes and adverse effects on reproductive cells; therefore, patient who is pregnant or planning pregnancy (including men) should avoid use.

- Topically, the volatile plant oil is an irritant. Monitor affected site for adverse effects and improvement.
- Monitor patient for sedative effects and GI complaints.
- Instruct patient to consult a health care provider for a thorough medical evaluation before using St. John's wort.
- Encourage patient to discuss depression and to seek regular psychiatric help, as indicated.
- Tell patient that St. John's wort may cause increased sensitivity to direct sunlight. Recommend protective clothing, sunscreen, and limited sun exposure.
- Inform patient that a sufficient washout period is needed after stopping a drug before switching to St. John's wort.
- Tell patient to report adverse effects to a health care provider.
- Warn patient to keep all herbal products away from children and pets.
- Tell patient to remind prescriber and pharmacist of any herbal and dietary supplements that he's taking when obtaining a new prescription.
- Advise patient to consult his health care provider before using an herbal preparation because a treatment with proven efficacy may be available.

Research summary

The concepts behind the use of St. John's wort and the claims made regarding its effects haven't yet been validated scientifically.

stone root

Citronella, Collinsonia canadensis, *hardback, hardhack, heal-all, horseweed, knob grass, knob root, knobweed, richleaf, richweed*

Stone root is available as a dried root or rhizome, tea, liquid extract, and tincture.

Stone root is obtained from *Collinsonia canadensis.* It contains volatile oils,

tannins, saponins, resin, mucilage, and caffeic acid derivatives.

Reported uses

Stone root is used for bladder inflammation, kidney stones, water retention, hyperuricuria, edema, GI disorders, headaches, and indigestion. In homeopathic medicine, stone root is used for hemorrhoids and constipation.

Administration

- Dried root: 1 to 4 g in 150 ml boiling water, steeped 5 to 10 minutes, and then strained; taken three times a day
- Liquid extract (1:1 in 25% alcohol): 1 to 4 ml by mouth three times a day
- Tincture (1:5 in 40% alcohol): 2 to 8 ml by mouth three times a day.

Hazards

Adverse effects associated with stone root include dizziness, numbness with ingestion of large quantities, irritation, abdominal pain, nausea, and painful urination.

Possible additive effects may occur if stone root is used with diuretics, including acetazolamide, furosemide, and hydrochlorothiazide. Advise patient to use with caution with other diuretics.

Possible additive effects may also occur if stone root is used with other herbs with diuretic action, such as gum acacia, Chinese cucumber, ginkgo, or sassafras. Advise patient to use with caution with other diuretics.

Pregnant or breast-feeding women should avoid this herb.

 SAFETY RISK *Stone root "citronella" isn't the same as true citronella oil* (Cymbopogon), *which is used as an insect repellent.*

Clinical considerations

- Because stone root may have diuretic effects, caution should be used when patient takes it with other herbs or drugs that have diuretic effects.
- Although no chemical interactions have been reported in clinical studies,

consider the pharmacologic properties of the herb and their potential to interfere with therapeutic effects of conventional drugs.

- Monitor patient's response to herbal therapy.
- Inform patient that stone root normally has a strong, unpleasant odor.
- Advise pregnant or breast-feeding patient not to take stone root.
- If patient takes a diuretic herb or drug, tell him to consult a health care provider before using stone root.
- Warn patient not to take herb for urinary or abdominal complaints before seeking medical attention because doing so may delay diagnosis of a potentially serious medical condition.
- Instruct patient to promptly notify health care provider about adverse effects or new symptoms.
- Advise patient to keep all herbal products away from children and pets.
- Tell patient to remind prescriber and pharmacist of any herbal and dietary supplements that he's taking when obtaining a new prescription.
- Advise patient to consult his health care provider before using an herbal preparation because a treatment with proven efficacy may be available.

Research summary

The concepts behind the use of stone root and the claims made regarding its effects haven't yet been validated scientifically.

sundew

Dew plant, Drosera ramentacea, D. rotundifolia, *lustwort, red rot, ros solis, round-leafed sundew, sonnenthau, youthwort*

Sundew is obtained from *Drosera ramentacea, D. rotundifolia, D. intermedia, D. anglica,* and others. It contains naphtho-quinone, thought to have antitussive, antimicrobial, secretolytic, and bronchospasmolytic effects. It may also have immunostimulant effects. Sundew is available as dried herb, tea, liquid extract, and tincture, and in products such as B&T Natural Relief – Cough.

Reported uses

Sundew is used orally for bronchitis, asthma, pertussis, coughing fits, and dry cough. May be used topically for warts.

Administration

- Average daily dose: 3 g dried plant by mouth
- Liquid extract (1:1 in 25% alcohol): 0.5 to 2 ml by mouth three times a day
- Tea: 1 to 2 g in 150 ml boiling water, steeped for 5 to 10 minutes, strained, and taken three times a day
- Tincture (1:5 in 60% alcohol): 0.5 to 1 ml by mouth three times a day.

Hazards

There are no known adverse effects associated with sundew. Herbal products that contain alcohol may cause a disulfiram-like reaction. Advise patient to avoid using together.

Pregnant or breast-feeding women shouldn't use this herb.

Clinical considerations

- Although few chemical interactions have been reported in clinical studies, consider the pharmacologic properties of the herb and its potential to interfere with therapeutic effects of conventional drugs.
- Warn patient not to take herb before seeking medical attention because doing so may delay diagnosis of a potentially serious medical condition.
- Advise patient not to use this herb while pregnant or breast-feeding.
- Warn patient that herb has a bitter, sour, hot taste.
- Warn patient not to take herb for persistent cough or difficulty breathing be-

fore seeking medical attention because doing so may delay diagnosis of a potentially serious medical condition.
- Instruct patient to promptly notify a health care provider about adverse effects or changes in symptoms.
- Warn patient to keep all herbal products away from children and pets.
- Tell patient to remind prescriber and pharmacist of any herbal and dietary supplements that he's taking when obtaining a new prescription.
- Advise patient to consult his health care provider before using an herbal preparation because a treatment with proven efficacy may be available.

Research summary
The concepts behind the use of sundew and the claims made regarding its effects haven't yet been validated scientifically.

sweet cicely

British myrrh, cow chervil,
Myrrhis odorata, *shepherd's needle, smooth cicely, sweet bracken, sweet chervil, sweet-cus, sweet-fern, sweet-humlock, sweets, the Roman plant*

Sweet cicely is obtained from *Myrrhis odorata*. Volatile oils and flavonoids may act as a digestive aid, an expectorant, and a carminative. Sweet cicely is available as ground root as a tonic or infusion. Also available as a salve.

Reported uses
Sweet cicely is used orally for asthma, trouble breathing, intestinal gas and colic, and for urinary tract, chest, and throat complaints. It's also used as an expectorant, a blood purifier, and a digestive aid. It's used topically to treat gout pain and acute wounds and sores.

Administration
The fresh herb salve is applied topically, as needed, to treat wounds, sores, and the pain associated with gout.

Hazards
There are no known adverse effects or interactions associated with sweet cicely. Pregnant or breast-feeding women shouldn't use this herb.

Clinical considerations
- Herb is generally thought to be harmless in typical quantities.
- Although no chemical interactions have been reported in clinical studies, consider the pharmacologic properties of the herb and its potential to interfere with therapeutic effects of conventional drugs.
- Warn patient not to take herb for breathing problems before seeking medical attention because doing so may delay diagnosis of a potentially serious medical condition.
- Advise pregnant or breast-feeding patient not to use this herb.
- Tell patient to promptly notify health care provider about adverse effects or changes in symptoms.
- Warn patient to keep all herbal products away from children and pets.
- Tell patient to remind prescriber and pharmacist of any herbal and dietary supplements that he's taking when obtaining a new prescription.
- Advise patient to consult his health care provider before using an herbal preparation because a treatment with proven efficacy may be available.

Research summary
The concepts behind the use of sweet cicely and the claims made regarding its effects haven't yet been validated scientifically.

sweet flag

Acorus calamus, *bacc*, *beewort*,
calamus, *cinnamon sedge*, *gladdon*,
myrtle-flag, *myrtle-grass*, *myrtle sedge*,
rat root, *sweet cane*, *sweet grass*,
sweet myrtle, *sweet root*, *sweet rush*,
sweet sedge, *vakhand*

Sweet flag is obtained from *Acorus calamus* or *A. gramineus*. There are four types of sweet flag, based on their content of asarone, a carcinogen. The North American type (*A. calamus* var. *americanus*) contains none of this component, but varieties from India do. Sweet flag also contains acorin, choline, resin, starch, calcium oxalate, tannins, mucilage, and asarone. Asarone is chemically related to reserpine. Sweet flag is available as an oil, extract, tincture, and dried and powdered rhizome.

Reported uses

Sweet flag is used orally for childhood colic, digestive complaints, fever, and sore throat. It's also used as a sweat inducer. It's used topically to treat rheumatism, angina, and gingivitis. Use of sweet flag as a flavoring agent in dental products, drinks, and medicines has been banned in the United States.

Administration

- Average daily dose: 1 to 3 g by mouth three times a day
- Liquid extract (1:1 in 60% alcohol): 1 to 3 ml by mouth three times a day
- Tea: One cup of tea by mouth three times a day; made from 1 to 3 g rhizome in 150 ml boiling water, steeped for 5 to 10 minutes, and strained
- Tincture (1:5 in 60% alcohol): 2 to 4 ml by mouth three times a day
- Wash: 250 to 500 g added to bath water.

Hazards

Adverse effects associated with sweet flag include sedation, tremors, seizures, and kidney damage.

Possible additive adverse reactions may occur if sweet flag is used with CNS depressants or MAO inhibitors. If sweet flag is used with histamine-2 (H_2)-receptor antagonists or proton pump inhibitors, decreased effect may be caused by acidifying effect of herb. Additive effects may occur if sweet flag is used with other herbs that cause sedation, including calendula, California poppy, capsicum, catnip, celery, couch grass, elecampane, German chamomile, golden seal, gotu kola, hops, Jamaica dogwood, kava, lemon balm, sage, sassafras, shepherd's purse, Siberian ginseng, skullcap, stinging nettle, St. John's wort, valerian, wild carrot, wild lettuce, withania root, and yerba maté. Possible additive sedative effects may occur if sweet flag is used with alcohol.

Pregnant or breast-feeding women shouldn't use this herb.

SAFETY RISK *Because of its potential cancer-causing properties, sweet flag is banned by the FDA for use in foods, medicine, and beverages in the United States. The cancer-causing component of sweet flag, asarone, usually isn't found in the North American variety; however, sweet flag from India contains large amounts of this chemical.*

Clinical considerations

- Chemical content of the supplement and its safety cannot be assured.
- If a patient is taking sweet flag, other sedative herbs or drugs should be avoided because of possible additive effects.
- Advise patient to avoid this herb in any form because of its cancer-causing potential.
- Inform patient taking sweet flag that other herbs or drugs that cause drowsiness should be avoided because of possible additive effects.
- Caution patient to avoid hazardous tasks until full sedative effects of herb are known.
- Tell patient to avoid alcohol while taking sweet flag because of possible additive sedative effects.

■ Advise pregnant or breast-feeding patient to avoid using this herb.
■ Instruct patient to promptly notify health care provider about adverse effects or change in symptoms.
■ Warn patient to keep all herbal products away from children and pets.
■ Tell patient to remind prescriber and pharmacist of any herbal and dietary supplements that he's taking when obtaining a new prescription.
■ Advise patient to consult his health care provider before using an herbal preparation because a treatment with proven efficacy may be available.

Research summary
The concepts behind the use of sweet flag and the claims made regarding its effects haven't yet been validated scientifically.

sweet violet

Garden violet, sweet violet herb,
Viola odorata, *violet*

Sweet violet is obtained from *Viola odorata*. It contains saponins that, in high doses, can irritate mucous membranes. In low doses, they act as expectorants. Also contains salicylic acid, methyl esters, and alkaloids. Herb has antimicrobial and bronchosecretolytic effects caused by saponin content. Sweet violet is available as dried or fresh root, dried flowers, and leaves, and in products such as Acnetonic, Herbal Pumpkin, and Sweet Violet Lotion.

Reported uses
Sweet violet is used as an expectorant in acute and chronic bronchitis, bronchial asthma, cough and cold symptoms, and late flu symptoms. It's also used as a sedative or relaxant, for urinary incontinence, and for GI complaints, such as heartburn, flatulence, and digestion problems.

Administration
■ Decoction: 1 tablespoon in boiling water in proportion to make a 5% w/v preparation, steeped for 10 to 15 minutes, and then strained; 1 tablespoon taken by mouth five to six times every day
■ Tea: 2 teaspoons herb in 250 ml boiling water, steeped for 10 to 15 minutes, then strained. Taken by mouth two to three times a day.

Hazards
There are no known adverse effects or interactions associated with sweet violet.

Clinical considerations
■ Sweet violet is often used in combination preparations for oral and topical use.
■ Although no chemical interactions have been reported in clinical studies, consider the pharmacologic properties of the herb and its potential to interfere with therapeutic effects of conventional drugs.
■ If patient takes sweet violet for respiratory problems, tell him to seek medical attention if it fails to relieve symptoms.
■ Instruct patient not to use more than recommended amounts because higher amounts can irritate the lining of the mouth, stomach, intestines, and lungs.
■ Urge pregnant or breast-feeding patient to consult a health care provider before using sweet violet.
■ Warn patient to keep all herbal products away from children and pets.
■ Tell patient to remind prescriber and pharmacist of any herbal and dietary supplements that he's taking when obtaining a new prescription.
■ Advise patient to consult his health care provider before using an herbal preparation because a treatment with proven efficacy may be available.

Research summary
The concepts behind the use of sweet violet and the claims made regarding its effects haven't yet been validated scientifically.

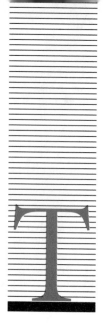

Tai chi chuan

*tai chi, t'ai chi,
t'ai chi ch'uan,*

A form of exercise based on the mind-body connection, tai chi chuan (or tai chi) combines physical movement, meditation, and breathing to induce relaxation and tranquility of mind and improve balance, posture, coordination, endurance, strength, and flexibility. The name means "Absolute fist." Practiced in China for centuries — as both a martial art and a form of slow, graceful, and rhythmic exercise — tai chi allows the individual to assume an active role in health promotion and disease prevention. Regular practice of these exercises can result in long life, good health, physical and mental vigor, and enhanced creativity.

There are numerous forms of tai chi, involving up to 108 different postures and controlled movements. Most of the forms have been passed down from generation to generation and have assumed the name of a particular family (such as Wu style or Yang style). Although each style is distinctive, the basic principles are the same.

It's possible for men and women of all ages, sizes, and physical abilities to practice tai chi because it relies more on technique than strength. Participants learn a series of rhythmic and coordinated movement patterns, which are performed slowly and methodically, with one motion leading into the next. The movements have descriptive names, such as "Grasp the Bird's Tail" and "White Crane Spreads Its Wings." During practice of the movements, close attention is paid to breathing, which is focused in the diaphragm rather than the chest. Abdominal breathing is believed to enhance the flow of energy, called *qi* or *chi*, throughout the body.

One of the primary purposes of tai chi is to restore balance so that chi flows freely. Like acupuncture, *qigong*, and other components of traditional Chinese medicine, tai chi is based on the Taoist principles of *yin* and *yang,* which form the basis for the Chinese understanding of health and sickness. *Yin* and *yang* refer to the opposing forces in nature, such as positive and negative, active and passive, light and dark. Good health, in the Taoist view, requires a balance of these opposing forces within the body. If one or the other predominates, the result is sickness.

Tai chi movements are carried out in pairs of opposites to balance negative *(yin)* forces and positive *(yang)* forces. For example, a movement that begins on the left will typically end with a move to the right. The movements themselves are simple, involving the bending and straightening of the knees while raising or lowering the arms. The coordination of movement and breathing pattern is what constitutes tai chi. The ultimate goal is to achieve harmony between body, mind, and spirit.

Reported uses

Tai chi can be used to complement physical therapy programs aimed at improving balance, posture, coordination, flexibility, and endurance. Cardiovascular indications include heart disease, hypertension, and deconditioning. Tai chi can also benefit patients who suffer from anxiety, stress, restlessness, and depression. However, tai chi's greatest benefit may be the promotion of health and wellness. It's especially well suited for elderly and frail people because its movements are slow

and controlled and do not involve impact. By incorporating all of the motions that typically become restricted with aging, tai chi improves respiratory status, trunk control, balance, and coordination. By improving physical balance, tai chi decreases the risk of falls. Done in a group setting, tai chi also provides an opportunity for socialization. A patient can benefit from the physical elements of tai chi without understanding its spiritual dimension.

How the treatment is performed

Tai chi requires a carpeted room with adequate floor space to permit participants to move their arms and bodies without interfering with one another. The room should be well lit to allow participants to see the leader. Participants should wear loose-fitting clothing and fitted sneakers or aerobic sneakers.

Although the guidance of a knowledgeable teacher is needed to master tai chi, careful practice of the basic steps still provides many of the benefits. Before patients begin a session, the practitioner assesses their physical health, looking for endurance, balance, and mobility. The purpose of the session is explained, with special emphasis on tai chi's focus on slow, nonstressful movements. Group members are encouraged to participate to the extent that they feel comfortable — not to the point of pain.

The session begins with some simple stretching exercises to loosen muscles and prevent injury. Then the teacher describes and demonstrates the first posture. In the first session, the patients may learn only the first few postures. New movements as well as breathing instructions can be added with each session. The teacher reminds group members that they can skip any movement they find too difficult. Most routines take approximately 20 minutes. The session closes with additional stretching exercises that allow the patients' muscles to cool down. The session and the participants' responses to it are documented.

Hazards

As with any physical exercise, patients performing tai chi can experience sprains or strains. Most practitioners believe that constantly shifting weight prevents the feeling of straining. Stretching before and after the session with warm-up and cool-down exercises, and changing positions slowly during the session, can prevent most injuries.

Falls and fractures are another possible complication, especially when one is performing postures that require standing on one leg. Again, proper use of stretching and slow movements should lessen the risk.

Clinical considerations

■ Instruct your patients to stop exercising if they experience pain or shortness of breath.

■ Make sure your patients are wearing appropriate footwear to reduce the risk of slipping and falling.

■ If a patient injures a muscle, isolate the body part to restrict movement, and try to elevate it to reduce swelling. Notify a health care provider and administer cold or heat therapy as ordered. Document the incident, your assessment, the patient's condition, any interventions, and the patient's response.

■ If a patient falls, perform your assessment while he's still lying down. Ask him to remain still for a moment, and ascertain whether he has any pain. Ask him to move all of his extremities. Check for any head injuries. If he can move without pain, gently assist him to a chair. Notify a health care provider and document the incident, your assessment, the patient's condition, any interventions, and the patient's response.

Research summary

Studies appearing in several major medical journals have shown that this exercise program can improve stamina, agility, muscle tone, and flexibility.

tansy

Bitter buttons, buttons, chrysanthemum vulgare, daisy, hindheal, parsley fern, scented fern, stinking Willie, Tanacetum vulgare

Tansy has been used extensively in traditional medicine and as a popular herb for centuries. The useful constituents of tansy are obtained from the above-ground parts of *Tanacetum vulgare*. Volatile oil derived from the plant contains thujone, a neurotoxin. Other components include sesquiterpenes and flavones. Caffeic acid may have bile-inducing effects. It's thought that thujone has a mind-altering effect, similar to tetrahydrocannabinol, an active component in marijuana. There have been reports of potential toxicity to tansy. The plant's activity and toxicity vary greatly among subtypes. Tansy is available as oil and an extract, in products such as T-HRT and T-Jaun.

Reported uses

Tansy is used orally to stimulate menstrual flow, induce abortion, improve digestion, and treat migraines. It's also used to treat GI worm infestations in children. Tansy is also used orally for neuralgia, epilepsy, and rheumatism; as an antispasmodic; and for treating flatulence, bloating, stomach and duodenal ulcers, noninflammatory gallbladder conditions, palpitations, sciatica, edema associated with a weak heart, colds, fever inducing sweating, hysteria, nervousness, gout, kidney problems, and tuberculosis.

Tansy is used topically to treat scabies, sunburn, toothache, sores, and sprains. It's also used for pruritus, bruises, swelling, and freckles. The dried leaves are said to be an effective insect repellent, and have been used as teas and food flavorings. The extracts have been used in perfumes and dyes.

Administration

The average daily dose of tansy is 0.1 g by mouth.

Hazards

Tansy can cause seizures, tremors, vertigo, restlessness, loss of consciousness, tonic-clonic spasms, tachycardia, irregular heartbeat, dilated pupils, pupillary rigidity, vomiting, gastroenteritis, abdominal pain, liver toxicity, kidney damage, uterine bleeding, and abortion. Externally, it can cause local mucous membrane irritation, contact dermatitis, severe facial flushing, and allergic reactions.

Tansy can cause altered control of blood glucose level and can increase the effect of hypoglycemics. There is risk of increased toxicity when tansy is combined with other herbs that may contain thujone, including cedar leaf oil, oak moss, oriental arborvitae, sage, tree moss, and wormwood. Because of the thujone component, tansy may increase and change the effects of alcohol.

Pregnant or breast-feeding women shouldn't use tansy. Tansy products shouldn't be used by patients allergic to ragweed, chrysanthemums, arnica, sunflowers, yarrow, marigolds, daisies, and similar plants.

 SAFETY RISK *Death has occurred from as little as 10 gtt of tansy oil taken orally.*

Clinical considerations

- Take a careful history if patient uses tansy. It's especially important to note if the patient has also taken any other herbs containing thujone, a potent toxin.
- Monitor patient's blood glucose level closely.
- Tansy poisoning may cause a weak tachycardic pulse, severe gastritis, violent spasms, and seizures.
- Gastric lavage and emesis have been used to treat symptomatic toxicity.
- Don't confuse with tansy ragwort (*Senecio jacoboea*).

- Warn patient that tansy is toxic at very low doses and is unsafe for any medicinal use.
- If patient takes tansy, caution him to watch for signs of toxicity, such as a rapid and weak pulse, severe abdominal pain, and seizures. Urge patient to seek emergency care immediately if adverse effects or toxic reactions develop.
- Advise patient that tansy may cause severe dermatitis.
- If patient has a history of allergy to any member of the Compositae family, such as arnica, yarrow, or sunflower, tell him not to take tansy because a cross-reaction may occur.
- Warn patient to keep all herbal products away from children and pets.
- Tell patient to remind pharmacist of any herbal and dietary supplements that are being taken when obtaining a new prescription.
- Advise patient to consult his health care provider before using an herbal preparation because a conventional treatment with proven efficacy may be available.

Research summary

The concepts behind the use of tansy and the claims made regarding its effects have not been validated scientifically.

tea tree

Melaleuca alternifolia, *paperbark tree*

Tea tree oil has been used in the United States in surgery and dentistry since the 1920s. Its healing properties were also used during World War II for skin injuries to munitions factory workers. It has become a popular addition to soaps, shampoos, and lotions. The useful constituents of the tea tree are extracted as oil by steam distillation from the leaves and branch tips of *Melaleuca alternifolia*. The main component is terpinene-4-ol, active against numerous pathogenic bacteria and fungi. Alpha-terpinene and linalool may also contribute to its antimicrobial activity. Tea tree oils with high cineole content are of lower quality and are more likely to cause skin irritation. Therapeutic concentrations range from 0.25% to 0.5%, but may contain up to 10% essential oil. Tea tree is available as essential oil, cream, lotion, ointment, suppositories, soap, and shampoo.

Reported uses

Tea tree oil is used as a topical antiseptic that's more effective than phenol for superficial skin infections, minor burns, cuts, sore throats, ingrown or infected toenails, sunburn, tinea pedis (athlete's foot), Candida species (including *C. albicans*), ulcers, cold sores, pimples, and acne. It's also used in aromatherapy and as a mouthwash and shampoo. Added to a sitz bath, it's used to treat vaginal infections. It can also be added to vaporizers for respiratory disorders.

Administration

- Skin and nail conditions: Apply 70% to 100% tea tree oil to affected areas at least twice a day
- Acne: Apply 5% to 15% concentration two to three times a day
- Vaginal douche: Concentrations as strong as 40% have been used as an additive to sitz bath water.

Hazards

Tea tree may cause ataxia, drowsiness, weakness, confusion, itching, burning, neutrophil leukocytosis, contact dermatitis, and rash. Tea tree may alter the effects of drugs that affect histamine release.

Patients shouldn't apply tea tree products to dry skin, cracked or broken skin, open wounds, or areas affected by rash that's not fungal.

Clinical considerations

- Because of systemic toxicity, tea tree oil shouldn't be used internally.
- Tea tree essential oil should be used externally only after being diluted, especially when used by people with sensitive skin.
- Tea tree oil may cause burns or itching in tender areas and shouldn't be used around nose, eyes, and mouth.
- Diluted essential oil, even as low as 0.25% to 0.5%, is active against microbes.
- Vaginal douches using concentrations as strong as 40% require extreme caution; stress to the patient the need for supervision by a health care provider.
- Pure (100%) essential tea tree oil is rarely used and only with close supervision by a health care provider.
- Other related *Melaleuca* species, such as *M. cajeputi*, *M. dissitiflora*, and *M. linariiflora*, are also known as tea trees, but tea tree oil can be obtained only from *M. alternifolia*.
- Tell patient to use very dilute tea tree oil (0.25% to 0.5%) as a topical anti-infective.
- Explain that a few drops are sufficient in mouthwash, shampoo, or sitz bath.
- Caution patient not to apply oil to wounds or to skin that is dry or cracked.
- Warn patient to keep all herbal products away from children and pets.
- Tell patient to remind pharmacist of any herbal and dietary supplements that are being taken when obtaining a new prescription.
- Advise patient to consult his health care provider before using an herbal preparation because a conventional treatment with proven efficacy may be available.

Research summary

The antimicrobial and healing properties of tea tree oil have been well documented since the 1920s. It has also been shown that tea tree oil is therapeutic for skin infections, respiratory disorders, and aromatherapy. However, the oil shouldn't be ingested by mouth.

Therapeutic Touch

Therapeutic Touch is a widely used complementary therapy developed by nurses in the 1970s in an attempt to bring a more humane and holistic approach to their practice. Rooted in the ancient art of "laying on of hands," this technique focuses on "healing" rather than "curing" and is built on the belief that all healing is basically self-healing.

Central to Therapeutic Touch is the concept of a universal life force (similar to the Ayurvedic concept of *prana* and the Chinese concept of *qi*) that practitioners believe permeates space and sustains all living organisms. In healthy people, this vital energy flows freely in and through the body in a balanced way that nourishes all body organs; when people get sick, it's because this energy field is out of equilibrium.

By using their hands to manipulate the energy field above the patient's skin, practitioners say they can restore equilibrium, thereby reactivating the mind-body-spirit connection and empowering the patient to fully participate in his own healing. Although the existence of a human energy field has not been proven scientifically, nurses claim that they can actually feel something best described as energy when performing this technique. (See *Human energy field*, page 476.) Despite its name, therapeutic touch does not require actual physical contact during a treatment. In most cases, the nurse's hands remain several inches above the patient's body.

Therapeutic Touch was developed in the early 1970s by Dolores Krieger, a nursing professor at New York University (NYU), and Dora Kunz, a healer. The two women had been studying the work of well-known healers who practiced the laying on of hands. In 1971, Krieger did a study comparing 19 people who received treatment from a world-famous healer and 9 people who received routine nursing care. All those who were treated by the healer had an increased hemoglobin count; the 9 in the control group had no increase. When this study was replicated with a group of Krieger's nursing students, it yielded the same results.

Krieger developed a formal instruction method for this healing process, which she called Therapeutic Touch, and began teaching it at NYU. The publication of Krieger's experiment in the *American Journal of Nursing* in 1975 marked the beginning of the acceptance of Therapeutic Touch as a recognized clinical method. In the early 1980s, Martha Rogers, dean of NYU's nursing school, postulated her human energy field theory, which complemented Krieger and Kunz's theory that Therapeutic Touch could interact in a specific way within the human energy field to promote healing.

Today, Therapeutic Touch is widely used by practitioners of holistic nursing and other health professionals and is practiced in many hospitals, hospices, long-term care facilities, and other settings. It's offered at more than 100 colleges and universities worldwide and has been taught to more than 40,000 health care providers. The North American Nursing Diagnosis Association recognizes "energy field disturbance" as a nursing diagnosis, and professional organizations, such as the American Nurses Association and the National League for Nursing, have supported Therapeutic Touch as a nursing intervention.

The Nurse Healers–Professional Association is the official organization representing nurses who practice Therapeutic Touch. (The American Holistic Nurses Association endorses Healing Touch, an offshoot of Therapeutic Touch developed in the 1980s that combines it with the practices of other energetic healers, including Rev. Roselyn Bruyere, Rev. Rudy Noel, Brugh Joy, and Barbara Brennan.) Although most practitioners are nurses, other health care professionals (massage therapists, physical therapists, dentists, medical doctors) and nonprofessionals have incorporated this therapy in their practices. Practitioners say that anyone

HUMAN ENERGY FIELD

Practitioners of Therapeutic Touch and other energy-based therapies believe that the human body emits several energy fields, as indicated in the illustration below. The layers aren't as separate as the illustration suggests; rather, each successive layer encompasses some of the preceding one

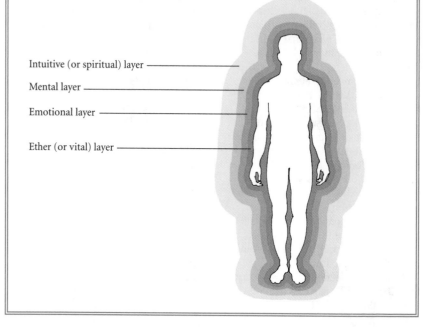

Intuitive (or spiritual) layer ————————

Mental layer ————————

Emotional layer ————————

Ether (or vital) layer ————————

can study the technique and apply it to themselves or others.

Reported uses

Therapeutic Touch is used as a complementary therapy for virtually all medical and nursing diagnoses, as well as for surgical procedures. Practitioners say it's especially helpful for patients with wounds or infections because it eases discomfort and speeds up the healing process. However, the technique is best known for its ability to relieve pain and anxiety.

Because it helps reduce anxiety and promote relaxation, proponents say Therapeutic Touch is helpful in treating stress-related disorders such as tension headaches, hypertension, ulcers, and emotional problems. It's also used in Lamaze classes and delivery rooms to in-

duce relaxation and in neonatal intensive care units to help speed the growth of premature infants.

How the treatment is performed

Therapeutic Touch treatment requires no equipment beyond the nurse's hands. An environment conducive to relaxation in the patient and inward-focused concentration in the nurse may include a comfortable chair, bed, or massage table for the patient and, possibly, soothing music.

Therapeutic Touch incorporates the nursing process, beginning with assessment and continuing through diagnosis, treatment, and evaluation. In a typical session, the patient usually lies fully clothed on a massage table or a hospital bed. The nurse begins by "centering" — achieving a calm, meditative state that increases sensitivity to whatever signs and symptoms the patient presents. This heightened sensitivity is also necessary to enable perception of subtle changes in the patient's energy field.

After becoming centered, the practitioner begins the assessment. The practitioner proceeds by moving his hands slowly above the patient's body — at a distance of 2″ to 4″ (5 to 10 cm) away from the patient's skin surface — to detect any alterations in the energy field, such as feelings of cold or heat, vibration, or blockage. Depending on what this assessment reveals, the practitioner then performs interventions aimed at balancing the energy field and removing any obstructions. These may include *unruffling* a chaotic and tangled field, eliminating *congestion*, or acting as a conduit to direct the life energy from the environment into the patient. Techniques may be altered based on the patient's response to treatment or changes in his condition.

Throughout the treatment, the patient remains quiet and relaxed. He or she may actually feel the practitioner's hands even though they aren't touching his body. According to practitioners, the patient does not have to consciously believe in the power of the procedure. However, in order to be effective in channeling energy into the patient, the practitioner must have *conscious intent* — that is, the intent to be a calm, focused instrument of healing, thereby enabling the patient's body to ultimately heal itself.

Hazards

Complications from Therapeutic Touch treatments are rare. Practitioners are careful to moderate the length and strength of the treatment for small children and elderly people because of their more fragile physiology. A common sign of overtreatment in these age groups is restlessness during or after the treatment.

Clinical considerations

■ Respect patient's personal preferences. People have differing tolerances for touch, and some people regard energy work as an invasion of their personal space and boundaries. Always obtain consent for this procedure before proceeding.

■ Certain patients, such as infants, the elderly, pregnant women (especially during the last trimester), patients with head injuries or psychosis, emaciated patients, and patients in shock, warrant extra sensitivity and shorter treatment periods.

Research summary

Since Krieger's 1971 experiment on patients treated by laying on of hands, numerous other studies have been done on this technique. Studies have shown that, similar to meditation and yoga, Therapeutic Touch produces signs of the relaxation response, including slower and deeper breathing, decreased muscle tension and heart rate, and altered brain wave activity. Other studies have reported benefits in reducing headache pain, promoting wound healing, easing breathing in asthmatic patients, decreasing fever and inflammation, and reducing postoperative pain.

In April 1998, a study by a fourth grade Colorado girl debunking Therapeutic Touch received widespread media attention when it was published in *JAMA*. To test proponents' claims that they can detect another person's energy field with their hands, the girl had 21 practitioners place their hands through holes cut in a cardboard partition and then placed her own hand over the subjects' right or left hand. The therapists were asked to say which hand could detect the girl's energy field. The average correct score was 44%, no more than would be expected by guessing. Proponents of Therapeutic Touch criticized the study's premise and setup. They also condemned the study as biased because the girl's mother, a registered nurse, had been a vocal opponent of the practice for years.

thuja

Arborvitae, hackmatack, swamp cedar,
Thuja occidentalis, *tree of life,*
white cedar

Thuja is obtained by steam distillation of leaves and twigs of *Thuja occidentalis*. It contains glycoproteins and polysaccharides, which have antiviral and immunostimulating properties. It also has uterine-stimulant activity. Thuja also contains the neurotoxin thujone. Thuja is available as oil, extract, ointment, and homeopathic products.

Reported uses

Thuja is used orally as an immune stimulant, expectorant, and diuretic. It's also used as an abortifacient. Other uses include treatment of trigeminal neuralgia, strep throat, gout, pruritus, blepharitis, conjunctivitis, otitis media, pertussis, tracheitis, kidney and bladder complaints, psoriasis, enuresis, amenorrhea, and cardiac insufficiency.

Thuja is used topically as an insect repellent and a treatment for skin diseases, infected wounds and burns, joint pain, arthritis, rheumatism, condylomata, warts, and cancers. It's also used as a fragrance in personal care items and as a flavoring; however, thuja is used in food items in the United States only if it's certified thujone-free.

 SAFETY RISK *Thuja preparations intended for oral or topical use shouldn't contain the neurotoxin thujone. Some thuja and thuja oil preparations are said to be thujone-free. If thujone toxicity is suspected, call a poison control center immediately.*

Administration

- Extract (1:1 in 50% alcohol, 1:10 in 60% alcohol): 1 to 2 ml by mouth three times a day
- Tincture (mix 100 parts thuja powder into 1,000 parts diluted spirit of wine).

Hazards

Thuja may cause seizures, neurotoxicity, hypotension, tachycardia, nausea, vomiting, diarrhea, uterine stimulation and cramping, fetal loss, and mucous membrane hemorrhaging.

There's an increased risk of toxicity when thuja is combined with other herbs that contain thujone, such as oak moss, oriental arborvitae, sage, tansy, tree moss, and wormwood. Additive central nervous system (CNS) effects may result when thuja is combined with alcohol.

Pregnant or breast-feeding women shouldn't use thuja. It shouldn't be used by transplant patients or those with a history of seizures or immune-related diseases, such as lupus, rheumatoid arthritis, or acquired immunodeficiency syndrome (AIDS) because it may accelerate the disease.

Clinical considerations

- Thujone is considered safe for oral use in concentrations up to 1.25 mg/kg of body weight.
- For homeopathic thuja preparations, patient must not eat or drink for 15 minutes before and after taking the remedy to prevent its dilution.
- Monitor patient's response to thuja; monitor patient for adverse effects.
- Don't confuse this *Thuja* species with *T. orientalis*, the Oriental arborvitae.
- Caution patient not to take thuja if he has a history of seizures.
- Warn patient that thuja leaf oil taken orally should be certified thujone-free.
- If patient takes a form that contains alcohol, caution to avoid hazardous activities until full CNS effects of the herb are known.
- Advise patient about signs of thujone toxicity and advise him to contact a poison control center or seek emergency treatment immediately if he becomes ill after taking thuja orally.
- Warn patient to keep all herbal products away from children and pets.
- Tell patient to remind pharmacist of any herbal and dietary supplements that

are being taken when obtaining a new prescription.

■ Advise patient to consult his health care provider before using an herbal preparation because a conventional treatment with proven efficacy may be available.

Research summary

The concepts behind the use of thuja and the claims made regarding its effects have not been validated scientifically.

thunder god vine

Huang-t'engken (yellow vine root), lei gong teng (Chinese), lei-kung t'eng, threewingnut, Tripteryigium wilfordii, *tsao-ho-hua (early rice flower), yellow vine*

Thunder god vine has been used for centuries in traditional Chinese medicine to treat fever, boils, abscesses, and inflammation. It's also used as an insecticide to kill maggots or larvae and as a rat and bird poison. The useful constituents of thunder god vine are obtained from the leaves and roots of *Tripteryigium wilfordii*. It contains tripochlorolide, tribromoline, and demethylzeylesteral constituents, which have immunosuppressive effects. Triptolide and tripdiolide may have male antifertility effects — by depressing spermatogenesis without affecting testosterone levels — and may also exert anti-inflammatory and immunosuppressive effects. Low doses of triptolide show evidence of antitumor and antileukemic effects. Demethylzeylesteral has antiangiogenic effects.

Reported uses

Thunder god vine is used for male antifertility effects. It's also used to treat rheumatoid arthritis, inflammation, abscesses and boils, heavy menstrual periods, and autoimmune diseases.

Administration

■ For rheumatoid arthritis: 30 mg extract by mouth once a day
■ Male antifertility effects: 10 mg extract by mouth once a day.

Hazards

Thunder god vine may cause rash, hypotension, shock, stomach upset, vomiting, diarrhea, amenorrhea, infertility, renal failure, and decreased white blood cell and lymphocyte count.

Thunder god vine may enhance the effects of immunosuppressants. Patients who take immunosuppressive drugs or have cardiovascular disease, a previous transplant, or immune disorders should avoid taking this herb. Men who wish to maintain optimum fertility and women who are pregnant or breast-feeding shouldn't use thunder god vine.

 SAFETY RISK *Thunder god vine may cause death in patients with a history of myocardial infarction (MI), coronary artery disease, or heart failure.*

Clinical considerations

■ Men considering conception shouldn't use thunder god vine because of its antifertility effect.
■ Fertility usually returns to normal 6 weeks after thunder god vine is stopped.
■ Caution patients with a history of heart disease, MI, or heart failure not to use thunder god vine.
■ Advise pregnant patients, those trying to become pregnant, and those not using adequate contraception to avoid thunder god vine. Tell patient to make sure she isn't pregnant before use.
■ Advise against using thunder god vine if patient has a disease or condition that alters the immune system, or if he takes other herbs or drugs that suppress the immune system.
■ Warn patient to keep all herbal products away from children and pets.
■ Tell patient to remind pharmacist of any herbal and dietary supplements that

are being taken when obtaining a new prescription.

■ Advise patient to consult his health care provider before using an herbal preparation because a conventional treatment with proven efficacy may be available.

Research summary

Most research studies to date have focused on autoimmune diseases such as rheumatoid arthritis. Recently, antifertility effects in men have been of interest. Thunder god vine has been shown to possess antiviral and antitumor actions.

thyme

Common thyme, French thyme, garden thyme, rubbed thyme, Spanish thyme, thymi herba,
Thymus serpyllum, T. vulgaris, T. zygis

The useful portions of thyme are obtained from the aerial parts of *Thymus serpyllum* or *T. vulgaris*. It contains thymol, flavonoids, and carvacrol, which have expectorant, antispasmodic, and antitussive effects. Thymol and carvacrol may also have antibacterial and antifungal effects. Rosmarinic acid may have antiedema and macrophage-inhibiting effects. Thyme may also act as a menstrual stimulant. Common thyme (*T. vulgaris*) contains more oil than wild thyme (*T. serpyllum*) or Spanish thyme (*T. zygis*). Thyme is available as 100% oil, dry herb, powder, liquid extract, and dry extract, in products such as Candistroy, Dentarone Plus Toothpaste, Fenu-Thyme (combination product), Respirtonic, Thyme Beautiful Skin Tea, and Ultimate Respiratory Cleanse.

Reported uses

Thyme is used to treat cough, bronchitis, pertussis, sore throat, laryngitis, tonsillitis, colic, dyspnea, dyspepsia, diarrhea, rheumatic diseases, and pediatric enuresis. It's also used as a diuretic, an antibac-

terial, and an antiflatulent. Thyme is used externally to treat wounds resistant to healing and as a mouthwash and gargle for mouth and throat inflammation, and stomatitis. It's also used for rheumatic and skin disorders. Thyme is a popular spice and flavoring agent.

Administration

■ Average daily dose: 1 to 2 g dried leaf or flower by mouth several times a day; maximum, 10 g of dried leaf every day
■ Thyme oil (oral): 2 to 3 drops on a sugar cube, two or three times a day
■ Bath: 0.004 g thyme oil (the minimum dose) added to 1 L water, filtered, and then added to 95° to 100.4° F (35° to 38° C) bath water; or 500 g of herb added to 4 L boiling water, filtered, and then added to bath water as directed above
■ Liquid extract: 1 to 2 g by mouth up to three times a day
■ Tea (1 to 2 g dried leaf or flower in 150 ml boiling water, steeped for 10 minutes, strained): taken several times every day
■ Topical: 5 g in 100 ml boiling water (5% infusion), steeped for 10 minutes, strained, cooled slightly, and used as gargle or applied as compress
■ Ointment: 1% to 2% ointment applied as needed.

Hazards

Thyme may cause irritation, mild sensitivity reactions, nausea, vomiting, gastric pain, seizures, headache, dizziness, coma, cardiac arrest, respiratory arrest, mucous membrane irritation, cheilitis, and glossitis. No drug interactions are known.

Pregnant or breast-feeding women should avoid thyme, as should patients allergic to oregano. Patients with GI disorders, such as ulcers, and those with urinary tract inflammation should use thyme with caution. Patients with widespread skin injuries or skin disease, high fever, infectious disease, or cardiac problems should be very cautious when using any herb as an ingredient in a whole-body bath.

Clinical considerations
■ Advise pregnant or breast-feeding patient not to use thyme in medicinal quantities.
■ Tell patient who uses thyme as an expectorant that increased benefit may be received by adding honey as a sweetener, if he has no sugar restrictions in his diet.
■ If patient is allergic to oregano, explain that thyme may cause mild allergic reactions.
■ Warn patient not to take thyme for persistent bronchitis or cough before seeking medical attention because doing so may delay diagnosis of a potentially serious medical condition.
■ Instruct patient to contact a health care provider if a skin reaction develops.
■ If patient has urinary tract inflammation, urge caution because thyme may aggravate it.
■ If patient has widespread skin injuries or skin disease, high fever, infectious disease, or cardiac problems, caution must be used when using any herb as an ingredient in a whole-body bath.
■ Instruct patient to promptly notify a health care provider about adverse effects or changes in symptoms.
■ Warn patient to keep all herbal products away from children and pets.
■ Tell patient to remind pharmacist of any herbal and dietary supplements that are being taken when obtaining a new prescription.
■ Advise patient to consult his health care provider before using an herbal preparation because a conventional treatment with proven efficacy may be available.

Research summary
The concepts behind the use of thyme and the claims made regarding its effects have not been validated scientifically.

tonka bean

Coumarouna odorata, curmaru,
Dipteryx odorata, *Dutch tonka,*
English tonka, tonca seed, tongo bean,
tonquin bean, torquin bean

Tonka is obtained from the seeds of *Dipteryx odorata (Coumarouna odorata).* It contains 1% to 3% coumarin, but possibly as much as 10%. Coumarin may increase venous and lymphatic return, thus reducing edema and inflammation. Tonka also contains a fatty oil.

Reported uses
Tonka is used orally as a tonic, and to treat cachexia, cramps, lymphedema, spasms, and tuberculosis. Some people have claimed the beans have aphrodisiac properties. Coumarin is used as a flavoring for cakes, tobacco, preserves, and soaps. In Chinese medicine, seed extracts are used rectally to treat schistosomiasis.

Tonka is also used topically to treat ulcers, earache, and sore throat.

Administration
Tonka beans aren't used medicinally, and are no longer available in the United States.

 SAFETY RISK *High doses or long-term consumption of tonka bean should be avoided because of the risk of liver damage and cardiac arrest.*

Hazards
Tonka may cause insomnia, dizziness, stupor, headache, nausea, vomiting, diarrhea, testicular atrophy, hepatotoxicity, elevated liver enzymes, liver damage, and growth retardation. Cardiac arrest may occur with large doses.

There is potential for coagulation disturbances when tonka is used with anticoagulants or antiplatelets such as aspirin, clopidogrel bisulfate, and warfarin. Tonka may also cause coagulation disturbances when used with angelica, anise, arnica, asafoetida, bogbean, boldo, capsicum, celery, chamomile, clove, danshen, fenugreek, feverfew, garlic, ginger, ginkgo, ginseng, horse chestnut, horseradish, licorice, meadowsweet, onion, papain, passion flower, poplar, prickly ash, quassia, red clover, turmeric, wild carrot, wild lettuce, and willow.

Pregnant patients, breast-feeding patients, and patients with a history of liver disease shouldn't use tonka.

Clinical considerations

■ Advise patient not to use tonka if he's taking antiplatelet drugs or anticoagulants.

■ Don't confuse coumarin with such anticoagulants as warfarin, dicumarol, or bishydroxycoumarin, but do recognize the potential for additive antiplatelet or anticoagulant effects.

■ Warn patient that vanilla extract and possibly other flavoring extracts purchased in foreign countries may contain coumarin impurities and are unsafe for consumption.

■ Monitor patient for signs of bleeding, such as easy bruising and gum bleeding.

■ Warn pregnant and breast-feeding patients to avoid tonka bean.

■ Explain the signs of bleeding, and urge patient to promptly notify a health care provider if this or any other adverse effect develops.

■ Tell patient to avoid high doses and long-term use of tonka bean.

■ Instruct patient to seek emergency medical care if he develops cardiac symptoms (chest pain, shortness of breath, diaphoresis) while taking tonka bean.

■ Tell patient to remind pharmacist of any herbal and dietary supplements that are being taken when obtaining a new prescription.

■ Advise patient to consult his health care provider before using an herbal preparation because a conventional treatment with proven efficacy may be available.

Research summary

There are no well-controlled studies describing the pharmacologic effects of tonka, but coumarin is toxic when ingested in high doses. The FDA Code states that tonka beans or foods containing any coumarin as a constituent of tonka extracts are deemed to be impure. The concepts behind the use of tonka beans and the claims made regarding its effects have not been validated scientifically.

tormentil

Biscuits, bloodroot, cinquefoil, earthbank, English sarsaparilla, ewe daisy, flesh and blood, potentilla, Potentilla erecta, septfoil, shepherd's knapperty, shepherd's knot, thormantle, tormentilla, tormentillae rhizoma

The useful constituents of tormentil are obtained from the rhizome of *Potentilla erecta*. It contains tannins, flavonoids, resins, ellagic acid, and kinovic acid. Tannins are probably responsible for pharmacologic actions. Extracts of tormentil root have been shown to have antiallergic, antihypertensive, antiviral, immunostimulant, and interferon-inducing actions. Tormentil is available as root, powder, tincture, and fluid extract, in products such as Immune Master.

Reported uses

Tormentil is used orally to treat diarrhea, mild gastroenteritis, and fever. It's used in combination with galangal, marshmallow root, and powdered ginger to treat diarrhea and dysentery.

Tormentil is used topically as a mouth rinse for mild oral inflammation and mild superficial bleeding. The fluid extract is also used to promote wound healing.

Administration

■ Tea (2 to 3 g of rhizome in 150 ml boiling water, steeped for 10 to 15 minutes, and then strained): 1 cup two to four times a day for diarrhea (1 teaspoon powdered rhizome is approximately equal to 4 g of herb)

■ Tincture: 10 to 20 gtt (1:10) in a glass of water by mouth, swished as a mouth rinse once to several times every day.

Hazards

Tormentil may cause nausea, vomiting, abdominal complaints, kidney damage, and liver necrosis. When alcohol-containing herbal extracts are taken with disulfiram or metronidazole, a disulfiram-like reaction may occur. When tormentil is taken with milk products, its antidiarrheal effect may be decreased.

Pregnant or breast-feeding women should avoid this herb, as should alcoholic patients and those with liver disease.

Clinical considerations

■ Do not confuse with potentilla (*Potentilla anserina*).

■ Tell pregnant and breast-feeding patients not to use tormentil.

■ Inform patient that milk products may bind the active ingredient in tormentil when used to treat diarrhea, thus reducing its effectiveness.

■ Urge patient to stop using tormentil and to contact a health care provider if diarrhea gets worse or continues for longer than 2 days.

■ Tell patient to promptly notify a health care provider about adverse effects or changes in symptoms.

■ Warn patient to keep all herbal products away from children and pets.

■ Tell patient to remind pharmacist of any herbal and dietary supplements that are being taken when obtaining a new prescription.

■ Advise patient to consult his health care provider before using an herbal preparation because a conventional treatment with proven efficacy may be available.

Research summary

The concepts behind the use of tormentil and the claims made regarding its effects have not yet been validated scientifically.

Traditional Chinese medicine

Traditional Chinese medicine is a sophisticated and complex system of health care that has been practiced for longer than 3,000 years and is rooted in Chinese culture. Its practice spread throughout Asia, and today it's used by about a quarter of the world's population. Japan, Vietnam, and Korea have developed strong variations that also have influenced practitioners of Chinese medicine around the world.

Over the centuries, Chinese medicine has expanded to embrace many theories, methods, and approaches, an abundance that is often missed by Westerners, who assume that Chinese medicine is a monolithic structure similar to that of modern Western medicine. Some of Chinese medicine's theories are contradictory, yet none is rejected outright. Instead, all the additions and accretions have remained in the main body of knowledge, awaiting new discoveries that may warrant their integration into the dynamic system of medicine.

This ancient system's approach to health and illness — from its basic understanding of human physiology to its methods of diagnosis and treatment — is very different from that of modern Western medicine. The focus of traditional Chinese medicine is prevention. According to ancient tradition, there are three levels of doctors: Physicians at the lowest level cure a disease after it manifests; those at the middle level cure disease before it begins to manifest; and those at the highest level — the ideal doctors — prevent disease by teaching patients to maximize good health through living correctly.

Traditional Chinese theory holds that good health depends, to a large extent, on the patient's lifestyle, thoughts, and emotions. This means that the patient bears much responsibility for his own well-being. The doctor serves as a guide and role model on the patient's journey to good health and long life by recommending measures to modify behavior and by offering help, when needed, in the administration of herbs, acupuncture, and massage.

The fundamental concepts underlying traditional Chinese medicine evolved from the metaphysical world views of Taoism, Confucianism, and Buddhism, and are thus based on 3,000 years of observation and philosophy rather than on the scientific method underlying Western medicine. Whereas Western philosophy and medicine view the body, mind, and spirit as separate entities, Eastern philosophy and medicine see them as interrelated elements that are intertwined with nature and the cosmos as a whole.

The cornerstone of Chinese theory is the concept of *qi* (pronounced "chee"). This concept, foreign to Western thought, is best described as a vital life force, or energy, that flows through the body along channels known as meridians. According to Chinese belief, qi is necessary to maintain life. A balance of qi — neither too much nor too little — is necessary to maintain health; an imbalance or blockage of qi can cause disease.

Another fundamental element in Chinese medicine is the concept of *yin* and *yang*, the interaction of opposing forces (such as male-female, hot-cold, light-dark). These complementary elements must be in balance for a person to maintain good health.

Reported uses

Because traditional Chinese medicine looks at illness in an entirely different way than Western medicine, it's difficult to discuss therapeutic uses in the usual Western biomedical framework. Treatment and dosage are determined not by a specific disease but by the patient's overall pattern of signs and symptoms.

For example, in the West, a person diagnosed with an acute infectious disease is treated with a standard course of antibiotics, and two people with the same condition typically receive the same type of treatment. In Chinese medicine, the treatment varies, depending on such factors as the state of the person's qi and the balance of yin and yang. For example, a person with a severe infectious disease whose qi is strong is able to receive a stronger treatment than a person with a milder case whose qi is impaired. That's because the person with impaired qi needs a gentler treatment to nourish and support his weakened physiologic and qi status.

How the treatment is performed

In traditional Chinese medicine, diagnosis focuses on detecting the pattern of imbalances in a particular patient, rather than labeling the person's disease state. This is a fundamentally different approach from that of Western medicine. Whereas a Western doctor typically will make the same diagnosis for two patients with the same symptoms, a doctor of Chinese medicine might arrive at two very different diagnoses (and treatment plans) based on different types of imbalances in the two patients.

To make a diagnosis, the doctor of Chinese medicine uses his own senses to gather data. By looking, questioning, listening, checking body sounds and odors, and palpating, the doctor can gather the essential information needed for diagnosis. Laboratory tests may be useful but only to provide corroborating data. The doctor may use a variety of diagnostic frameworks to identify a pattern of imbalance, depending on the particular patient. In addition to assessing the patient's qi through the techniques mentioned above, he evaluates body functions using the following methods:

■ Eight Principles (or Eight Parameters): These principles are hot versus cold, interior versus exterior, excessive versus deficient, and yin versus yang. Based on the patient's symptoms and the results of the physical examination, the doctor detects a pattern of illness that he describes in terms of these eight parameters. For example, whereas a Western doctor might diagnose a patient with pneumonia (the name of a condition), the Chinese doctor's diagnosis might be "excessive heat in the lung and insufficient qi."

■ Pathogenic factors: These factors include the Six Evils (or Six Excesses) — wind, cold, heat, dampness, dryness, and fire (which can either invade the body from outside or be generated internally) — and the Seven Moods — joy, anger, anxiety, obsession, sorrow, horror, and fear. Disease is seen as resulting from the struggle between qi and these pathogenic factors. If the body has sufficient qi, it can resist even the most dangerous pathogenic factors; if not, even a minor pathogenic factor can lead to disease.

■ Lifestyle factors: The idea that health is influenced by behavior and thought is fundamental to Chinese medicine. According to this philosophy, leading a balanced lifestyle can improve one's ability to prevent (or combat) illness. On the other hand, intemperate practices, such as poor diet, excessive alcohol intake, insufficient sleep, and too much or too little sexual activity, can cause alterations in the physical body or disruptions in the qi, blood, body fluids, or organ systems, with disease as the result.

■ Six Stages: This pattern, which consists of the three yin and the three yang, attempts to identify the location of disease within the meridians, the 12 channels of the body along which qi is said to flow. Each of the 12 major organs is associated with a channel bearing the organ name. Any abnormality that appears along the pathway may indicate an imbalance in that channel.

■ The Four Levels of Disease: These levels are qi, defense, construction, and blood. They are used to indicate the depth at which a pathogenic factor is affecting the body and are applied to infectious febrile disease (also called an attack of external wind-heat).

■ The Three Burners: This diagnostic pattern, referring to the division of the abdomen into upper, middle, and lower burners, is often used as a metaphor for the processes of metabolism.

■ Five Phases theory: This diagnostic system is based on the premise that each organ either enhances or inhibits the function of another organ, just as the five elements — fire, earth, metal, water, and wood — affect each other adversely or beneficially.

The art and skill of the traditional Chinese doctor lie in knowing which combination of signs and symptoms should be interpreted and which of these diagnostic frameworks is appropriate. In making the diagnosis, the doctor considers the presenting complaint within the context of the patient's emotional state, medical history, family and home environment, and social environment, and any other factors that may help provide a fuller understanding of the patient.

Therapies

Once a diagnosis is made, the doctor prescribes the appropriate therapy in an attempt to restore the balance of elements within the patient. Therapies include herbal remedies, acupuncture, acupressure, dietary recommendations, moxibustion, massage, cupping, and qigong (pronounced "chee-gong").

HERBAL REMEDIES. Developed over the centuries, herbal remedies are the backbone of traditional Chinese therapy; their use far outweighs that of acupuncture and massage. The herbal formulary consists of more than 3,000 herbs, as well as animal and mineral substances such as deer antlers and oyster shells. A typical herbal preparation contains a dozen or so herbs, roots, powders, or animal substances and may be prepared for administration in a number of ways. A traditional Chinese herbalist must be able to recall thousands of combinations and know the best way to administer them. It's important to note that herbalists require more training than other practitioners.

The most common administration form is decoction — the herbs are boiled in water and then drunk as an herbal tea in several doses throughout the day. Herbs may also be prepared as powders, pills, syrups, liniments, suppositories, and enemas. Although many of the formulas are prescribed for specific diagnostic patterns, the dosages — percentages of particular herbs included in the formula — are adjusted for each patient. What is appropriate for one person may be toxic for another, even though both may have the same illness using Western diagnostic criteria.

ACUPUNCTURE. Acupuncture involves the insertion of thin metal needles at specific points on the body that relate to the qi meridians. This therapy is commonly used to relieve pain.

ACUPRESSURE. Acupressure involves the stimulation of acupuncture points by applying direct pressure on them with the hands or fingertips, rather than using needles. This therapy is also typically used for pain relief.

DIET. Traditional Chinese practitioners view food as a type of medicine. According to this outlook, all foods are primarily yin or yang by nature; consequently, each has an effect on various imbalances in the body. Depending on the specific patient, certain foods should be avoided but other foods can have a therapeutic effect.

Foods are further organized into groups based on their energetic qualities, such as heating, cooling, and moistening. Special importance is also given to eating in harmony with seasonal shifts and life activities.

MOXIBUSTION. Moxibustion involves the burning of a mound of the plant moxa (*Artemisia vulgaris*) on specific points of the body near qi meridians. The moxa may be burned directly on the skin or on acupuncture needles, which are then implanted in the skin. The heat produced by this procedure is believed to penetrate deep into the body, stimulating or inhibiting certain target points, and thereby restoring the balance of qi.

MASSAGE. Like acupuncture and moxibustion, massage and manipulation are practiced on specific parts of the body associated with meridians in an attempt to restore the balance of qi in areas where it's lacking, excessive, or blocked. Massage is often used in combination with other therapies, such as acupuncture. *Tui na,* a combination of massage, manipulation, and acupressure, has been practiced in China for nearly 2,000 years.

CUPPING. In the cupping technique, suction is created by warming the air inside a glass jar and placing the overturned jar over the part of the body requiring treatment. The vacuum created by the heat is believed to dispel dampness, warm the qi, and reduce swelling. Cupping is commonly used to relieve bronchial congestion and to treat chronic conditions, such as arthritis and bronchitis.

QIGONG. There are hundreds of forms of *qigong,* a therapy consisting of exercise, breathing techniques, and meditation, which is also aimed at balancing qi. The medical form of qigong is similar to Therapeutic Touch (see page 475).

Clinical considerations

■ Be sure the patient isn't allergic to the prescribed herbs.

■ Obtain a medication history to ensure that the herbal remedy does not interact with previously prescribed medications or herbs.

■ Warn the patient about the risks involved in sharing his individually prescribed remedies with others.

■ Advise the patient that a combination of Western and Chinese medicine may be the best course when life-threatening illnesses are being treated.

■ Instruct the patient to discontinue the therapy and notify a health care provider if signs or symptoms worsen.

■ Advise recovering alcoholics to make sure that herbal tinctures are mixed with water, not alcohol.

Research summary

At least one therapy—acupuncture for pain relief—has undergone considerable scientific testing, with positive results. Extensive studies have been done on acupuncture for other ailments, and on some of the more common herbal remedies used in traditional Chinese medicine. However, the fundamentally different methods of diagnosis and treatment have made it difficult to prove the efficacy of Chinese medicine in treating specific diseases or conditions.

Most of the studies done in China involve empirical methods—observing the results of various treatments—rather than the double-blind, placebo-controlled studies used in Western research. Traditional Chinese medicine isn't conducive to Western-style research because of the great variations in treatment for similar symptoms. Yet, despite this lack of scientifically proven evidence, Chinese medicine is used to treat the full range of human illnesses—from asthma, allergies, and headaches to cancer and infertility.

tragacanth

Astragalus gummifer, *goat's thorn, green dragon, gum dragon, gum tragacanth, gummi tragacanthae, hog gum, Syrian tragacanth*

Tragacanth has been used since ancient times as an emulsifier, thickening agent, and suspending agent. Today it's used extensively in foods (such as ice cream). The useful constituents are obtained from the latex that's found beneath the bark of the *Astragalus gummifer* tree. Tragacanth contains tragacanthine and bassorin, which form a colloidal solution and a thick gel, respectively, when wet.

Tragacanth promotes peristaltic movement, has adhesive properties, and may inhibit cancer cell growth. It's available in products such as Normacol and Tragacanth Mucilage.

Reported uses

Tragacanth is used orally for diarrhea and constipation. It's also used as a stabilizer, a thickener, a suspending agent in food and pharmaceutical products, a binder, an emulsifier, and an ingredient in denture adhesives. The mucilage is used as an adjunct for burns.

Administration

The average daily dose of tragacanth is 1 teaspoon granulated herb (approximately 3 g) added to 250 to 300 ml liquid, by mouth.

Hazards

Tragacanth may cause esophageal pain or blockage, obstructed ileus, and contact dermatitis. No interactions are known.

Patients allergic to quillaja bark (*Quillaja saponaria*) may be sensitive to tragacanth preparations and should avoid its use. Pregnant or breast-feeding women should avoid tragacanth, as should patients with esophageal stricture or intestinal obstruction.

Clinical considerations

■ Instruct patient to drink full glass of water with each dose of tragacanth to avoid expansion of the compound in the esophagus and possible blockage or damage.

■ Tragacanth may inhibit absorption of oral drugs, herbs, and foods. Doses of preparations that contain large amounts of tragacanth should be separated from other oral intake by 2 hours.

■ Monitor patient for adverse effects, including difficulty swallowing and esophageal pain.

■ Warn the patient to seek medical help immediately if unable to swallow, or if significant pain, vomiting, or esophageal bleeding occurs.

- Warn patient to keep all herbal products away from children and pets.
- Tell patient to remind pharmacist of any herbal and dietary supplements that are being taken when obtaining a new prescription.
- Advise patient to consult his health care provider before using an herbal preparation because a conventional treatment with proven efficacy may be available.

Research summary

To date, tragacanth has a safe use profile. It does not appear to have any beneficial influence on serum lipid or glucose levels as do other soluble gums. However, the concepts behind the use of tragacanth and the claims made regarding its effects have not yet been validated scientifically.

Trager approach

Like the Alexander (see page 35) and Feldenkrais (see page 203) techniques, the Trager approach is a gentle method of movement reeducation intended to help people recognize and unlearn mental and physical habits that limit their movement, cause muscle pain and tension, and prevent them from functioning optimally. This technique has two components: gentle, rhythmic body work designed to loosen stiff joints and muscles, increase range of motion, and enhance relaxation (known as Psychophysical Integration), and dancelike exercises (known as Mentastics, or mental gymnastics) designed to increase awareness of how the body moves and teach people how to move more freely and pleasurably.

The method was developed by Milton Trager, an American doctor who became a follower of Maharishi Mahesh Yogi, the founder of Transcendental Meditation. Trager believed that the subconscious mind transfers the stresses of daily life into musculoskeletal tension, which dictates the way we hold and move our bod-

ies. To alleviate this physical tension, Trager focused on gentle movement as a way of repatterning the brain by loosening the body.

Rather than using set exercises, the Trager approach involves gently pushing, pulling, stretching, and rocking the body to loosen tense muscles and stiff joints. The emphasis isn't on moving particular muscles and joints, but on using movement to produce pleasant sensations of lightness, limberness, and deep relaxation. Eventually, Trager believed, the unconscious mind would mimic movements that produced these pleasurable sensations.

SAFETY RISK *Founded in 1980, the Trager Institute in Mill Valley, California, provides training and certification in this technique. There are more than 1,000 certified Trager practitioners worldwide.*

Reported uses

The Trager approach is viewed as a learning experience rather than a medical treatment. It's believed that anyone can benefit. Trager used it to improve the condition of people suffering from serious musculoskeletal disorders, such as multiple sclerosis, muscular dystrophy, and polio. Proponents say it has also benefited people with back problems, asthma, and emphysema. Athletes have also reported improved performance and increased stamina as a result of Trager work, which releases tension, thereby allowing the body to function at full capacity.

How the treatment is performed

This technique requires only a well-padded table and a room big enough to allow free movement. The practitioner begins by entering a relaxed, meditative state (which Trager called "hook-up") that allows him to connect with the patient and remain aware of the patient's slightest responses. In this state, the practitioner begins touching, rocking, pulling, and otherwise gently manipulating the patient's trunk and limbs, helping to induce a state of total relaxation. As the patient's body relaxes, the therapist continues performing the gentle, rhythmic movements to extend range of motion, as if demonstrating to the patient's body that movements beyond its previous limits are not only possible but also pleasurable. In addition to the Psychophysical Integration, the patient receives instruction in the use of Mentastics; this system of effortless, dancelike movements is intended to enhance the sense of lightness, freedom, and flexibility produced by the table work. A typical session lasts 60 to 90 minutes, and therapy is repeated as often as necessary.

Hazards
The gentle movements used in the Trager method are unlikely to cause any complications.

Clinical considerations
The Trager method isn't recommended for people who are uncomfortable with physical contact.

Research summary
The concepts behind the use of the Trager approach and the claims made regarding its effects have not yet been validated scientifically.

tree of heaven

Ailanthus altissima, *ailanto,
a-lan-thus, Chinese sumach, copal tree,
heaven tree, paradise tree,
varnish tree, vernis de Japon*

The useful constituents of tree of heaven are obtained from the bark of the *Ailanthus altissima* tree. Tannins and alkaloids may have astringent, antipyretic, and antispasmodic properties. Herb also has cardiac depressant activity and purgative action, and it may have antimalarial properties. Quassinoid constituents such as ailanthone and quassin may have antihelmintic, antileukemic, and cytotoxic effects. It's available as trunk or root bark, tincture, tea, or infusion, in products such as Chun Pi.

Reported uses
Tree of heaven is used for pathologic leukorrhea, diarrhea, chronic dysentery, dysmenorrhea, cramps, asthma, tachycardia, gonorrhea, epilepsy, and tapeworm infestation.

Administration
- Infusion (add 50 g bark to 75 g hot water, strain, and then cool): 1 teaspoon twice a day, for a total daily dose of 6 to 9 g of herb
- Tincture: 5 to 60 gtt (about 7 to 20 grains) per dose by mouth two to four times a day, for a total daily dose of 6 to 9 g of herb.

Hazards
Tree of heaven may cause headache, tingling in the limb, dizziness, decreased cardiac function, nausea, and diarrhea. Dermatitis may occur after contact with leaves. Tree of heaven products that contain alcohol may cause a disulfiram-like reaction.

Pregnant or breast-feeding women should avoid this herb. Children and patients with compromised cardiac function, such as heart failure, coronary artery disease, or a history of myocardial infarction, should also avoid its use.

Clinical considerations
- Tree of heaven bark preparations have an offensive smell commonly described as burnt peanuts.
- Monitor patient carefully for adverse GI or central nervous system effects.
- If patient has diarrhea, monitor intake and output as indicated.
- Don't confuse tree of heaven (*Ailanthus altissima*) with tree of life (*Thuja occidentalis*).
- Advise patient to avoid use of tree of heaven while pregnant or breast-feeding.

■ Caution parents not to give tree of heaven to children.

■ Warn patient not to take tree of heaven for diarrhea, dysmenorrhea, or other symptoms before seeking medical attention because doing so may delay diagnosis of a potentially serious medical condition.

■ Tell patient to store herb in a dry, well-ventilated area away from moths.

■ Warn patient to keep all herbal products away from children and pets.

■ Tell patient to remind pharmacist of any herbal and dietary supplements that are being taken when obtaining a new prescription.

■ Advise patient to consult his health care provider before using an herbal preparation because a conventional treatment with proven efficacy may be available.

Research summary

The concepts behind the use of tree of heaven and the claims made regarding its effects have not yet been validated scientifically.

true unicorn root

Ague grass, ague-root, Aletris farinosa, *aloe-root, bettie grass, bitter grass, black-root, blazing star, colic-root, crow corn, devil's bit, star grass, starwort, star-grass, unicorn root, whitetube stargrass*

The useful constituents of true unicorn root are obtained from *Aletris farinosa.* True unicorn contains some steroidal components that may have estrogenic properties. It also contains alkaloids, oil, saponin, and resins. It's available as powdered or dried root, fluid extract, and infusion, in products such as Extraction Aletridis Alcoholicum, Aletris compound, Fem-H, FemTone, and Femtrol.

Reported uses

True unicorn root is used for rheumatism, gynecologic disorders (particularly dysmenorrhea and amenorrhea), habitual miscarriage, and symptoms caused by a prolapsed vagina. It's also used as a sedative, general tonic, laxative, antiflatulent, antidiarrheal, diuretic, and antispasmodic.

Administration

■ Fluid extract (1:1 in 45% alcohol): 0.3 to 0.6 g by mouth three times a day
■ Infusion (1.5 g of herb to 100 ml water): 0.3 to 0.6 g by mouth three times a day.

Hazards

True unicorn root may cause vertigo and colic. It may cause increased gastric acidity and reduced drug effects when used with antacids, histamine H_2 antagonists, proton pump inhibitors, and sucralfate. Herbal products that contain alcohol may cause a disulfiram-like reaction. True unicorn root may have additive effects when used with estrogens and hormonal contraceptives. It may antagonize the effects of oxytocin.

Pregnant or breast-feeding women should avoid this herb, as should patients being treated for alcoholism or liver disease. Because of its possible estrogenic effects, women with hormone-sensitive conditions (breast, uterine, and ovarian cancer, as well as endometriosis and uterine fibroids) should avoid using unicorn root.

Clinical considerations

■ Patient taking true unicorn root with estrogens and hormonal contraceptives may need dosage adjustment or a change to nonhormonal birth control.
■ Some patients may use true unicorn for repeated miscarriage despite repeated warnings against such use.
■ Advise patient that true unicorn root may increase stomach acid and interfere with the action of antacids and other

drugs used to limit or stop stomach acid production.
- Caution women of childbearing age and those attempting to conceive that using herb while pregnant or breast-feeding may have adverse effects.
- Warn patient not to take herb before seeking medical attention because doing so may delay diagnosis of a potentially serious medical condition.
- Instruct patient to promptly notify a health care provider about adverse effects or changes in symptoms.
- Tell patient to remind pharmacist of any herbal and dietary supplements that are being taken when obtaining a new prescription.
- Advise patient to consult his health care provider before using an herbal preparation because a conventional treatment with proven efficacy may be available.

Research summary
The concepts behind the use of true unicorn root and the claims made regarding its effects have not yet been validated scientifically.

turmeric

Amomum curcuma, Curcuma domestica, C. longa, C. rotunda, *Indian saffron*

Turmeric is a primary component of curry powders and some mustards. It's obtained from *Curcuma longa* and other species. The root contains volatile oils and diaryl heptanoids thought to have anti-inflammatory effects. Diaryl heptanoids may also have bile-stimulating and liver-protecting effects. Antispasmodic activity has also been noted. Other components include turmerone, atlantone, zingiberene, and more than six minor components of the oil. Two compounds, ukonon A and ukonon D, may possess anticancer activity via activation of phagocytosis and the reticuloendothelial system. Turmeric-containing products include Inflam-Aid, Lipolytics Plus, Phyto Quench Supreme, Pitta Balancing Elixir, Stone Free, and Turmeric Catechu Supreme.

Reported uses
Turmeric is used orally for dyspepsia, abdominal bloating, flatulence, liver and gallbladder complaints, headaches, and chest infections. It's also used as a flavoring and coloring agent in foods. Turmeric is used topically for analgesia, inflammation of the oral mucosa, inflammatory skin conditions, and ringworm.

Administration
- Average daily dose is 0.5 to 1 g of powdered root by mouth several times a day between meals; the usual maximum dose is 1.5 to 3.0 g by mouth every day
- Tincture: 10 to 15 gtt by mouth taken two or three times a day
- An infusion may be made by scalding 0.5 to 1 g powdered root in boiling water, covering and steeping for 5 minutes, and then straining. (Infusion isn't the preferred method of administration because turmeric contains volatile oils that aren't water soluble.) If used, 2 to 3 cups are taken by mouth between meals.

Hazards
Turmeric may cause indigestion, increased weight of sexual organs, increased sperm motility, decreased white and red blood cell counts, and depression of clotting factors.
  Turmeric may cause additive effects when taken with antiplatelet drugs, such as aspirin, clopidogrel bisulfate, and dipyridamole. It may also cause additive antiplatelet activity when taken with angelica, anise, arnica, asafoetida, bogbean, boldo, capsicum, celery, chamomile, clove, danshen, fenugreek, feverfew, garlic, ginger, ginkgo, ginseng, horse chestnut, horseradish, licorice, meadowsweet, onion, papain, passion flower, poplar,

prickly ash, quassia, red clover, wild carrot, wild lettuce, and willow.

Patients with bile duct obstruction, gallstones, gastric ulcers, or hyperacidity shouldn't use turmeric. Turmeric should be used with caution in patients who take other herbs or drugs that have antiplatelet activity.

Clinical considerations

- Patients who take indomethacin or reserpine may have a reduced risk of drug-induced gastric or duodenal ulcers when they also take turmeric.
- If patient takes an antiplatelet drug with turmeric, advise him to do so with caution.
- Tell patient to contact a health care provider immediately if frequent nosebleeds or other evidence of excessive anticoagulation develops.
- Warn patient not to take herb before seeking medical attention because doing so may delay diagnosis of a potentially serious medical condition.
- Instruct patient to protect turmeric from light and to keep all herbal products away from children and pets.
- Tell patient to remind pharmacist of any herbal and dietary supplements that are being taken when obtaining a new prescription.
- Advise patient to consult his health care provider before using an herbal preparation because a conventional treatment with proven efficacy may be available.

Research summary

Recent investigations indicate that the strong antioxidant effects of several components of turmeric result in an inhibition of carcinogenesis, and extracts may play a role as chemoprotectants, which limit the development of cancers.

Urine therapy

Amaroli, auto-urine therapy,
shivambu kalpa vidhi

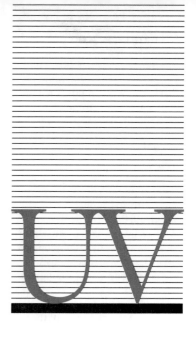

Urine has been used as a therapeutic agent for thousands of years. It is referred to as shivambu kalpa vidhi ("the method of drinking urine in order to rejuvenate") in Ayurvedic texts written over 5,000 years ago. Yogic texts refer to urine therapy as Amaroli ("the practice of ingesting one's own urine.") The Greeks and Romans were acquainted with the use of urine as a medicine. Hippocrates, the father of western medicine, mentioned the effectiveness of urine therapy. A major German encyclopedia includes various tips concerning the use of urine as medicine. John Armstrong is considered a modern urine therapy pioneer because of his famous book *The Water of Life*. He was exceptionally persistent in his conviction and enthusiasm concerning urine therapy, because he cured himself of tuberculosis which had been declared "incurable" through urine therapy. Perhaps the most difficult aspect of urine therapy is the psychological barrier.

Urine contains minute quantities of numerous chemicals, including agglutins and preciptins, which have a neutralizing effect on poliovirus and other viruses; antineoplastons, which selectively prevent the growth of cancer cells; and urokinase, a vasodilator that is extracted from urine and sold as medicine. A person normally excretes an average of 25 to

30 grams of urea per day. Some of the urea is converted into glutamine, and intestinal bacteria decompose urea into ammonia. Urea and ammonia have strong antibacterial and antiviral effects.

Reported uses

Urine therapy is reported to be a useful treatment for conditions including aging, acquired immunodeficiency syndrome, allergies, arthritis, bronchitis, burns, cancer, dandruff, diarrhea, depression, fatigue, fever, headache, leukemia, morning sickness, muscular dystrophy, obesity, poliomyelitis, syphilis, tuberculosis, varicose veins, vertigo, and warts, among others.

How the treatment is performed

- Drinking: Several ounces of the midstream, first morning excretion are drunk
- Gargling: Urine is gargled and is said to help with gum disease or other oral problems
- Drops: 2 to 3 drops are applied to the eye or ear
- Soaking: Urine is used to soak the feet in cases of athlete's foot
- Packing: Cotton gauze saturated with urine is applied topically to minor wounds, snake bites, bee stings, pest bites
- Massage: Fresh urine is massaged into the skin or hair for topical application
- Capsules: The purified ingredients from 700 ml of urine are packed into a 500-mg capsule which is taken orally with cold water
- Injection: One bottle containing 5 g in 100 ml of purified ingredients from 7,000 ml urine is mixed with Ringer's solution and administered by I.V. infusion
- Homeopathic preparation: A homeopathic preparation of urine is made by sequentially diluting it in water. The remedy is potentized by succussing (vigorously striking the bottle against a hard surface) the mixture between each dilution. A commonly used potency is a 6X, in which a 1 in 10 dilution is made 6 times (a $1 \div 1,000,000$ solution). Several drops of the remedy are applied to the tongue a few times each day for a week.

Hazards

Urine therapy should not be used when there is an active bladder infection or venereal disease. Caution should be used if the patient is taking prescription or recreational drugs. Many drugs are metabolized and secreted in urine. Patients with diabetes and kidney disease can have very low pH readings. In this case, it is important to check for acidity.

Some people experience a "healing crisis" or "recovery reaction." Common symptoms include diarrhea, itching, pain, fatigue, shoulder soreness, and fever. These symptoms appear more frequently in patients suffering long-term or serious illnesses, and symptoms may repeat several times. Each episode may last 3 to 7 days, but sometimes it may last for a month, or worsen over 6 months. Urine therapists should make patients aware of such reactions, and should stress that they are considered to be normal responses as the body initiates healing.

Clinical considerations

Urine therapy has been used for centuries. It is important that clinicians be aware of such therapies in case their patients have questions. There is a significant psychological barrier associated with its use.

Research summary

The concepts behind the use of urine therapy and the claims made regarding its effects have not yet been validated scientifically.

valerian

All-heal, amantilla, baldrian,
capon's tail, garden heliotrope, radix,
setewale, setwall, Valeriana officinalis,
vandal root

The useful constituents of valerian are
obtained from the underground parts
and roots of *Valeriana officinalis.* Many of
its constituents, including the essential
oils, seem to contribute to sedative properties of valerian. Valeric acid, the main
component of the root, inhibits the enzyme system responsible for breaking
down the neurotransmitter gamma-
aminobutyric acid (GABA), thus increasing its level in the brain. Valerian has
been used as a sedative and a perfume for
centuries. It is still used widely in Europe
as a sleep aid. Valerian may also have
mild pain relief properties and some hypotensive effects. Valerian is available as
dried root, essential oil, tea, tincture, extract, capsules, and tablets, in products
such as Herbal Sure Valerian Root, Nu-
Veg Valerian Root, and Quanterra Sleep.

Reported uses

Valerian is used to treat menstrual
cramps, restlessness, sleep disorders from
nervous conditions, and other symptoms
of psychological stress, such as anxiety,
nervous headaches, and gastric spasms.
It's used topically as a bath additive to
treat restlessness and sleep disorders.

Administration

■ Bath additive: Mix 100 g of root with
2 L of hot water, then add to the bath water
■ For restlessness: 220 mg of extract is
taken by mouth three times a day
■ Tea (steep 2 to 3 g root in 150 ml boiling water for 5 to 10 minutes, then
strain): 1 cup may be taken by mouth
two to three times a day, and before bedtime
■ Valerian tincture (1:5 solution in 45%
to 50% alcohol): 15 to 20 gtt in water

several times every day, or 1 to 3 ml several times a day
■ For hastening sleep and improving
sleep quality: 400 to 800 mg root is taken
by mouth up to 2 hours before bedtime.
Some patients need 2 to 4 weeks of use
for significant improvement. The maximum dosage is 15 g every day.

Hazards

Valerian may cause headache, morning
drowsiness, uneasiness, restlessness,
cardiac disturbances, GI complaints, contact allergies, and withdrawal symptoms,
including increased agitation and decreased sleep.

Valerian may enhance the effects of
barbiturates and benzodiazepines. Sedative effects of herbs such as catnip, hops,
kava, passion flower, and skullcap may be
potentiated by the use of valerian. Valerian may potentiate sedative effects of alcohol.

Pregnant or breast-feeding women
should avoid valerian. Patients with acute
or major skin injuries, fever, infectious
diseases, cardiac insufficiency, or hypertonia shouldn't bathe with valerian products.

 SAFETY RISK *Signs of valerian*
toxicity include ataxia, hypother-
mia, increased muscle relaxation,
chest tightness, abdominal cramps, and
tremor.

Clinical considerations

■ Valerian seems to have a more pronounced effect on those with disturbed
sleep or sleep disorders.
■ Evidence of valerian toxicity includes
difficulty walking, hypothermia, and increased muscle relaxation.
■ Withdrawal symptoms, such as increased agitation and decreased sleep, can
occur if valerian is abruptly stopped after
prolonged use.
■ Caution patient taking valerian for an
extended period to gradually decrease the
amount taken to avoid withdrawal.

- Valerian should be taken 1 to 2 hours before the desired sleep time. Explain that herb may take 2 to 4 weeks to act.
- Inform patient that most adverse effects occur only after long-term use.
- Instruct patient to promptly notify a health care provider about adverse effects.
- Warn patient not to take herb for insomnia before seeking medical attention because doing so may delay diagnosis of a potentially serious medical condition.
- Instruct patient to avoid hazardous activities until full central nervous system effects of herb are known.
- Tell patient to protect herb from light and to keep tincture in a tightly closed plastic container at room temperature.
- Warn patient to keep all herbal products away from children and pets.
- Tell patient to remind pharmacist of any herbal and dietary supplements that are being taken when obtaining a new prescription.
- Advise patient to consult his health care provider before using an herbal preparation because a conventional treatment with proven efficacy may be available.

Research summary
There is evidence that valerian is effective as a sleep aid and as a mild antianxiety agent. It has also been studied in combination with other herbs such as hops and St. John's wort. These have shown statistically significant effects. Valerian has been approved by the German Commission E for restlessness and sleep disorders, and is officially listed in the European Pharmacopoeia.

Valerian has been classified as generally recognized as safe in the United States for food use; extracts and the root oil are used as flavorings in foods and beverages.

Although it appears to be safe and effective as a sleep aid, further research is required.

Vegetarianism

Vegetarianism is the practice of avoiding animal flesh and fish in the diet. More than a simple dietary option, vegetarianism is a complex and varied lifestyle choice. Some, like Seventh Day Adventists and vegans, adhere to the diet for ideological reasons; others may adopt it strictly for nutritional benefits.

There are many subcategories of vegetarians: lacto-ovo vegetarians (eat only dairy and egg products), lactovegetarians (eat dairy but no egg products), vegans (avoid all animal-derived products), fruitarians (eat only fruits and nuts) and living foodists (eat only germinated seeds, cereals, sprouts, vegetables, fruits, berries, and nuts). The macrobiotic diet (see page 317) is sometimes incorrectly included under the heading of vegetarianism, but because it includes fish, it isn't truly vegetarian. Differentiating among vegetarians is significant as it demonstrates the varying degrees of nutrition available in the subcategories. For instance, an ovolactovegetarian will generally derive more protein, calcium, and B_{12} from his diet than a vegan. This is not to suggest that those adopting a living foods or vegan diet may not get adequate nutrition; rather, they must be more conscientious in their dietary choices to ensure proper nutrition.

Reported uses
Vegetarianism is used both as a lifestyle choice and as a specific treatment plan. Patients with cancer, cardiovascular disease, cerebrovascular disease, chronic renal failure, type II diabetes (non-insulin–dependent diabetes mellitus), obesity, ocular macular degeneration, and rheumatoid arthritis have all been shown to benefit from the vegetarian diet in general or one of its subcategories.

How the treatment is performed
Because vegetarianism is a lifestyle rather than a specific medication, there is no specific treatment plan. Rather, there are

general guidelines for the particular health conditions previously cited.

Hazards

Vegetarianism is a safe and effective adjunct treatment for many conditions. However, in certain subgroups such as vegans, fruitarians, and living foods vegetarians, it is prudent to check for nutrient deficiency states, such deficiencies in B_{12}, iron, calcium, zinc, and protein. Ovolacto- and lactovegetarians do not seem to have these deficiencies. One adverse effect, increased intestinal gas production, is common at the onset of adoption of a vegetarian diet.

As in the nonvegetarian pregnant woman, it is important to observe overall health and to ascertain if the woman is supplementing her diet with vitamins, minerals, and other nutrients. This will give the clinician an idea of the nutritional status of the diet. With pregnant women who appear less healthy, check for iron, fatty acid, and B_{12} deficiencies. Vitamin B_{12} deficiencies during pregnancy may lead to myelination dysfunction in the newborn or other neurological problems that may or may not resolve with the administration of B_{12} to the newborn. These same considerations should be addressed with the lactating vegetarian mother.

In a child's early developmental years, a strict vegetarian diet such as vegan, living foods, or fruitarian may not provide sufficient fatty acids, protein, and specific nutrients. In some instances, rickets, osteoporosis, anemia, and growth retardation have occurred. Supplementation with vitamins and minerals may avert these conditions.

As with the nonvegetarian child, the overall health of a vegetarian child depends on the quality of nutrition. Like their nonvegetarian counterparts, vegetarian children may resist eating vegetables. Creative parents can usually overcome these objections by encouraging the child to take part in grocery shopping and meal preparation. Calcium may be-

come a critical issue with the vegan subtype; adequate fatty acids may be more of concern with the raw or living foods vegetarian than with the ovolacto- or lactovegetarian. There is conflicting information concerning the growth and maturation of a vegetarian child; however, a lower body mass index is found consistently. The growth and maturation status of the vegetarian population is within the normal to low range.

Some adolescents adopt a vegetarian lifestyle as a passing fad, and others adopt it to lose weight. This particular group is often unaware of the need for beans, grains, and vegetables in their diets. They may frequently subsist on simple carbohydrates, convenience foods, and dairy products. Diets and supplementation should be reviewed carefully for adequate protein, calcium, and iron.

There are conflicting results in the various studies of bone mineral density (BMD) comparing vegetarian and nonvegetarian premenopausal and postmenopausal women. Some results indicate that the BMD at the spine is similar between vegetarians and omnivores, but that the BMD at the hip can be significantly lower in vegetarians. In other studies, which used the Wilcoxon signed-rank test, there was no significant difference in bone measurements between vegetarians and omnivores at any site except the skull. Between vegans and lactovegetarians, there was no significant difference in BMD. Calcium supplementation is essential in the vegetarian female at this life stage.

Clinical considerations

It is important to determine three factors about vegetarian patients: the type of vegetarianism the patient practices; whether the diet was adopted for ideological or health reasons; and whether the patient supplements his diet. This information gives the clinician a better idea of the nutritional value of the diet. Some vegetarians adhere to the diet for religious reasons and are less concerned about the nutritional value. Some sub-groups, such as vegans and living food vegetarians, may be reluctant to take food supplementation for ideological reasons. Suggest the addition of kelp, an easily obtainable seaweed and a source of B_{12}, for these patients.

In 1999, the Department of Nutrition at Loma Linda University in California presented an alternative food pyramid for vegetarians as a guide for a healthier diet. The pyramid consists of six levels. On the bottom level are whole grains (40%) and legumes (60%). The second level from the bottom recommends fruits (40%) and vegetables (60%); the third level contains nuts and seeds. In the vegetarian food pyramid, the top three layers are considered optional. The top layer is sweets, the second, dairy and eggs, and the third, vegetable oils. This new framework may be beneficial for advising vegetarians how to balance the various components of their diet.

Research summary
Dean Ornish, a cardiologist and an advocate of a low-fat vegan diet, has established the efficacy of the diet in reversing cardiovascular disease. His groundbreaking study first appeared in *JAMA* in 1983, and in *Lancet* in 1990.

Another important dietary study, the China Project, shows a connection between diet and the risk of developing disease. Researchers studied over 10,000 Chinese, in both villages and urban settings, who maintained the same diet, lifestyle, and locality of residence for their entire lives. The first survey was taken in 1983 to 1984, the second in 1989 to 1990. One of the main conclusions derived from the study is that the vegetarian diet, and a vegan diet in particular, lead to fewer risks of cancer, obesity, and cardiovascular disease.

Another group frequently studied to research vegetarianism are the members of the Seventh Day Adventist Church. Approximately 50% of these church members practice vegetarianism as part

of their religion, thus presenting an opportunity for researchers to study the long-term effects of the vegetarian diet. Loma Linda University in California and the Sydney Adventist Hospital in Australia have done most of the research on this group. Their conclusions support the vegetarian diet for prevention of coronary heart disease, diabetes mellitus, hypertension, arthritis, and some forms of cancer.

vervain

Eisenkraut, enchanter's plant, herb of Grace, herb of the cross, holywort, Juno's tears, pigeon's grass, pigeonweed, verbena,
Verbena officinalis

The useful parts of vervain are obtained from the above-ground parts of *Verbena officinalis*. It contains iridoid glycosides, including verbascoside, verbenalin, and verbenin. Vervain's actions are many and varied. Small amounts of verbenin appear to stimulate sympathetic activity; larger amounts inhibit it. Verbenin may also stimulate milk secretion. Verbenalin may be a uterine stimulant and abortifacient. Verbascoside may have analgesic and antihypertensive action and may enhance the antitremor action of levodopa. Vervain is available as tablets, liquid extract, and tincture, in products such as Quanterra Sinus and Sinupret.

Reported uses
Vervain is used to treat sore throats and other oral and pharyngeal inflammation, asthma, whooping cough, and sinusitis. It's also used to stimulate secretion of breast milk. Vervain is used topically to treat wounds, abscesses, arthritis pain, contusions, itching, and minor burns. It's also used as a gargle for cold symptoms.

Administration
- Liquid extract (1:1 in 25% alcohol): 2 to 4 ml by mouth every day
- Tea (add 2 to 4 g dried herb to 150 ml boiling water): 1 cup by mouth three times a day
- Tincture (1:1 in 40% alcohol): 5 to 10 ml by mouth three times a day.

Hazards
Vervain may cause paralysis, stupor, seizures, sedation, hypertension, hypotension, vomiting, and uterine stimulation.

Excessive amounts of vervain can interfere with hormone therapy. Vervain may reduce the effect of hypertensive and hypotensive drugs. Herbal products that contain alcohol may cause a disulfiram-like reaction. When vervain is combined with alcohol, there may be additive sedative effects.

Pregnant or breast-feeding women should avoid vervain, as should patients on hypertensive, hypotensive, or hormone therapies.

Clinical considerations
- Monitor patient closely for adverse central nervous system (CNS) effects and response to herb.
- Evidence of excessive intake of the verbenalin component includes CNS paralysis, stupor, and seizures.
- If patient takes hormone therapy, a hypertensive drug, or a hypotensive drug, warn against using this herb.
- Tell patient to refrain from alcohol and other sedatives because they may cause increased sedative effects.
- Caution patient taking disulfiram about possible adverse reactions.
- Advise patient that taking excessive amounts of vervain can cause CNS depression.
- Warn patient to keep all herbal products away from children and pets.
- Tell patient to remind pharmacist of any herbal and dietary supplements that are being taken when obtaining a new prescription.
- Advise patient to consult his health care provider before using an herbal preparation because a conventional treatment with proven efficacy may be available.

Research summary
The concepts behind the use of vervain and the claims made regarding its effects have not yet been validated scientifically.

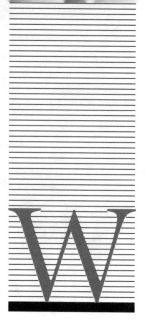

wahoo

Arrow wood, bitter ash, bleeding heart, burning bush, bursting heart, Euonymus atropurpureus, *fish wood, fusanum, fusoria, gatten, Indian arrowroot, pigwood, spindle tree*

The medicinal parts of wahoo are obtained from the stems, root bark, and berries of *Euonymus atropurpureus*. Its seeds and bark contain cardioactive steroid glycosides similar to digoxin, as well as various alkaloids, caffeine, and theobromine. Wahoo is thought to stimulate bile flow and to have laxative and diuretic effects. In larger amounts, it can affect the heart. It's available as fresh or dried herb, juice, and capsules.

 SAFETY RISK *Wahoo is poisonous. Reportedly, ingesting just 36 berries can be fatal. Signs of toxicity include upset stomach, bloody diarrhea, fever, shortness of breath, collapse, stupor increasing to unconsciousness, severe tonic-clonic spasms with locked jaw muscles, and coma.*

Reported uses
Wahoo bark is used orally to treat indigestion and to stimulate bile production. It's also used as a laxative, a diuretic, and a tonic.

Administration
Use of wahoo isn't recommended.

Hazards

Wahoo shouldn't be used by anyone. It is poisonous even in small amounts. It causes stupor, severe tonic-clonic spasms with lockjaw, coma, circulatory collapse, upset stomach, severe bloody diarrhea, dyspnea, and fever.

If wahoo is used with digoxin or other cardioactive drugs, there's an increased risk of cardiac or cardiac glycoside toxicity. If used with macrolide antibiotics or tetracyclines, there may be an increased risk of cardiac glycoside toxicity. Increased risk of cardiac glycoside toxicity occurs when wahoo is used with potassium-depleting diuretics, as well. Glycoside toxicity may increase when wahoo is used with stimulant laxatives. Wahoo may also increase risk of cardiac toxicity (through potassium depletion) if used in conjunction with horsetail, licorice, or stimulant laxative herbs, such as aloe, cascara bark, and yellow dock.

Clinical considerations

- Wahoo interacts with many drugs.
- Warn patient of potential dangers of using wahoo, and discourage its use.
- Warn patient not to take herb before seeking medical attention because doing so may delay diagnosis of a potentially serious medical condition.
- Warn patient to keep all herbal products away from children and pets.
- Tell patient to remind pharmacist of any herbal and dietary supplements that are being taken when obtaining a new prescription.
- Advise patient to consult his health care provider before using this herbal preparation because a conventional treatment with proven efficacy may be available.

Research summary

Wahoo is poisonous even in small amounts, and shouldn't be used.

watercress

Agrao, berro, brunnenkressenkraut, crescione di fonte, Indian cress, mizu-garushi, nasilord, nasturtii herba, Nasturtium officinale, *oranda-garashi, scurvy grass, selada-air*

The useful parts of watercress are obtained from the above ground parts of *Nasturtium officinale*. It contains mustard oil, vitamin C, beta carotene, minerals, and vitamins B_1, B_2, E, and K. Watercress has diuretic and slight antibiotic activity, which may also result from mustard oil.

Reported uses

Watercress is used for treating catarrh (an inflammation of the air passages usually involving the nose, throat, or lungs), chronic bronchitis, and mucous membrane inflammation of the respiratory tract. It's also used as a poultice for skin irritation, a detoxifying agent, a diuretic, a spring tonic, and an appetite stimulant. Watercress is also widely cultivated as a salad herb.

Administration

- The average daily dose is 4 to 6 g of dried herb, 20 to 30 g fresh herb, or 60 to 150 g freshly pressed juice
- The average daily dose of watercress tea is 2 to 3 cups, taken by mouth. The tea is prepared by pouring 150 ml boiling water over 2 g of drug (about 1 to 2 teaspoons), covering for 10 to 15 minutes, and then straining.

Hazards

Watercress may cause GI irritation, kidney damage, and skin irritation. It may potentiate the effects of drugs such as chlorzoxazone and orphenadrine citrate. There may be additive effects if watercress is used with diuretics. Watercress may antagonize the anticoagulant effects of warfarin because of its high vitamin K content.

Pregnant or breast-feeding women should avoid watercress, as should children younger than age 4 years and patients with gastric ulcers, intestinal ulcers, or inflammatory kidney disease.

Clinical considerations
- Consuming large amounts of watercress may cause GI irritation.
- Watercress can be used topically as a poultice or compress, but watch for skin irritation.
- Caution patient about possible GI irritation from the effects of mustard oil on mucous membranes.
- Use caution if patient also takes an anticoagulant. Warn the patient that watercress has a vitamin K content and instruct him to watch for signs of bleeding, such as easy bruising and bleeding gums.
- Warn patient not to take watercress before seeking medical attention because doing so may delay diagnosis of a potentially serious medical condition.
- Warn patient to keep all herbal products away from children and pets.
- Tell patient to remind pharmacist of any herbal and dietary supplements that are being taken when obtaining a new prescription.
- Advise patient to consult his health care provider before using an herbal preparation because a conventional treatment with proven efficacy may be available.

Research summary
The concepts behind the use of watercress and the claims made regarding its effects have not yet been validated scientifically.

wild cherry

Black cherry, black choke, choke cherry, Prunus serotina, P. virginiana, rum cherry bark, Virginian prune, wild black cherry

The useful constituents of the wild cherry are obtained from the stem bark of *Prunus serotina* or *P. virginiana*. It contains prunasin, a cyanogenic glycoside that's hydrolyzed to toxic hydrocyanic acid (HCN) and benzaldehyde. Wild cherry has astringent, antitussive, and sedative effects. Bark collected in the fall has higher HCN content than bark collected in the spring. Wild cherry is available as dried bark and liquid extract, and in combination products.

Reported uses
Wild cherry is widely used in cough syrups because of its sedative, expectorant, and antitussive effects. It's also used to treat colds, bronchitis, whooping cough, other lung problems, nervous digestive disorders, and diarrhea. It's used in foods and beverages as a flavoring agent.

Administration
The average dose of the liquid extract (alcohol 12% to 14% by volume) is 5 to 12 gtt in water by mouth two to three times a day.

Hazards
Fatal poisoning may occur with ingestion of large amounts of wild cherry. No drug interactions are known. Pregnant or breast-feeding women shouldn't use wild cherry because prunasin, one of its constituents, may be teratogenic.

 SAFETY RISK *Wild cherry should be avoided because of its HCN content. Keep wild cherry plant parts out of reach of children; indeed, deaths have occurred among children who ate fruit or leaves.*

Clinical considerations

- Wild cherry is best used only in very small amounts as a component of cough syrups because of the risk of poisoning at larger doses.
- Instruct patient to use wild cherry only in combination cough syrups, as directed by a health care provider or pharmacist.
- Caution patient about dangers of excessive use of wild cherry.
- Warn patient not to take wild cherry for respiratory problems before seeking medical attention because doing so may delay diagnosis of a potentially serious medical condition.
- Warn patient to keep all herbal products away from children and pets.
- Tell patient to remind pharmacist of any herbal and dietary supplements that are being taken when obtaining a new prescription.
- Advise patient to consult his health care provider before using an herbal preparation because a conventional treatment with proven efficacy may be available.

Research summary

The concepts behind the use of wild cherry and the claims made regarding its effects have not yet been validated scientifically, with the exception of chemical interactions that have been reported in clinical studies.

wild ginger

Asarabacca, Asarum canadense, A. europaeum, *cat's foot, false coltsfoot, hazelwort, Indian ginger, public house plant, snakeroot, wild nard*

The useful constituents of wild ginger are obtained from *Asarum canadense* or *A. europaeum.* It contains phenylpropanol, trans-isoasarone, and aristolochic acid. Mode of action is unknown, but constituents of rhizome may have antibiotic, antiseptic, antispasmodic, anti-inflammatory, expectorant, and sedative properties. Phenylpropanol may be responsible for effects on bronchitis and bronchial asthma. Some products are standardized for this constituent. Trans-isoasarone may cause emetic and spasmolytic effects. Aristolochic acid may be carcinogenic and nephrotoxic. Wild ginger is available as dried root, dried rhizome, and liquid extract, in products such as Bronchaid and Immunaid.

Reported uses

Asarum canadense is used to treat GI spasms, gas, and chronic pulmonary conditions such as bronchitis. It's also used to produce sweating and promote menstruation. Wild ginger may be added to multiple-ingredient products and is promoted for chronic cough, bronchitis, or immune system support.

Extract of *A. europaeum* is used in Europe for acute and chronic bronchitis, bronchial spasms, and bronchial asthma. It's also used as a menstrual stimulant and antitussive and to treat angina pectoris, migraines, liver disease, jaundice, and pneumonia.

Administration

- Typical doses of *A. canadense*: 1½ oz of powdered root in 1 pint boiling water as tea; taken hot
- Typical doses of *A. europaeum*: 30 mg dry extract by mouth for adults and children older than age 13.

Hazards

Wild ginger may cause partial paralysis, burning of tongue, nausea, vomiting, gastroenteritis, diarrhea, acute renal failure, and dermatitis. Herbal products that contain alcohol may cause a disulfiram-like reaction.

Pregnant or breast-feeding women should avoid wild ginger, as should patients with a kidney disorder or an infectious or inflammatory GI condition.

Clinical considerations
- Monitor patient's kidney function with long-term use of wild ginger.
- Monitor patient's response to wild ginger.
- Don't confuse wild ginger with bitter milkwort (*Polygala amara*) or senega (*P. senega*), both of which are also known as snakeroot.
- Caution patient against long-term use because of possible kidney problems and carcinogenic effects of aristolochic acid in the wild ginger.
- Warn patient to keep all herbal products away from children and pets.
- Tell patient to remind pharmacist of any herbal and dietary supplements that are being taken when obtaining a new prescription.
- Advise patient to consult his health care provider before using an herbal preparation because a conventional treatment with proven efficacy may be available.

Research summary
The concepts behind the use of wild ginger and the claims made regarding its effects have not yet been validated scientifically.

wild indigo

American indigo, Baptisia tinctoria, *false indigo, horse-fly weed, indigo broom, rattlebush, rattleweed, yellow broom, yellow indigo*

The useful parts of wild indigo are obtained from the root of *Baptisia tinctoria*. It contains polysaccharides, glycoproteins, quinolizidine alkaloids, isoflavonoids, and hydroxycoumarins. Wild indigo may have immunostimulant properties and a mild estrogenic effect. It's available as dried root, root powder, capsules, tablets, suppositories, drops, homeopathic injection, and liquid extracts, in products such as Esberitox, Immune Boost, and Re-Zist.

Reported uses
Wild indigo is used to treat infections, such as typhoid, diphtheria, malaria, and scarlet fever. Large doses induce bowel evacuation and vomiting. It's also used to treat ear, nose, and throat infections and for inflamed lymph glands and fever. It's commonly combined with other herbs, such as echinacea, which are thought to stimulate the immune system. In homeopathic medicine, wild indigo is used to treat confusion and blood poisoning. Wild indigo is used as a mouthwash to treat mouth sores and gum disease. It's used topically for wound cleaning.

Administration
- Decoction (½ to 1 teaspoon of root in a cup of water, boiled, and then simmered 10 to 15 minutes): by mouth three times a day
- Homeopathic dosing: 5 to 10 gtt, 1 tablet, or 5 to 10 globules by mouth up to three times a day; for injection solution, 1 ml twice weekly subcutaneously
- Liquid extract or tincture (1:1 in 60% alcohol): 1 to 2 ml by mouth three times a day
- Ointment (1:8 parts liquid extract to ointment base): applied topically to affected area.

Hazards
Wild indigo may cause vomiting, diarrhea, inflammation of the GI tract, spasms, and skin irritation. Herbal products that contain alcohol may cause a disulfiram-like reaction.

Pregnant or breast-feeding women should avoid wild indigo, as should patients with inflammatory GI conditions. Long-term use (by mouth or topical) is contraindicated owing to potential toxicity.

Clinical considerations

■ Do not confuse wild indigo with the root of false blue indigo (*B. australis*) or *B. alba*.

■ Warn patient not to take wild indigo before seeking medical attention because doing so may delay diagnosis of a potentially serious medical condition.

■ Tell patient to watch for adverse effects such as local reactions if wild indigo is used topically as an ointment. Urge him to promptly notify health care provider about any change in symptoms.

■ Wild indigo may be toxic, and the use of it isn't advised.

■ Warn patient to keep all herbal products away from children and pets.

■ Tell patient to remind pharmacist of any herbal and dietary supplements that are being taken when obtaining a new prescription.

■ Advise patient to consult his health care provider before using an herbal preparation because a conventional treatment with proven efficacy may be available.

Research summary

The concepts behind the use of wild indigo and the claims made regarding its effects have not yet been validated scientifically.

wild lettuce

Acrid lettuce, bitter lettuce, green endive, Lactuca canadensis, L. virosa, *lactucarium, lettuce opium, poison lettuce*

Wild lettuce is obtained from the dried latex and leaves of *Lactuca canadensis* and *L. virosa*. The milky latex can cause mydriasis. Lactucin, a component of the latex, may have sedative and central nervous system (CNS) depressant properties. Trace amounts of morphine have been found in *Lactuca* species, but not enough to exert pharmacologic ef-

fects. Wild lettuce is available as dried or powdered herb, oil, dried sap, and extracts, in products such as Hypericum Pro (contains multiple ingredients), Hydro, Sahivah Blend, Turkhash, Spirit Walk, and Vision Quest.

Reported uses

Wild lettuce is typically used as an antiseptic. The latex is also used as a sedative and as a treatment for colic and cough. The seed oil is used for arteriosclerosis and as a substitute for wheat germ oil. The leaf is used for insomnia, restlessness, dry irritated cough, and muscle or joint pain. The latex and leaf are used for excitability in children, priapism, painful menses, swollen genitals, and as an opium substitute in cough preparations. The leaf and dried sap of wild lettuce are smoked recreationally as legal substitutes for marijuana and hashish. The crude extract has been injected intravenously for the same purpose. Wild lettuce is also used as an analgesic and a GI aid.

Administration

■ Infusion (1 or 2 teaspoons [0.5 to 3 g] dried leaves in 150 ml of boiling water, steeped for 10 to 15 minutes): by mouth three times a day

■ Tincture: 1 to 2 ml by mouth three times a day

■ Liquid extract (1:1 in 25% alcohol— 0.5 to 3.0 ml) three times a day

■ Dried latex extract: 0.3 to 1 g three times a day.

Hazards

Wild lettuce may cause dizziness, ringing in ears, somnolence, coma, tachycardia, pupil dilation, tachypnea, contact dermatitis, and allergic reaction.

Wild lettuce may have additive sedative effects when used with antihistamines, nonprescription cold drugs, and sedatives. There's increased risk of bleeding when wild lettuce is used with herbs that have anticoagulant or antiplatelet effects. Wild lettuce may enhance the therapeutic and adverse effects of herbs with sedative effects. Herbal products that contain alcohol may cause a disulfiram-like reaction. Wild lettuce may add to the CNS effects of alcohol.

Pregnant or breast-feeding women should avoid wild lettuce, as should patients hypersensitive to members of the Compositae family and patients with a history of glaucoma or benign prostatic hypertrophy.

 SAFETY RISK *Large doses of wild lettuce can cause stupor, depressed respiration, and death.*

Clinical considerations

■ Monitor patient for bleeding, and check prothrombin time and International Normalized Ratio, if indicated.

■ Advise the patient to use caution if combining wild lettuce with other sedating drugs or with alcohol.

■ Caution patient to avoid hazardous activities until CNS effects of wild lettuce are fully known.

■ Warn patient not to take wild lettuce before seeking medical attention because doing so may delay diagnosis of a potentially serious medical condition.

■ Tell patient to promptly notify a health care provider about adverse effects or changes in symptoms.

■ Warn patient to keep all herbal products away from children and pets.

■ Tell patient to remind pharmacist of any herbal and dietary supplements that are being taken when obtaining a new prescription.

■ Advise patient to consult his health care provider before using an herbal preparation because a conventional treatment with proven efficacy may be available.

Research summary

The concepts behind the use of wild lettuce and the claims made regarding its effects have not yet been validated scientifically.

wild yam

Atlantic yam, barbasco,
China root, colic root, devil's bones,
Dioscorea composita, D. villosa,
Mexican wild yam, rheumatism root,
yuma

Wild yam was popularized in the 19th century for its supposed antispasmodic properties and was prescribed for biliary colic and spasm of the bowel. More recently, it has been promoted for the relief of nausea in pregnancy, for amenorrhea, and for dysmenorrhea. Wild yam is obtained from the rhizome and roots of *Dioscorea composita* or *D. villosa*. It contains a glycoside, diosgenin, saponins, and tannins. Diosgenin is a steroid precursor used in the first commercial production of oral contraceptives, topical hormones, estrogens, progestogens, androgens, and other sex hormones. However, compounds in wild yam can't be used as hormones by the human body. Diosgenin may have some weak estrogenic effects, but not progesterogenic actions. Progesterogenic effects are sometimes obtained from wild yam cream by adding "natural" (that is, produced synthetically but derived from natural sources such as soybeans or other plant sources) progesterone, which is absorbed through the skin. Diosegenin prevents estrogen-induced bile flow suppression. It may stimulate the growth of mammary tissue.

Wild yam is available as capsules, creams, gels, and liquid extracts. Common trade names include combination products such as Bone Strengthener Formula, Super Female Formula, Ultra Diet Pep, and Yam Extract Plus 30. It's also available in creams such as Born Again Wild Yam Gel, Resolve, and Yamcon Vaginal. Wild yam creams with progesterone include FemPro, Progesterone Plus, Yam Complex, Wild Yamcon, Wild Yam EFX, and Yamcon Pro. Oral products include MexiYam.

Reported uses

Commercial wild yam cream and oral preparations are used to relieve menopausal symptoms, premenstrual syndrome (PMS), and other gynecologic symptoms. Wild yam doesn't, however, contain hormones or compounds such as dihydroepiandrosterone (DHEA), which are converted into hormones in the human body. Orally, wild yam is used as a "natural alternative" for estrogen replacement, postmenopausal vaginal dryness, PMS, osteoporosis, increasing energy and libido in men and women, and breast enlargement. It may also be used for diverticulosis, gallbladder colic, painful menstruation, cramps, rheumatoid arthritis, and urinary tract infection. Wild yam cream with progesterone added from other sources exerts physiologic effects from the absorbed progesterone. Progesterone cream may be useful for treating menopausal symptoms. However, progesterone has been shown to be an ineffective treatment for PMS even at much higher doses.

Wild yam is also used in multiple-ingredient commercial formulas promoted for treatment of menopause symptoms and PMS, prevention of osteoporosis and threatened abortion, andenhancement of weight loss, women's general health, and men's prostate health. Diosgenin, a yam constituent, is promoted as a natural precursor to DHEA to improve athletic performance and slow the aging process.

Administration

No consensus exists for either oral or topical dosage of wild yam. See manufacturer's product labels for instructions.

Hazards

Wild yam may cause dizziness, headache, fatigue, nausea, vomiting, diarrhea, abdominal pain, breast pain, and infection. It may cause abnormal menstrual flow, including amenorrhea, spotting, and breakthrough bleeding.

Wild yam may increase blood levels and enhance adverse effects of prescribed progestins. When taken with indomethacin, wild yam may decrease the drug's anti-inflammatory effect. Herbal products that contain alcohol may cause a disulfiram-like reaction.

The addition of progesterone and the amount added may not be obvious on package labeling. Pregnant or breast-feeding women should avoid wild yam. Progesterone-containing products shouldn't be used by patients with breast cancer, liver disease, liver cancer, or undiagnosed uterine or urinary tract bleeding.

Clinical considerations

- Topical creams that contain progesterone may increase the adverse effects of prescribed progestins.
- Topical progesterone alone may not reduce the risk of osteoporosis.
- Breast examinations should be performed routinely, especially with prolonged progestin use.
- Instruct patient to have appropriate medical evaluation before beginning any new herbal or dietary supplement.
- Urge patient to talk to a health care provider before using progesterone-containing products.
- Warn patient not to take wild yam before seeking medical attention because doing so may delay diagnosis of a potentially serious medical condition.
- Instruct patient to apply cream to alternate body areas daily to ensure optimum absorption.
- Tell patient to promptly notify a health care provider about adverse effects or changes in symptoms.
- Caution pregnant and breast-feeding woman that effects of wild yam are unknown.
- Warn patient to keep all herbal products away from children and pets.
- Tell patient to remind pharmacist of any herbal and dietary supplements that are being taken when obtaining a new prescription.

- Advise patient to consult his health care provider before using an herbal preparation because a conventional treatment with proven efficacy may be available.

Research summary

Wild yam root is currently being used for the treatment of menstrual dysfunction; however, little scientific evidence supports its use in medicine. The potential for toxicity is modest, but in the absence of evidence of benefit, it cannot be recommended.

willow

Bay willow, black willow, brittle willow, crack willow, Daphne willow, laurel willow, purple osier, pupurweide, Salix alba, S. nigra, *violet willow, white willow*

For centuries, willow bark has was used to treat fevers, headache and other pain, and arthritis. In the late 19th century, salicylic acid was widely used in place of willow bark, and its derivative, aspirin, was discovered to be less irritating to the mouth and stomach. The useful constituents of willow are obtained from *Salix alba* or *S. nigra*. The bark contains 2% to 11% salicin, which is converted by the body into salicylic acid — similar to aspirin in its analgesic, anti-inflammatory, and fever-reducing properties. It also contains flavonoids, and 10% to 20% tannins, which have astringent properties. Willow is available as crude inner bark, capsules, and dry and liquid extract. Extracts are often combined with root powder in commercial products. Common trade names include Willowprin, and combination products include Allerelief, Arth Plus, Cold-Control, Coldrin, Congest Ease, Menstrual-Ease, and Migracin.

Reported uses

Willow is used to reduce fever, treat inflamed joints, ease GI disorders, and relieve pain. It's also used in combination products for colds, flu, allergies, menstrual pain, premenstrual syndrome, migraines, arthritis, and inflammation.

Administration

- Bark equivalent: 600 to 3,000 mg up to six times a day
- Decoction (1 or 2 teaspoons [1 to 3 g] of bark added to 1 cup water, boiled, simmered 10 to 15 minutes, then strained): by mouth three times a day
- Liquid extract (1:1 in 25% alcohol) 1 to 3 ml three times a day.

Hazards

Willow may cause stomach upset, esophageal cancer, kidney damage, liver necrosis, skin rash, and bleeding episodes. There is increased risk of bleeding if willow is taken with anticoagulants. Herbal products that contain alcohol may cause a disulfiram-like reaction. GI bleeding and ulceration may occur if willow is taken with nonsteroidal anti-inflammatory drugs, including aspirin and ibuprofen. Use of willow with other herbal products should be avoided because of the risk that the tannin component will precipitate alkaloids.

Willow shouldn't be used by patients hypersensitive to aspirin or salicylates or by those with gastritis, peptic ulcer disease, or kidney or liver dysfunction. It shouldn't be given to feverish children or adolescents because salicylates may cause Reye's syndrome. Pregnant women shouldn't use willow because it contains salicylates similar to aspirin, which are usually contraindicated in pregnancy.

 SAFETY RISK *Willow bark products may be marketed as aspirin-free but may cause some of the same adverse reactions as aspirin, such as Reye's syndrome and salicylate hypersensitivity.*

Clinical considerations

■ Problems in breast-fed infants with usual analgesic doses of aspirin or willow haven't been documented. However, salicylates appear in breast milk and may cause macular rashes in breast-fed infants.

■ Monitor patient for adverse reactions and signs of bleeding. Routinely check prothrombin time and International Normalized Ratio, as indicated.

■ Watch for sedative effects if patient takes a form of willow that contains alcohol.

■ Ask whether patient has had adverse reactions to aspirin.

■ Advise pregnant and breast-feeding women that effects of this herb are unknown and that aspirin, which is similar to some components in willow, is usually contraindicated in pregnancy.

■ Caution parents not to give willow-containing products to feverish children or adolescents.

■ Tell patient that taking willow with meals may reduce stomach upset.

■ Instruct patient to separate doses of willow from intake of other oral drugs to avoid interactions.

■ Urge patient to have an appropriate medical evaluation before beginning to take an herbal supplement.

■ Warn patient not to take willow before seeking medical attention because doing so may delay diagnosis of a potentially serious medical condition.

■ Tell patient to promptly notify a health care provider about adverse effects or changes in symptoms.

■ Warn patient to keep all herbal products away from children and pets.

■ Tell patient to remind pharmacist of any herbal and dietary supplements that are being taken when obtaining a new prescription.

■ Advise patient to consult his health care provider before using an herbal preparation because a conventional treatment with proven efficacy may be available.

Research summary

Willow bark is approved by the German Commission E for diseases accompanied by fever, rheumatic ailments, and headaches. It is monographed in British literature, and is due to be published in the American Herbal Pharmacopeia shortly.

wintergreen

Boxberry, Canada tea, checkerberry, deerberry, gaultheria oil,
Gaultheria procumbens, *ground berry, hillberry, mountain tea, partridge berry, spiceberry, teaberry, wax cluster*

The useful portions of wintergreen are obtained from *Gaultheria procumbens.* Wintergreen oil is obtained by steam distillation of the warmed, water-soaked leaves. It is used interchangeably with sweet birch oil or methylsalicylate for flavoring foods and candies. The plant and its oil are used in traditional medicine as an anodyne and analgesic, carminative, astringent, and topical rubefacient. Teas made from wintergreen are used to relieve cold symptoms and muscle aches. Wintergreen contains a volatile oil, 96% to 98% of which is methyl salicylate, and during steam distillation of the leaves, the monotropitoside, gaultherin, is enzymatically hydrolyzed to methyl salicylate. Topical counterirritant and analgesic effects result from methyl salicylate, which is percutaneously absorbed and inhibits prostaglandin synthesis. Wintergreen is available as oil, cream, lotion, gel, and liniment, in products such as Koong Yick Hung Fa Oil and Olbas Oil.

Reported uses

Wintergreen is used as an anodyne, analgesic, antasthmatic, digestive stimulant, antiseptic, and aromatic. It's also used to treat neuralgia, gastralgia, pleurisy, pleurodynia, ovarialgia, orchitis, epididymitis, diaphragmitis, uratic arthritis, and dysmenorrhea. Wintergreen is used topically as an antiseptic and to treat musculo-skeletal pain and rheumatoid arthritis. It's also used as a flavoring agent in candies and foods.

Administration

- Tea: 1 teaspoon dried leaves added to 1 cup boiling water by mouth every day
- Gels, lotions, ointments, liniments containing 10% to 60% methyl salicylate: For adults and children older than age 2, these products are applied topically to the affected area three to four times a day.

Hazards

Wintergreen may cause confusion, pulmonary edema and collapse, tinnitus, GI distress, nausea, vomiting, renal failure, liver failure, metabolic acidosis, rhab-domyolysis, hyperventilation, respiratory alkalosis, contact dermatitis, and diaphoresis.

There's increased risk of bleeding when wintergreen is used with anticoag-ulants or antiplatelet drugs. Large doses of topical or oral wintergreen may increase hypoglycemia if used with antidia-betics or salicylates. Use of oral winter-green with alcohol may increase the risk for GI irritation.

Women who are pregnant or wish to become pregnant and those who are breast-feeding should avoid wintergreen, as should patients with severe asthma, nasal polyps, peptic or duodenal ulcers, or allergy to salicylates. Because methyl salicylate may play a role in Reye's syn-drome, wintergreen shouldn't be used in infants, children, or adolescents during or after flulike symptoms.

 SAFETY RISK *One teaspoon win-tergreen oil is the equivalent of about 7,000 mg salicylate or 21.5 adult aspirin (325 mg) tablets. Ingestion of more than small amounts of methyl sali-cylate is hazardous. Although the average lethal dose of methyl salicylate is estimated to be 10 ml for children and 30 ml for adults, death has resulted after intake of as little as 4 ml in infants and 5 ml in chil-dren. Because of this toxicity, no drug product may contain more than 5% methyl salicylate or it will be regarded as misbranded. The FDA requires child-resistant containers for liquid forms that contain more than 5% methyl salicylate.*

Clinical considerations

- The highest concentration of methyl salicylate used in candy flavoring is 0.04%.
- Monitor serum glucose level in patients who take large doses of winter-green.
- Advise patient to inform health care provider before using wintergreen.
- Caution patient not to use a heating pad with topical wintergreen and not to apply topical wintergreen after strenuous exercise, especially on a hot, humid day. These conditions increase transdermal absorption of wintergreen.
- Warn parents not to use wintergreen in infants, children, or adolescents during or after flulike symptoms.
- Instruct diabetic patient to closely monitor serum glucose level and to re-port changes to a health care provider.
- If patient is taking wintergreen oil orally, stress the importance of proper dosing, because amounts from 4 to 10 ml of the oil have been fatal.
- Explain the evidence of salicylism, in-cluding tinnitus, nausea, vomiting, sweating, and hyperventilation. Tell pa-tient to seek medical attention immedi-ately if symptoms occur.
- Caution patient not to consume alco-hol while taking wintergreen.
- Warn patient to keep all herbal prod-ucts away from children and pets.
- Tell patient to remind pharmacist of any herbal and dietary supplements that are being taken when obtaining a new prescription.
- Advise patient to consult his health care provider before using an herbal preparation because a conventional treat-ment with proven efficacy may be avail-able.

Research summary

To date there is very limited research on the uses of wintergreen, and what research has been done has focused on the potential dangers from wintergreen oil. The counterirritant and analgesic effects are well documented. Other claims made for the use of wintergreen oil have not yet been validated scientifically.

witch hazel

Hamamelis virginiana,
*hamamelis water, hazel nut,
snapping hazel, spotted alder,
striped alder, tobacco wood,
winter bloom*

Witch hazel is a widely known plant with a long history of use in the Americas. It was known to native North American people as a treatment for tumor and eye inflammation. It was used internally for hemorrhaging. Eighteenth century settlers came to value its astringency, and it is still used today for this and other purposes. Witch hazel is obtained from dried or fresh bark, leaves, and roots of *Hamamelis virginiana*. It contains flavonoids such as kaempferol and quercitrin, tannins (up to 12%), and a volatile oil (about 0.5%). The oil contains small amounts of safrole and eugenol, sesquiterpenes, resin, wax, and choline. Witch hazel's astringent and hemostatic properties result from high levels of tannins in the leaf, bark, and extract. Extracts may cause vasoconstriction, decrease vascular permeability, tighten distended vessels, restore vessel tone, and stop bleeding immediately. Hamamelis water, or witch hazel water, doesn't contain tannins, so its astringent properties may result from other constituents or from alcohol content. Witch hazel is available as poultices, medicated pads and toilettes, soap, shampoo, aftershave, ointment and gel, decoction, suppositories, liquid, liquid extract, and gargle, in products such as Grandpa

Soap Witch Hazel, Superhazl Medicated Pads, Thayer's Herbal Astringent, and Tucks Medicated Pads.

Reported uses

Witch hazel is primarily used topically for itching, insect bites, minor burns, local inflammation of skin and mucous membranes, varicose veins, hemorrhoids, and bruises. It's also used rectally as an enema for bleeding hemorrhoids. Witch hazel may enhance solar protection factor (SPF) when combined with other skin protective agents. Witch hazel is an approved ingredient in many over-the-counter products for topical use. It may also be used orally to treat diarrhea, mucous colitis, hematemesis, and hemoptysis.

Administration

- Suppository: One suppository is inserted rectally one to three times a day
- Tea (150 ml boiling water poured over 2 to 3 g drug and strained after 10 minutes): Taken by mouth three times a day
- Hamamelis liquid extract (1:1 in 45% alcohol): Dosage is 2 to 4 ml by mouth three times a day
- Hamamelis water in 14% to 15% alcohol: For anorectal disorders, witch hazel may be applied up to six times every day, or after each bowel movement. For minor cuts, burns, and wounds, the affected area is soaked two to four times a day for 15 to 30 minutes, or a compress is applied, soaked in the solution, and reapplied every few minutes for 20 to 30 minutes, four to six times every day.

Hazards

Witch hazel may cause nausea, vomiting, constipation, fecal impaction, liver damage, and contact allergy. Herbal products that contain alcohol may cause a disulfiram-like reaction.

Pregnant or breast-feeding women shouldn't use witch hazel. Although extracts of witch hazel are available commercially, internal use isn't recommended because of tannin and safrole content.

Clinical considerations

- Witch hazel water (hamamelis water) isn't intended for internal use.
- In doses of 1 g, witch hazel has caused nausea, vomiting, or constipation, possibly leading to fecal impaction.
- Advise pregnant or breast-feeding patient to avoid oral use of witch hazel.
- Warn patient against taking more than 1 g of witch hazel to reduce the risk of nausea, vomiting, or constipation, possibly leading to fecal impaction.
- Inform patient that long-term oral use may lead to liver damage, possibly because of herb's tannin content.
- Warn patient not to take witch hazel before seeking medical attention because doing so may delay diagnosis of a potentially serious medical condition.
- Tell patient to promptly notify a health care provider about adverse effects or changes in symptoms.
- Warn patient to keep all herbal products away from children and pets.
- Tell patient to remind pharmacist of any herbal and dietary supplements that are being taken when obtaining a new prescription.
- Advise patient to consult his health care provider before using an herbal preparation because a conventional treatment with proven efficacy may be available.

Research summary

The concepts behind the use of witch hazel and the claims made regarding its effects have not yet been validated scientifically, especially for oral ingestion. Witch hazel has a low toxicity profile, but internal use isn't recommended. Topically, the astringent and hemostatic properties have been demonstrated and are well known.

wormwood

Absinth, absinthe, absinthii herba, absinthium, ajenjo, armoise, Artemisia absinthium, *green ginger, herbe d'absinthe, wurmkraut, wermut, wermutkraut*

The name wormwood is derived from the ancient use of the plant and its extracts as an intestinal anthelmintic. The leaves and flowering tops were used as a bitter aromatic tonic, sedative, and flavoring. A tea was used as a diaphoretic. Wormwood is obtained from fresh or dried shoots and leaves of *Artemisia absinthium*. It contains the bitter principles absinthine, anabsinthine, artabsine, and others; a volatile oil containing up to 12% thujone; and flavones. Bitter principles may stimulate receptors in the taste buds, triggering increased stomach acid secretion. Flavones may have spasmolytic activity. Thujone acts as an anthelmintic, causing expulsion of roundworms. It also acts on the same receptor in the brain as tetrahydrocannabinol, the active principle of marijuana. Interaction with these receptors may contribute to appetite stimulation and to the central nervous system (CNS) toxicity seen with higher doses. Wormwood is available as fresh or dried herb, powder, extract, and tincture.

Reported uses

Wormwood is used orally for anthelmintic and diaphoretic effects and to treat appetite loss, dyspepsia, bloating, and biliary dyskinesia. It's used topically for wounds, skin ulcers, and insect bites. Wormwood is also used as a flavoring agent for foods and aromatic alcoholic beverages such as vermouth. Extracts have been investigated for antimalarial, antimicrobial, and antifungal properties. The FDA has classified wormwood as an unsafe herb, although thujone-free derivatives have been approved for use in foods.

Administration
- Liquid extract: 1 or 2 ml by mouth three times a day
- Tea: 1 g of herb in 1 cup of water, by mouth 30 minutes before each meal
- Tincture: 10 to 30 gtt in sufficient water, by mouth three times a day.

Hazards
Wormwood may cause headache, dizziness, restlessness, vertigo, trembling of the limbs, numbness of extremities, loss of intellect, paralysis, seizures, delirium, unconsciousness, vomiting, stomach and intestinal cramping, thirst, renal dysfunction, and topical eruptions.

Wormwood causes increased stomach acidity and decreased drug action when used with acid inhibitors, such as antacids, histamine H_2 antagonists, proton pump inhibitors, or sucralfate. It may increase bleeding risk when used with anticoagulants and antiplatelet drugs. Wormwood may decrease the effectiveness of anticonvulsants. Herbal products that contain alcohol may cause a disulfiram-like reaction. Wormwood may potentiate hypoglycemic effect. Thujone-containing herbs, such as oak-moss, oriental arborvitae, sage, tansy, thuja, and yarrow, may increase risk of CNS toxicity when used with wormwood. Wormwood may cause CNS toxicity if used with alcohol, especially with large doses or continuous use.

Because of thujone content, consumption of large doses or continuous use of wormwood isn't recommended. Pregnant or breast-feeding women should avoid wormwood, as should children, patients allergic to members of the Compositae family (such as sunflower seeds, chamomile, pistachios, hazelnuts, ragweed, chrysanthemums, marigolds, daisies), and patients with seizure disorders, bile duct obstruction, gallbladder inflammation, gallstones, liver disease, renal dysfunction, or gastric or duodenal ulcers.

 SAFETY RISK *The FDA has classified wormwood as an unsafe herb, although thujone-free derivatives have been approved for use in foods.*

Clinical considerations
- Many tinctures contain significant levels of alcohol, up to 20%, and may not be suitable for children, alcoholic patients, patients with liver disease, or patients who take disulfiram or metronidazole.
- Monitor International Normalized Ratio and prothrombin time closely if patient takes an anticoagulant.
- Monitor serum glucose level and check for signs of hypoglycemia.
- If patient has a seizure disorder, watch for lack of anticonvulsant effectiveness and lack of seizure control.
- Monitor patient for adverse effects, such as absinthism, a CNS disorder characterized by vertigo, restlessness, and delirium.
- Tell patient not to use wormwood in large doses or for continuous periods.
- Caution pregnant and breast-feeding women to avoid wormwood.
- Warn patient not to drink alcohol with wormwood.
- Tell patient to promptly notify a health care provider about adverse effects or changes in symptoms.
- Instruct patient to store wormwood in a sealed container, protected from light.
- Warn patient to keep all herbal products away from children and pets.
- Warn patient that if he's allergic to ragweed, marigolds, or daisies, he'll probably also be allergic to wormwood.
- Tell patient to remind pharmacist of any herbal and dietary supplements that are being taken when filling a new prescription.
- Advise patient to consult with a health care provider before using an herbal preparation because a conventional treatment with proven efficacy may be available.

Research summary
The concepts behind the use of worm-wood and the claims made regarding its effects have not been validated scientifically.

woundwort

Anthyllis vulneraria, *kidney vetch, ladies' fingers, lamb's toes, staunchwort*

The useful parts of woundwort are obtained from the flowers of *Anthyllis vulneraria*. It contains tannins, saponins, flavonoids, isoflavonoids, and lectins. Tannins provide astringent, hemostatic, anti-inflammatory, and antibacterial properties. Tannins may also exert vasoconstriction, decrease vascular permeability, tighten distended vessels, restore vessel tone, and stop bleeding immediately. The alcohol extract may have anti-herpetic properties. Flavonoids in other herbs have been found to exert spasmolytic properties, which may account for woundwort's effect in controlling vomiting. Woundwort is available as dried flowers and extract.

Reported uses
Woundwort is used internally to treat oral-pharyngeal disorders and both externally and internally for ulcers and wounds. It's also used for cramps, dizziness, fever, gout, and menstrual disorders. Woundwort is combined with other herbs to purify blood and to treat coughs and vomiting.

Administration
■ Extract or poultice: Applied externally
■ Tea: 9 ml flowers to 250 ml of water, 1 cup three times a day.

Hazards
Woundwort may cause digestive complaints, nausea, vomiting, constipation, fecal impaction, and liver toxicity. No drug interactions are known. Because of its tannin content, excessive ingestion of woundwort isn't recommended. Woundwort shouldn't be taken by children or patients who are pregnant, planning to become pregnant, or breast-feeding.

Clinical considerations
■ Monitor patient for GI symptoms, including nausea, vomiting, and constipation.
■ Do not confuse woundwort with herbs such as *Stachys palustris* (marsh woundwort) or *S. sylvatica* (hedge woundwort). Other plants called woundwort include *Prunella vulgaris* and *Achillea millefolium*.
■ Tell patient to consult with health care provider before using woundwort.
■ Inform patient that if woundwort is taken orally in large amounts, the tannin content may lead to nausea, vomiting, constipation, and possible fecal impaction.
■ Warn patient not to take woundwort before seeking medical attention because doing so may delay diagnosis of a potentially serious medical condition.
■ Inform patient that long-term use of herbs containing tannins may lead to liver toxicity.
■ Warn patient to keep all herbal products away from children and pets.
■ Tell patient to remind pharmacist of any herbal and dietary supplements that are being taken when filling a new prescription.
■ Advise patient to consult with a health care provider before using an herbal preparation because a conventional treatment with proven efficacy may be available.

Research summary
The concepts behind the use of woundwort and the claims made regarding its effects have not been validated scientifically.

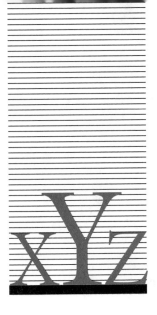

yarrow

Achilee, achillea, Achillea millefolium,
acuilee, band man's plaything,
bauchweh, birangasifa, bloodwort,
carpenter's weed, civan percemi,
devil's plaything, erba da cartentieri,
erba da falegname, gemeine schafgarbe,
green arrow, herbe aux charpentiers,
katzenkrat, milefolio, milfoil,
millefolium, millefuille, nose bleed,
old man's pepper, roga mari,
sanguinary, soldier's woundwort,
staunchweed, tausendaugbram,
thousand-leaf, woundwort

The use of yarrow in food and medicine
dates back to the Trojan War, when it was
used to stanch bleeding wounds. Yarrow
leaves are used to make tea, and young
leaves and flowers are used in salads. Infusions of yarrow are used in cosmetic
cleansers and medicines. It's also used as
a tonic and astringent. The useful constituents of yarrow are obtained from the
dried flowers and dried or fresh above-
ground parts of *Achillea millefolium*. It
contains a volatile oil (0.2% to 1.0%)
composed of sesquiterpene lactones,
terpinen-4-ol, polyenes, alkamids, flavonoids, tannins, thujone, and betaines.
The sesquiterpene lactones found in the
volatile oil are azulenes and chamazu-
lenes. Azulenes may have antispasmodic
and anti-inflammatory effects; tannins
may have astringent effects. Terpinen-4-
ol may have diuretic effects. Alcohol ex-

tracts and chamazulene may be active against *Staphylococcus aureus, Bacillus subtilis, Candida albicans, Mycobacterium smegmatis, Escherichia coli,* and both *Shigella sonnei* and *S. flexneri.* These properties may explain the benefit of yarrow in controlling diarrhea and dysentery. Bitter principles found in yarrow may stimulate receptors in the taste buds, triggering increased stomach acid secretion. Thujone, found in small amounts in yarrow, may contribute to appetite stimulation. The antipyretic and hypotensive effects of yarrow may be caused by alkaloids. Yarrow's volatile oil may exert central nervous system (CNS) depressant effects. Yarrow is available as dried flower or herb, liquid extract, tincture, tea, or capsules.

Reported uses

Yarrow is used orally to induce sweating and to treat fever, common cold, hypertension, amenorrhea, dysentery, dyspepsia, diarrhea, loss of appetite, and mild or spasmodic GI tract discomfort. It's used specifically for thrombotic conditions with hypertension, including cerebral and coronary thromboses. Yarrow is used topically for its antibacterial and astringent properties in wound healing, to treat bleeding hemorrhoids, and as a bath to remove perspiration.

In the United States, yarrow is approved for use only in alcoholic beverages, and the finished product must be thujone-free. The German Commission E approves the use of yarrow in sitz baths for "painful, lower pelvic, cramp-like conditions of psychosomatic origin in women and in oral dosage forms for dyspeptic complaints."

Administration

- Liquid extract (1:1 in 25% alcohol): 2 to 4 ml by mouth three times a day
- Tea (steep 2 g of herb in boiling water for 10 to 15 minutes, and then strain): 1 cup freshly made tea, taken three to four times a day between meals

- Tincture (1:5 in 45% alcohol): 2 to 4 ml by mouth three times a day
- Total oral daily dose not to exceed 4.5 g of yarrow herb, 3 g of yarrow flower, or 3 teaspoons of pressed juice from fresh plants
- Sitz bath: 100 g of herb in 20 L water.

Hazards

Yarrow may cause sedation, CNS toxicities, headache, dizziness, vomiting, stomach and intestinal cramping, diuresis, renal dysfunction, hypoglycemia, and contact dermatitis.

Increased stomach acid resulting from yarrow may decrease the effectiveness of acid-inhibiting drugs, such as antacids, histamine H_2 antagonists, proton pump inhibitors, and sucralfate. Yarrow may decrease the effectiveness of anticoagulants. It may potentiate the hypoglycemic effect of antidiabetics. Yarrow may reduce the effects of antihypertensives and hypotensives. It may increase the sedative effects of barbiturates and benzodiazepines. Herbal products that contain alcohol may cause a disulfiram-like reaction. Yarrow may increase the sedative effect of hypnotics and sedative herbs. Thujone-containing herbs, such as oak moss, oriental arborvitae, sage, tansy, thuja, and wormwood, may increase the risk of CNS toxicity if taken with yarrow. Combining alcohol with yarrow may increase CNS toxicity.

Pregnant or breast-feeding women should avoid yarrow, as should patients allergic to members of the Compositae family such as wormwood, honey, sunflower seeds, chamomile, pistachios, hazelnuts, ragweed, chrysanthemums, marigolds, and daisies.

Clinical considerations

- Closely monitor International Normalized Ratio and prothrombin time in patients who take anticoagulants with yarrow.
- Closely monitor patient's serum electrolytes, blood pressure, and serum glucose level.

■ Caution patient not to drink alcohol with yarrow.

■ Caution patient that taking yarrow with sedatives or other CNS depressant drugs may cause increased sedation or lethargy.

■ Tell patient to avoid hazardous activities until full CNS effects of yarrow are known.

■ Advise patient to protect yarrow from light and moisture and not to store essential oil in a synthetic container.

■ Warn patient to keep all herbal products away from children and pets.

■ Tell patient to remind pharmacist of any herbal and dietary supplements that are being taken when filling a new prescription.

■ Advise patient to consult with a health care provider before using an herbal preparation because a conventional treatment with proven efficacy may be available.

Research summary
The concepts behind the use of yarrow and the claims made regarding its effects have not been validated scientifically.

yellow root

Parsley-leaved yellow root,
shrub yellow root, yellow wort,
Xanthorrhiza simplicissima

Yellow root is used in the southern United States for treating hypertension and diabetes. It was popular in folk medicine and has been used for mouth infections and sore throat, diabetes, and childbirth. It's obtained from the roots of *Xanthorrhiza simplicissima*. Yellow root contains several alkaloids, including berberine, jatrorhizine, and mognoflorine. Berberine is the most abundant. Two isoquinoline alkaloids, iriodenine and palmitin, also have been identified. Yellow root's pharmacologic activity arises primarily from berberine, which may have antihyperten-

sive, antitumor, antibacterial, antifungal, and antiprotozoal effects. It's available as an alcoholic tincture.

Reported uses
Yellow root is used to treat diabetes, hypertension, and infections.

Administration
Dosage & administration: Not well documented.

Hazards
Yellow root may cause reflex tachycardia, tremors, sedation, GI irritation, vomiting, and arsenic poisoning. It may reduce the effectiveness of heparin. It may also reduce the effectiveness of paclitaxel.

Pregnant or breast-feeding women shouldn't use yellow root. Patients with cardiac conditions or diabetes should use it with caution.

Clinical considerations
■ Tell patient about the berberine content of yellow root and its effects on blood pressure and blood clotting.

■ Warn patient not to take yellow root before seeking medical attention because doing so may delay diagnosis of a potentially serious medical condition.

■ Caution patient not to confuse yellow root with other herbs with similar names, such as goldenseal, which also contains berberine.

■ Tell patient to promptly notify a health care provider about adverse effects or changes in symptoms.

■ Warn patient to keep all herbal products away from children and pets.

■ Tell patient to remind pharmacist of any herbal and dietary supplements that are being taken when filling a new prescription.

■ Advise patient to consult with a health care provider before using an herbal preparation because a conventional treatment with proven efficacy may be available.

Research summary

Recent studies documenting antineoplastic effects may lead to expanded interest in berberine-containing plants, such as yellow root, in treating cancer; however, current research has focused only on the in vitro antineoplastic effects of berberine alkaloids. The concepts behind the traditional uses of yellow root and the claims made regarding its effects have not been validated scientifically.

yerba maté

Bartholomew's tea, campeche, gaucho, ilex, Ilex paraguariensis, *jaguar, Jesuit's tea, la hoja, la mulata, mate, oro verde, Paraguay tea, payadito*

The useful parts of yerba maté are obtained from the leaves of *Ilex paraguariensis.* Its leaves contain several methylxanthines, chiefly caffeine (0.2% to 2.0%), theobromine (0.1% to 0.2%), and theophylline (0.05%). The leaves also contain the flavonoids kaempferol and quercetin, as well as terpenoids, ursolic acid, beta-amyrin, ilexides A and B, and tannins (4% to 16%). Carotene, vitamins A and D, riboflavin, ascorbic acid, and nicotinic acid are present as well. Hepatotoxic pyrrolizadine alkaloids have also been reported. Most pharmacologic effects, including diuresis, appetite suppression, smooth muscle relaxation, and central nervous sytem (CNS), respiratory, skeletal, and cardiac muscle stimulation, are caused by the methylxanthines, especially caffeine. Yerba maté is available as dried leaves and liquid extract.

Reported uses

Yerba maté is used as a CNS stimulant for drowsiness or fatigue, and as a mild analgesic for headaches caused by fatigue. It's also used as a diuretic and an appetite suppressant.

Administration

- Infusion (1 teaspoon or 2 to 4 g dried leaves steeped in 1 cup hot water for 5 to 10 minutes, and then strained): 3 cups taken by mouth every day
- Tincture (1:1 in 25% alcohol): 2 to 4 ml by mouth three times a day.

Hazards

Yerba maté may cause sleeplessness, restlessness, irritability, anxiety, tremor, headache, sleep disturbances, and palpitations. It may cause esophageal cancer, bladder cancer, and liver toxicity.

Yerba maté may cause additive stimulatory and diuretic effects when taken with other CNS stimulants or with caffeine. When taken with grapefruit juice, yerba maté interacts with caffeine metabolism and can increase caffeine levels, effects, and risk of adverse reactions.

Pregnant or breast-feeding women should avoid yerba maté, as should patients with cardiovascular disease (such as hypertension), ischemic heart disease, or chronic liver disease.

Clinical considerations

- Monitor patient for evidence of excessive stimulation, such as hypertension, restlessness, and sleeplessness.
- Consumption of caffeine-containing products may cause additive effects.
- Inform patient that yerba maté is a source of caffeine and theophylline, and combining with other caffeine-containing beverages or other stimulants could lead to excessive stimulation.
- Caution patient about possible liver toxicity and possible increased cancer risk.
- If evidence of excessive stimulation arises, suggest that patient decrease or eliminate consumption of yerba maté.
- Urge patient to promptly notify a health care provider about adverse effects or changes in symptoms.
- Tell patient that he may have withdrawal symptoms, such as headache and sleep disturbances, when discontinuing yerba maté.

- Warn patient to keep all herbal products away from children and pets.
- Tell patient to remind pharmacist of any herbal and dietary supplements that are being taken when filling a new prescription.
- Advise patient to consult with a health care provider before using an herbal preparation because a conventional treatment with proven efficacy may be available.

Research summary
The effects of the methylxanthines caffeine, theobromine, and theophylline have been well documented. The concepts behind the use of yerba maté and the claims made regarding its effects have not been validated scientifically.

yerba santa

Bear's weed, consumptive's weed, Eriodictyon californicum, *gum bush, holy weed, mountain balm, sacred herb, tarweed*

The name yerba santa ("holy weed") was given by the Spanish priests who learned from native American Indians of the medicinal value of the shrub. It has a long tradition of use in the United States. Yerba santa is obtained from *Eriodictyon californicum*. It contains at least 12 flavonoids, including eriodictyonin (6%), eriodictyol (0.5%), and eriodictine. It also contains four flavones — cirsimaritin, chrysoeriol, hispidulin, and chrysin. Eriodictyol is a mild expectorant. Resins in the plant have a pleasant taste and aroma, explaining why yerba santa is used to mask the bitter taste of certain drugs and as a flavoring in foods and beverages. Several flavones and flavonoids inhibit formation of active metabolites of the carcinogen benzo[a]pyrene, thus showing chemopreventive potential. Yerba santa is also a mild diuretic. It's available as fresh or dried herb, powdered herb, liquid, and ointment, in products such as Feminease and Respirtone.

Reported uses
Yerba santa is used orally to treat coughs, colds, asthma, and bronchitis. It's used topically to treat bruises, sprains, skin wounds, poison ivy, and insect bites.

Administration
- Fresh leaves: Chewed as needed
- Tea (1 teaspoon dried or fresh leaves added to 1 cup hot water): taken by mouth 30 minutes before bedtime.

Hazards
Yerba santa causes a sticky residue on teeth after fresh leaves are chewed. No drug interactions are reported. Pregnant or breast-feeding women shouldn't use yerba santa because effects of herb are unknown.

Clinical considerations
- Monitor patient's response to yerba santa.
- Advise patient that chewing the fresh leaves will leave a sticky residue on his teeth.
- Warn patient not to take yerba santa for a chronic cough or cold before seeking medical attention because doing so may delay diagnosis of a potentially serious medical condition.
- Instruct patient to promptly notify a health care provider about adverse effects or changes in symptoms.
- Warn patient to keep all herbal products away from children and pets.
- Tell patient to remind pharmacist of any herbal and dietary supplements that are being taken when filling a new prescription.
- Advise patient to consult with a health care provider before using an herbal preparation because a conventional treatment with proven efficacy may be available.

Research summary
The concepts behind the use of yerba santa and the claims made regarding its effects have not been validated scientifically.

yew

American yew, chinwood, English yew, globe-berry, Japanese yew, Oregon yew, Pacific yew, Taxus baccata, T. brevifolia, T. canadenis, T. cuspidata, T. cuspididata, T. floridana, *Western yew*

The ancient Celts coated their arrows with yew sap as a nerve toxicant. The alkaloid taxine has been used as an antispasmodic. A tincture of the leaves had been used to treat rheumatism and liver and urinary tract conditions. Yew is obtained from bark and branch tips of *Taxus brevifolia*. It contains a mixture of about 19 taxane-type diterpene esters, referred to as taxines; most prominent of these are paclitaxel and taxine A and B. Other constituents include taxicatin, milossine, and ephedrine. Paclitaxel inhibits cell division by binding to the β-tubulin subunit of microtubules, which prevents the disassembly of microtubules. Cells are thus arrested in mitosis. Yew is available as a tincture, capsules, and a salve of yew bark.

Reported uses
Yew is used to promote menstruation, eliminate tapeworms, and treat tonsillitis. Taxol, the trade name for the drug paclitaxel, is isolated from the bark of *T. brevifolia*. Taxotere is the trade name of docetaxel, a more potent analogue of paclitaxel. Paclitaxel is FDA-approved for treating metastatic, ovarian, and breast cancers.

Administration
- For cancers: Optimal doses and administration protocols are still being determined in ongoing clinical trials
- Infusion (bark or needles are added to 1 cup hot water): The infusion is taken by mouth once every day
- Tinctures: Doses of yew bark tinctures vary widely.

SAFETY RISK *Most parts of the yew plant are highly poisonous. Ingestion of 50 to 100 g of yew needles or berries has been fatal and is especially dangerous in children. Treatment includes digoxin-specific fragment antigen-binding antibodies and gastric lavage followed by administration of charcoal. Supportive measures to treat cardiac effects and other symptoms may also be indicated.*

Hazards
Yew may cause dizziness, unconsciousness, bradycardia, tachycardia, hypotension, cardiac failure, mydriasis, dry mouth, reddened lips, abdominal cramps, nausea, vomiting, dyspnea, respiratory failure, rash, pallor, and cyanosis. It may also cause miscarriage.

Potentiation of myelosuppression and interactions occurs when yew is taken with other chemotherapeutic drugs. Advise patient to use together only with extreme caution and only under direct supervision of a health care provider.

Women who are pregnant or breastfeeding shouldn't use yew. Because of the potential extreme toxicity of multiple constituents, herbal formulations of the yew tree should be used only with extreme caution, if at all.

Clinical considerations
- Monitor vital signs and electrocardiogram if large amounts of yew are ingested.
- Because of the potential extreme toxicity of yew, only prescription forms of paclitaxel should be used, and then only under the careful guidance of an oncologist.

- Some common hypersensitivity reactions to paclitaxel have been reduced by giving the drug as a slow infusion over 6 to 24 hours.
- Advise patient of the need for regular follow-up care with an oncologist if taking yew for a cancerous condition.
- Urge patient to report adverse effects promptly to a health care provider.
- Tell patient to seek emergency medical care if he develops adverse effects or a toxic response.
- Warn patient of the danger of taking yew without medical supervision.
- Warn patient to keep all herbal products away from children and pets.
- Tell patient to remind pharmacist of any herbal and dietary supplements that are being taken when filling a new prescription.
- Advise patient to consult with a health care provider before using an herbal preparation because a conventional treatment with proven efficacy may be available.

Research summary
Clinical trials in the use of the FDA-approved drug paclitaxel are ongoing to determine treatment approval for other cancers, and optimal dose and administration protocols.

Yoga

One of the oldest known health practices, yoga (which means "union" in Sanskrit) is the integration of physical, mental, and spiritual energies to promote health and wellness. Yoga is based on the Hindu principle of mind-body unity: a chronically restless or agitated mind will result in poor health and decreased mental clarity. Practitioners believe that practicing yoga techniques can combat these effects and restore good mental and physical health.

The basic components of yoga are proper breathing, movement, meditation, and postures. While performing specific postures, the practitioner pays close attention to his breathing, which is correlated with the postures, exhaling at certain times and inhaling at others. The breathing techniques are believed to help maintain the postures as well as promote relaxation and enhance the flow of vital energy known as *prana*, similar to the Chinese concept of *qi*.

As with tai chi chuan (see page 470), there are many styles of yoga. The type most widely taught in the West today is Hatha yoga. A unique combination of physical postures and exercises (known as *asanas*), breathing techniques (known as *pranayamas*), relaxation, diet, and proper thinking, Hatha yoga aims to cleanse the body of toxins, clear the mind, energize and realign the body, release muscle tension, and increase flexibility and strength.

The *asanas*, meaning "ease" in Sanskrit, fall into two categories: meditative and therapeutic. Meditative asanas align the head and spine to promote relaxation, concentration, and proper blood flow through the body. They are also believed to keep the heart, glands, and lungs properly energized. The therapeutic asanas are commonly prescribed to treat specific ailments, such as neck, back, and joint pain.

According to Hindu belief, the goal of a properly executed asana is to create a balance between movement and stillness, which is the state of a healthy body. Although many of these postures require little movement, they all require concentration on the body's postures and movements. Eventually, as with meditation, practitioners say they can learn to regulate their autonomic functions, such as heartbeat and respiratory rate, while reducing physical tensions.

Although it was originally developed as part of a spiritual belief system aimed at achieving a higher state of consciousness (known as *samadhi*), yoga in the West is more often practiced for its physical and psychological benefits, such as improving strength and flexibility, maintaining physical fitness, and inducing relaxation.

Reported uses

Aside from promoting relaxation and enhancing feelings of well-being, yoga is also widely used as a complementary therapy to relieve the pain and anxiety that often accompany certain chronic illnesses, such as heart disease (as in Dean Ornish's program to reverse cardiovascular disease), diabetes, migraine headaches, hypertension, and arthritis.

Yoga has also been credited with decreasing serum cholesterol levels and increasing histamine levels to fight allergies. Its ability to help the user regulate blood flow is being studied for possible use in cancer therapy. Scientists are eager to see whether restricted blood flow to the tumor region will slow tumor growth.

Yoga techniques can fit the needs of people in almost any physical condition. It can be practiced by children as young as 5 years old, and by the elderly. Individuals unable to perform some of the more physically demanding postures can still benefit from the breathing or meditation techniques.

How the treatment is performed

Minimal supplies are needed to practice yoga. The most important element is a private, quiet environment that is free from distractions, with enough room for the participants to move without touching or distracting each other. A small blanket, a large towel, or a mat is necessary for some of the postures. The participants should wear loose clothing and slippers or sneakers.

Yoga programs vary with the teacher, the experience of the participants, and the goal of the treatment. A balanced program of postures will help most participants achieve positive effects on their overall health.

Prior to beginning, the instructor explains to the participants the purpose of the session and describes the planned exercises and their benefits. He then answers any questions, and reminds the participants that they don't have to engage in any posture that may be uncomfortable.

The yoga teacher talks the group through the positions and breathing techniques, demonstrating each one. After everyone has assumed the position or begun the breathing pattern, the teacher circulates among the members to adjust their technique as needed. At the end of the session, the teacher instructs the participants to take a few slow, deep breaths. The session is documented, including the techniques used and the patients' responses.

Hazards

Some of the more physical aspects of yoga can cause muscle injury if they aren't properly performed or if the individual tries to force his body into position.

Clinical considerations

■ Because some of the postures used in yoga can be stressful to people with certain health problems, advise your patients to consult their health care provider before undertaking a yoga program.

■ Remind patients that yoga is a complementary therapy, not a cure for disease. They will still need to continue their conventional medical treatments.

■ Advise patients to attempt the different postures with caution, and remind them that very few people can perform all the movements in the beginning.

■ Inform them that yoga requires regular repetition and practice to perform the positions effectively.

Research summary

Numerous studies have demonstrated the effectiveness of yoga in alleviating stress and anxiety, lowering blood pressure and respiratory rate, relieving pain, improving motor skills and balance, increasing auditory and visual perception, improving metabolic and respiratory function, and producing brain wave activity associated with relaxation. The breath control aspect has also been shown to aid digestion, regulate cardiac function, and reduce the frequency of asthma attacks.

yohimbe

Aphrodien, Corynanthe yohimbi, corynine, Pausinystalia yohimbe, yohimbehe, yohimbine

The bark of the West African yohimbe tree (*Pausinystalia yohimbe*) is rich in the alkaloid yohimbine, and both the crude bark and purified compound have long been hailed as aphrodisiacs. The bark has been smoked as a hallucinogen and has been used in traditional medicine to treat angina and hypertension. Today the drug is being investigated for the treatment of organic impotence. Yohimbe contains tannins and 2.7% to 5.9% indole alkaloids, especially yohimbine. Other alkaloids include ajamalicine, dihydroyohimbine, corynantheine, and others. Effects of yohimbine are mediated mostly via selective blockade of alpha$_2$ receptors, primarily in the central nervous system (CNS). At higher levels, yohimbine acts as an agonist at alpha$_1$, serotonin, and dopamine receptors. Yohimbine may also inhibit monoamine oxidase (MAO) and slow L-type calcium channels in heart and blood vessels.

Yohimbe increases penile cavernous blood flow in men with erectile dysfunction. It also increases autonomic nerve activity from the brain to genital tissues and increases reflex excitability in the sacral region of the spinal cord. It's available as tablets and tinctures, in products such as Aphrodyne, Dayto Himbin, Potensan, Yobinol, Yocon, Yohimbine HCL, Yohimbe Power MAX for Women, and Yohimmex.

Reported uses

Yohimbe is primarily used as an aphrodisiac and to treat organic and psychogenic erectile dysfunction in men. It's also used at higher doses to treat orthostatic hypotension.

Administration

For erectile dysfunction, dosage is 5.4 mg by mouth three times a day. Doses of 20 to 30 mg have been shown to significantly increase blood pressure. Yohimbe bark alcoholic extracts are usually standardized to contain a certain amount of yohimbine.

Hazards

Yohimbe may cause nervousness, anxiety, irritability, increased motor activity, headache, anorexia, dizziness, insomnia, manic or psychotic episodes, paralysis, tachycardia, hypotension, hypertension, abdominal discomfort, diarrhea, nausea, and acute renal failure.

Yohimbe may precipitate clonidine withdrawal hypertensive crisis when used with antihypertensives, including adrenergics and clonidine. It may block the action of anxiolytics. Yohimbe may enhance the effects of CNS-stimulating drugs, including tricyclic antidepressants and selective serotonin reuptake inhibitors. Naltrexone may increase the patient's sensitivity to yohimbe, potentiating adverse reactions. Yohimbe may enhance the effects of caffeine. Because of its reported weak MAO-inhibiting activity, yohimbe may interact with tyramine-containing foods. There may be additive effects if yohimbe is used with alcohol.

Yohimbe shouldn't be used by children, geriatric patients, pregnant women, breast-feeding women, and people with psychiatric disorders, liver disease, kidney disease, hyperthyroidism, angina pectoris, or cardiovascular disease, especially hypertension.

Clinical considerations

- Yohimbe is used mainly by men to help with impotence, but some women may take it for an aphrodisiac effect.
- Be alert for possible CNS and blood pressure changes.
- Yohimbe can significantly increase blood pressure in patients with orthostatic hypotension caused by autonomic failure or multisystem atrophy.
- Follow patient's vital signs and electrocardiogram closely.
- Monitor patient for adverse effects or changes in condition.
- Inform patient that yohimbe is considered by many to have a high risk-to-benefit ratio.
- Instruct patient not to take caffeine products while also taking yohimbe.
- Warn patient not to take yohimbe for erectile dysfunction before seeking medical attention because doing so may delay diagnosis of a potentially serious medical condition.
- Instruct patient to report adverse effects promptly to a health care provider.
- Warn patient to keep all herbal products away from children and pets.
- Tell patient to remind pharmacist of any herbal and dietary supplements that are being taken when filling a new prescription.
- Advise patient to consult with a health care provider before using an herbal preparation because a conventional treatment with proven efficacy may be available.

Research summary

Yohimbe is currently approved by the FDA as a drug, but has no FDA sanctioned indications. Some types of impotence have successfully been treated with yohimbine, but data are sparse and adverse reactions can be severe. Herbal use of yohimbe is potentially more dangerous owing to varying amounts of the alkaloid yohime in different preparations.

Appendices

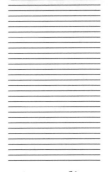

Appendix 1
Herbal resource list

Alternative Medicine.com
www.alternativemedicine.com
1650 Tiburon Blvd., Suite 2
Tiburon, CA 94920
Phone (800) 515-4325

American Botanical Council
www.herbalgram.org
P.O. Box 144345
Austin, TX 78714-4345
Phone (512) 926-4900

American Herbal Pharmacopoeia
www.herbal-ahp.org
Box 5159
Santa Cruz, CA 95063
Phone (831) 461-6317

American Holistic Health Association
www.ahha.org
P.O. Box 17400
Anaheim, CA 92817-7400
Phone (714) 779-6152

Association of Natural Medicine
    Pharmacists
www.anmp.org
P.O. Box 150727
San Rafael, CA 94915-0727
Phone (415) 453-3534

Botanical Society of America
www.botany.org
Office of Publications
1735 Neil Avenue
Columbus, OH 43210-1293
Phone (614) 292-3519

Centers for Disease Control and
    Prevention
www.cdc.gov
1600 Clifton Road
Atlanta, GA 30333
Phone (404) 639-3311

Healthy Alternatives
www.health-alt.com
4532 W. Kennedy Blvd. #312
Tampa, FL 33609-3042

Herb Research Foundation
www.herbs.org
1007 Pearl Street, Suite 200
Boulder, CO 80302
Phone (800) 748-2617 or (303) 449-2265

Office of Dietary Supplements
http://ods.od.nih.gov
National Institutes of Health
Building 31, Room 1B29
31 Center Drive, MSC 2086
Bethesda, MD 20892-2086
Phone (301) 435-2920

MedHerb.com
www.medherb.com
Bergner Communications
P.O. Box 20512
Boulder, CO 80308

National Center for Homeopathy
www.homeopathic.org
801 N. Fairfax Street, Suite 306
Alexandria, VA 22314
Phone (877) 624-0613 or (703) 548-7790

The Richard and Hinda Rosenthal Center
   and the Center for Complementary
   and Alternative Medicine (CAM)
   Research in Women's Health
http://cpmcnet.columbia.edu/dept/
   rosenthal
Columbia University, College of
   Physicians and Surgeons
630 W. 168th Street
P.O. Box 75
New York, NY 10032
Phone (212) 543-9542

The Special Nutritionals Adverse Event
   Monitoring System
http://vm.cfsan.fda.gov/~dms/aems.html
United States Food and Drug
   Administration
Center for Food Safety and Applied
   Nutrition
200 C Street, SW
Washington, DC 20204
Phone (888) SAFEFOOD (723-3366)

United States Department of Agriculture
www.usda.gov/welcome.html
14th and Independence Avenue, SW
Washington, DC 20250
Phone (202) 720-2791

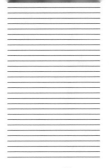

Appendix 2
Alternative therapies for specific conditions

The list below gives a sampling of alternative and complementary therapies that practitioners may use for specific conditions, diseases, and signs and symptoms. In many cases, these therapies are used as adjuncts to conventional therapies. Because some of these therapies remain experimental, advise your patients to research any therapy they're considering before beginning it.

Allergies, hay fever
- Environmental medicine
- Homeopathy
- Hypnotherapy
- Juice therapy
- Naturopathic therapy
- Pancreatic enzyme therapy
- Plant enzyme therapy
- Vitamin therapy

Alzheimer's disease
- Art therapy
- Chelation therapy
- Dance therapy
- Music therapy
- Sound therapy
- Vitamin therapy

Anemia
- Plant enzyme therapy

Anxiety
- Biofeedback
- Herbal/vitamin therapy
- Meditation
- Transcranial electrostimulation

Arthritis
- Apitherapy
- Bioelectromagnetic therapy
- Detoxification therapy
- Diet (eliminate foods such as potatoes, tomatoes, peppers, eggplant, and tobacco)
- Nutritional supplements (boron, zinc, copper, selenium, manganese, proteolytic enzymes, flavonoids, glucosamine sulfate, evening primrose oil)
- Environmental medicine
- Fasting
- Herbal therapy
- Juice therapy
- Osteopathic manipulation
- Vitamin therapy (vitamins A, B_1, B_6, C, E)
- Yoga

Asthma
- Ayurvedic remedies
- Biofeedback/relaxation and breathing therapy
- Chiropractic treatment
- Guided imagery
- Herbal therapy (ephedra, mullein tea, passion flower tea)
- Homeopathy
- Hydrotherapy
- Hypnotherapy
- Juice therapy
- Naturopathic therapy
- Nutritional therapy
- Osteopathic manipulation
- Yoga

Atherosclerosis
- Chelation therapy
- Vitamin therapy

Autism
- Music therapy
- Sound therapy

Back pain
- Bioelectromagnetic therapy
- Osteopathic manipulation

Benign prostatic hyperplasia (BPH)
- Herbal therapy (nettles, *Pygeum africanum*, saw palmetto)
- Nutritional/vitamin therapy (lycopene)

Bone fractures
- Pulsed electromagnetic fields
- Vitamin therapy (chondroitin sulfate)

Brain injuries
- Music therapy

Cancer (all types)
- Antineoplaston therapy
- Antioxidants (vitamins A, C, E, and trace mineral selenium)
- Bioelectromagnetic therapy
- Cell-specific cancer therapy-200
- Coley's toxins
- Dance therapy
- Detoxification therapy
- Diet (organic foods, avoid sugar)
- Guided imagery
- Homeopathy
- Hydrazine sulfate
- Juice therapy
- Meditation
- Naturopathic therapy
- Pancreatic enzyme therapy
- Shark cartilage
- Vitamin/nutritional therapy
- 714X therapy

Cancer (breast)
- Bioelectromagnetic therapy
- Diet (organic foods, avoid sugar)
- Vitamin/nutritional therapy

Cancer (colon)
- Diet (high-fiber)

Cardiovascular disorders
- Bioelectromagnetic therapy
- Biofeedback
- Dance therapy
- Detoxification therapy
- Humor therapy
- Meditation
- Osteopathic manipulation
- Tai chi chuan
- Vitamin/nutritional therapy
- Yoga

Carpal tunnel syndrome
- Acupressure
- Bioelectromagnetic therapy
- Vitamin therapy (B_6)

Cerebral palsy
- Biofeedback

Cerebrovascular disease
- Chelation therapy
- Music therapy
- Vitamin therapy

Childbirth
- Hypnosis
- Imagery
- Massage
- Music therapy

Circulation, impaired
- Herbal therapy (butcher's broom, cayenne, and, for brain and extremities, ginkgo biloba)
- Phytoestrogens (found in soy products, lentils, chickpeas, kidney beans, wheat, corn, and rice)

Colds and flu
- Guided imagery
- Herbal therapy
- Homeopathy
- Vitamin/nutritional therapy

Constipation
- Colonic irrigation
- Diet (high-fiber, drink plenty of water)
- Herbal therapy

Coronary artery disease
- Ayurvedic medicine
- Chelation therapy
- Diet (for example, macrobiotic or low-fat)
- Meditation, stress-control program
- Polyphenols (found in onions, apples, wine, and coffee)
- Antioxidants (trace mineral selenium)

Decubitus ulcers
- Bioelectromagnetic therapy

Dental disorders
- Bioelectromagnetic therapy
- Hypnosis

Depression
- Auriculotherapy (See *Acupuncture*, page 30.)
- Herbal therapy (Saint John's wort)
- Vitamin therapy

Diabetes
- Bioelectromagnetic therapy
- Detoxification therapy
- Vitamin therapy
- Yoga

Diabetic neuropathy
- Bioelectromagnetic therapy
- Vitamin therapy (B_{12} prevents neuropathies)

Digestive disorders
- Biofeedback
- Herbal therapy
- Homeopathy
- Juice therapy
- Osteopathic manipulation
- Pancreatic enzyme therapy
- Yoga

Drug and alcohol addiction
- Acupuncture
- Meditation
- Music therapy
- Yoga

Dyslexia
- Auriculotherapy (See *Acupuncture*, page 30.)

Emphysema
- Diet (avoid mucus-producing foods, such as dairy products, salt, and "junk" food)
- Herbal therapy (coltsfoot tea, comfrey or ephedra tea, licorice root)
- Hydrotherapy

Fatigue, chronic
- Bioelectromagnetic therapy
- Biofeedback
- Osteopathic manipulation

Fibrocystic breast disease
- Antineoplaston therapy
- Vitamin E

Fibromyalgia
- Bioelectromagnetic therapy

Genital warts
- Antineoplaston therapy

Glucose, unstable levels
- CO-Q-10
- Garlic
- Spirulina

Gout
- Apitherapy
- Bioelectromagnetic therapy
- Diet (low purine diet)

Hay fever
- Diet (avoid common allergenic foods, such as dairy products, wheat, eggs, chocolate, and peanuts)
- Herbal therapy (nettle, tincture of licorice, comfrey tea)
- Hydrotherapy (hot and cold compresses, steam inhalation)
- Juice therapy
- Vitamin therapy

Headaches
- Bioelectromagnetic therapy
- Biofeedback
- Colon hydrotherapy
- Fasting
- Herbal therapy
- Homeopathy
- Imagery
- Meditation
- Naturopathic therapy
- Osteopathic manipulation
- Yoga

Head trauma
- Music therapy

Hemoglobin, increased
- Spirulina
- Therapeutic Touch

Hemophilia
- Hypnotherapy

Hemorrhoids
- Diet (high-fiber)
- Hydrotherapy
- Qigong
- Reflexology
- Yoga

Hepatitis
- Herbal therapy
- Juice therapy
- Magnetic field therapy
- Oxygen therapy
- Vitamin therapy

Herpes zoster
- Bioelectromagnetic therapy
- Vitamin therapy

Human immunodeficiency virus (HIV) infection
- Dance therapy
- Homeopathy
- I.V. ozone therapy
- Meditation
- Vitamin/nutritional therapy
- Yoga

Hyperactivity
- Biofeedback
- Vitamin/nutritional therapy

Hypertension
- Bioelectromagnetic therapy
- Biofeedback
- Fasting
- Herbal therapy
- Meditation
- Osteopathic manipulation
- Relaxation therapy
- Sound therapy
- Tai chi chuan
- Vitamin/nutritional therapy
- Yoga

Ichthyosis
- Hypnotherapy

Immune disorders (general)
- Enzyme therapy
- Sound therapy
- Vitamin/nutritional therapy

Incontinence (urinary)
- Biofeedback
- Relaxation therapy

Infection
- Herbal therapy (echinacea)
- Nutritional therapy

Inflammatory diseases
- Fasting
- Flavonoids

Insomnia
- Aromatherapy
- Biofeedback
- Herbal therapy (kava kava and valerian)
- Magnetic field therapy
- Melatonin
- Relaxation therapy
- Vitamin therapy (calcium before bed)

Jet lag
- Melatonin

Menstrual disorders
- Herbal therapy
- Naturopathic therapy
- Osteopathic manipulation
- Relaxation therapy

Migraines
- Bioelectromagnetic therapy
- Biofeedback
- Colonic irrigation
- Hypnotherapy
- Yoga

Motion sickness
- Acupressure
- Biofeedback
- Herbal therapy (ginger)
- Reflexology
- Relaxation therapies

Multiple sclerosis
- Apitherapy
- Bioelectromagnetic therapy
- Feldenkrais method
- Pancreatic enzyme therapy
- Vitamin therapy

Muscle and joint pain
- Acupressure
- Alexander technique
- Apitherapy
- Bioelectromagnetic therapy
- Feldenkrais method
- Juice therapy
- Reflexology
- Vitamin therapy

Obesity
- Detoxification therapy
- Diet (high fiber)
- Vitamin therapy (fat metabolism and endocrine support)

Optic nerve atrophy
- Bioelectromagnetic therapy

Osteoporosis
- Bioelectromagnetic therapy

Pain
- Acupuncture
- Auriculotherapy (See *Acupuncture*, page 30.)
- Bioelectromagnetic therapy
- Biofeedback
- Breath therapy
- Electroacupuncture
- Herbal/vitamin therapy
- Hypnotherapy
- Imagery
- Meditation
- Music therapy
- Osteopathic manipulation
- Radiofrequency diathermy
- Relaxation therapies
- Sound therapy
- Stress control classes
- Transcutaneous electrical nerve stimulation (TENS)
- Yoga

Pancreatitis
- Detoxification therapy
- Enzyme therapy
- Fasting
- Juice therapy
- Magnetic field therapy
- Oxygen therapy
- Qigong

Parasitic infection
- Herbal/vitamin therapy
- Light-beam generator therapy

Parkinson's disease
- Auriculotherapy (See *Acupuncture*, page 30.)
- Bioelectromagnetic therapy
- Music therapy

Phantom limb pain
- Bioelectromagnetic therapy

Pneumonia
- Acupuncture
- Diet (eliminate common allergenic foods, such as dairy products, wheat, eggs, chocolate, and peanuts)
- Herbal therapy (lobelia, hydrastis)
- Hydrotherapy

Prostate disorders
- Herbal/vitamin therapy
- Juice therapy

Psychological disorders (all types)
- Art therapy
- Biofeedback
- Fasting
- Hypnotherapy
- Meditation
- Music therapy
- Psychotherapy

Sciatica
- Acupressure
- Applied kinesiology
- Chiropractic treatment
- Hydrotherapy
- Osteopathic manipulation
- Reflexology
- Vitamin therapy

Scoliosis
- Chiropractic treatment
- Osteopathic manipulation

Seizures
- Bioelectromagnetic therapy
- Vitamin therapy

Sinusitis
- Herbal therapy (ephedra, goldenseal, poke root, yarrow)
- Homeopathy
- Hydrotherapy (nasal lavage, hot and cold compresses, steam inhalation)

Sore throat
- Aromatherapy
- Herbal therapy (soothing and astringent gargles)
- Hydrotherapy
- Light therapy
- Pancreatic enzyme therapy
- Reflexology
- Vitamin therapy

Spinal cord injuries
- Art therapy

Sprains and strains
- Bioelectromagnetic therapy
- Herbal/vitamin therapy

Temporomandibular joint syndrome
- Bioelectromagnetic therapy
- Biofeedback
- Vitamin therapy

Trigeminal neuralgia
- Bioelectromagnetic therapy

Ulcerative colitis
- Enzyme therapy
- Relaxation therapies

Ulcers (gastric)
- Herbal therapy
- Pancreatic enzyme therapy

Urinary problems (chronic)
- Acupressure
- Aromatherapy
- Herbal therapy
- Juice therapy
- Magnetic field therapy

Viral illness
- Detoxification therapy
- Fasting
- Herbal therapy
- Juice therapy
- Magnetic field therapy
- Oxygen therapy
- Pancreatic enzyme therapy

Warts
- Herbal therapy (bloodroot paste)
- Hypnotherapy
- Moxibustion (See *Traditional Chinese Medicine*, page 483.)
- Vitamin therapy

Whiplash
- Bioelectromagnetic therapy
- Osteopathic manipulation

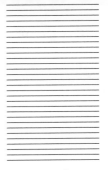

Appendix 3
Therapeutic monitoring guidelines

Herbal product	Monitoring guidelines	Explanation
Aloe	■ Serum electrolytes ■ Weight patterns ■ BUN and creatinine ■ Urinalysis	Aloe possesses cathartic properties, which inhibit water and electrolyte reabsorption, thus leading to possible potassium depletion, weight loss, and diarrhea. Long-term use may lead to nephritis, albuminuria, hematuria, and cardiac disturbances.
Bilberry	■ Weight patterns ■ CBC ■ Blood glucose ■ Triglycerides ■ Liver function	Bilberry contains flavonoids and chromium, which are thought to have blood glucose– and triglyceride-lowering effects. Continued intoxication may lead to wasting, anemia, and jaundice.
Capsicum	■ Liver function ■ BUN and creatinine	Oral administration of capsicum can lead to gastroenteritis and hepatic or renal damage.
Cat's claw	■ Blood pressure ■ Lipid panel ■ Serum electrolytes	Cat's claw can potentially cause hypotension through inhibition of the sympathetic nervous system and its diuretic properties. May also lower cholesterol.
Chamomile (German, Roman)	■ Menstrual changes ■ Pregnancy	German chamomile has been reported to cause changes in menstrual cycle and is a known teratogen in animals. Roman chamomile is thought to be an abortifacient.
Echinacea	■ Temperature	Echinacea can cause fever, nausea, and vomiting.
Ephedra	■ Blood pressure ■ Heart rate ■ Weight patterns	Ephedra's active ingredient, ephedrine, stimulates the CNS in a manner similar to amphetamine. Adverse effects include hypertension, tachycardia, cardiac arrest, stroke, and death.
Evening primrose	■ Pregnancy ■ Lipid profile	Evening primrose oil can reduce elevated plasma lipids and platelet aggregation. It may increase the risk of pregnancy complications, including rupture of membranes, oxytocin augmentation, arrest of descent, and vacuum extraction.

Herbal product	Monitoring guidelines	Explanation
Fennel	■ Liver function	Fennel contains trans-anethole and estragole. Trans-anethole has estrogenic activity, whereas estragole is a procarcinogen with the potential to cause liver damage. Adverse effects include photodermatitis and allergic reactions, particularly in individuals sensitive to carrots, celery, and mugwort.
Feverfew	■ Pregnancy ■ Sleep patterns	Feverfew may inhibit blood platelet aggregation and decrease neutrophil and platelet secretory activity. It can cause uterine contractions in full-term, pregnant women. Adverse effects include mouth ulceration, tongue irritation and inflammation, abdominal pain, indigestion, diarrhea, flatulence, nausea, and vomiting. "Post-feverfew syndrome" includes nervousness, headache, insomnia, joint pain, stiffness, and fatigue.
Flaxseed	■ Lipid panel	Flaxseed possesses weak estrogenic and anti-estrogenic activity. May cause a reduction in platelet aggregation and serum cholesterol. Oral administration with inadequate fluid intake can cause intestinal blockage.
Garlic	■ Blood pressure ■ Lipid panel ■ Blood glucose ■ CBC ■ PT and INR	Garlic has been associated with hypotension, leukocytosis, inhibition of platelet aggregation, decreased blood glucose, and decreased cholesterol. Postoperative bleeding and prolonged bleeding time have also occurred.
Ginger	■ Blood glucose ■ Blood pressure ■ Heart rate ■ Respiratory rate ■ Lipid panel ■ ECG (overdose)	Ginger contains gingerols, which have demonstrated positive inotropic properties. Adverse events include platelet inhibition, hypoglycemia, hypotension, hypertension, and stimulation of respiratory centers. Overdoses have caused CNS depression and arrhythmias.
Ginkgo biloba	■ Respiratory rate ■ Heart rate	Consumption of ginkgo *seed* may cause difficulty breathing, weak pulse, seizures, loss of consciousness, and shock. Ginkgo *leaf* has been associated with male and female infertility, as well as GI upset, headache, dizziness, palpitations, restlessness, lack of muscle tone, and weakness.
Ginseng (American, Panax, Siberian)	■ Blood pressure ■ Liver function ■ Blood glucose ■ Heart rate ■ Sleep patterns ■ Menstrual changes ■ Weight patterns ■ PT, PTT, INR	Ginseng contains ginsenosides and eleutherosides that can have effects on blood pressure, CNS activity, platelet aggregation, and coagulation. Reductions in glucose and hemoglobin A_{1C} levels have also been reported. Adverse effects include insomnia, mastalgia, vaginal bleeding, tachycardia, mania, cerebral arteritis, Stevens-Johnson syndrome, cholestatic hepatitis, amenorrhea, decreased appetite, diarrhea, edema, hyperpyrexia, pruritus, hypotension, palpitations, headache, vertigo, euphoria, and neonatal death.

Herbal product	Monitoring guidelines	Explanation
Goldenseal	<ul><li>Respiratory rate</li><li>Heart rate</li><li>Blood pressure</li><li>Mood patterns</li></ul>	Adverse effects from oral use of goldenseal include digestive disorders, constipation, excitatory states, hallucinations, delirium, GI upset, nervousness, depression, dyspnea, and bradycardia. Goldenseal contains berberine and hydrastine. Berberine has been shown to improve bile secretion and bilirubin, correct cirrhosis, increase coronary blood flow, and stimulate or inhibit cardiac activity. Hydrastine has caused hypotension, hypertension, increased cardiac output, exaggerated reflexes, convulsions, paralysis, and death from respiratory failure. However, berberine and hydrastine are poorly absorbed when given orally; most of these effects occur only in overdose or with parenteral administration.
Kava kava	<ul><li>Weight patterns</li><li>CBC</li><li>Mood changes</li></ul>	Kava kava can cause drowsiness and may impair motor reflexes, affecting the patient's ability to drive or operate machinery. Long-term use may lead to weight loss, hematuria, increased red blood cell volume, decreased platelets, decreased lymphocytes, reduced protein levels, puffy face, pulmonary hypertension, and kava dermopathy (dry, flaking skin, reddened eyes, yellow discoloration of skin, hair, and nails).
Milk thistle	<ul><li>Liver function</li></ul>	Milk thistle contains flavanolignans, which exhibit liver-protective and antioxidant effects.
Nettle	<ul><li>Blood glucose</li><li>Blood pressure</li><li>Weight patterns</li><li>BUN and creatinine</li><li>Serum electrolytes</li><li>Heart rate</li></ul>	Nettle contains significant amounts of vitamin C, vitamin K, potassium, and calcium. Nettle may cause hyperglycemia, decreased blood pressure, decreased heart rate, weight loss, and diuretic effects.
Passionflower	<ul><li>Liver function</li><li>Amylase</li><li>Lipase</li></ul>	Passionflower may contain cyanogenic glycosides, potentially causing liver and pancreas toxicity.
St. John's wort	<ul><li>Vision</li><li>Menstrual changes</li></ul>	Changes in menstrual bleeding have been noted, primarily in women taking oral contraceptives. Such changes may be a result of drug interaction. Other adverse events include GI upset, fatigue, dry mouth, dizziness, headache, delayed hypersensitivity, phototoxicity, and neuropathy. St. John's wort may also increase the risk of cataracts.
SAM-e	<ul><li>Blood pressure</li><li>Heart rate</li><li>BUN and creatinine</li></ul>	SAM-e contains homocysteine, which requires folate, cyanocobalamin, and pyridoxine for metabolism. Increased levels of homocysteine have been associated with cardiovascular and renal disease.

Herbal product	Monitoring guidelines	Explanation
Valerian	■ Blood pressure ■ Sleep patterns ■ Liver function	Valerian contains valerenic acid, which increases gamma-butyric acid and decreases CNS activity. Adverse effects include cardiac disturbances, insomnia, tight chest, and hepatotoxicity. Extended use can cause benzodiazepine-like withdrawal syndrome.

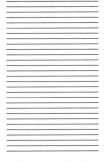

Appendix 4
Supplemental vitamins and minerals

Supplement and dietary reference intakes (DRI)	Uses	Special considerations
Vitamin A/retinol ***DRI:*** *Adult men:* 1,000 mcg retinol equivalents (RE) or 5,000 IU *Adult women:* 800 mcg RE or 4,000 IU *Pregnancy:* Supplement with beta-carotene to form necessary retinol	■ Maintains good vision (rod and cone function; adaptation to light changes) ■ Promotes growth, differentiation, and maintenance of epithelial tissue in GI and respiratory tracts ■ Enhances immune function ■ Aids in bone and teeth formation ■ Promotes wound healing ■ Acts as an antioxidant; used for cancer prevention	■ Only food sources are liver, fish liver oil, tuna, mackerel, eggs, cheese, fortified milk ■ Best if taken with B-complex; vitamins C, D, and E; calcium; phosphorus; and zinc ■ Mineral oil may decrease GI absorption of vitamin A ■ Supplementation of over 6,000 IU daily of retinol, but not of beta-carotene, is associated with birth defects ■ Should be taken during or shortly after a meal ■ Vitamin A and isotretinoin enhance the toxicity of each ■ Patients taking cholestyramine resin may need more vitamin A ■ Use of oral contraceptives increases vitamin A levels
Beta-carotene ***DRI:*** Amount of beta-carotene needed to meet the vitamin A requirement is roughly double that of retinol: 6 mcg beta-carotene = 1 mcg RE = 3.33 IU	■ Same as retinol ■ Forms vitamin A when retinol isn't present in the diet. Beta-carotene is an excellent antioxidant; therefore, probably functions in cancer prevention with a network of other antioxidants ■ Enhances function of immune system	■ Best food sources include dark green and yellow fruits and vegetables, such as carrots, cantaloupe, sweet potato, papaya, apricots, squash ■ Best if taken with a meal, because fat facilitates absorption ■ Water-soluble nutrient ■ Safe supplementation range is 5-25,000 IU ■ Should be taken with a network of other antioxidants: vitamin E, vitamin C, selenium, and zinc ■ Hypercarotenemia produces a yellowing of the palms, nasolabial folds, and soles of the feet, but, unlike jaundice, not the sclerae

Supplement and dietary reference intakes (DRI)	Uses	Special considerations
Vitamin B₁/thiamine **DRI:** *Adult men:* 1-1.5 mg *Adult women:* 1-1.1 mg *Pregnancy:* 1.5 mg	■ Aids digestion, especially carbohydrates ■ Improves mental attitude and maintains a healthy nervous system ■ Stimulates good muscle tone and appetite ■ Prevents beriberi	■ Best food sources include brewer's yeast, whole grain brown rice, soybeans/tofu, whole wheat, oatmeal, wheat germ, milk, and most vegetables ■ Best if taken with B-complex, vitamin C, and manganese ■ Increased physical activity combined with carbohydrate loading may promote depletion ■ Allicin, a substance in onions and garlic, promotes the absorption of vitamin B_1
Vitamin B₂/ riboflavin **DRI:** *Adult men:* 1.2-1.5 mg *Adult women:* 1.2-1.3 mg *Pregnancy:* 1.6 mg	■ Necessary for carbohydrate, protein, and fat metabolism ■ Aids in RBC formation ■ Promotes healthy vision, nails ■ Necessary for tissue repair	■ No known toxic ranges with oral supplementation, as B vitamins are water soluble ■ Chronic alcoholism inhibits absorption of vitamin B_1 from the intestinal lumen ■ Long-term use of loop diuretics and oral contraceptives depletes the body of vitamin B_1 ■ Best food sources include milk, brewer's yeast, liver, cheese, fish, eggs, leafy green vegetables, broccoli, beef, and pork ■ Riboflavin needs gastric acids to be released from foods ■ Best if taken with B-complex, folic acid, and vitamin C ■ Urine turns yellow with high doses of riboflavin, which can affect urinalysis results ■ Absorption slowed by psyllium, alcohol, and oral contraceptives ■ Deficiency results in cracking of the skin on the lips and at the corners of the mouth and increased sensitivity of the eyes to light
Vitamin B₃/ niacin, nicotinic acid **DRI:** *Adult men:* 19-20 mg *Adult women:* 15 mg *Pregnancy:* 17 mg	■ Improves circulation and reduces cholesterol ■ Necessary for carbohydrate, fat, and protein metabolism ■ Needed for healthy skin, nervous system, and digestive tract	■ Best food sources include eggs, organ meats, fortified grains, nuts, brewer's yeast, cottage cheese, broccoli, peas, mushrooms, rice, and wheat bran ■ Best if taken with B-complex, vitamin C, magnesium, and potassium ■ Hepatotoxicity is more likely with high-dose, sustained-release niacin; such therapy shouldn't be used long-term or without a doctor's supervision ■ Should be taken with food

Supplement and dietary reference intakes (DRI)	Uses	Special considerations
Vitamin B$_5$/ pantothenic acid **DRI:** *Adult men:* 4-7 mg *Adult women:* 4-7 mg *Pregnancy:* 4-7 mg	■ Aids in stress resistance ■ Assists in use of carbohydrates, fat, and protein for energy ■ Needed for healthy skin, nervous system, digestive tract, and adrenal gland function	■ Best food sources include organ meats, whole grain cereals, chicken, milk, nuts, eggs, beans, sweet potatoes, broccoli ■ Best if taken with B-complex and vitamin C
Vitamin B$_6$/ pyridoxamine **DRI:** *Adult men:* 2.0 mg *Adult women:* 1.6 mg	■ Necessary for carbohydrate, fat, and protein metabolism ■ Aids in antibody and RBC formation ■ Helps maintain balance of sodium and phosphorus ■ Acts as a natural diuretic ■ Essential for neurotransmitter synthesis ■ Maintains immune function ■ Prevents atherosclerosis	■ Best food sources include brewer's yeast, liver, bananas, soybeans, lentils, brown rice, avocado, cauliflower, seeds, and nuts ■ Best if taken with B-complex, vitamin C, magnesium, and potassium ■ Oral contraceptives, theophylline, isoniazid, cycloserine, penicillamine, and hydralazine are drugs that interfere with vitamin B$_6$ metabolism and lower B$_6$ levels ■ Reduces homocysteine levels to lower cholesterol ■ Caution must be used when prescribing large daily doses for premenstrual syndrome, and nausea and vomiting of pregnancy because of potential risk of neurotoxicity
Vitamin B$_9$/folic acid **DRI:** *Adult men:* 150-200 mcg *Adult women:* 150-180 mcg *Pregnancy:* 400 mcg	■ Helps prevent birth defects and improve lactation ■ Important in RBC formation ■ Necessary for growth and division of body cells and proper function of the nervous system ■ May relieve depression and certain headaches ■ Protects against osteoporosis and cervical dysplasia ■ Indicated, with B$_{12}$ for macrocytic anemia	■ Best food sources include green leafy vegetables, beans, liver, egg yolk, brewer's yeast, whole wheat, peanuts, beef liver, soybean flour ■ Best if taken with B-complex, B$_{12}$, vitamin C, and biotin vitamin C helps reduce the amount of folic acid lost to excretion ■ Estrogens, alcohol, some chemotherapy drugs, sulfasalazine, barbiturates, and anticonvulsants decrease folate absorption ■ High-dose folic acid supplementation should be used with extreme caution in those with epilepsy. It may increase seizure activity ■ Folic acid supplementation can mask vitamin B$_{12}$ deficiency, which can lead to irreversible neurologic damage. Therefore, folic acid supplementation should always include vitamin B$_{12}$

Supplement and dietary reference intakes (DRI)	Uses	Special considerations
Vitamin B$_{12}$/ cyanocobalamin **DRI:** *Adult men:* 2.0 mcg *Adult women:* 2.0 mcg *Pregnancy:* 2.2 mcg	▪ Essential for all blood cell formation and a healthy nervous system ▪ Helps to improve the appetite and increase energy ▪ Necessary for carbohydrate, fat, and protein metabolism ▪ Together with folic acid and vitamin B$_6$, vitamin B$_{12}$ has been shown to reduce high plasma levels of homocysteine, which is an independent risk factor for CV disease	▪ Best food sources include liver, kidney, milk, eggs, fish, cheese, yogurt ▪ Best if taken with B-complex, folic acid, vitamin C, potassium, and calcium ▪ Vegetarians are at a higher risk for low B$_{12}$ levels than nonvegetarians ▪ Adequate gastric intrinsic factor is necessary to convert oral vitamin B$_{12}$ to its active form ▪ Parenteral cyanocobalamin given for B$_{12}$ deficiency caused by malabsorption should be given I.M. or by deep S.C. route but never I.V. ▪ Nitrous oxide, anticonvulsants, and alcohol decrease vitamin B$_{12}$ levels in the blood
B-complex **DRI:** Group of vitamins; no DRI	▪ Helps nervous system function and maintains a healthy digestive tract ▪ Necessary for carbohydrate, fat, and protein metabolism ▪ Maintains healthy eyes, skin, hair, and liver	▪ Best food sources include brewer's yeast, liver, wheat germ, whole grains, nuts, beans ▪ A balanced B-complex helps to ensure proper absorption of all the B vitamins and minimizes the risk of toxicity from individual B vitamins ▪ Best if taken with vitamin C, vitamin E, calcium, phosphorus, and magnesium
Vitamin C **DRI:** *Adult men:* 60 mg *Adult women:* 60 mg *Pregnancy:* 70 mg	▪ Helps heal wounds and burns, and prevents hemorrhage ▪ Reduces serum cholesterol ▪ Aids in preventing many bacterial and viral infections by enhancing immune function ▪ Fights toxins caused by smoke pollution ▪ Maintains healthy blood vessels and joints ▪ Useful in treating allergies ▪ Aids in iron absorption ▪ Antioxidant effect protects against cancer ▪ Prevents scurvy	▪ Best food sources include citrus fruits, berries, tomatoes, broccoli, green and red pepper, dark leafy greens, kiwi, papaya, strawberries, brussels sprouts, potatoes ▪ More effective with all other vitamins and minerals ▪ Interferes with blood tests for vitamin B$_{12}$; inform your provider if you're having these tests and taking extra vitamin C ▪ In high doses of more than 2,000 mg daily, can cause diarrhea, gas, or stomach upset ▪ Buffered vitamin C is available if regular vitamin C upsets the stomach ▪ Cooking vegetables will decrease their vitamin C content ▪ Stress increases the requirement for vitamin C

Supplement and dietary reference intakes (DRI)	Uses	Special considerations
Vitamin D **DRI:** *Adult men:* 200 IU *Adult women:* 200 IU *Pregnancy:* 400 IU *Adults ages 51-70:* 400 IU	■ Needed for absorption and utilization of calcium and phosphorus, which are essential for strong bones and teeth ■ Helps maintain normal heart action and stable nervous system ■ Helps to control serum glucose level ■ Reduces cartilage damage in people with osteoarthritis and may decrease the severity of rheumatoid arthritis	■ Best food sources include fortified milk, fish liver oil, sardines, tuna, salmon, mackerel ■ Sunlight is the most common natural source: 20 to 30 minutes per day for fair-skinned people, about 3 hours per day for dark-skinned people ■ More than 1,000 IU of vitamin D daily can cause illness. Symptoms include dry mouth, muscle and bone pain, nausea vomiting, weakness, headache, constipation ■ Drug interactions that may lead to mineral imbalances include digoxin, verapamil, and thiazide diuretics
Vitamin E **DRI:** *Adult men:* 15 IU *Adult women:* 12 IU *Pregnancy:* 15 IU The DRI for disease prevention and treatment for adults is 400-800 IU/day	■ Potent antioxidant that, along with vitamin C, helps protect cells from damage by free radicals and prevents heart disease, cancer, and stroke ■ Helps wounds heal faster ■ Decreases LDL peroxidation ■ Decreases platelet aggregation	■ Best food sources include wheat germ, soybeans, nuts, leafy greens, sunflower, walnut, safflower oils, sweet potato, whole wheat, liver ■ Best if taken with B-complex, vitamin C, magnesium, and selenium ■ Natural vitamin E (d-alpha-tocopherol) is the preferred form, as it's absorbed best and most actively ■ Chronic alcoholism depletes vitamin E stores in the liver ■ May prolong bleeding time and enhance blood thinning or antiplatelet drugs ■ High doses may interfere with vitamin K activity ■ Cholestyramine and colestipol may decrease absorption of vitamin E ■ Selenium enhances vitamin E's antioxidant activity ■ Improves vitamin A effectiveness ■ Considered generally nontoxic. In high doses of more than 1,200 IU daily, it can cause nausea, gas, diarrhea, and heart palpitations
Vitamin H/biotin **DRI:** *Adult men:* 30-100 mcg *Adult women:* 30-100 mcg *Pregnancy:* 30-100 mcg	■ Necessary for carbohydrate, fat, and protein metabolism ■ Helps fatty acid and amino acid synthesis ■ Improves serum glucose control in diabetics by enhancing insulin sensitivity	■ Best food sources include liver, almonds, peanuts, pecans, walnuts, mushrooms, cooked egg, cauliflower, brewer's yeast, oat bran, unpolished rice, cheese ■ Because biotin is synthesized in the intestinal microflora, deficiency is rare ■ Works best when taken with B-complex and vitamin C

Supplement and dietary reference intakes (DRI)	Uses	Special considerations
Vitamin H/biotin *(continued)*	■ Needed for healthy hair, skin, and nails	■ Isn't absorbed in the presence of raw egg whites ■ Requirements may rise if a person takes sulfa drugs or estrogen, or drinks alcohol ■ Deficiency may result from prolonged use of alcohol (inhibits absorption) or long-term antibiotic therapy (destroys biotin-producing microflora in the gut) ■ Biotin is nontoxic; no adverse effects have been noted, even at high doses ■ Food processing can destroy biotin
Vitamin K/ phytomenadione **DRI:** *Adult men:* 80 mcg *Adult women:* 65 mcg *Pregnancy:* 65 mcg	■ Necessary for pro-thrombin formation and blood coagulation ■ Essential for normal liver functioning ■ Essential for healthy bones ■ Vitamin K is needed for the bones to use calcium ■ May prevent osteoporosis ■ Water-soluble forms are used to treat skin wounds	■ Best food sources include dark green leafy vegetables, especially kale, spinach, turnip greens, broccoli, and cabbage; beef liver; egg yolk; safflower oil ■ Natural vitamin K taken orally is generally nontoxic ■ Large doses of the synthetic form of vitamin K, which are usually given to prevent bleeding in certain conditions, may cause anemia and liver damage ■ Vitamin K can interfere with the action of anticoagulants such as warfarin ■ X-rays and radiation can raise vitamin K requirements ■ Extended use of antibiotics can result in vitamin K deficiency ■ Aspirin, cholestyramine, or mineral oil laxatives may decrease vitamin K levels ■ Freezing foods may destroy vitamin K, but heating doesn't affect it ■ Phenytoin increases vitamin K metabolism and can decrease levels ■ As with all drugs and supplements, check with a health care provider before giving vitamin K to a child
Calcium **DRI:** *Adult men:* 800-1,200 mg *Adult women:* 800-1,200 mg *Pregnancy:* 1,200 mg	■ Calcium is critical in the development and maintenance of bones and teeth ■ Plays important role in maintaining heartbeat and proper blood pressure, and transmitting nerve impulses ■ Reduces risks of pregnancy, such as high blood pressure and preeclampsia	■ Best food sources include milk, yogurt, cottage cheese, cheese, broccoli, dark leafy greens, canned salmon, mackerel, sardines, fortified orange juice, soymilk, soybean nuts, hard or mineral water, almonds, Brazil nuts ■ Vitamin D and magnesium enhance the absorption of calcium ■ Exercise increases absorption of calcium ■ Ideally, supplements should be taken in small doses throughout the day ■ High-protein diets increase calcium excretion

Supplement and dietary reference intakes (DRI)	Uses	Special considerations
Calcium *(continued)*	■ Helps to maintain proper cholesterol levels ■ Used to treat rickets and osteoporosis ■ May be useful in preventing colon cancer	■ Increased calcium loss through the urine is also caused by sodium, phosphorus, sugar, saturated fats, caffeine, alcohol, aluminum-containing antacids, aspartame ■ Excess calcium can interfere with the absorption of iron, zinc, magnesium, iodine, manganese, and copper ■ Doses of 5,000 mg daily are toxic ■ Doses above 2,000 mg daily may increase the risk of kidney stones and soft-tissue calcification ■ There are several types of calcium supplements; check dosage for the type of calcium ingested
Magnesium ***DRI:*** *Adult men: 270-400 mg* *Adult women: 280-300 mg* *Pregnancy: 320 mg*	■ Necessary for protein synthesis and amino acid activation ■ Autonomic control of the heart; may correct heart arrhythmia and lower blood pressure ■ Nerve transmission ■ Muscle contractility/relaxation ■ Essential for development and maintenance of teeth and bones ■ Essential to many metabolic reactions, with its primary function as an enzyme cofactor, thus producing energy, synthesizing lipids and proteins, regulating calcium flow, forming urea, and relaxing muscles ■ May prevent premenstrual syndrome and non–insulin-dependent diabetes mellitus	■ Best food sources include tofu, legumes, whole grains, green leafy vegetables, Brazil nuts, almonds, cashews, pumpkin and squash seeds, pine nuts, oatmeal, bananas, baked potatoes with skins on ■ Vitamin B_6 assists in the body's accumulation of magnesium and works with magnesium in many enzyme systems ■ Magnesium and calcium don't inhibit each other's absorption, but increased magnesium intake may result in excess calcium excretion ■ Magnesium should be taken with a full glass of water with each dose to avoid diarrhea ■ Some foods, drinks, and drugs can cause magnesium loss, including sodium, sugar, caffeine, alcohol, fiber, riboflavin in high doses, insulin, diuretics, and digitalis ■ Magnesium supplements shouldn't be taken by those with severe heart or kidney disease without consultation with a health care provider
Potassium ***DRI:*** *Adult men: 3,500 mg/ day* *Adult women: 3,500 mg/ day* *Pregnancy: 3,500 mg/day*	■ The most important use of potassium is to treat symptoms of hypokalemia, which include weakness, lack of energy, mental confusion, stomach disturbances, an irregular heartbeat, and an abnormal electrocardiogram	■ Best food sources include fresh, unprocessed meats, fish, vegetables (especially potatoes); fruits (especially avocados; and citrus juices), milk, cereals ■ Potassium in food is lost through cooking ■ Potassium supplements, other than what is in a multivitamin, shouldn't be taken unless recommended by a health care provider

Supplement and dietary reference intakes (DRI)	Uses	Special considerations
Potassium *(continued)*	▪ To control or prevent hypertension ▪ To reduce the mortality associated with acute myocardial infarction ▪ To treat muscle weakness ▪ To protect against stroke	▪ Patients with renal insufficiency should use with caution. Care should be taken when prescribing potassium supplements to geriatric patients because of decreased renal functions ▪ Potassium-depleting drugs include thiazides, furosemide, bumetanide, and ethacrynic acid ▪ Other drugs interacting with potassium include potassium-sparing diuretics, NSAIDs, ACE inhibitors, beta blockers, heparin, digoxin, trimethoprim
Iron **DRI:** *Adult men:* 10 mg *Adult women:* 15 mg *Pregnancy:* 30 mg	▪ The most important use of iron supplements is to improve the symptoms of iron-deficient anemia ▪ Chronic blood loss resulting in anemia ▪ Increased iron requirement caused by expanded blood volume, such as occurs in infancy, adolescence, pregnancy ▪ Iron helps to deliver oxygen from the lungs to all parts of the body	▪ Best food sources include liver, lean red meat, poultry, fish, dried beans, fruits, vegetables ▪ Iron supplements should be kept in childproof bottles and away from children ▪ Children between the ages of 12 and 24 months are at highest risk of iron poisoning from accidental ingestion ▪ Vitamin C enhances absorption of iron from the diet ▪ Antacids can reduce the absorption of iron supplements ▪ The absorption of antibiotics ciprofloxacin, norfloxacin, ofloxacin, and tetracycline is reduced by iron ▪ The major adverse effects of supplemental oral iron are GI disturbances, such as nausea, diarrhea, constipation, heartburn, upper gastric discomfort
Selenium **DRI:** *Adult men:* 70 mcg *Adult women:* 50 mcg *Pregnancy:* 65 mcg	▪ Along with being a necessary trace mineral, selenium is an important antioxidant, acting to boost the immune system and prevent age-related diseases such as cancer ▪ Helps with reproductive health and is essential for proper fetal development ▪ Studies show that selenium prevents heart attacks and stroke by lowering low-density lipoprotein (LDL) cholesterol	▪ Best food sources include brewer's yeast, wheat germ, liver, butter, fish, shellfish, sunflower seeds, Brazil nuts ▪ The amount of selenium in foodstuffs corresponds directly to selenium levels in the soil ▪ Deficiencies are noted in parts of China and the U.S. where soil selenium levels are low ▪ Food-source selenium is destroyed during processing ▪ Selenium should be taken with vitamin E, as the two act synergistically ▪ Vitamin C may increase risk of selenium toxicity ▪ Although rare, extended high intake, exceeding 1,000 mcg daily, may lead to toxicity

Supplement and dietary reference intakes (DRI)	Uses	Special considerations
Selenium *(continued)*	■ Required for antioxidant protection of the eye lens; helps prevent cataract formation ■ Promotes proper liver and metabolic function	■ Chemotherapy drugs may increase selenium requirements
Zinc **DRI:** *Adult men:* 15 mg *Adult women:* 12 mg *Pregnancy:* 15 mg	■ Zinc is an essential trace mineral and antioxidant ■ An important part of more than 200 enzymatic reactions in the body ■ Essential for proper growth and development, especially in early life ■ Necessary to maintain proper vision, taste, and smell ■ Improves wound healing ■ Improves immune system function ■ Helps maintain a healthy prostate ■ Required for hormone production, including insulin and growth and sex hormones	■ Best food sources include red meats, lima beans, pinto beans, soybeans, whole grains, miso, tofu, brewer's yeast, cooked greens, pumpkin seeds, and oysters, shrimp, crab, and other shellfish ■ Zinc sulfate can cause GI irritation with nausea and vomiting ■ Supplemental dosage ranges from 20 to 50 mg daily ■ Zinc toxicity is rare, usually occurring only after a dose of 2,000 mg or more has been ingested ■ High doses of zinc will interfere with the assimilation of other trace minerals, such as copper and iron ■ Alcohol, steroids, oral contraceptives, and diuretics decrease zinc levels ■ Calcium may interfere with zinc absorption at high doses ■ Because of the multiple interactions zinc has with other nutrients, it's advisable to take a balanced multiple vitamin/mineral preparation that contains zinc as well as copper, iron, and folate to help prevent deficiencies of these nutrients
Manganese **Estimated safe and adequate DRI:** *Adults:* 2-5 mg	■ Aids in forming connective tissue, fats, and cholesterol, bones, blood clotting factors, and proteins ■ Necessary for normal brain function ■ Is a component of manganese superoxide dismutase (MnSOD), an antioxidant that protects the body from toxic substances ■ Required by multiple enzyme systems ■ Helps prevent osteoporosis	■ Best food sources include Brazil nuts, pecans, almonds, wheat germ, whole grains, leafy vegetables, liver, kidney, legumes, dried fruits ■ There's no RDA for manganese ■ Manganese deficiency has been induced in animals, but not in humans ■ Manganese is the least toxic of the trace elements. Toxicity is more common in humans exposed to manganese dust found in steel mills and mines and certain chemical industries ■ Excess manganese may produce iron-deficient anemia

Supplement and dietary reference intakes (DRI)	Uses	Special considerations
Copper ***Estimated safe and adequate DRI:*** *Adults:* 1.5-3.0 mg	■ Copper is an essential nutrient required for hemoglobin formation, the main component of RBCs ■ Involved in many reactions to produce and release energy ■ Essential for the development and maintenance of skeletal structures ■ Plays a role in proper functioning of the immune system ■ May help prevent atherosclerosis	■ Ideally, manganese supplements should be taken in divided doses to increase absorption ■ Best food sources include seafood, organ meats, nuts, legumes, chocolate, fruits and vegetables, black pepper, blackstrap molasses, water that flows through copper piping ■ Copper supplements should be kept away from children. A dose as little as 3.5 g may be lethal ■ Excess copper can interfere with absorption of zinc ■ Copper absorption may be decreased by calcium, iron, manganese, zinc, vitamin B_6, high levels of vitamin C, antacids in high amounts ■ Copper deficiency may be aggravated by alcohol, eggs, and fructose ■ Copper deficiency in human beings is rare ■ High doses can cause nausea and vomiting

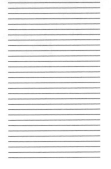

Appendix 5
Herb-drug interactions

Herb	Drug	Possible effects
Aloe	Cardiac glycosides, antiarrhythmics	Ingestion of aloe juice may lead to hypokalemia, which may potentiate cardiac glycosides and antiarrhythmics.
	Thiazide diuretics, licorice, and other potassium-wasting drugs	Additive effect of potassium wasting with thiazide diuretics, and other potassium-wasting drugs.
	Orally administered drugs	Potential for decreased absorption of drugs because of more rapid GI transit time.
Bilberry	Antiplatelets, anticoagulants	Decreases platelet aggregation.
	Insulin, hypoglycemics	May increase serum insulin levels, causing hypoglycemia; additive effect with diabetes drugs.
Capsicum	Antiplatelets, anticoagulants	Decreases platelet aggregation and increases fibrinolytic activity, prolonging bleeding time.
	NSAIDs	Stimulates GI secretions to help protect against NSAID-induced GI irritation.
	ACE inhibitors	May cause cough.
	Theophylline	Increases absorption of theophylline, possibly leading to higher serum levels or toxicity.
	MAO inhibitors	Decreased effects resulting from the increased catecholamine secretion by capsicum.
	CNS depressants such as opioids, benzodiazepines, barbiturates	Increased sedative effect.

Herb	Drug	Possible effects
Capsicum (continued)	H2 blockers, proton pump inhibitors	Potential for decreased effectiveness because of increased acid secretion by capsicum.
Chamomile	Drugs requiring GI absorption	May delay drug absorption.
	Anticoagulants	Warfarin constituents may enhance anticoagulant therapy and prolong bleeding time.
	Iron	Tannic acid content may reduce iron absorption.
Echinacea	Immunosuppressants	Echinacea may counteract immunosuppressant drugs.
	Hepatotoxics	Hepatotoxicity may increase with drugs known to elevate liver enzyme levels.
	Warfarin	Increased bleeding time without an increased INR.
Evening primrose	Anticonvulsants	Lowered seizure threshold.
Feverfew	Antiplatelets, anticoagulants	May decrease platelet aggregation and increase fibrinolytic activity.
	Methysergide	May potentiate methysergide.
Garlic	Antiplatelets, anticoagulants	Enhances platelet inhibition, leading to increased anticoagulation.
	Insulin, other drugs causing hypoglycemia	May increase serum insulin levels, causing hypoglycemia, an additive effect with antidiabetics.
	Antihypertensives	Potential for additive hypotension.
	Antihyperlipidemics	May have additive lipid-lowering properties.
Ginger	Chemotherapy	Ginger may reduce nausea associated with chemotherapy.
	H_2 blockers, proton pump inhibitors	Potential for decreased effectiveness because of increased acid secretion by ginger.
	Antiplatelets, anticoagulants	Inhibits platelet aggregation by antagonizing thromboxane synthetase and enhancing prostacyclin, leading to prolonged bleeding time.
	Calcium channel blockers	May increase calcium uptake by myocardium, leading to altered drug effects.
	Antihypertensives	May antagonize antihypertensive effect.

Herb	Drug	Possible effects
Ginkgo	Antiplatelets, anticoagulants	May enhance platelet inhibition, leading to increased anticoagulation.
	Anticonvulsants	May decrease effectiveness of anticonvulsants.
	Drugs known to lower seizure threshold	Potential further reduction of seizure threshold.
Ginseng	Stimulants	May potentiate stimulant effects.
	Warfarin	Antagonism of warfarin, resulting in a decreased INR.
	Antibiotics	Siberian ginseng may enhance effects of some antibiotics.
	Anticoagulants, antiplatelets	Decreased platelet adhesiveness.
	Digoxin	Ginseng may falsely elevate digoxin levels.
	MAO inhibitors	Potentiates action of MAO inhibitors.
	Hormones, anabolic steroids	May potentiate effects of hormone and anabolic steroid therapies. Estrogenic effects of ginseng may cause vaginal bleeding and breast nodules.
	Alcohol	Increases alcohol clearance, possibly by increasing activity of alcohol dehydrogenase.
	Furosemide	May decrease diuretic effect with furosemide.
	Antipsychotics	Because of CNS stimulant activity, avoid use with antipsychotics.
Goldenseal	Heparin	May counteract anticoagulant effect of heparin.
	Diuretics	Additive diuretic effect.
	H_2 blockers, proton pump inhibitors	Potential for decreased effectiveness because of increased acid secretion by goldenseal.
	General anesthetics	May potentiate hypotensive action of general anesthetics.
	CNS depressants, such as opioids, barbiturates, benzodiazepines	Increased sedative effect.

Herb	Drug	Possible effects
Grapeseed	Warfarin	Increased effects and INR caused by tocopherol content of grapeseed.
Green tea	Warfarin	Antagonism resulting from vitamin content of green tea.
Hawthorn berry	Digoxin	Additive positive inotropic effect, with potential for digitalis toxicity.
Kava	CNS stimulants or depressants	May hinder therapy with CNS stimulants.
	Benzodiazepines	Use with benzodiazepines has resulted in comalike states.
	Alcohol	Potentiates depressant effect of alcohol and other CNS depressants.
	Levodopa	Decreased effectiveness caused by dopamine antagonism by kava.
Licorice	Digoxin	Licorice causes hypokalemia, which predisposes to digitalis toxicity.
	Oral contraceptives	Increased fluid retention and potential for increased blood pressure resulting from fluid overload.
	Corticosteroids	Additive and enhanced effects of the corticosteroids.
	Spironolactone	Decreases the effects of spironolactone.
Ma huang	MAO inhibitors	Potentiates MAO inhibitors.
	CNS stimulants, caffeine, theophylline	Additive CNS stimulation.
	Digoxin	Increased risk of arrhythmias.
	Hypoglycemics	Decreased hypoglycemic effect because of hyperglycemia caused by ma huang.
Melatonin	CNS depressants (such as opioids, barbiturates, benzodiazepines)	Increased sedative effect.
Milk thistle	Drugs causing diarrhea	Increases bile secretion and often causes loose stools. May increase effect of other drugs commonly causing diarrhea. Liver membrane-stabilization and antioxidant effects leading to protection from liver damage from various hepatotoxic drugs such as acetaminophen, phenytoin, ethanol, phenothiazines, butyrophenones.

Herb	Drug	Possible effects
Nettle	Anticonvulsants	May increase sedative adverse effects; may increase risk of seizure.
	Narcotics, anxiolytics, hypnotics	May increase sedative adverse effects.
	Warfarin	Antagonism resulting from vitamin K content of aerial parts of nettle.
	Iron	Tannic acid content may reduce iron absorption.
Passion flower	CNS depressants (such as opioids, barbiturates, benzodiazepines)	Increased sedative effect.
St. John's wort	SSRIs, MAO inhibitors, nefazodone, trazodone	Additive effects with SSRIs, MAO inhibitors, and other antidepressants, potentially leading to serotonin syndrome, especially when combined with SSRIs.
	Indinavir; HIV protease inhibitors (PIs); nonnucleoside reverse transcriptase inhibitors (NNRTIs)	Induces cytochrome P450 metabolic pathway, which may decrease therapeutic effects of drugs using this pathway for metabolism. Use of St. John's wort and PIs or NNRTIs should be avoided because of the potential for subtherapeutic antiretroviral levels and insufficient virologic response that could lead to resistance or class cross-resistance.
	Narcotics, alcohol	Enhances the sedative effect of narcotics and alcohol.
	Photosensitizing drugs	Increases photosensitivity.
	Sympathomimetic amines (such as pseudoephedrine)	Additive effects.
	Digoxin	May reduce serum digoxin concentrations, decreasing therapeutic effects.
	Reserpine	Antagonizes effects of reserpine.
	Oral contraceptives	Increases breakthrough bleeding when taken with oral contraceptives; also decreases contraceptive's effectiveness.
	Theophylline	May decrease serum theophylline levels, making the drug less effective.
	Anesthetics	May prolong effect of anesthesia drugs.

Herb	Drug	Possible effects
St. John's wort (continued)	Cyclosporine	Decreased cyclosporine levels below therapeutic levels, threatening transplanted organ rejection.
	Iron	Tannic acid content may reduce iron absorption.
	Warfarin	Potential to alter INR. Reduces effectiveness of anticoagulant, requiring increased dosage of drug.
Valerian	Sedative hypnotics, CNS depressants	Enhances effects of sedative hypnotic drugs.
	Alcohol	Claims no risk for increased sedation with alcohol, although debated.
	Iron	Tannic acid content may reduce iron absorption.

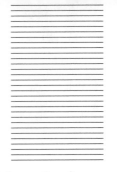

Selected references

Note: References are grouped under the following headings:
General references
Alternative systems of medical practice
Bioelectromagnetic therapies
Diet and nutrition therapies
Herbal medicines
Manual healing therapies
Mind-body therapies
Pharmacologic and biological therapies

General references

Alternative Medicine: Expanding Medical Horizons. A Report to the National Institutes of Health on Alternative Medical Systems and Practices in the United States. NIH Pub. #94-066. Washington, D.C.: U.S. Government Printing Office, 1994.

Alternative Therapies in Health and Medicine. Larry Dossey, MD, Ed., Innovision Communications, Encinitas, CA.

Booth. "Complementary Medicine: Nutritional Therapies," *Nursing Times* 89(37): 44-46, 1993.

Burton Goldberg Group. *Alternative Medicine: The Definitive Guide.* Fife, Washington: Future Medicine Publishing, 1994.

Cassileth, B.R. *The Alternative Medicine Handbook: The Complete Reference Guide to Alternative and Complementary Therapies.* New York: W.W. Norton, 1998.

Davis, C.M. *Complementary Therapies in Rehabilitation: Holistic.Approaches for Prevention and Wellness.* Thorofare, N.J.: Slack Incorporated, 1997.

Decker, G.M. *An Introduction to Complementary and Alternative Therapies.* Pittsburgh, Pa.: Oncology Nursing Press, Inc., 1999.

Dunn, L., and Perry, B.C. "Complementary and Alternative Therapies in Primary Care," *Primary Care Clinics in Office Practice* 24(4):715-721, 1997.

Eliopoulous, C. *Integrating Conventional and Alternative Therapies.* St. Louis, Mo.: Mosby, 1999.

Goldberg, B. *Alternative Medicine: The Definitive Guide.* Tiburon, Calif.: Future Medicine Publishing, Inc., 1999.

Krieger, D. *Foundations of Holistic Nursing Practices.* Philadelphia: J.B. Lippincott, 1981.

Jonas, W.B., and Levin, J.S. Essentials of Complementary and Alternative Medicine. Baltimore: Lippincott Williams & Wilkins, 1999.

Micozzi, M.S. *Fundamentals of Complementary and Alternative Medicine.* New York: Churchill Livingstone, Inc., 1995.

Novey, D.W. *Clinician's Complete Reference to Complementary and Alternative Medicine.* St. Louis, Mo.: Mosby, 2000.

Null, G. *Clinicians Handbook of Natural Healing.* Kensington Publishing, 1997.

Nurse's Handbook of Alternative & Complementary Therapies. Springhouse, Pa.: Springhouse Corp., 1999.

Rosenfeld, I. *Dr. Rosenfeld's Guide to Alternative Medicine: What Works, What Doesn't, and What's Right for You.* New York: Random House, 1996.

Southwest Naturopathic Medical Center, 8010 E. McDowell Road, Suite 205; Scottsdale, AZ 85257; Tel. 480-970-0000

Stone, J. "Regulating Complementary Medicine," *British Medical Journal* 312(7045):1492-93, 1996.

Alternative systems of medical practice

Beasley, J.D., and Swift, J. *The Kellog Report: The Impact of Nutrition, Environment, and Lifestyle on the Health of Americans.* Annandale-on-Hudson, NY: The Institute of Health Policy and Practice, The Bard College Center, 1989.

Reilly, D.T., et al. "Is Homeopathy a Placebo Response?" *Lancet* 2(8518):1272, November 29, 1986.

Vithoulkas, G. *The Science of Homeopathy.* New York: Grove Press, 1980.

Bioelectromagnetic therapies

American Polarity Therapy Association available at: http://www.polaritytherapy.org. Accessed 2000.

Ballentine, R. *Radical Healing.* New York: Harmony Books, 1999.

Beaulieu, J. *Polarity Therapy Workbook.* New York: BioSonic Enterprises, 1994.

Becker, R.O. *Cross Currents: The Perils of Electropollution, the Promise of Electromedicine.* Los Angeles: Putnam Publishing Group, 1990.

Becker, R.O., and Selden, G. *The Body Electric: Electromagnetism and the Foundation of Life.* New York: William Morrow, 1987.

Benford, M.S., et al. "Gamma Radiation Fluctuations During Alternative Healing Therapy," *Alternative Therapies in Health and Medicine.* 5(4):51-56, 1999.

Berbari, P., et al. "Antiantigenic Effects of the Oral Administration of Liquid Cartilage Extract in Humans," *Journal of Surgical Research* 87:108-13, 1999.

Bourgault, L. *The American Indian Secrets of Crystal Healing.* London: Foulsham, 1997.

Bradford, M. *The Healing Energy of Your Hands.* Freedom, Calif.: Crossing Press, 1995.

Bronzino, J.D., ed. *The Biomedical Engineering Handbook.* Hartford, Conn.: CRC Press, 1995.

Bruyere, R.L. *Wheels of Light.* New York: Fireside Books, Simon & Schuster, 1994.

Capra, F. *The Tao of Physics.* Boulder, Colo.: Bantam Books with Shambhala Publications, Inc., 2000.

Davies, B. *The 7 Healing Chakras.* Berkley, Calif.: Ulysses Press, 2000.

Dossey, L. *Reinventing Medicine: Beyond Mind-Body to a New Era of Healing.* San Francisco: HarperCollins Publishers, 1999.

Dossey, L. "Distant Nonlocal Awareness." *Alternative Therapies* 6(6):10-14, 102-110, 2000.

Gerber, R. *Vibrational Medicine for the 21st Century.* New York: Eagle Brook 2000.

Kirschvink, J.L., et al. "Magnetite Biomineralization in the Human Brain," *Proceedings of the National Academy of Sciences USA* 89(16):7683-87, August 15, 1992.

Kirschvink, J.L., et al. "Magnetite in Human Tissues: A Mechanism for the Biological Effects of Weak ELF Magnetic Fields," *Bioelectromagnetics* (suppl 1):101-13, 1992.

Klinger-Omenka, U. *Reiki with Gemstones.* Twin Lakes, Wis.: Lotus Light Publications, 1997. (Germany, Schneebwe Verlagsberattung 1990.)

Krieger, D. *The Therapeutic Touch: How To Use Your Hands to Help or to Heal.* Englewood Cliffs, N.J.: Prentice-Hall, Inc., 1979.

Leadbeater, C.W. *The Chakras.* Wheaton, Ill.: Theosophical Publishing House, 1997.

Levitt, B.B. *Electromagnetic Fields.* San Diego: Harcourt Brace, 1995.

Malmivuo, J., and Plonsey, R. *Bioelectromagnetism: Principles and Applications of Bioelectric and Biomagnetic Fields.* New York: Oxford University Press, 1995.

Nakagawa, K. "Magnetic Field Deficiency Syndrome and Magnetic Treatment," *Japan Medical Journal* (2475):1-12, 1976.

Niehans, P. *Introduction to Cellular Therapy.* New York, Pageant Books, 1960.

Oschman, J.L.. *Energy Medicine: The Scientific Basis.* New York: Churchill Livingstone, 2000.

Philpott, W.H. "Cancer Prevention and Reversal: The Magnetic Answer," *Magnetic Health Quarterly* 2(4):1-26, 1996.

Philpott, W.H. "Magnetic Resonance Bio-Oxidative Therapy for Major Mental Disorders," *Magnetic Health Quarterly* 3(3):1-44, 1997.

Philpott, W.H., and Taplin, S. *Biomagnetic Handbook.* Choctaw, Okla.: Enviro-Tech, 1990.

Roeder, D. *Crystal Co-creators.* Sedona, Ariz.: Light Technology Publishing, 1994.

Roffey, L.E. "Why Magnetic Therapy Works," *Massage* (44):34-36, July-August, 1993.

Rosenfeld, I. *Dr. Rosenfeld's Guide to Alternative Medicine: What Works, What Doesn't, and What's Right for You.* New York: Random House, 1996.

Rubik, B. "Can Western Science Provide a Foundation for Acupuncture?" *Alternative Therapies* 1(4):41-47, 1995.

Sullivan, K. *The Crystal Handbook.* NY: Armadillo Press, Signet Book (Penguin Putnam, Inc.), 1987.

Tierra, M. *Biomagnetic and Herbal Therapy.* Twin Lakes, Wis.: Lotus Press, 1997.

Ulett, G.A. "Conditioned Healing with Electroacupuncture," *Alternative Therapies in Health and Medicine* 2(5):56-60, 1996.

Vallbona, C. "Response of Pain to Static Magnetic Fields in Postpolio Patients: A Double-Blind Pilot Study," *Archives of Physical Medicine and Rehabilitation* 78(11):1200-03, November 1997.

Zimmerman, J.T. "An Explanation About the Assignment of North and South Magnetic Polarities," *BEMI Currents:* *Journal of the Bio-Electro-Magnetics Institute* 2(3):5, 1990.

Zimmerman, J.T. "Comparisons Between Different Brands of Magnetic Bed Products," *BEMI Currents: Journal of the Bio-Electro-Magnetics Institute* 4(1):11, 1995.

Zimmerman, J.T., and Hinrichs, D. "Magnetotherapy: An Introduction," *BEMI Currents: Journal of the Bio-Electro-Magnetics Institute* 4(1):3-7, 1995.

Zukav, G. *The Dancing Wu Li Masters: An Overview of the New Physics.* New York: Bantam Books with William Morrow & Co., Inc., 1979.

Diet and nutrition therapies

Adams, A.K., et al. "Antioxidant Vitamins and the Prevention of Coronary Heart Disease," *American Family Physician* 60(3):895-904, 1999.

Anderson, J.J.B., and Garner, S.C. "The Effects of Phytoestrogens on Bone," *Nutrition Research* 17(10):1617-32, 1997.

Apfeldorf, R., and Infante, P. "Review of Epidemiologic Study with Result of Vinyl Chloride Related Compounds," *Environmental Health Perspective* 41:221-26, 1981.

Appleby, P.N., et al. "The Oxford Vegetarian Study: An Overview," *American Journal of Clinical Nutrition* 70(suppl 3): 525S-531S, 1999

Arts I.C., Hollman P.C., and Kromhout D. "Chocolate as a Source of Tea Flavonoids," *Lancet* 354:488, 1999.

Baird, D.D., et al. "Dietary Intervention Study to Assess Estrogenicity of Dietary Soy Among Postmenopausal Women." *Journal of Clinical Endocrinology and Metabolism* 80(5):1685-90, 1995.

Balch, J.F., and Balch, P.H. *Prescriptions for Nutritional Healing,* 2nd ed. Garden City, N.Y.: Avery Pubs., 1997.

Beall, J.R., and Ulsamer, A. G. "Formaldehyde and Hepatotoxicity: A Review." *Journal of Toxicology and Environmental Health* 13:1, 1984.

Bertelli, A.A., et al. "Resveratrol, a Natural Stilbene in Grapes and Wine, Enhances Intraphagocytosis in Human Promonocytes: A Cofactor in Anti-inflammatory and Anticancer Chemopreventive Activity." *International Journal of Tissue Reactions* 21(4):93-104, 1999.

Bland, J.S. "Food and Nutrient Effects on Detoxification." *Townsend Letter for Doctors and Patients* December:40-44, 1995.

Brzezinski, A., et al. "Short Term Effects of Phytoestrogen-Rich Diet on Postmenopausal Women." *Menopause: The Journal of the North American Menopause Society* 4(2):89-94, 1997.

Butler, R.N., et al. "Anti-aging Medicine Efficiency and Safety of Hormones and Antioxidants," *Geriatrics* 55(7):48-52, 55-56, 58, 2000.

Ciani, F., et al. "Prolonged Exclusive Breast-feeding from Vegan Mother Causing an Acute Onset of Isolated Methylmalonic Aciduria Due to a Mild Mutase Deficiency." *Public Health and Nutrition* 1(1):33-41, 1998. [Published erratum appears in *American Journal of Clinical Nutrition* 56(5):954, 1992.]

Cross, C.E., et al. "Micronutrient Antioxidants and Smoking," *British Medical Bulletin* 55(3):691-704, 2000.

Damianaki, A.,et al. "Potent Inhibitory Action of Red Wine Polyphenols on Human Breast Cancer Cells, "*Journal of Cellular Biochemistry* 78(3):429-41, 2000.

Das, D.K., et al. "Cardioprotection of Red Wine: Role of Polyphenolic Antioxidants," *Drugs Under Experimental and Clinical Research* 25(2-3):115-20, 1999.

Dees, C. "Dietary Estrogens Stimulate Human Breast Cells to Enter the Cell Cycle," *Environmental Health Perspectives* 105(suppl 3):633-36, 1997.

Divi, R.L., et al. "Anti-thyroid Isoflavones from Soybean: Isolation, Characterization and Mechanism of Action," *Biochemical Pharmacology* 54(10):1087-96, 1997.

Douglas, R.M., et al. *Vitamin C for the Common Cold. The Cochrane Collaboration.* Issue 2. Oxford: The Cochane Library Update Software; 1998.

Fernades, C.F., and Shahani, K.M. "Therapeutic Role of Dietary Lactobacilli and Lactobacilli Fermented Dairy Products," *FEMS Microbiology Reviews* 46:343-56, 1987.

Fontaine, K.L. "Herbs and Nutritional Supplementals," in *Healing Practices: Alternative Therapies for Nursing.* Upper Saddle River, N.J.: Prentice Hall, 2000.

Fortin, P.R., "Validation of a Meta-analysis: The Effects of Fish Oil in Rheumatoid Arthritis," *Journal of Clinical Epidemiology* 48:1379-90, 1995.

Fraser, G.E. "Associations Between Diet and Cancer, Ischemic Heart Disease, and All-Cause Mortality in Non-Hispanic White California Seventh-Day Adventists," *American Journal of Clinical Nutrition* 70(suppl 3):532S-538S, 1999.

Fugh-Berman, A. "Clinical Trials of Herbs," *Complementary and Alternative Therapies in Primary Care* 24(4):889-903, 1997.

Garrison, M.B. *A Cancer Therapy: Results of Fifty Cases and the Cure of Advance Cancer by Diet Therapy.* Barrytown, N.Y.: Station Hill Press, 1990.

George, D. "Antioxidants: Can They Reverse the Aging Process?" *Clinical Excellence for Nurse Practitioners* 1(5):299-903, 1997.

Gerson, M.B. *A Cancer Therapy: Results of Fifty Cases and the Cure of Advanced Cancer by Diet Therapy.* Barrytown, NY: Station Hill Press, 1990.

Gries, F., and Ziegler, D. "Alpha-lipoic Acid in the Treatment of Diabetic Peripheral and Cardiac Autonomic Neuropathy," *Diabetes* 46(9):62-66, 1997.

Hackett, A., et al. "Is a Vegetarian Diet Adequate for Children?" *Journal of Nephrology* 10(1):41-5, 1997.

Hanninen, O., et al. "Vegan Diet in Physiological Health Promotion," *Acta Physiologica Hungarica* 86(3-4):171-180, 1999.

Hebbelinck, M., et al. "Growth, development, and physical fitness of Flemish vegetarian children, adolescents, and young adults," *American Journal of Clinical Nutrition* 70(suppl 3):579S-585S, 1999.

Hertog, M., et al. "Dietary Antioxidant Flavonoids and Risk of Coronary Heart Disease: The Zutphen Elderly Study," *Lancet* 342:1007-11, 1993.

Hollman, P.C., et al. "Role of Dietary Flavonoids in Protection Against Cancer and Coronary Heart Disease." *Biochemicat Society Transitions* 24:785-89, 1996.

Hsieh, C.Y., "Estrogenic Effects of Genistein on the Growth of Estrogen Receptor—Positive Human Breast Cancer (MCF-7) Cells In Vitro and In Vivo." *Cancer Research* 58(17):3833-3838, 1998

Ingram, D., "Case Control Study of Phytoestrogens and Breast Cancer," *Lancet* 350(9083):990-94, 1997.

Jakoby, W.B., et al., eds. *Metabolic Basis of Detoxification: Metabolism and Functional Groups.* New York: Academic Press Inc., 1980.

Jibani, M.M., et al. "Predominantly Vegetarian Diet in Patients with Incipient and Early Clinical Diabetic Nephropathy: Effects on Albumin Excretion Rate and Nutritional Status," *Nephron* 79(2):173-80, 1998.

Johansson, G., et al. *One Answer to Cancer.* Pomeroy, Wash: Health Research, 1994.

Johnston, P.K., Haddad, E., Sabate, J. "The Vegetarian Adolescent," *Adolescent Medicine* 3(3):417-438, 1992

Kjeldsen-Kragh, J. "Rheumatoid Arthritis Treated with Vegetarian Diets," *American Journal of Clinical Nutrition* 70(suppl 3):579S-585S, 1999.

Knekt, P., "Flavonoid Intake and Coronary Mortality in Finland: A Cohort Study," *British Medical Journal* 312:478-81, 1996.

Kondo, K., "Inhibition of LDL Oxidation by Cocoa," *Lancet* 348:1514, 1996.

LaLonde, C., et al. "Antioxidants Prevent the Cellular Deficit Produced in Response to Burn Injury," *Burn Care and Rehabilitation* 17(5):383-97, 1996.

Lau, E.M., et al. "Bone Mineral Density in Chinese Elderly Female Vegetarians, Vegans, Lacto-Vegetarians and Omnivores," *European Journal of Clinical Nutrition* 74(2):390-4, 1996.

Lazarus, S., et al. "Chocolate Contains Additional Flavonoids Not Found in Tea," *Lancet* 354:1825, 1999.

Leblanc, J.C., et al. "Nutritional Intakes of Vegetarian Populations in France." 53(6):459-85, 1999.

Lentze, M.J. *Vegetarian and Outsider Diets in Childhood.* Bonn: Zentrum fur Kinderheilkunde, 1999.

Lin. J.K., and Liang, Y.C. "Cancer Chemoprevention by Tea Polyphenols." *Proceedings of the National Science Council, Republic of China. Part B, Life Sciences* 24(1):1-13, 2000.

Lloyd, T., et al. *Urinary Hormonal Concentrations and Spinal Bone Densities of Premenopausal Vegetarian and Nonvegetarian Women.* Hershey, Pa.: Department of Obstetrics and Gynecology, Pennsylvania State University College of Medicine, Milton S Hershey Medical Center, 1999.

Lovblad, K., et al. "Retardation of Myelination Due to Dietary Vitamin B_{12} Deficiency: Cranial MRI Findings," *Pediatric Radiology* 19(2):137-9, 2000.

McCarty, M.F. "Nutrition 21/AMBI, San Diego, CA, USA." *American Journal of Clinical Nutrition* 70(3 suppl):615S-19S, 1999.

McCarty, M.F. "Vegan Proteins May Reduce Risk of Cancer, Obesity, and Cardiovascular Disease by Promoting Increased Glucagon Activity," *Medical Hypotheses* 53:459-485, 1999.

McCarty, M.F. "The Origins of Western Obesity: A Role for Animal Protein," San Diego, Calif.: Helicon Foundation, 54:488-494, 2000.

McKeown, N. "Antioxidants and Breast Cancer," *Nutrition Reviews* 57(10):321-24, 1999.

Meydani, M. "Effect of Functional Food Ingredients: Vitamin E Modulation by Cardiovascular Diseases and Immune System in the Elderly," *American Journal of Clinical Nutrition* 71(suppl 6):1665S-1668S, 2000.

Meyerowitz, S. *Power Juices, Super Drinks*, Summertown, Tenn: Book Publishing, 2000.

Monzani, G., et al. "Lp(a) Levels: Effects of Progressive Chronic Renal Failure and Dietary Manipulation," *Medical Hypotheses* 10(1):41-45, 1997.

Murkies, A.L., et al. "Dietary Flour Supplementation Decreases Post-Menopausal Hot Flushes: Effect of Soy and Wheat," *Maturitas* 21(3):189-95, 1995.

Nenonen, M.T., et al. "Uncooked, Lactobacilli-Rich, Vegan Food and Rheumatoid Arthritis," *British Journal of Rheumatology* 17(4):269-270, 1998.

Nicholson, A.S., et al. "Toward Improved Management of NIDDM: A Randomized, Controlled, Pilot Intervention Using a Lowfat, Vegetarian Diet," *European Journal of Clinical Nutrition* 52(1):60-4, 1998.

Okubo, S., et al. "Effects of a 5-Day Fast on Clinical Laboratory Data from Patients with Rheumatoid Arthritis," *Proceedings of the Nutrition Society* 58(2):271-5, 1999.

Pauling, L. "Orthomolecular Psychiatry." *Science.* 160:265-71, April 1968.

Peterson, J., and Dwyer, J. "Taxonomic Classification Helps Identify Flavonoid-Containing Foods on a Semiquantitive Food Frequency Questionnaire," *Journal of the American Dietetic Association* 98:682-85, 1998.

Richelle, M., et al. "Plasma Kinetics in Man of Epicatechin From Black Chocolate," *European Journal of Clinical Nutrition* 53(1):22-26, 1999.

Ross, R., and Epstein, F.H. "Atherosclerosis: An Inflammatory Disease," *New England Journal of Medicine* 340:115-26, 1999.

Sabate, J. "Nut Consumption, Vegetarian Diets, Ischemic Heart Disease Risk, and All-Cause Mortality: Evidence from Epidemiologic Studies," *Nutrition and Health* 12(3):189-95, 1998.

Schramm, D.D., et al. "Chocolate Procyanidins Mediate Cardioprotective Effects in Humans." Abstract presented at the 219th Annual Meeting of the American Chemical Society (ACS), San Francisco, California, March 2000. 81(9):254-8, 1992.

Segasothy, M., and Phillips, P.A. "Vegetarian Diet: Panacea for Modern Lifestyle Diseases?" *QJM* 92(9):531-544, 1999.

Setchell, K.D.R., et al. "Exposure of Infants to Phytoestrogens from Soy-Based Infant Formula," *Lancet* 350(9070):23-27, 1997.

Sheehan, D.M. "Herbal Medicines, Phytoestrogens and Toxicity: Risk-Benefit Considerations," *Proceedings of the Society for Experimental Biology and Medicine* 217(3):379-85, 1998.

Soroka, N., et al. "Comparison of vegetable-based (soya) and animal-based low-protein diet in predialysis chronic renal failure patients," *Nephron* 79(2):173-180, 1998.

Surh, Y. "Molecular Mechanisms of Chemopreventive Effects of Selected Dietary and Medicinal Phenolic Substances," *Mutation Research* 428(1-2):305-27, 1999.

Tansey, G., et al. "Effects of Dietary Soybean Estrogens on the Reproductive Tract in Female Rats," Proceedings of the Society for Experimental Biology and Medicine, 1998.

Tesar, R., et al. "Axial and Peripheral Bone Density and Nutrient Intakes of Postmenopausal Vegetarian and Omnivorous Women," *International Journal of Obesity and Related Metabolic Disorders* 22(5):454-60, 1998.

The ALSPAC Study Team. "Avon Longitudinal Study of Pregnancy and Childhood. A Maternal Vegetarian Diet in

Pregnancy Is Associated with Hypospadias," *Pediatric Radiology* 27(2):155-58, 1997.

Van Het Hof, K.H., et al. "Plasma and Lipoprotein Levels of Tea Catechins Following Repeated Tea Consumption," *Proceedings of the Society for Experimental Biology and Medicine* 220:203-9, 1999.

Wang, C.F., and Kurzer, M.S. "Phytoestrogen Concentration Determines Effects on DNA Synthesis in Human Breast Cancer Cells," *Nutrition and Cancer: An International Journal.* 28(3):236-47, 1997.

Waterhouse, A., et al. "Antioxidants in Chocolate," *Lancet* 348:834, 1996.

West, P.S. *History of Hoxsey Treatment.* The Office of Technology Assessment (OTA) of the United States Congress, Contract Report, 1988.

Wyatt, K.M., et al. "Efficacy of Vitamin B$_6$ in the Treatment of Premenstrual Syndrome: Systematic Review," *British Medical Journal* 318:1375-81, 1999.

Herbal medicines

Abuja, P.M., et al. "Antioxidant and Prooxidant Activities of Elderberry (*Sambucus nigra*) Extract in Low-Density Lipoprotein Oxidation," *Journal of Agricultural and Food Chemistry* 46:4091, 1998.

Agarwal, C. "Anticarcinogenic Effect of a Polyphenolic Fraction Isolated from Grape Seeds in Human Prostate Carcinoma DU145 Cells: Modulation of Mitogenic Signaling and Cell-Cycle Regulators and Induction of G1 Arrest and Apoptosis," *Molecular Carcinogenesis* 28(3):129-38, 2000.

Agrawal, P., et al. "Randomized Placebo Controlled Single-Blind Trial of Holy Basil Leaves in Patients with Non-Insulin Dependent Diabetes Mellitus," *International Journal of Clinical Pharmacology and Therapeutics* 34:406-09, 1996.

Ahmad, N., et al. "Effect of *Momordica charantia* (Karolla) Extracts on Fasting and

Postprandial Serum Glucose Levels in NIDDM Patients," *Bangladesh Medical Research Council Bulletin* 25:11-13, 1999.

Ajabnoor, M.A. "Effect of Aloes on Blood Glucose Levels in Normal and Alloxan Diabetic Mice," *Journal of Ethnopharmacology* 28:215-20, 1990.

Alderman, S., et al. "Cholestatic Hepatitis after Ingestion of Chaparral Leaf: Confirmation by Endoscopic Retrograde Cholangiopancreatography and Liver Biopsy," *Journal of Clinical Gastroenterology* 19(3):242-47, 1994.

Anderson, D.M., et al. "Specifications for Gum Arabic (*Acacia senegal*); Analytical Data for Samples Collected Between 1904 and 1989," 7(3):303-21, May-June 1990.

Anonymous. "Jimson Weed Poisoning—Texas, New York, and California, 1994," *Journal of the American Medical Association* 273:532-3, 1995.

Anonymous. "Poisoning from Elderberry Juice—California," *Morbidity and Mortality Weekly Report* 33:173, 1984.

Anpalahan, M., and LeCouteur, D.G. "Deliberate Self-Poisoning with Eucalyptus Oil in an Elderly Woman" (letter), *Australian and New Zealand Journal of Medicine* 28:58,1998.

Aquino, R., et al. "Plant Metabolites. New Compounds and Anti-Inflammatory Activity of *Uncaria tomentosa*," *Journal of Natural Products* 54(2):453-59, 1991.

Arlt, W., et al. "Biotransformation of Oral Dehydroepiandrosterone in Elderly Men: Significant Increase in Circulating Estrogens," *Journal of Clinical Endocrinology and Metabolism* 84(6):2170-6, 1999.

Arlt, W., et al. "Dehydroepiandrosterone Replacement in Women with Adrenal Insufficiency," *New England Journal of Medicine* 341(14):1013-20, 1999.

Arpaia, M.R., et al. "Effects of *Centella asiatica* Extract on Mucopolysaccharide Metabolism in Subjects with Varicose Veins," *International Journal of Clinical Pharmacology Research* 10:229-33, 1990.

Arts, I.C., et al. "Chocolate as a Source of Tea Flavonoids," *Lancet* 354(9177):488, 1999.

Atawodi, S.E., et al. "Nitrosatable Amines and Nitrosamide Formation in Natural Stimulants: *Cola acuminata, C. nitida,* and *Garcinia cola,*" *Food and Chemical Toxicology* 33(8):625-30, 1995.

Avorn, J., et al. "Reduction of Bacteriuria and Pyuria after Ingestion of Cranberry Juice," *Journal of the American Medical Association* 271(10):751-4, 1994.

Babu, T.D. "Cytotoxic and Anti-Tumour Properties of Certain Taxa of Umbelliferae with Special Reference to *Centella asiatica* (L.) Urban." *Journal of Ethnopharmacology* 48(1):53-7, 1995.

Bach, N., et al. "Comfrey Herb Tea—Induced Hepatic Veno-occlusive Disease," *American Journal of Medicine* 87:97-9, 1989.

Bagchi, D., "Oxygen Free Radical Scavenging Abilities of Vitamins C and E, and a Grape Seed Proanthocyanidin Extract in Vitro," *Research Communications in Molecular Pathology and Pharmacology* 95(2):179-89, 1997.

Bagchi, D., et al. "Free Radicals and Grape Seed Proanthocyanidin Extract: Importance in Human Health and Disease Prevention," *Toxicology* 7;148(2-3):187-97, 2000.

Bagchi, D., et al. "Protective Effects of Grape Seed Proanthocyanidins and Selected Antioxidants Against TPA-Induced Hepatic and Brain Lipid Peroxidation and DNA Fragmentation, and Peritoneal Macrophage Activation in Mice," *General Pharmacology* 30(5):771-6, 1998.

Baldazzi, C., et al. "Effects of the Major Alkaloid of *Hydrastis Canadensis* L., Berberine, on Rabbit Prostate Strips," *Phytotherapy Research* 12:589-91, 1998.

Barnhart, K.T. "The Effect of Dehydroepiandrosterone Supplementation to Symptomatic Perimenopausal Women on Serum Endocrine Profiles, Lipid Parameters, and Health-Related Quality of Life," *Journal of Clinical Endocrinology and Metabolism* 84(11): 3896-902, 1999.

Barrette, E.P. "Creatine Supplementation for Enhancement of Athletic Performance," *Alternative Medicine Alert* 7:73-84, 1998.

Bauer, R., et al. "TLC and HPLC Analysis of *Echinacea pallida* and *E angustifolia* Roots," *Planta Medica* 54:426, 1988.

Bauer, V., et al. "Immunologic In Vivo and In Vitro Examinations of *Echinacea* Extracts," *Arzneimittelforschung* 38:276, 1988.

Baulieu, E.E., et al. "Dehydroepiandrosterone (DHEA), DHEA Sulfate, and Aging: Contribution of the DHEAge Study to a Sociobiomedical Issue," *Proceedings of the National Academy of Sciences of the United States of America* 97:4279–84, 2000.

Belcaro, G.V., et al. "Improvement of Capillary Permeability in Patients with Venous Hypertension after Treatment with TTFCA," *Angiology* 41:533-40, 1990.

Bempong, D.K., and Houghton, P.J. "Dissolution and Absorption of Caffeine from Guarana," *Journal of Pharmacy and Pharmacology* 44(9):769-71, 1992.

Benoni, H., et al. "Studies on the Essential Oil from Guarana," *Zeitschrift fur Lebensmittel-Untersuchung und-Forschung* 203(1):95-8, 1996.

Bensky, D., and Gamble, A. *Chinese Herbal Medicine,* Revised Edition. Materia Medica, Seattle:1993.

Ben-Yehuda, A., et al. "The Influence of Sequential Annual Vaccination and of DHEA Administration on the Efficacy of the Immune Response to Influenza Vaccine in the Elderly," *Mechanisms of Ageing and Development* 102(2-3):299-306, 1998.

Berkan, T., et al. "Anti-Inflammatory, Analgesic, and Antipyretic Effects of an Aqueous Extract of *Erythaea centaurium,*" *Planta Medica* 57:34-37, 1991.

Berthold, H.K., et al. "Effect of a Garlic Oil Preparation on Serum Lipoproteins and Cholesterol Metabolism," *Journal of the*

American Medical Association 279: 1900-02, 1998.

Bickel, U., et al. "Pharmacokinetics of Galanthamine in Humans and Corresponding Cholinesterase Inhibition," *Clinical Pharmacology and Therapeutics* 50: 420-28, 1991.

Bierenbaum, M.L., et al. "Reducing Atherogenic Risk in Hyperlipemic Humans with Flax Seed Supplementation: A Preliminary Report," *Journal of the American College of Nutrition* 12:501, 1993.

Bilbao, I., et al. "Allergic Contact Dermatitis from Butoxyethyl Nicotinic Acid and *Centella asiatica* Extract," *Contact Dermatitis* 33(6):435-6, 1995.

Bland, J.S. "Food & Nutrient Effects on Detoxification," *Townsend Letter for Doctors and Patients* December:40-4, 1995.

Bloch, M., et al. "Dehydroepiandrosterone Treatment of Midlife Dysthymia," *Biological Psychiatry* 45(12): 1533-41, 1999.

Blumenthal, M., et al. *Herbal Medicine Expanded Commission E Monographs.* Integrative Medicine Communications, 2000.

Blumenthal, M., et al., eds. *The Complete German Commission E Monographs: Therapeutic Guide to Herbal Medicines.* [Translated by S. Klein.] Boston: Integrated Medicine Communications, 1998.

Bock, S.A. "Anaphylaxis to Coriander: A Sleuthing Story," *Journal of Allergy and Clinical Immunology* 91:1232-33, 1993.

Bogacheva, A.M., et al. "A New Subtilisin-like Proteinase from Roots of the Dandelion *Taraxacum officinale*," Webb S.L. *Biochemistry (Moscow)* 64(9):1030-7, 1999.

Bolle, P., et al. "Response of Rabbit Detrusor Muscle to Total Extract and Major Alkaloids of *Hydrastis Canadensis*," *Phytotherapy Research* 12(suppl 1):S86-8, 1998.

Bone, K. "Bilberry—The Vision Herb," *MediHerb Professional Review* 59:1-4, 1997.

Bordia, A. "Garlic and Coronary Heart Disease. The Effects of Garlic Extract Therapy Over Three Years on the Reinfarction and Mortality Rate," [translated from German], *Deutsch Apothecary Ztg* 129(suppl 15):16–17, 1989.

Boulin, D.J. "Garlic as a Platelet Inhibitor" (letter), *Lancet* i:776, 1981.

Bouskela, E., et al. "Effects of Ruscus Extract on the Internal Diameter of Arterioles and Venules of the Hamster Cheek Pouch Microcirculation," *Journal of Cardiovascular Pharmacology* 22:221-24, 1993.

Bouskela, E., et al. "Inhibitory Effect of the Ruscus Extract and of the Flavonoid Hesperidine Methylchalcone on Increased Microvascular Permeability Induced by Various Agents in the Hamster Cheek Pouch," *Journal of Cardiovascular Pharmacology* 22:225-30, 1993.

Bradwejn, J., et al. "A Double-Blind, Placebo-Controlled Study on the Effects of Gotu Kola (*Centella asiatica*) on Acoustic Startle Response in Healthy Subjects," *Journal of Clinical Psychopharmacology* 20(6):680-4, 2000.

Brinker, F. "*Larrea tridentata* (D.C.) Coville (Chaparral or Creosote Bush)," *British Journal of Phytotherapy* 3(1):10-31, 1993/1994.

Brinkhaus, B., et al. "Chemical, Pharmacological and Clinical Profile of the East Asian Medical Plant *Centella asiatica*," *Phytomedicine* 7(5):427-48, 2000.

Brzeski, M., et al. "Evening Primrose Oil in Patients with Rheumatoid Arthritis and Side-Effects of Non-steroidal Anti-inflammatory Drugs," *British Journal of Rheumatology* 30:370-2, 1991.

Budavari, S., et al. *The Merck Index,* 12th ed. Rahway, N.J.: Merck & Co., 1996.

Bunyapraphatsara, N., et al. "Antidiabetic Activity of Aloe Vera L. Juice II. Clinical Trial in Diabetes Mellitus Patients in Combination with Glibenclamide," *Phytomedicine* 3:245-48, 1996.

Bushunow, P., et al. "Gossypol Treatment of Recurrent Adult Malignant Gliomas,"

Journal of Neuro-Oncology 43:79-86, 1999.

Bussin, A., and Schweizer, K. "Effects of a Phytopreparation from *Hellebore niger* on Immunocompetent Cells In Vitro," *Journal of Ethnopharmacology* 59(3):139-46, 1998.

Bydlowski, S.P., et al. "A Novel Property of an Aqueous Guarana Extract (*Paullinia cupana*): Inhibition of Platelet Aggregation In Vitro and In Vivo," *Brazilian Journal of Medicine and Biological Research* 21(3):535-8, 1988.

Bydlowski, S.P., et al. "An Aqueous Extract of Guarana (*Paullinia cupana*) Decreases Platelet Thromboxane Synthesis," *Brazilian Journal of Medical and Biological Research* 24(4):421-4, 1991.

Cantrell, C.L., et al. "Antimycobacterial Eudesmanolides from *Inula helenium* and *Rudbeckia subtomentosa*," *Planta Medica* 65:351, 1999.

Caplan, R.M. "Chaulmoogra Oil," *Iowa Medicine* 75(5):223, 1985.

Carini, M., et al. "UVB-Induced Hemolysis of Rat Erythrocytes: Protective Effect of Procyanidins from Grape Seeds," *Life Sciences* 67(15):1799-814, 2000.

Castleman, M. *The Healing Herbs. The Ultimate Guide to the Curative Power of Nature's Medicines.* Emmaus, Pa.: Rodale Press, 1991.

Cauffield, J.S., and Forbes, H.J. "Dietary Supplements Used in the Treatment of Depression, Anxiety, and Sleep Disorders," *Primary Care: Clinics in Office Practice* 3(3):290-304, 1999.

Cerri, R., et al. "New Quinoic Acid Glycosides from *Uncaria tomentosa*," *Journal of Natural Products* 51(2):257, 1988.

Cesarone, M.R., et al. "The Microcirculatory Activity of Centella asiatica in Venous Insufficiency. A Double-Blind Study," *Minerva Cardioangiologica* 42(6):299-304, 1994.

Chapman, E. "Grand Round: Hellebore niger," *Journal of the American Institute of Homeopathy* 85(2):74-7, 1992.

Chaudhuri, S.K., and Ghosh, S. "Review on Chaulmoogra Oil," *Indian Journal of Dermatology* 18(3):55-61, 1973.

Chavez, M.L., and Chavez, P.I. "Echinacea," *Hospital Pharmacy* 33:180, 1998.

Chavez, M.L., and Chavez, P.I. "Feverfew," *Hospital Pharmacy* 34:436-61, 1999.

Chen, Y.J., et al. "The Effect of Tetrandrine and Extracts of *Centella asiatica* on Acute Radiation Dermatitis in Rats," *Biological and Pharmaceutical Bulletin* 22(7):703-6, 1999.

Cheng, C.L., and Koo, M.W. "Effects of *Centella asiatica* on Ethanol Induced Gastric Mucosal Lesions in Rats," *Life Sciences* 67(21):2647-53, 2000.

Chitra, V., and Leelamma, S. "Hypolipidemic Effect of Coriander Seeds (*Coriandrum sativum*): Mechanism of Action," *Plant Foods for Human Nutrition* 51(2):167-72, 1997.

Chrubasik, S., et al. "Effectiveness of Harpagophytum Extract WS 1531 in the Treatment of Exacerbation of Low Back Pain: A Randomized, Placebo-Controlled, Double-Blind Study," *European Journal of Anaesthesiology* 16(2):118-29, 1999.

Clark, I.M., et al. "Spatially Distinct Expression of Two New Cytochrome P450s in Leaves of *Nepeta racemosa*: Identification of a Trichrome-Specific Soform," *Plant Molecular Biology* 33(5):875-85, 1997.

Clarke, J.A., and Yermanos, D.M. "Effects of Ingestion of Jojoba Oil on Blood Cholesterol Levels and Lipoprotein Patterns in New Zealand White Rabbits," *Biochemical and Biophysical Research Communications* 102:1409-15, 1981.

Cohen, S.H., et al. "Acute Allergic Reaction after Composite Pollen Ingestion," *Journal of Allergy and Clinical Immunology* 64(4):270-4, 1979.

Cometa, M.F., et al. "Spasmolytic Activities of *Hydrastis canadensis* L. on Rat Uterus and Guinea-Pig Trachea," *Phytotherapy Research* 12(suppl 1):S83-5, 1998.

da Fonseca, C.A., et al. "Genotoxic and Mutagenic Effects of Guarana (*Paullinia cupana*) in Prokaryotic Organisms," *Mutatation Research* 321(3):165-73, 1994.

Danese, P., et al. "Allergic Contact Dermatitis Due to *Centella asiatica* Extract," *Contact Dermatitis* 31(3):201, 1994.

Dao, V., et al. "Synthesis and Cytotoxicity of Gossypol Related Compounds," *European Journal of Medical Chemistry* 35(9):805-13, 2000.

Darzynkiewicz, Z., et al. "Effects of Derivatives of Chrysophanol, a New Type of Potential Antitumor Agent of Anthraquinone Family, on Growth and Cell Cycle of L1210 Leukemic Cells," *Cancer Letters* 46(3):181-87, 1989.

Dawe, R.S., et al. "Daisy, Dandelion and Thistle Contact Allergy in the Photosensitivity Dermatitis and Actinic Reticuloid Syndrome," *Contact Dermatitis* 35(2):109-10, 1996.

Degelau, J., et al. "The Effect of DHEAS on Influenza Vaccination in Aging Adults," *Journal of the American Geriatric Society* 45(6):747-51, 1997.

Delaveau, P., et al. "Stimulation of the Phagocytic Activity of R.E.S. by Plant Extracts," *Planta Medica* 40(1):49-54, 1980.

DerMarderosian, A., et al., eds. *Facts and Comparisons: The Review of Natural Products*. St. Louis, Mo.: Wolters Kluwer Co., 1999.

Desmarchelier, C., et al. "Evaluation of the In Vitro Antioxidant Activity in Extracts of *Uncaria tomentosa* (Willd.) DC," *Phytotherapy Research* 11(3):254-56, 1997.

Didry, N., et al. "Components and Activity of *Tussilago farfara*," *Annales Pharmaceutiques Francaises* 40(1):75-80, 1982.

Donadio, V., et al. "Myoglobinuria After Ingestion of Extracts of Guarana, Ginkgo Biloba and Kava," *Neurological Sciences* 21(2):124, 2000.

Dove, D, and Johnson, P. "Oral Evening Primrose Oil: Its Effect on Length of Pregnancy and Selected Intrapartum Outcomes in Low-Risk Nulliparous Women," *J Nurse-Midwifery* 44:320-24, 1999.

Duke, J. *The Green Pharmacy*. Emmaus, Pa.: Rodale Press, 1997.

Ellis, C.N., et al. "A Double Blind Evaluation of Topical Capsaicin in Pruritic Psoriasis," *Journal of the American Academy of Dermatology* 29(3):438-42, 1993.

Englisch, W., et al. "Efficacy of Artichoke Dry Extract in Patients with Hyperlipoproteinemia," *Arzneimittelforschung* 50:260-65, 2000.

Espinola, E.B., et al. "Pharmacological Activity of Guarana (*Paullinia cupana* Mart.) in Laboratory Animals," *Journal of Ethnopharmacology* 55(3):223-9, 1997.

European Scientific Cooperative on Phytotherapy. *Harpagophyti radix* (devil's claw). Exeter, UK: ESCOP; 1996-1997. [Monographs on the Medicinal Uses of Plant Drugs. Fascicule 2.]

Evans, T.G., et al. "The Use of Oral Dehydroepiandrosterone Sulfate as an Adjuvant in Tetanus and Influenza Vaccination of the Elderly," *Vaccine* 14(16):1531-7, 1996.

Fam, A. "Use of Titrated Extract of *Centella asiatica* (TECA) in Bilharzial Bladder Lesions," *International Surgery* 58(7):451-2, 1973 passim.

Fernades, C.F., and Shahani, K.M. "Therapeutic Role of Dietary Lactobacilli and Lactobacilli Fermented Dairy Products," *FEMS Microbiology Reviews* 46:343-56, 1987.

Fidler, P., et al. "Prospective Evaluation of a Chamomile Mouthwash for Prevention of 5-FU-Induced Mucositis," *Cancer* 77(3):522-25, 1996.

Finkelstein, E. "An Outbreak of Phytophotodermatitis Due to Celery," *International Journal of Dermatology* 33(2):116-18, 1994.

Flack, M.R., et al. "Oral Gossypol in the Treatment of Metastatic Adrenal Cancer," *Journal of Clinical Endocrinology and Metabolism* 76:1019-24, 1993.

Foster, S. "Black Cohosh (*Cimicifuga racemosa*): A Literature Review," *Herbalgram* 45:35-50, 1999.

Foster, S. *Goldenseal:* Hydrastic canadensis. Botanical Series No. 309. Austin, Tex.: American Botanical Council, 1991.

Foster, S., and Tyler, V.E. *Tyler's Honest Herbal: A Sensible Guide to the Use of Herbs and Related Remedies,* 4th ed. New York: The Haworth Herbal Press, 1999.

Fotisch, K., et al. "Involvement of Carbohydrate Epitopes in the IgE Response of Celery-Allergic Patients," *International Archives of Allergy and Immunology* 120(1):30-42, 1999.

Freeman, G.L. "Allergy to Fresh Dill," *Allergy* 54(5):531-2, 1999.

Frohne, V.D. "The Urinary Disinfectant Effect of Extract From Leaves Uva Ursi," [in German; English abstract] *Planta Medica* 18:1-25, 1970.

Fugh-Berman, A. "Herb-Drug Interactions," *Lancet* 355:134-38, 2000.

Galduroz, J.C., and Carlini, E.A. "Acute Effects of the *Paulinia cupana,* "Guarana," on the Cognition of Normal Volunteers," *Revista Paulista de Medicina* 112(3):607-11, 1994.

Galduroz, J.C., and Carlini, E.A. "The Effects of Long-Term Administration of Guarana on the Cognition of Normal, Elderly Volunteers," *Revista Paulista de Medicina* 114(1):1073-8, 1996.

Garbacki, N., et al. "Anti-Inflammatory and Immunological Effects of *Centaurea cyanus* Flower-Heads," *Journal of Ethnopharmacology* 68(1-3):235-41, 1999.

Gatley, C.A., et al. "Drug Treatments for Mastalgia: 17 Years Experience in the Cardiff Mastalgia Clinic," *Journal of the Royal Society of Medicine* 85:12-5, 1992.

Geyman, J.P. "Anaphylactic Reaction After Ingestion of Bee Pollen," *Journal of the American Board of Family Practice* 7(3):250-52, 1994.

Ghannam, N., et al. "The Antidiabetic Activity of Aloes: Preliminary Clinical and Experimental Observations," *Hormone Research* 24:288-94, 1986.

Ghazaly, M., et al. "Study of the Anti-inflammatory Activity of *Populus tremula, Solidago virgaurea* and *Fraxinus excelsior,*" *Arzneimittelforschung* 42(3):333-6, 1992.

Gibson, D. "Hellebore niger," *Homeopathy* 7(2):79-83, 1987.

Glowania, H.J., et al. "The Effect of Chamomile on Wound Healing—-A Controlled Clinical-Experimental Double-Blind Trial," *Z Hautkr* 62:1262-71, 1987.

Goldberg, A., et al. "Asthma Responses to Pollen of Ornamental Plants: High Incidence in the General Atopic Population and Especially Among Flower Growers," *Journal of Allergy and Clinical Immunology* 102:210-14, 1998.

Goldberg, M. "Dehydroepiandrosterone, Insulin-like Growth Factor, and Prostate Cancer," *Annals of Internal Medicine* 129(7): 587-88, 1998.

Gonzalo Garijo, M.A., et al. "Allergic Contact Dermatitis due to *Centella asiatica:* A New Case," *Allergologia et Immunopathologia (Madrid)* 24(3):132-4, 1996.

Gordon, D.W., et al. "Chaparral Ingestion. The Broadening Spectrum of Liver Injury Caused by Herbal Medications," *Journal of the American Medical Association* 273(6):489-90, 1995.

Grando, L.J., et al. "In Vitro Study of Enamel Erosion Caused by Soft Drinks and Lemon Juice in Deciduous Teeth Analysed by Stereomicroscopy and Scanning Eelectron Microscopy," *Caries Research* 30(5):373-8, 1996.

Gray, A.M., and Flatt, P.R. "Actions of the Traditional Antidiabetic Plant, *Agromony Eupatoria* (Agromony)—Effects on Hyperglycaemia, Cellular Glucose Metabolism and Insulin Secretion," *British Journal of Nutrition* 80(1):109-14, 1998.

Gray, A.M., and Flatt, P.R. "Insulin-Releasing and Insulin-Like Activity of the Traditional Anti-Diabetic Plant *Coriandrum sativum* (Coriander)," *British Journal of Nutrition* 81(3):203-09, 1999.

Greally, P., et al. "Gaviscon and Carobel Compared with Cisapride in Gastroesophageal Reflux," *Archives of Disease in Childhood* 67(5):618-21, 1992.

Greenfield, S.M., et al. "A Randomized Controlled Study of Evening Primrose Oil and Fish Oil in Ulcerative Colitis," *Alimentary Pharmacology and Therapeutics* 7:159-66, 1993.

Grieve, M., and Leyel, C.F., eds. *A Modern Herbal.*. New York: Dover Publications Inc., 1978.

Grognet, J. "Catnip: Its Uses and Effects, Past and Present," *Canadian Veterinary Journal* 31(6):455-56, 1990.

Gruenwald, J., et al. "Acacia Senegal," in *PDR for Herbal Medicines*, 2nd ed. Montvale, N.J.: Medical Economics Company, 2000.

Guin, J.D., and Skidmore, G. "Compositae Dermatitis in Childhood," *Archives of Dermatology* 123(4):500-2, 1987.

Gurley, B.J., et al. "Ephedrine Pharmacokinetics after the Ingestion of Nutritional Supplements Containing *Ephedra sinica* (*ma huang*)," *Therapeutic Drug Monitoring* 20:439, 1998.

Harvey, S.C. "Topical Drugs," in *Remington's Pharmaceutical Sciences*, 18th ed. Edited by Gennaro, A.R., et al. Pennsylvania: Mack, 1990.

Hausen, B.M. "*Centella asiatica* (Indian Pennywort), an Effective Therapeutic But a Weak Sensitizer," *Contact Dermatitis* 29(4):175-9, 1993.

Healing Herbs. Edited by Cassidy, C.M. Prevention Health Specials, 1996.

Henry, D.Y., et al. "Isolation and Characterization of 9-Hydroxy-10-trans,12-cis-octadecadenoic Acid, a Novel Regulator of Platelet Adenylate Cyclase from *Glechoma hederacea* L. Labiatae," *European Journal of Biochemistry* 30;170(1-2):389-94, 1987.

Herbal Medicinals: A Clinician's Guide. Edited by Miller, L.G., and Murray, W.J. New York, NY: Pharmaceutical Products Press, 1998.

Herbert, D., et al. "In Vitro Experiments with *Centella asiatica*: Investigation to Elucidate the Effect of an Indigenously Prepared Powder of This Plant on the Acid-Fastness and Viability of *M. tuberculosis*," *Indian Journal of Leprosy* 66(1):65-8, 1994.

Herbs and Supplements: Eyebright. The *Natural Pharmacist* (www.tnp.com)

Hernandez, M.M., et al. "Biological Activities of Crude Plant Extracts from *Vitex trifolia*," *Journal of Ethnopharmacology* 67(1):37-44, 1999.

Hilton, E., et al. "Efficacy of Lactobacillus GG as a Diarrheal Preventive in Travelers," *Journal of Travel Medicine* 4:41-43, 1997.

Hirata, J.D., et al. "Does Dong Quai Have Estrogenic Effects in Postmenopausal Women? A Double-Blind Placebo-Controlled Trial," *Fertility and Sterility* 68:981, 1997.

Hirono, I., et al. "Carcinogenic Activity of Coltsfoot, *Tussilago farfara l.*," *Gann* 67(1):125-29, 1976.

Hirono, I., et al. "Safety Examination of Some Edible Plants, Part 2," *Journal of Environmental Pathology and Toxicology* 1(1):71-4, 1978.

Hoffman, D. *The Complete Illustrated Holistic Herbal. A Safe and Practical Guide to Making and Using Herbal Remedies*. Rockport, Mass.: Element Books, 1996.

Hoffman-Sommergruber, K., et al. "IgE Reactivity to Api g 1, a Major Celery Allergen, in a Central European Population Is Based on Primary Sensitization by Bet v 1," *Journal of Allergy and Clinical Immunology* 104(2I):478-84, 1999.

Hostettler, M., et al. "Efficacy and Tolerance of Insoluble Carob Fraction in the Treatment of Traveler's Diarrhea," *Journal of Diarrhoeal Diseases Research* 13(3):155-58, 1995.

Howell, A.B., et al. "Inhibition of the Adherence of P-fimbrinated *Escherichia coli* to Uroepithelial Cell Surfaces by Proanthrocyanidin Extracts from Cranberries," *New England Journal of Medicine* 339:1005-06, 1998.

Huang, Y.T., et al. "*Fructus aurantii* Reduced Portal Pressure In Portal Hypertensive Rats," *Life Sciences* 57:2011-20, 1995.

Iannuzzi, J. "Pollen: Food for Honey Bee - and Man?" *American Bee Journal* 133(9):633-37, 1993.

Iverson, T., et al. "The Effect of NaO Li Su on Memory Functions and Blood Chemistry in Elderly People," *Journal of Ethnopharmacology* 56:109-16, 1997.

Jackson, B., and Reed, A. "Catnip and the Alteration of Consciousness," *Journal of the American Medical Association* 207(7):1349-50, 1969.

Jaffe, A.M., et al. "Poisoning Due to Ingestion of *Veratrum viride* (False Hellebore)," *Journal of Emergency Medicine* 8(2):161-67, 1990.

Jakoby, W. B., et al., eds. *Metabolic Basis of Detoxification: Metabolism and Functional Groups*. New York: Academic Press Inc., 1980.

Jayasooriya, A.P., et al. "Effects of *Momordica charantia* Powder on Serum Glucose Levels and Various Lipid Parameters in Rats Fed with Cholesterol-Free and Cholesterol-Enriched Diets," *Journal of Ethnopharmacology* 72:331-36, 2000.

Jefferson, J.W. "Lithium Tremor and Caffeine Intake: Two Cases of Drinking Less and Shaking More," *Journal of Clinical Psychiatry* 49(2):72-3, 1988.

Jellin, J.M., et al. *Pharmacist's Letter/Prescriber's Letter Natural Medicines Comprehensive Database*, 3rd ed. Stockton, Calif.: Therapeutic Research Faculty, 2000.

Jeng, J.H., et al. "Effects of Areca Nut, Inflorescence *Piper betle* Extracts and Arecoline on Cytotoxicity, Total and Unscheduled DNA Synthesis in Cultured Gingival Keratinocytes," *Journal of Oral Pathology and Medicine* 28:64-71, 1999.

Jensen-Jarolim, E., et al. "Fatal Outcome of Anaphylaxis to Chamomile-Containing Enema During Labor: A Case Study,"

Journal of Allergy and Clinical Immunology 102(6):1041-42, 1998.

Jones, C.L.A. "Fight Fungus with Five Topical Herbs," *Nutrition Science News* 3(12):630-35, 1998.

Katz, M., and Saibil, F. "Herbal Hepatitis: Subacute Hepatic Necrosis Secondary to Chaparral Leaf," *Journal of Clinical Gastroenterology* 12(2):203-06, 1990.

Katzung, W. ["Guarana—-A Natural Product with High Caffeine Content"] (review, German), *Medizinische Monatsschrift fur Pharmazeuten* 16(11):330-3, 1993.

Kay, M.A. *Healing with Plants in the American and Mexican West*. Tucson, Ariz.: University of Arizona Press, 1996.

Kedzia, B., et al. "Antibacterial Action of Urine Containing Arbutine Metabolism" [in Polish; English summary], *Medycyna Doswiadczalna Mikrobiologia* 27:305-14, 1975.

Keeler, R.F., et al. "Concentration of Galegine in *Verbesina encelioides* and *Galega officinalis* and the Toxic and Pathologic Effects Induced by the Plants," *Journal of Environmental and Pathological Toxicology and Oncology* 11:11-17, 1992.

Keeler, R.F., et al. "Toxicosis from and Possible Adaptation to *Galega officinalis* in Sheep and the Relationship to *Verbesina encelioides* Toxicosis," *Veterinary and Human Toxicology* 28:309-15, 1986.

Kemper, K.J. "Rhubarb Root (*Rheum officinale* or *R. palmatum*)," Longwood Herbal Task Force. Revised September 24, 1999. Available at http://www.mcp.edu/herbal/default.htm. Accessed Jan 27, 2000.

Keplinger, K., et al. "*Uncaria tomentosa* (Willd.) DC - Ethnomedicinal Use and New Pharmacological, Toxicological and Botanical Results," *Journal of Ethnopharmacology* 64(1):23-34, 1999.

Kerr, K.G. "Cranberry Juice and Prevention of Recurrent Urinary Tract Infection," *Lancet* 353(9153):673, 1999.

Kim, H.M., et al. "Activation of Inducible Nitric Oxide Synthase by *Taraxacum of-*

ficinale in Mouse Peritoneal Macrophages," *General Pharmacology* 32(6):683-8, 1999.

Kim, H.M., et al. *"Taraxacum officinale* Restores Inhibition of Nitric Oxide Production by Cadmium in Mouse Peritoneal Microphages,"*Immunopharmacology and Immunotoxicology* 20(2):283-97, 1998.

Kim, Y.N., et al. "Enhancement of the Attachment on Microcarriers and tPA Production by Fibroblast Cells in a Serum-Free Medium by the Addition of the Extracts of *Centella asiatica,"* *Cytotechnology* 13(3):221-6, 1993.

Kline, M.D., and Jaggers, E.D. "Mania Onset While Using Dehydroepiandrosterone," *American Journal of Psychiatry* 156(6):971, 1999.

Koyama, M., et al. "Intercalculating Agents with Covalent Bond Forming Capabilities. A Novel Type of Potential Anticancer Agents," *Journal of Medicinal Chemistry* 32(7):1594-99, 1989.

Kraft, K. "Artichoke Leaf Extract—Recent Findings Reflecting Effects on Lipid Metabolism, Liver and Gastrointestinal Tracts," *Phytomedicine* 4:369-78, 1997.

Krustak, D., et al. "The Composition of the Volatile Oil of *Vitex agnus castus,"* *Planta Medica* 58(suppl 1):A681, 1992.

Kupke, D., et al. "An Evaluation of the Choleretic Activity of a Plant-Based Cholagogue" [translated from German], *Z Allgemeinmed* 67:1046-58, 1991.

Lanhers, M.C., et al. "Anti-inflammatory and Analgesic Effects of an Aqueous Extract of *Harpagophytum procumbens,"* *Planta Medica* 58(2):117-23, 1992.

Lauritzen, C.H., et al. "Treatment of Premenstrual Tension Syndrome with *Vitex agnus castus*—-Controlled, Double-Blind Study Versus Pyridoxine," *Phytomedicine* 4:183-89, 1997.

Leatherdale, B.A., et al. "Improvement in Glucose Tolerance Due to *Momordica charantia* (Karela)," *British Medical Journal (Clinical Research Edition)* 282:1823-24, 1981.

Lecomte, A., et al. "Harpagophytum Dans l'Arthrose: Etude en Double Insu Contre Placebo," *Le Magazine* 15:27–30, 1992.

Leenders, N., et al. "Creatine Supplementation and Swimming Performance," *International Journal of Sport Nutrition* 9:251-62, 1999.

Leitner, A., et al. "Allergens in Pepper and Paprika: Immunologic Investigation of the Celery-Birch-Mugwort-Spice Syndrome," *Allergy* 53(1):36-41, 1998.

Leung, A.Y., and Foster, S. *Encyclopedia of Common Natural Ingredients.* New York: John Wiley & Sons, Inc., 1995.

Levy, L. "The Activity of Chaulmoogra Acids Against *Mycobacterium leprae,"* *American Review of Respiratory Disease* 111(5):703-05, 1975.

Liao, Y.L., et al. "Contact Leukomelanosis Induced by the Leaves of *Piper betle* L. (Piperaceae): A Clinical and Histopathologic Survey," *Journal of the American Academy of Dermatology* 40:583-89, 1999.

Lininger, S., et al. *The Natural Pharmacy.* Prima Health, Virtual Health, 1998.

Lis-Balchin, M., and Hart, S. "A Preliminary Study of the Effect of Essential Oils on Skeletal and Smooth Muscle In Vitro," *Journal of Ethnopharmacology* 58(3):83-7, 1997.

Ljunggren, B. "Severe Phototoxic Burn Following Celery Ingestion," *Archives of Dermatology* 126(10):1334-36, 1990.

Lovell, C.R., and Rowan, M. "Dandelion Dermatitis," *Contact Dermatitis* 25(3):185-8, 1991.

Lowthian, P. "'Last-Resort' Dressings for Intractable Pressure Sores," *British Journal of Nursing* 4:1183-9, 1995.

Lust, J. *The Herb Book.* New York: Bantam Books, 1974.

Mabey, R. *The New Age Herbalist. How to Use Herbs for Healing, Nutrition, Body Care, and Relaxation.* New York: Simon & Schuster Inc., 1988.

Macdonald, H.G. *A Dictionary of Natural Products.* Medford N.J.: Plexus Publishing, 1997.

Maquart, F.X., et al. "Triterpenes from *Centella asiatica* Stimulate Extracellular Matrix Accumulation in Rat Experimental Wounds," *European Journal of Dermatology* 9(4):289-96, 1999.

Marcus, D.A., et al. "A Double-Blind Provocative Study of Chocolate as a Trigger of Headache," *Cephalalgia* 17:855-62, 1997.

Marks, D.R., et al. "A Double-Blind, Placebo-Controlled Trial of Intracranial Capsaicin for Cluster Headaches," *Cephalalgia* 13:114-66, 1993.

Mascolo, N., et al. "Biological Screening of Italian Medicinal Plants for Anti-Inflammatory Activity," *Phytotherapy Research* 1:28-31, 1987.

Massoco, C.O., et al. "Behavioral Effects of Acute and Long-Term Administration of Catnip (*Nepta cataria*) in Mice," *Veterinary and Human Toxicology* 37(6):530-33, 1995.

Mattei, R., et al. "Guarana (*Paullinia cupana*): Toxic Behavioral Effects in Laboratory Animals and Antioxidant Activity In Vitro," *Journal of Ethnopharmacology* 60(2):111-6, 1998.

May, B., et al. "Efficacy of a Fixed Peppermint Oil/Caraway Oil Combination in Non-Ulcer Dyspepsia," *Arznzeimittelforschung* 46(12):1149-53, 1996.

McFarlin, B.L., et al. "A National Survey of Herbal Preparations Used by Nurse-Midwives for Labor Stimulation: Review of the Literature and Recommendations for Practice," *Journal of Nurse-Midwifery* 44:205-16, 1999.

McGuffin, M., et al. *American Herbal Products Association's Botanical Safety Handbook.* New York: CRC Press, 1997.

McGuffin, M., et al. *Botanical Safety Handbook.* CRC Press, 1997.

Meinwald, J., et al. "Cyclopentanoid Terpene Biosynthesis in a Phasmid Insect and in Catmint," *Science* 151(706):79-80, 1966.

Melchart, D., et al. "Immunomodulation with Echinacea—Systematic Review of Controlled Clinical Trials," *Phytomedicine* 1:245, 1994.

Mengs, U., et al. "Toxicity of *Echinacea purpurea*: Acute, Subacute and Genotoxicity Studies," *Arzneimittelforschung* 41:1076, 1991.

Meyer, B., et al. "Antioxidative Properties of Alcoholic Extracts from *Fraxinus excelsior, Populus tremula* and *Solidage virgaurea*," *Arzneimittelforschung* 45:174-76, 1995.

Micklefield, G.H., et al. "Effects of Peppermint Oil and Caraway Oil on Gastroduodenal Motility," *Phytotherapy Research* 14:20-23, 2000.

Milewicz, A., et al. "*Vitex agnus castus* Extract in the Treatment of Luteal Phase Defects Due to Latent Hyperprolactinaemia. Results of a Randomized Placebo-Controlled Double-Blind Study," *Arzneimittelforschung* 43(II):752-56, 1993.

Miller, L.G. "Herbal Medicinals: Selected Clinical Considerations Focusing on Known or Potential Drug-Herb Interaction," *Archives of Internal Medicine* 158:2200-11, 1998.

Miura, T., et al. "Effect of Guarana on Exercise in Normal and Epinephrine-Induced Glycogenolytic Mice," *Biological and Pharmaceutical Bulletin* 21(6):646-8, 1998.

Miyase, T., and Mimatsu, A. "Acylated Iridoid and Phenylethanoid Glycosides from the Aerial Parts of *Scrophularia nodosa*," *Journal of Natural Products* 62(8):1079-84, 1999.

Mok, J.S., et al. "Cardiovascular Response in the Normotensive Rate Produced by Intravenous Injection of Gambarine Isolated from *Uncaria callophylla* BL ex Korth," *Journal of Ethnopharmacology* 36(3):219, 1992.

Moore, M. *Herbal Materia Medica*, 5th ed. Albuquerque, N.M.: Southwest School of Botanical Medicine, 1995.

Morales, A.J., et al. "The Effect of Six Months Treatment with a 100 mg Daily Dose of Dehydroepiandrosterone (DHEA) on Circulating Sex Steroids, Body Composition and Muscle Strength in Age-Advanced Men and

Women," *Clinical Endocrinology* 49(4):421-32, 1998.

Morganti, P., et al. "Extraction and Analysis of Cosmetic Active Ingredients from an Anti-cellulitis Transdermal Delivery System by High-Performance Liquid Chromatography," *Journal of Chromatographic Science* 37(2):51-5, 1999.

Morton, J.F. "Widespread Tannin Intake Via Stimulants and Masticatories, Especially Guarana, Kola Nut, Betel Vine, and Accessories" (review), *Basic Life Sciences* 59:739-65, 1992.

Mossik, G., et al. "Small Doses of Capsaicin Given Intragastrically Inhibit Gastric Basal Acid Secretion in Healthy Human Subjects," *Journal of Physiology, Paris* 93:433-6, 1999.

Moussard, C., et al. "A Drug Used in Traditional Medicine, *Harpagophytum procumbens*: No Evidence for NSAID-like Effects on Whole Blood Eicosanoid Production in Humans," *Prostaglandins Leukotrienes and Essential Fatty Acids* 46(4):283-6, 1992.

Mowrey, D.B., and Clayson, D.E. "Motion Sickness, Ginger, and Psychophysics," *Lancet* March 20:655-57, 1982.

Mueller, B.A., et al. "Noni Juice (*Morinda citrifolia*): Hidden Potential for Hyperkalemia?" *American Journal of Kidney Disease* 35(2):310, 1999.

Murphy, J.J., et al. "Randomized, Double-Blind, Placebo-Controlled Trial of Feverfew in Migraine Prevention," *Lancet* 2:189-92, 1988.

Murrar, M., and Pizzorno, J. *Encyclopedia of Natural Medicine*, 2nd ed. Rocklin, Calif.: Prima Publishing, 1998.

Murray, M, and Pizzorno, J. *The Encyclopedia of Natural Medicine*. Prima Publishing, 1997.

Natarajan, S., and Paily, P.P. "Effect of Topical *Hydrocotyle asiatica* in Psoriasis," *Indian Journal of Dermatology* 18:82-85, 1973.

Nemecz, G. "Chamomile," *US Pharamacist* 3:104-16, 1998.

Nemecz, G., and Lee, T.J. "Kava-Kava," *US Pharmacist* June:53-61, 1999.

Newhall, C.A., et al. *Herbal Medicines: A Guide for Health Care Professionals.* London: The Pharmaceutical Press, 1996.

Norton, S.A. "Useful Plants of Dermatology. I. Hydnocarpus and Chaulmoogra," *Journal of the American Academy of Dermatology* 31(4):683-86, 1994.

Odes, H.S., and Madar, Z. "A Double-Blind Trial of a Celandine Aloevera and Psyllium Laxative Preparation in Adult Patients with Constipation," *Digestion* 49(2):65-71, 1991.

Oliwiecki, S., and Burton, J.L. "Evening Primrose Oil and Marine Oil in the Treatment of Psoriasis," *Clinical and Experimental Dermatology* 19:127-9, 1994.

Oommen, S.T., et al. "Effect of Oil of Hydnocarpus on Wound Healing," *International Journal of Leprosy and Other Mycobacterial Diseases* 67(2):154-58, 1999.

Page, R.L., and Lawrence, J.D. "Potentiation of Warfarin by Dong Quai," *Pharmacotherapy* 19:870, 1999.

Palit, P., et al. "Novel Weight-Reducing Activity of *Galega officinalis* in Mice," *Journal of Pharmacy and Pharmacology* 51:1313-19, 1999.

Patel, S., and Wiggins, J. "Eucalyptus Oil Poisoning," *Archives of Diseases in Childhood* 55:405-6, 1980.

Patil, S.P., et al. "Allergy to Fenugreek (*Trigonella foenum graecum*)," *Annals of Allergy and Asthma Immunology* 78:297-300, 1997.

Pattrick, M., et al. "Feverfew in Rheumatoid Arthritis: A Double-Blind, Placebo-Controlled Study," *Annals of Rheumatic Disease* 48:547-9, 1989.

Patzelt-Wenczler, R., and Ponce-Poschl, E. "Proof of Efficacy of Kamillosan® Cream in Atopic Eczema," *European Journal of Medical Research* 5:171-75, 2000.

Pauli, G. "Celery Allergy: Clinical and Biological Study of 20 Cases," *Annals of Allergy* 60(3):243-46, 1988.

PDR for Herbal Medicines, 1st ed. Montvale, N.J.: Medical Economics Co., 1999.

Peana, A.T., et al. "Chemical Composition and Antimicrobial Action of the Essential Oils of *Salvia desoleana* and *S. sclarea*," *Planta Medica* 65(8):752, 1999.

Pearn, J. "Corked Up: Clinical Hyoscine Poisoning with Alkaloids of the Native Corkwood, Duboisia," *Medical Journal of Australia* 2:422-23, 1981.

Peirce, A. *The American Pharmaceutical Association. Practical Guide to Natural Medicines.* New York: The Stonesong Press, Inc., 1999.

Pepping J. "Kava: *Piper methysticum*," *American Journal of Health-System Pharmacists* 56:957-60, 1999.

Pepping, J. "Black Cohosh: *Cimicifuga racemosa*," *American Journal of Health-System Pharmacists* 56:1400-03, 1999.

Pepping, J. "Coenzyme Q10," *American Journal of Health System Pharmacists* 56(6):519-21, 1999.

Pepping, J.P. "Alternative Therapies: Melatonin," *American Journal of Health System Pharmacists* 56:2520-27, 1999.

Pereira, F., et al. "Contact Dermatitis from Chamomile Tea," *Contact Dermatitis* 36(6):307, 1997.

Petersik, J.T., et al. "Of Cats, Catnip, and Cannabis," *Journal of the American Medical Association* 208(2):360, 1969.

Petit, P.R., et al. "Steroid Saponins from Fenugreek Seeds—-Extraction, Purification, and Pharmacological Investigation of Feeding Behavior and Plasma Cholesterol," *Steroids* 60:674-80, 1995.

Petrowicz, O., et al. "Effects of Artichoke Leaf Extract (ALE) on Lipoprotein Metabolism In Vitro and In Vivo," *Atherosclerosis* 129:147, 1997.

Pfutzner, W., et al. "Anaphylactic Reaction Elicited by Condurango Bark in a Patient Allergic to Natural Rubber Latex," *Journal of Allergy and Clinical Immunology* 101:281-82, 1998.

Philippi, A.F., et al. "Glucosamine, Chondroitin, and Manganese Ascorbate for Degenerative Joint Disease of the Knee or Low Back: A Randomized, Double-Blind, Placebo-Controlled Pilot Study," *Military Medicine* 164(2):85-91, 1999.

Pierce, A. *The American Pharmaceutical Association: Practical Guide to Natural Medicines.* New York: Stronesong Press, 1999.

Pinheiro, C.E., et al. ["Effect of Guarana and Stevia Rebaudiana Bertoni (Leaves) Extracts, and Stevioside, on the Fermentation and Synthesis of Extracellular Insoluble Polysaccharides of Dental Plaque"] (Portuguese), *Review of Odontology at the University of Sao Paulo* 1(4):9-13, 1987.

Pointel, J.P., et al. "Titrated Extract of *Centella asiatica* (TECA) in the Treatment of Venous Insufficiency of the Lower Limbs," *Angiology* 38:46-50, 1987.

Quintana, P.J., et al. "Gossypol-Induced DNA Breaks in Rat Lymphocytes Are Secondary to Cytotoxicity," *Toxicology Letters* 117(1-2):85-94, 2000.

Ramadan, W., et al. "Oil of Bitter Orange: New Topical Antifungal Agent," *International Journal of Dermatology* 35(6):448-9, 1996.

Ratsula, K., et al. "Vaginal Contraception with Gossypol: A Clinical Study," *Contraception* 27:571-6, 1983.

Ray, S.D., et al. "A Novel Proanthocyanidin IH636 Grape Seed Extract Increases In Vivo Bcl-XL Expression and Prevents Acetaminophen-Induced Programmed and Unprogrammed Cell Death in Mouse Liver," *Archives of Biochemistry and Biophysics* 369(1):42-58, 1999.

Rehman, J., et al. "Increased Production of Antigen-Specific Immunoglobulins G and M Following In Vivo Treatment with the Medicinal Plants *Echinacea angustifolia* and *Hydrastis Canadensis*," *Immunology Letters* 68:391-5, 1999.

Reiter, W.J., et al. "Dehydroepiandrosterone in the Treatment of Erectile Dysfunction: A Prospective, Double-Blind, Randomized, Placebo-Controlled Study," *Urology* 53:590-95, 1999.

Rekka, E.A., et al. "Investigation of the Effect of Chamazulene on Lipid Peroxidation and Free Radical Processes," *Research Communications in Molecular*

Pathology and Pharmacology 92(3):361-64, 1996.

Ribes, G., et al. "Antidiabetic Effects of Subfractions from Fenugreek Seeds in Diabetic Dogs," *Proceedings of the Society for Experimental Biology and Medicine* 182:159-66, 1986.

Ridker, P.M., and McDermott, W.V. "Comfrey Herb Tea and Hepatic Veno-Occlusive Disease," *Lancet* 1(8235):657-58, 1989.

Ridker, P.M., and McDermott, W.V. "Comfrey Herb Tea and Hepatic Veno-Occlusive Disease," *Lancet* 1(8235):657-58, 1989.

Rizzi, R., et al. "Mutagenic and Antimutagenic Activities of *Uncaria tomentosa* and Its Extract," *Journal of Ethnopharmacology* 38(1):63, 1993.

Robbers, J.E., et al. *Pharmacognosy and Pharmacobiotechnology*. Baltimore: Williams & Wilkins, 1996.

Rodriguez-Serna, M., et al. "Allergic and Systemic Contact Dermatitis from *Matricaria chamomilla* Tea," *Contact Dermatitis* 39(4):192-93, 1998.

Roman-Ramos, R., et al. "Experimental Study of the Hypoglycemic Effect of Some Antidiabetic Plants," *Archives of Investigative Medicine (Mexico)* 22:87-93, 1991.

Royer, R.E., et al. "Comparison of the Antiviral Activities of 3?-Azido-3?-deoxythymidine (AZT) and Gossylic Iminolactone (GIL) Against Clinical Isolates of HIV-1," *Pharmacology Research* 31:49-52, 1995.

Rubino, S., et al. "Neuroendocrine Effect of a Short-Term Treatment with DHEA in Postmenopausal Women," *Maturitas* 28(3):251-7, 1998.

Rudenskaya, G.N., et al. "Taraxalisin—-A Serine Proteinase from Dandelion *Taraxacum officinale* Webb S.L.," *FEBS Letters* 437(3):237-40, 1998.

Sahelian, R., and Stuart, B. "Dehydroepiandrosterone and Cardiac Arrhythmia," *Annals of Internal Medicine* 129(7):588, 1998.

Santa Maria, A., et al. "Evaluation of the Toxicity of Guarana with In Vitro Bioassays," *Ecotoxicology and Environmental Safety* 39(3):164-7, 1998.

Sato, M., et al. "Cardioprotective Effects of Grape Seed Proanthocyanidin Against Ischemic Reperfusion Injury," *Journal of Molecular and Cellular Cardiology* 31(6):1289-97, 1999.

Scarpignato, C., and Rampal, P. "Prevention and Treatment of Traveler's Diarrhea: A Clinical Pharmacological Approach," *Chemotherapy* 41(suppl 1):48-81, 1995.

Schatzle, M., et al. "Allergic Contact Dermatitis from Goldenrod (*Herba solidaginis*) after Systemic Administration," *Contact Dermatitis* 39(5):271-74, 1998.

Schauenberg, P., and Paris, F. *Guide to Medicinal Plants*. New Canaan, Conn.: Keats Publishing, 1997.

Schiedermayer, D. "Evening Primrose Oil in the Treatment of Atopic and Irritant Contact Dermatitis," *Alternative Medicine Alert* January, 1999.

Schmidt, U., et al. "Efficacy of the Hawthorn (*Crataegus*) Preparation LI 132 in 78 Patients with Chronic Congestive Heart Failure Defined as NYHA Functional Class II," *Phytomedicine* 1:17-24, 1994.

Schulz, V., et al. *Rational Phytotherapy: The Physician's Guide to Herbal Medicine*. Berlin: Springer-Verlag, 1998.

Schwartz, H.J., et al. "Occupational Allergic Rhinoconjunctivitis and Asthma Due to Fennel Seed," *Annals of Allergy and Asthma Immunology* 78:37-40, 1997.

Seedat, H.A., and Van Wyk, C.W. "The Oral Features of Betel Nut Chewers Without Submucous Fibrosis," *J Biol Buccale* 16:123-28, 1988.

Sengupta, A., et al. "The Component Fatty Acids of Chaulmoogra Oil," *Journal of Science, Food, and Agriculture* 24(6):669-74, 1973.

Sharma, R.D., et al. "Use of Fenugreek Seed Powder in the Management of Non-Insulin Dependent Diabetes Mellitus," *Nutrition Research* 16:1331-9, 1996.

Sheikh, N.M., et al. "Chaparral-Associated Hepatotoxicity," *Archives of Internal Medicine* 157(8):913-19, 1997.

Shelley, M.D., et al. "Stereo-Specific Cytotoxic Effects of Gossypol Enantiomers and Gossypolone in Tumour Cell Lines," *Cancer Letters* 135:171-80, 1999.

Sheng, Y., et al. "Enhanced DNA Repair, Immune Function and Reduced Toxicity of C-MED-100 (TM), a Novel Aqueous Extract from *Uncaria tomentosa*," *Journal of Ethnopharmacology* 69(2):115-26, 2000.

Shidaifat, F., et al. "Inhibition of Human Prostate Cancer Cell Growth by Gossypol Is Associated with Stimulation of Transforming Growth Factor-Beta," *Cancer Letters* 107:37-44, 1996.

Shukla, A., et al. "Asiaticoside-Induced Elevation of Antioxidant Levels in Healing Wounds," *Phytotherapy Research* 13(1):50-4, 1990.

Shukla, A., et al. "In Vitro and In Vivo Wound Healing Activity of Asiaticoside Isolated from *Centella asiatica*," *Journal of Ethnopharmacology* 65(1):1-11, 1999.

Simopoulos, A.P. "Omega 3-Fatty Acids in Health and Disease and in Growth and Development," *American Journal of Clinical Nutrition* 54:438-63, 1991.

Singh, H.B., et al. "Cinnamon Bark Oil, a Potent Fungitoxicant Against Fungi Causing Respiratory Tract Mycoses," *Allergy* 50(12):995-99, 1995.

Sivam, G.P., et al. "*Helicobacter pylori:* In Vitro Susceptibility to Garlic (*Allium sativum*) Extract," *Nutrition and Cancer* 27:118-21, 1997.

Snorrason, E., and Stefansson, J.G. "Galanthamine Hydrobromide in Mania" (letter), *Lancet* 337:557, 1991.

Soulimani, R., et al. "The Role of Stomachal Digestion on the Pharmacological Activity of Aqueous Extracts of Devil's-Claw," *Canadian Journal of Physiology and Pharmacology* 72(12):1532-6, 1994.

Srivastava, Y., et al. "Antidiabetic and Adaptogenic Properties of *Momordica charantia* Extract: An Experimental and Clinical Evaluation," *Phytotherapy Research* 7:285-89, 1993.

Steinberg, M. "Pharmacologic Treatment of Alzheimer's Disease: An Update on Approved, Unapproved Therapies," *Formulary* 34:41, 1999.

Stewart, J.J., et al. "Effects of Ginger on Motion Sickness Susceptibility and Gastric Function," *Pharmacology* 42(2):111-20, 1991.

Stoll, W. "Phytotherapeutic Agent Affects Atrophic Vaginal Epithelium. Double-Blind Study: *Cimicifuga* vs. an Estrogen Preparation" [translated from German], *Therapeutikon* 1:23-31, 1987.

Stomati, M., et al. "Endocrine, Neuroendocrine and Behavioral Effects of Oral Dehydroepiandrosterone Sulfate Supplementation in Postmenopausal Women," *Gynecologic Endocrinology* 13(1):15-25, 1999.

Subiza, J., et al. "Allergic Conjunctivitis to Chamomile Tea," *Annals of Allergy* 65:127-32, 1990.

Suguna, L., et al. "Effects of *Centella asiatica* Extract on Dermal Wound Healing in Rats," *Indian Journal of Experimental Biology* 34(12):1208-11, 1996.

Sunilkumar, K.B., et al. "Evaluation of Topical Formulations of Aqueous Extract of *Centella asiatica* on Open Wounds in Rats," *Indian Journal of Experimental Biology* 36(6):569-72, 1998.

Swanston-Flatt, S.K., et al. "Evaluation of Traditional Plant Treatments for Diabetes: Studies in Streptozotocin Diabetic Mice," *Acta Diabetalogica Latina* 26:51-5, 1989.

Swiatek, L., et al. "6-O-beta-D-xylopyranosylcatalpol, a New Iridoid Glycoside from *Verbascum thapsiforme*," *Planta Medica* 45(3):12, 1982.

Syed, T.A., et al. "Management of Genital Herpes in Men with 0.5% Aloe Vera Extract in a Hydrophilic Cream: A Placebo-Controlled Double-Blind Study,"

Journal of Dermatologic Treatment 8:99-102, 1997.

Tang, D.H. "Ephedra (Ma Huang)," *Clinical Toxicology Review* 18:1, 1996.

The New Age Herbalist. Edited by Mabey, R. New York: Simon & Schuster, 1988.

Tierra, L. *The Herbs of Life. Health and Healing Using Western and Chinese Techniques.* Freedom, Calif.: The Crossing Press, 1997.

Tiongson, J., and Salen, P. "Mass Ingestion of Jimson Weed by Eleven Teenagers," *Delaware Medical Journal* 70:471-6, 1998.

Tirillini, B. "Fingerprints of *Uncaria tomentosa* Leaf, Stem, and Root Bark Decoction," *Phytotherapy Research* 10(suppl 1):S67-8, 1996.

Tokuda, H., et al. "Inhibitory Effects of Ursolic and Oleanolic Acid on Skin Tumor Promotion by 12-O-tetradecanoylphorbol-13-acetate," *Cancer Letters* 33(3):279-85, 1986.

Turner, S., and Mills, S. "A Double-Blind Clinical Trial on an Herbal Remedy for Premenstrual Syndrome: A Case Study," *Complementary Therapies in Medicine* 1:73-77, 1993.

Tyler, V.E. *The Honest Herbal,* 3rd ed. New York: Haworth Press, 1993.

Tyler, V.E. *The Honest Herbal: A Sensible Guide to the Use of Herbs and Related Remedies,* 3rd ed. Binghamton, N.Y.: Pharmaceutical Products Press, 1993.

van der Bijl, P., and Thompson, I.O.C. "Effect of Aqueous Areca Nut Extract on the Permeability of Mucosa," *South African Journal of Science* 94:241-43, 1998.

van der Brempt, X., et al. "Rhinitis and Asthma Caused by Occupational Exposure to Carob Bean Flour," *Journal of Allergy and Clinical Immunol* 90(6):1008-1010, 1992.

van Vollenhoven, R.F., et al. "A Double-Blind, Placebo-Controlled, Clinical Trial of Dehydroepiandrosterone in Severe Systemic Lupus Erythematosus," *Lupus* 8(3):181-7, 1999.

van Vollenhoven, R.F., et al. "Treatment of Systemic Lupus Erythematosus with Dehydroepiandrosterone: 50 Patients Treated Up to 12 Months," *Journal of Rheumatology* 25(2):285-9, 1998.

Vanderhoff, B.T., and Mosser, K.H. "Jimson Weed Toxicity: Management of Anticholinergic Plant Ingestion," *American Family Physician* 46:526-30, 1992.

Vieths, S., et al. "Immunoblot Study of lgE Binding Allergens in Celery Roots," *Annals of Allergy* 75(1):48-55, 1995.

Viola, H., et al. "Apigenin, a Component of *Matricaria recutita* Flowers, Is a Central Benzodiazepine Receptor-Ligand with Anxiolytic Effects," *Planta Medica* 61(3):213-16, 1995.

Vogler, B.K., and Ernst, E. "Aloe Vera: A Systematic Review of Its Clinical Effectiveness," *British Journal of General Practitioners* 49:823-28, 1999.

von Kruedener, S., et al. "A Combination of *Populus tremula, Solidago virgaurea* and *Fraxinus excelsior* as an Anti-inflammatory and Antirheumatic Drug. A short review" (review), *Arzneimittelforschung* 45(2):169-71, 1995.

Wade, A., and Weller, P.J. *Handbook of Pharmaceutical Excipients,* 2nd ed. Washington, D.C.: The Pharmaceutical Press, 1994.

Wadworth, A.N., and Faulds, D. "Hydroxyethylrutosides: A Review of Its Pharmacology and Therapeutic Efficacy in Venous Insufficency and Related Disorders," *Drugs* 44:1013-32, 1992.

Wagner, W. "Karaya Gum Hypersensitivity in an Enterostomal Therapist" (letter), *Journal of the American Medical Association* 243:432, 1980.

Wakelin, S.H., et al. "Compositae Sensitivity and Chronic Hand Dermatitis in a Seven-Year-Old Boy," *British Journal of Dermatology* 137(2):289-91, 1997.

Wang, X., et al. "Cytotoxic Effect of Gossypol on Colon Carcinoma Cells," *Life Sciences* 67(22):2663-71, 2000.

Wantke, F., et al. "Contact Dermatitis from Jojoba Oil and Myristyl Lactate/Malenated Soybean Oil," *Contact Dermatitis* 34:71-2, 1996.

Warshafsky, S., et al. "Effect of Garlic on Total Serum Cholesterol," *Annals of Internal Medicine* 119:599-605, 1993.

Weiss, R.F. *Herbal Medicine.* Beaconsfield, U.K.: Beaconsfield Publishers Ltd., 1988.

Welhinda, J., et al. "Effect of *Momordica charantia* on the Glucose Tolerance in Maturity Onset Diabetes," *Journal of Ethnopharmacology* 17:277-82, 1986.

Welihinda, J., et al. "The Insulin-Releasing Activity of the Tropical Plant *Momordica charantia*," *Acta Biol Med Ger* 41:1229-40, 1982.

Whitaker, D.K., et al. "Evening Primrose Oil (Epogam®) in the Treatment of Chronic Hand Dermatitis: Disappointing Therapeutic Results," *Dermatology* 193:115-20, 1996.

Whitehouse, L.W., et al. "Devil's Claw (*Harpagophytum procumbens*): No Evidence for Anti-inflammatory Activity in the Treatment of Arthritic Disease," *Canadian Medical Association Journal* 129(3):249-51, 1983.

Wichtl, M.W. *Herbal Drugs and Phytopharmaceuticals.* Edited by Bisset, N.M. Stuttgart: Medpharm GmbH Scientific Publishers, 1994.

Wolf, O.T., et al. "Effects of a Two-Week Physiological Dehydroepiandrosterone Substitution on Cognitive Performance and Well-Being in Healthy Elderly Women and Men," *Journal of Clinical and Endocrinological Metabolism* 82(7):2363-7, 1997.

Wolkowitz, O.M., et al. "Dehydroepiandrosterone (DHEA) Treatment of Depression," *Biological Psychiatry* 41(3):311-8, 1997.

Wolkowitz, O.M., et al. "Double-Blind Treatment of Major Depression with Dehydroepiandrosterone," *American Journal of Psychiatry* 156(4):646-9, 1999.

Wu, D. "An Overview of the Clinical Pharmacology and Therapeutic Potential of Gossypol as a Male Contraceptive Agent and in Gynaecological Disease," *Drugs* 38:333-41, 1989.

Yaffe, K., et al. "Neuropsychiatric Function and Dehydroepiandrosterone Sulfate in Elderly Women: A Prospective Study," *Biological Psychiatry* 43(9):694-700, 1998.

Ye, X., et al. "The Cytotoxic Effects of a Novel IH636 Grape Seed Proanthocyanidin Extract on Cultured Human Cancer Cells," *Molecular and Cellular Biochemistry* 196(1-2):99-108, 1999.

Yongchaiyudha, S., et al. "Antidiabetic Activity of Aloe Vera L. Juice. I. Clinical Trial in New Cases of Diabetes Mellitus," *Phytomedicine* 3:241-43, 1996.

Yoosook, C., et al. "Anti-Herpes Simplex Virus Activities of Crude Water Extracts of Thai Medicinal Plants," *Phytomedicine* 6(6):411-9, 2000.

Young, G.L., and Jewell, D. "Creams for Preventing Stretch Marks in Pregnancy" (review), Cochrane Database System Review (2):CD000066, 2000.

Zain, R.B., et al. "Oral Mucosal Lesions Associated with Betel Quid, Areca Nut and Tobacco Chewing Habits: Consensus from a Workshop Held in Kuala Lumpur, Malaysia, November 25-27, 1996," *Journal of Oral Pathology and Medicine* 28:1-4, 1999.

Zakay-Rones, Z., et al. "Inhibition of Several Strains of Influenza Virus In Vitro and Reduction of Symptoms by an Elderberry Extract (*Sambucus nigra L.*) During an Outbreak of Influenza B Panama," *Journal of Alternative and Complementary Medicine* 1:361, 1995.

Zang, L.Y., et al. "Scavenging of Superoxide Anion Radical by Chaparral," *Molecular and Cellular Biochemistry* 196(1-2):157-61, 1999.

Zheng, G.Q., et al. "Anethofuran, Carvone, and Limonene: Potential Cancer Chemopreventive Agents from Dill Weed Oil and Caraway Oil," *Planta Medica* 58(4):338-41, 1992.

Zhu, P.D.Q. "Dong Quai," *American Journal of Chinese Medicine* 15:117, 1987.

Manual healing therapies

"Amebiasis Associated with Colonic Irrigation—Colorado," *MMWR Morbidity and Mortality Weekly Report* 30(9):101-02, 1981.

"Body Rebuilder," *New Age Journal,* Nov./Dec. 1989 (reprint).

"Bodywork: Choosing an Approach to Suit Your Needs," *Yoga Journal,* Jan./Feb. 1986:28-32.

Albright, G.L.; and Fischer, A.A. "Effects of Warming Imagery Aimed at Trigger-Point Sites on Tissue Compliance, Skin Temperature, and Pain Sensitivity in Biofeedback-Trained Patients with Chronic Pain: A Preliminary Study," *Perceptual Motor Skills* 71(3 Pt 2):1163-709, 1990.

Alexander Technique Web site. www.alexandertech.com Accessed 2/9/01.

Alexander, F.M. *The Use of Self.* London: Big Sur Tapes, 1996.

Aston Postural Assessment Workbook: Skills for Observing and Evaluating Body Patterns. Therapy Skill Builders, 1998.

Aston, J., and Low, J. "Your Three-Dimensional Body: The Aston System of Body Usage, Movement, and Fitness," *Physical Therapy Today* Fall, 1991.

Aston-Patterning. www.aston-patterning.com 2000.

Bergeron-Oliver, S., and Oliver, B. *Working Without Pain: Eliminate Repetitive Strain Injuries with Alexander Technique.* Chico, Calif.: Pacific Institute for the Alexander Technique, 1996.

Betz, J.M., et al. "Gas Chromatographic Determination of Yohimbine in Commercial Yohimbine Products," *J AOAC Int* 78(5):1189-94, 1995.

Bigos, S., et al. *Acute Low Back Problems in Adults: Clinical Practice Guideline Number 14.* Rockville, Md.: Agency for Health Care Policy and Research, Public Health Service, United States Department of Health and Human Services, 1994.

Boyle, W, and Saine, A. *Lessons in Naturopathic Hydrotherapy.* East Palestine, Ohio: Buckeye Naturopathic Press, 1988.

Briel, J.W., et al. "Clinical Value of Colonic Irrigation in Patients with Continence Disturbances," *Diseases of the Colon and Rectum* 40(7):802-05, 1997.

Cohen, D. *An Introduction to Craniosacral Therapy.* Berkeley, Calif.: North Atlantic Books, 1995.

Cross, J.R. *Acupressure: Clinical Applications in Musculo-skeletal Conditions.* Boston, Mass: Butterworth, 2000.

De Domenico, G., and Wood, E.C. *Beard's Massage,* 4th ed. Philadelphia: W.B. Saunders Co., 1997.

Easter, A. "The State of Research on the Effects of Therapeutic Touch," *Journal of Holistic Nursing* 15(2):158-75, June 1997.

Eisenberg, D., and Wright, T.L. *Encounters with Qi: Exploring Chinese Medicine.* New York: W.W. Norton & Co., 1995.

Ernst, E. "Colonic Irrigation and the Theory of Autointoxication: A Triumph of Ignorance Over Science" [editorial], *Journal of Clinical Gastroenterology* 24(4):196-98, 1997.

Fasano-Ramos, M.,Weintraub, M. "Alternative Medical Care: Shiatsu, Swedish muscle massage, and Trigger Point Suppression in Spinal Pain Syndrome," *American Journal of Pain Management* 2(2):74-78, 1992.

Feldenkrais, M. *Awareness Through Movement: Easy-to-Do Health Exercises to Improve Your Posture, Vision, Imagination, and Personal Awareness.* New York: Harper and Row, 1991.

Froehle, R.M. "Ear Infection: A Retrospective Study Examining Improvement from Chiropractic Care and Analyzing Influencing Factors," *Journal of Manipulation and Physiological Therapy* 19(3):169-77, 1996.

Gach, M.R. *Acupressure's Potent Points. A Bantam Book.* New York: Bantam, 1990.

Garvey, T.A., et al. "A Prospective, Randomized, Double-Blind Evaluation of Trigger-Point Injection Therapy for Low-Back Pain," *Spine* 14(9):962, 1989.

Hesse, J., et al. "Acupuncture Versus Metoprolol in Migraine Prophylaxis: A Randomized Trial of Trigger Point Inactivation," *Journal of Internal Medicine* 235(5):451-67, 1994.

Hover-Kramer, D. *Healing Touch: A Resource for Health Care Professionals.* Albany, N.Y.: Delmar Pubs., 1996.

Hunt, T. "Colonic Irrigation," *Nurs Mirror Midwives Journal* 139(1):76-77, 1974.

Istre, G.R., et al. "An Outbreak of Amebiasis Spread by Colonic Irrigation at a Chiropractic Clinic," *New England Journal of Medicine* 307(6):339-42, 1982.

Jaeger, B., and Reeves, J.L. "Quantification of Changes in Myofascial Trigger Point Sensitivity with the Pressure Algometer Following Passive Stretch," *Pain* 27(2):203-210, 1986.

Kadakia, S.C. "The Disappearing Colonic Irrigation Tube" [letter], *Gastrointestinal Endoscopy* 38(6):733-34, 1992.

Krieger, D. *Accepting Your Power to Heal: The Personal Practice of Therapeutic Touch.* Santa Fe, NM: Bear and Company, 1993.

Maisel, E., *Tai Chi for Health*, Englewood Cliffs, NJ: Prentice Hall, 1963.

Mennell, J "Myofascial Trigger Points as a Cause of Headaches," *Journal of Manipulative Physiology and Therapy* 12(4):308-13, 1989.

Murphy, G.J. "Physical Medicine Modalities and Trigger Point Injections in the Management of Temporomandibular Disorders and Assessing Treatment Outcome," *Oral Surgery, Oral Medicine, Oral Pathology, Oral Radiology and Endodontics* 83(1):118-226, 1997.

Peterson, K.B. "A Preliminary Inquiry Into Manual Testing Response in Phobic and Control Subjects Exposed to Threatening Stimuli," *Journal of Manipulation and Physiological Therapy* 19(5):310-16, 1996.

Pomeranz, B., and Gabriel, S. *Basics of Acupuncture—-Scientific Basis of Acupuncture.* New York: Springer, 1995.

Prudden, B. *Myotherapy: Bonnie Prudden's Complete Guide to Pain-Free Living.*

Garden City, New York: The Dial Press, Doubleday & Company, Inc., 1984.

Quaid, A. "The Mechanics of Motion: Interview with Judith Aston, Developer of Aston-Patterning," *PT Today* July 1995.

Richards, R.K. "Effects of Vitamin C Deficiency and Starvation Upon the Toxicity of Procaine," *Anesthesia and Analgesia* 26:22-29, 1947.

Rolf, I. *Rolfing: Reestablishing the Natural Alignment and Structural Integration of the Human Body for Vitality and Well-Being.* Rochester, Vt.: Inner Traditions, 1990.

Rosa, L., et al. "A Close Look at Therapeutic Touch," *Journal of the American Medical Association* 279(13):1005-10, April 1, 1998.

Rubin, D. "Myofascial Trigger Point Syndromes: An Approach to Management," *Archives of Physical Medicine and Rehabilitation* 62(3):107-10, 1981.

Serizawa, K. *Tsubo, Vital Points for Oriental Therapy.* Tokyo and New York: Japan Publications, Inc., 1976.

Shah, D. "Neural Correlates of Acupressure," University Scholar Thesis, University of Connecticut, 1999 .

Shealy, N., ed. *The Complete Family Guide to Alternative Medicine.* New York: Barnes and Noble, 1996.

Sieh, R. *Tai Chi Ch'uan: The Internal Tradition.* Berkeley, CA: North Atlantic Books, 1992.

Simons, D.G. "Electrogenic Nature of Palpable Bands and 'Jump Sign' Associated with Myofascial Trigger Points," Monograph 1977, Aug 12:913-8.

Takahashi, Y. "Local and Remote Sustained Trigger Point Therapy for Exacerbations of Chronic Low Back Pain" [letter; comment], *Spine* 15;23(8):959-960, 1998.

Tan, M.P., and Cheong, D.M. "Life-Threatening Perineal Gangrene from Rectal Perforation Following Colonic Hydrotherapy: A Case Report," *Annals of the Academy of Medicine of Singapore* 28(4):583-85, 1999.

Tivy, D. "Comments on the Side Effects of Myotherapy," in *Myotherapy.* Edited by Prudden, B. Garden City, New York: Doubleday & Company, Inc., 1984:22-24.

Trager, M. *Movement as a Way to Agelessness: A Guide to Trager Mentastics.* Barrytown, N.Y.: Station Hill Press, 1994.

Travell, J. "Identification of Myofascial Trigger Point Syndromes: A Case of Atypical Facial Neuralgia," *Archives of Physical Medicine and Rehabilitation* 62(3):100-613, 1981.

Travell, J., and Simons, D.G. *Myofascial Pain and Dysfunction: The Trigger Point Manual.* Baltimore: Williams & Wilkins, 1983

Tucker, P. *Tai Chi, Flowing Movements for Harmony and Balance.* New York: 1997.

Upledger, J.E., and Vredevoogd, M.F.A. *Craniosacral Therapy.* Vista, Calif.: Eastland Press, 1998.

Woods, J. "Forces of Nature in the Aston Paradigm: Key Concepts of Aston-Patterning," *Massage & Bodywork,* Spring 1997.

Mind-body therapies

Achterberg, J. *Imagery in Healing.* Boston: Shambala, 1995.

Basmajian, J.V., ed. *Biofeedback: Principles and Practice for Clinicians.* Baltimore: Williams & Wilkins, 1989.

Benjamin, S.A., et al. "Mind-Body Medicine: Expanding the Health Model," *Patient Care* 31(14):126-45, Sept. 15, 1997.

Benson, H. *The Relaxation Response.* New York: William Morrow & Co., 1975.

Debenedittis, G., et al. "Effects of Hypnotic Analgesia and Hypnotizability on Experimental Ischemic Pain," *International Journal of Clinical and Experimental Hypnosis* 37(1):55-69, January 1989.

Dossey, L. *Healing Words: The Power of Prayer and the Practice of Medicine.* New York: Harper Collins, 1995.

Goldberg, B. "Hypnosis and the Immune Response," *International Journal of Psychosomatics* 32(3):34-36, 1985.

Honest Abe's NLP Emporium: http://www3.mistral.co.uk/bradbury-ac/nlpfax.html#one

John Seymour and associates NLP training: www.johnseymour-nlp.co.uk/index.html

Kabat-Zinn, J. *Wherever You Go, There You Are: Mindfulness Meditation in Everyday Life.* New York: Hyperion, 1994.

Rossman, M. *Healing Yourself: A Step-by-Step Program for Better Health Through Imagery.* Mill Valley, Calif.: Awareness Press, 1999.

Schwartz, M.S., et al. *Biofeedback: A Practitioner's Guide.* New York: Guilford, 1987.

Tucker, P. *Tai Chi, Flowing Movements for Harmony and Balance.* New York: 1997.

Udolf, R. *Handbook of Hypnosis for Professionals.* Northvale, N.J.: Jason Aronson, 1995.

Vishnudevananda, S. *The Complete Illustrated Book of Yoga.* New York: Random House, 1995.

Weil, A. *Spontaneous Healing: How to Discover and Enhance Your Body's Natural Ability to Maintain and Heal Itself.* New York: Fawcett, 1996.

Pharmacologic and biological therapies

Alpers, B.J: "The Problem of Sciatica," *Medical Clinics of North America* (37):503, 1953.

Altman, N. *Oxygen Healing Therapies.* Rochester, Vt.: Healing Arts Press, 1998.

Bach, E., and Wheeler, F.J. *The Bach Flower Remedies.* Chicago: Keats Publishing, Inc., 1979.

Banks, A.R. "A Rationale for Prolotherapy," *Journal of Orthopedic Medicine* 3:54-59, 1991.

Blatteis, C. "Fever: Is It Beneficial?" *Yale Journal of Biology* 59:107-16, 1986.

Buckle, J. *Clinical Aromatherapy.* San Diego: Singular, 1997.

Buckner, J.C., et al. "Phase II Study of Anti-neoplastons A10 and AS2-1 in Patients with Recurrent Glioma," *Mayo Clinic Proceedings* 74(2):137-45, 1999.

Burzynski, S.R., et al. "Antineoplastin A in Cancer Therapy," *Physiology, Chemistry and Physics* 9:485, 1977.

Cabanac, M., and Brinnel, H. "The Pathology of Human Temperature Regulation," *Thermiatrics Experientia* 43:19-27, 1987.

Carbajal, D., et al. "Anti-ulcer Activity of Higher Primary Alcohols of Beeswax," *Journal of Pharmacy and Pharmacology* 47:731-33, 1995.

Centers for Disease Control. "Self-Induced Malaria Associated with Malariotherapy for Lyme Disease—-Texas," *Journal of the American Medical Association* 266(16):2199, 1991..

Chlebowski, R.T., et al. "Hydrazine Sulfate in Cancer Patients with Weight Loss," *Cancer* 59:406-10, 1987.

Chlebowski, R.T., et al. "Hydrazine Sulfate Influence on Nutritional Status and Survival in Non-Small Cell Lung Cancer," *Journal of Clinical Oncology* 8:9-15, 1990.

Chlebowski, R.T., et al. "Influence of Hydrazine Sulfate on Abnormal Carbohydrate Metabolism in Cancer Patients with Weight Loss," *Cancer Research* 44:857-61, 1984.

Coen van der Kroon. *The Golden Fountain: The Complete Guide to Urine Therapy.* Wishland, 1993.

Coley's Toxins. The University of Texas Center for Alternative Medicine Research (UT-CAM) www.sph.uth.tmc.edu/utcam/summary/coley_sum.htm. July 27, 1999.

Cram, J. "Flower Essences and Stress Profiling: A Matter Of Head and Heart," Unpublished research from Sierra health Institute. 1999.www.flowersociety.org/research

Cram, J. "Flower Essences Reduce Stress Reaction to Intense Environmental Stimulus," Unpublished research from

Sierra Health Institute. 1999. www.flowersociety.org/research.

Crinnion, Walter, N.D. "Results of a Decade of Naturopathic Treatment for Environmental Illnesses: A Review of Clinical Records," *The Journal of Naturopathic Medicine* 7(2):21-27, 1997.

Curt, G., et al. "Immunoaugmentative Therapy: A Primer on the Perils of Improved Treatments," *Journal of the American Medical Association* 255:505-07, 1986.

Done, A. "Uses and Abuses of Antipyretic Treatment," *Pediatrics* pp 774-80, 1959.

Duffy, M., et al. "Urokinase-Plasminogen Activator, A Marker for Aggressive Breast Carcinomas," *Cancer* 62(3):531-33, 1988.

Eaton, M., et al. "Virucidal (Rabies and Poliomyelitis) Activity of Aqueous Urea Solutions," *American Proceedings of the Society for Experimental Biology* 35:74-76, 1936.

Farr, C.H. *Protocol for the Intravenous Administration of Hydrogen Peroxide.* Oklahoma City: International Bio-Oxidative Medicine Foundation, 1993:29-31.

Filov, V.A., et al. "Experience of the Treatment with Sehydrin (Hydrazine Sulfate, hs) in the Advanced Cancer Patient," *Investigative New Drugs* 13:89-97, 1995.

Foulger, J.H. "The Action of Urea and Some of Its Derivatives on Bacteria" and "The Antiseptic and Bacterial Action of Urea," *Journal of Laboratory and Clinical Medicine*, University of Cincinnati, 1935.

Gard, Z.R., and Brown, E.J. "Literature Review and Comparison Studies of Sauna/Hyperthermia in Detoxification," *Townsend Letter for Doctors* 107:470-78, 1992.

Gold, J. "Anabolic Profiles in Late-Stage Cancer Patients Responsive to Hydrazine Sulfate," *Nutrition and Cancer* 3:13-19, 1981.

Gold, J. "Hydrazine Sulfate: A Current Perspective," *Nutrition and Cancer* 9:59-66, 1987.

Gold, J. "Use of Hydrazine Sulfate in Terminal and Preterminal Cancer Patients: Results of Investigational New Drug (IND) Study in 84 Evaluable Patients," *Oncology* 32:1-10, 1975.

Hackett, G.S. *Ligament and Tendon Relaxation Treated by Prolotherapy*, 3rd ed. Charles C Thomas Pubs., 1956.

Halstead, B., and Rozema, T. *The Scientific Chelation Therapy*, 2nd ed. Tyron, N.C.: TRC Publishing, 1997.

Hanson, L.A., et al. "Characterization of Antibodies in Human Urine," *Journal of Clinical Investigation* 44(5):703-15, 1965.

Harvey, M.A., et al. "Suggested Limits to the Use of the Hot Tub and Sauna by Pregnant Women," *Canadian Medical Association Journal* 125:50-53, 1981.

Haussinger, et al. *Glutamine Metabolism in Mammalian Tissues*. New York: Springer-Verlag, 1984.

Hender, S.S. *The Oxygen Breakthrough*. New York: Pocket Books, 1989.

Kaminski, P. "Touching the Soul: Using Flower Essences for Massage Therapy," *Massage and Bodywork* 13(1):71-74, 1998.

Kaye, D. "Antibacterial Activity of Human Urine," Cornell University Medical College, 1968.

Kief, H. "The Autohomologous Immune Therapy Monograph." (Ludwigshafen: Kief Clinic), 1992.

Klein, R.G., et al. "Proliferant Injections for Low Back Pain: Histologic Changes of Injected Ligaments and Objective Measurements of Lumbar Spine Mobility Before and After Treatment," *Journal of Neurologic and Orthopedic Medicine and Surgery* 10(2):141-44, 1989.

Klein, R.G., et al. "Randomized Double-Blind Trial of Dextrose-Glycerine-Phenol Injections for Chronic Low Back Pain," *Journal of Spinal Disorders* 6(1):23-33, 1993.

Konings, A. W. T. "Membranes as Targets for Hyperthermic Cell Killing," *Recent Results in Cancer Research* 109:9-2 1, 1988.

Lerner, A.M., et al. "Neutralizing Antibody to Polioviruses in Normal Human Urine," *Journal of Clinical Investigation* 41(4):805-15, 1962.

Liu, F.J., and Sun, D.M. "Studies on the Active Constituents Lowering Blood Lipids in Beeswax," *Journal of Chinese Material Medicine* 21:553-54, 1996.

Love, I.N. "Peroxide of Hydrogen as a Remedial Agent," *Journal of the American Medical Association* March 3, 1888:262-65.

Magro Filho, O., and de Carvalho, A.C. "Application of Propolis to Dental Sockets and Skin Wounds," *Journal of Nihon University School of Dentistry* 32(1):4-13, 1994.

McCarthy, P., et.al. "Predictive Value of Abnormal Physical Examination Findings in Ill-Appearing and Well-Appearing Febrile Children," *Pediatrics* 76:167-71, 1985.

Mirzoeva, O.K., and Calder, P.C. "The Effect of Propolis and Its Components on Eicosanoid Production During the Inflammatory Process," *Prostaglandins Leukotrienes and Essential Fatty Acids* 55:441-49, 1996.

Muldavis, L., and Holtzman, J.M. "Treatment of Infected Wounds with Urea," *The London Lancet*, 1938.

Nagappan, R., and Riddell, T. "Pyridoxine Therapy in a Patient with Severe Hydrazine Sulfate Toxicity," *Critical Care Medicine* 28(6):2116-8, 2000.

Nauts, H.C. *Giant Cell Tumor of Bone: End Results Following Immunotherapy (Coley Toxins) Alone or Combined With Surgery and/or Radiation, 66 Cases and Concurrent Infection, 4 Cases.* New York: New York Cancer Research Institute, Inc., 1976.

Neville, A. J., and Sauder, D. N. "Whole Body Hyperthermia (41-42 Degree C) Induces Interleukin-I In Vivo," *Lymphokine Research* 7(3):201-06, 1988.

Noble, R.C., and Parekh, M. "Bactericidal Properties of Urine for *Neisseria gonorrhoeae*," *Journal of Sexually Transmitted Disease*, 1987.

Ongley, M.J., et al. "A New Approach to the Treatment of Chronic Low Back Pain," *Lancet* 8551(2):143-46, 1987.

Ongley, M.J., et al: "Ligament Instability of Knees: A New Approach to Treatment," *Manual of Medicine* (3):152-54, 1988.

Park, M.M., et al. "The Effect of Whole Body Hyperthermia on the Immune Cell Activity of Cancer Patients," *Lymphokine Research* 9(2):213-23, 1990.

Park, Y.K., et al. "Antimicrobial Activity of Propolis on Oral Microorganisms," *Current Microbiology* 36:24-28, 1998.

Pheatt, N. "Nonherbal Dietary Supplements," *Pharmacist's Letter Continuing Education Booklet* 98(4):1-51, 1998.

Plesch, J. "Urine Therapy," *Medical Press (London)* 218:128-33, 1947.

Quinn-Nance, D. "Critical Care Extra: A Case History of Glioblastoma," *American Journal of Nursing* 99(12):24, 1999.

Richardson, M.A., et al. "Coley Toxins Immunotherapy: A Retrospective Review," *Alternative Therapies in Health and Medicine* 5(3):42-47, 1999.

Sawtell, N.M., and Thompson, R.L. "Rapid In Vivo Reactivation of Herpes Simplex Virus in Latently Infected Murine Ganglionic Neurons after Transient Hyperthermia," *Journal of Virology* 66(4):2150-56, 1992.

Schmitt, B. "Fever Phobia," *American Journal of Diseases of Childhood* 134:176-81, 1980.

Schroeder, S.A., et al. *Current Medical Diagnosis & Treatment*. Norwalk, Conn.: Appleton & Lange, 1989:899-1003.

Skibba, J.L., et al. "Oxidative Stress as a Precursor to the Irreversible Hepatocellular Injury Caused by Hyperthermia," *International Journal of Hyperthermia* 7(5):749-61, 1991.

Spire, B., et al. "Inactivation of Lymphadenopathy-Associated Virus by Heat, Gamma Rays, and Ultraviolet Light," *Lancet* I(8422):188-89, 1985.

Staff Reporter. "Antineoplastins: New Antitumor Agents With High Expectations," *Oncology News* 16(4)1:1990.

Staff Reporter. "Now Urine Business," *Hippocrates* (magazine), May 1988.

Standish, L., et al. "One Year Open Trial of Naturopathic Treatment of HIV Infection Class IV A in Men," *Journal of Naturopathic Medicine* 3(1):42-64, 1992.

Tayek, J.A., et al. "Altered Metabolism and Mortality in Patients with Colon Cancer Receiving Chemotherapy," *American Journal of Medical Science* 310:48-55, 1995.

Tayek, J.A., et al. "Effect of Hydrazine Sulfate on Whole-Body Protein Breakdown Measured by C-Lysine Metabolism in Lung Cancer Patients," *Lancet* 2:241-4, 1987.

Todd, J. "Childhood Infections," *American Journal of Diseases of Childhood* 127:810-6, 1974.

Toffoli, G., et al. "Effect of Hyperthermia on Intracellular Drug Accumulation and Chemosensitivity in Drug-Sensitive and Drug-Resistant P388 Leukaemia Cell Lines," *International Journal of Hyperthermia* 5(2):163-72, 1989.

Tresidder, A. "Flower Essences in General Practice," *Positive Health* 27:10-12, 1998.

Tyrrell, D., et al. "Local Hyperthermia Benefits Natural and Experimental Common Colds," *British Medical Journal* 298:1280-83, 1989.

Valnet, J. *The Practice of Aromatherapy: Holistic Health and the Essential Oils of Flowers and Herbs*. Vermont: Healing Arts Press, 1990.

van Haselen, R.A. "The Relationship Between Homeopathy and the Dr Bach System of Flower Remedies: A Critical Appraisal," *British Homoeopathic Journal* 88(3):121-7, 1999.

Vlamis, G. *Bach Flower Remedies to the Rescue*. Vermont: Healing Arts Press, 1990.

Waisbren, B.A. "Observations on the Combined Systemic Administration of Mixed Bacterial Vaccine, Bacillus Calmette-Guerin, Transfer Factor, and Lymphoblastoid Lymphocytes to patients with Cancer, 1974-1985," *Journal of Biological Response Modifiers* 6:1-19, 1987.

Waisbren, B.A. A Scientific Essay Regarding A Twenty-five Year Experience in the Treatment of Cancer with Multiple Immunotherapy Modalities, 2000.http://www.waisbrenclinic.com.

Warburg, O. *The Prime Cause and Prevention of Cancer.* Wurzburg: K. Triltsch, 1966.

Weatherburn, H. "Hyperthermia and Aids Treatment," *British Journal of Radiology* 61(729):862-63, 1988.

Weiman, B., and Starnes, C. "Coly's Toxins, Tumor Necrosis Factor, and Cancer Research, a Historical Perspective," *Pharmacologic Therapy* 64:529-64, 1994.

Index

H

Z

NOTES

NOTES

NOTES